Ebersole and Hess'

Gerontological Nursing & Healthy Aging

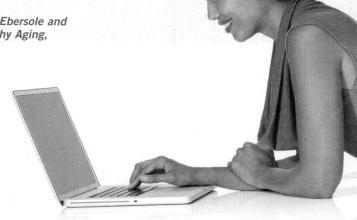

Ebersole and Hess'

Gerontological Nursing & Healthy Aging

FOURTH EDITION

THERIS A. TOUHY, DNP, CNS, DPNAP
Emeritus Professor
Christine E. Lynn College of Nursing
Florida Atlantic University
Boca Raton, Florida

KATHLEEN F. JETT, PhD, GNP-BC
Gerontological Nurse Practitioner
Oak Hammock at the University of Florida
Department of Aging and Geriatrics College of Medicine
Gainesville, Florida

Research Consultant
College of Nursing
University of Florida
Gainesville, Florida

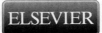

3251 Riverport Lane
St. Louis, Missouri 63043

EBERSOLE AND HESS' GERONTOLOGICAL NURSING
AND HEALTHY AGING

ISBN: 978-0-323-09606-5

Notices

Knowledge and best practice in this field are constantly changing. As new research and experience broaden our understanding, changes in research methods, professional practices, or medical treatment may become necessary.

Practitioners and researchers must always rely on their own experience and knowledge in evaluating and using any information, methods, compounds, or experiments described herein. In using such information or methods they should be mindful of their own safety and the safety of others, including parties for whom they have a professional responsibility.

With respect to any drug or pharmaceutical products identified, readers are advised to check the most current information provided (i) on procedures featured or (ii) by the manufacturer of each product to be administered, to verify the recommended dose or formula, the method and duration of administration, and contraindications. It is the responsibility of practitioners, relying on their own experience and knowledge of their patients, to make diagnoses, to determine dosages and the best treatment for each individual patient, and to take all appropriate safety precautions.

To the fullest extent of the law, neither the Publisher nor the authors, contributors, or editors, assume any liability for any injury and/or damage to persons or property as a matter of products liability, negligence or otherwise, or from any use or operation of any methods, products, instructions, or ideas contained in the material herein.

Library of Congress Cataloging-in-Publication Data

Touhy, Theris A.
    Ebersole and Hess' gerontological nursing & healthy aging / Theris A. Touhy, Kathleen F. Jett.—4th ed.
        p. ; cm.
    Gerontological nursing & healthy aging
    Includes bibliographical references and index.
    ISBN 978-0-323-09606-5 (pbk. : alk. paper)
    I. Jett, Kathleen Freudenberger. II. Ebersole, Priscilla. III. Title. IV. Title: Gerontological nursing
& healthy aging.
    [DNLM: 1. Geriatric Nursing. 2. Aged. 3. Aging. 4. Health Promotion. 5. Holistic Nursing. WY 152]

    618.97'0231—dc23

                                                2012047074

Content Manager: Michele D. Hayden
Associate Content Development Specialists: Sarah Jane Watson and Melissa Rawe
Publishing Services Manager: Jeff Patterson
Project Manager: Megan Isenberg
Design Direction: Paula Catalano

Printed in the United States of America

Last digit is the print number: 9   8   7   6   5   4   3   2

To my beautiful grandchildren, Colin, Molly, and Auden Touhy.
Being your Gramma TT makes growing older the best time of my life and I love you.
To my sons and daughters-in-law, thanks for surrounding me with love and family.
To my husband, just thanks for loving me for 45 years even though it's not always easy!
To the older people I have been privileged to nurse, and their caregivers, thanks
for making the words in this book a reality for the elders you care for and
for teaching me how to be a gerontological nurse.

Theris Touhy

To my husband Steve, who is a source of never-ending support.
Without his willingness to keep me supplied with food,
the long hours sitting in front of the computer and writing
would not have been possible.
To the older adults who have opened their lives to me so that I may learn.
To our four children and four wonderful grandchildren, Haley, Amelia, Emory, and Logan,
who always remind me that the best part of life is the time we spend together
and that the older we get, the more we have loved
and the more adventures we have shared.

Kathleen Jett

Reviewers

Patricia L. Buls, MSN, RN, BC
Assistant and Adjunct Professor
Allen College
Waterloo, Iowa

Patricia Burbank, DNSc, RN
Professor, College of Nursing
University of Rhode Island
Kingston, Rhode Island

Sarah Gilbert, RN, MSN, G-CNS, BC
Instructor, School of Nursing
Radford University
Radford, Virginia

Vickie Ann Grosso, PhD, RN
Professor, Department of Nursing
Essex County College
Newark, New Jersey

Colleen J. Hewes, RN, MSN, DC
Instructor of Nursing
Lake Washington Technical College
Kirkland, Washington

Laurie Kennedy-Malone, PhD, APRN-BC, FAAN
Professor, School of Nursing
University of North Carolina at Greensboro
Greensboro, North Carolina

Judy Kopka, RN, MSN
Clinical Associate Professor, Columbia College of Nursing
Columbia-St. Mary's, Inc.
Milwaukee, Wisconsin

Carla Lynch, MS, RN
Clinical Assistant Professor of Nursing
The University of Tulsa
Tulsa, Oklahoma

Marie Messier, BSN, MSN, MEd
Associate Professor of Nursing
Germanna Community College
Locust Grove, Virginia

Carmella M. Mikol, PhD, MN, BSN
Professor, Nursing Program
College of Lake County
Grayslake, Illinois

Claudia Mitchell, RN, MSN
Assistant Professor of Clinical Nursing
College of Nursing
University of Cincinnati
Cincinnati, Ohio

Margaret Moriarty-Litz, BSN, MNA
Instructor/Coordinator
St. Joseph School of Nursing
Nashua, New Hampshire

Lillian A. Rafeldt, RN, MA, CNE
Assistant Professor of Nursing
Three Rivers Community College
Norwich, Connecticut

Janine Ray, RN, MSN
Instructor, Nursing Program
Cisco Junior College
Abilene, Texas

Katherine Seibert, EdDc, RN
Associate Professor of Nursing, School of Nursing
Mercy College of Health Sciences
Des Moines, Iowa

Tracy A. Szirony, PhD, RNC, CHPN
Associate Professor of Nursing
College of Nursing
University of Toledo
Toledo, Ohio

Jane Tanking, RN, MSN
School of Nursing Lecturer
Washburn University
Topeka, Kansas

Judith Townsend Rocchiccioli, PhD, RN
Professor of Nursing
James Madison University
Harrisonburg, Virginia

Anne Van Landingham, RN, MSN, BSN
Nursing Instructor
Orlando Tech
Orlando, Florida

Anne Viviano, RN, MSN
Nursing Faculty
Baker College
Clinton Township, Michigan

Loretta Wack, RN, MSN
Associate Professor of Nursing
Blue Ridge Community College
Weyers Cave, Virginia

Tricia Wickers, RN, MSN
Associate Professor of Nursing
Los Angeles Harbor College
Wilmington, California

Preface

This text is about health, wellness, and aging. It is designed to provide nurses, faculty, and students with the most current information on evidence-based gerontological nursing, an area often neglected in basic nursing education and nursing texts. The fourth edition provides content consistent with the *Recommended Baccalaureate Competencies and Curricular Guidelines for the Nursing Care of Older Adults* developed by AACN in collaboration with the John A. Hartford Foundation Institute for Geriatric Nursing at New York University. The book sections have been revised with totally updated content and new chapters on metabolic and neurological disorders. The goals set forth by *Healthy People 2020* provide the framework for the study of healthy aging. Although Maslow's Hierarchy of Needs is the organizing framework, it includes additional frameworks for a range of situations.

Section 1, "Foundations of Healthy Aging," explores gerontological nursing history, education, and roles; care across the continuum; the impact of culture and health disparities; theories of aging and physical changes; and the social, psychological, spiritual, and cognitive aspects of aging. In Section 2, "Fundamentals of Caring," content ranges from assessment tools, skillful documentation, and safe medication use to evidence-based nursing responses to promote healthy nutrition, sleep, elimination, skin, and the maintenance of mobility and safety. Section 3, "Coping with Chronic Disorders in Late Life," focuses on common health problems seen in older adults and what nurses can do to help elders living with chronic illness to achieve optimum wellness. This section does not provide the in-depth coverage of the topics that one would find in a medical-surgical nursing textbook, but highlights the key aspects of the problems as they relate specifically to older adults. In Section 4, "Caring for Elders and Their Caregivers," we present discussions of the global topics that affect all of us as we age: economic and legal issues; relationships; caregiving; roles and transitions; coping with grief and loss; and dying and death.

The text is organized for optimal student learning experiences. Each chapter begins with the phenomenological consideration of the lived experience of an elder. Key concepts, glossaries, learning activities, and discussion questions summarize the important points presented and relate directly to the objectives of the chapter. For readers who wish to seek additional information, resources are provided at http://evolve.elsevier.com/Ebersole/gerontological.

Gerontological nurses have always assumed a leadership role in improving care for elders, ensuring fulfillment of all levels of Maslow's Hierarchy of Needs, and promoting healthy aging. Since the first edition of this text, there has been an explosion of knowledge, research, interest, and resources in gerontological nursing. The specialty continues to grow in importance, and gerontological nursing competencies are now recognized as basic education requirements for nurses in all specialties. Today, the expectation is that all nurses will be prepared to care for the growing number of diverse older adults and have the knowledge and skills to promote healthy aging for people of all ages around the globe. We can look forward to the coming years when aging in health will be the norm, and we hope this text will provide the knowledge nurses need to play a key role in making this happen.

Theris A. Touhy
Kathleen F. Jett

Ancillaries

Ancillaries are available at http://evolve.elsevier.com/Ebersole/gerontological.

For Instructors

- **TEACH for Nurses: A NEW resource for this edition,** **TEACH for Nurses** Lesson Plans for each book chapter include learning objectives; key terms; student and instructor resources; suggested classroom activities; answers to Critical Thinking Activities in the book; and clinical activities that can be used for classroom discussion, projects, and further study. Also included is an outline of nursing curriculum standards for each chapter that includes QSEN, Concepts, and BSN Essentials, and a unique Case Study for each book chapter.

- **PowerPoint Presentations:** PowerPoint slide presentations to accompany each chapter (approximately 480 slides total)
- **Test Bank:** Approximately 500 questions in the latest NCLEX® examination format (ExamView format)
- **Image Collection:** Over 50 illustrations and photos that can be used in a presentation or as visual aids

For Students

- **Animations:** Full-color animations that visually enhance the material in the text
- **NCLEX®-Style Review Questions:** Questions organized by chapter for additional help in preparing for the NCLEX® examination
- **Resources:** Additional resources organized by chapter for further study of concepts presented in the chapter

Acknowledgments

We would like to thank Priscilla Ebersole and Patricia Hess for the opportunity to author this book and to share their beautiful words and passion for gerontological nursing. We hope that our work honors them and the specialty we all love. It has been a real privilege for us to be a part of the work of two gerontological nurses from whom we have learned how to care for older people.

Theris A. Touhy
Kathleen F. Jett

Contents

Section 3　　Coping with Chronic Disorders in Late Life

Section 4   Caring for Elders and Their Caregivers

CHAPTER 1

Introduction to Healthy Aging

Kathleen F. Jett

evolve evolve.elsevier.com/Ebersole/gerontological

LEARNING OBJECTIVES

Upon completion of this chapter, the reader will be able to:
- Identify at least three factors that influence the aging experience.
- Define health and wellness within the context of aging and chronic illness.
- Describe the trends seen in global aging today.
- Apply Maslow's Hierarchy of Needs to gerontological nursing.

GLOSSARY

Cohort A Group in which members share some common experience.
Wellness A state of health that is optimal for the individual person at any point in time.
Centenarian A person who is at least 100 years of age.
Holistic health care That which considers the whole person and the interaction with and between the parts.

THE LIVED EXPERIENCE

I believe a human life is like a river, meandering through its course, rushing through rapids, flowing placidly over the plains, twisting and turning through countless bends until it spends itself. It is the same river; yet it looks very different from one place to another. So it is with our lives; circumstances vary from one time to another in the course of a life, but I think each stage has its own value.

Georgia, 35 years old

Caring for older adults gives us a unique opportunity to influence their quality of life in so many ways.

Nursing student, age 19

Providing nursing care to older persons is a rewarding, life-affirming vocation. Through this textbook we hope to provide students with the basics to begin a career as a gerontological nurse and care for older adults with more skill and sensitivity. We present an overview of aging, the most common health care needs of older adults, and the vital and exciting role of the nurse in facilitating healthy aging and wellness.

Aging in the United States

Although all of us begin aging at birth, both the meaning of aging and those who are identified as elders are determined by society and culture and influenced by history and gender. In the early American Puritan community of the 1600s, the process of aging was considered a sacred pilgrimage to God, and as such, persons in late life were revered. However, by the late 1800s, aging was devalued as youth became the symbol of growth and expansion. In 1935, with the establishment of Social Security, the time when one became "old" was set at 65. In the 2000s this age is creeping toward 70 along with the eligibility for retirement benefits.

Psychologists have traditionally divided the "old" into three groups: the young-old, roughly 65 to 74 years of age; the middle-old, 75 to 84 years of age; and the old-old, or those over 85. Those 100 years of age and older (centenarians) are the most rapidly growing group today; those over 110 are referred to as *supercentenarians* (Willcox et al., 2008) (Box 1-1). In 2009 about 12.9% of the population in the United States or 39.6 million persons were 65 and over, compared with 0.1% in 1901. The total number is expected to double between 2000 and 2030, increasing to about 72.1 million or 19% of the population (Administration on Aging [AOA], 2011).

Those born within the same decade and country may share a common historical context and are referred to as a *cohort.* For example, men born between 1920 and 1930 were very likely to have been active participants in World War II or the Korean War. In comparison, men born between 1940 and 1950 were likely to have been involved in the Vietnam conflict, an entirely different experience. It is not surprising that these two groups of men have different perspectives and different health problems. Likewise, privileged women born between 1920 and 1930 were raised with what are known as traditional values and roles and may have either never worked outside the home or been limited to what was considered "women's work," such as housekeeping, teaching, and nursing. In contrast, similar women born between 1940 and 1950 had pressure to work outside the home and had considerably more opportunities, partially as a result of the feminist revolution of the 1960s and 1970s.

Gender can have a significant effect on various aspects of aging. Women usually live longer than men and live alone after widowhood. Men who survive their wives often remarry and live alone significantly less often than women. Women usually have larger social networks outside the work environment than men, which could potentially reduce social isolation after the death of a spouse or companion (see Chapter 24).

Finally, the United States is experiencing a "gerontological explosion" of all persons over 65, including ethnically diverse older adults. Persons comprising groups that have been considered statistical minorities in the late 1900s can now be considered an emerging majority as the relative percentage of their numbers rises rapidly. See Figure 1-1 for the projected changes in the demographics of older adults by ethnicity and race by the year 2050. Although the health status of racial and ethnic groups has improved over the past century, disparities in major health indicators between white and nonwhite groups are growing (Box 1-2). Increasing the numbers of health care providers from different cultures as well as ensuring cultural competence of all providers is essential to meet the needs of a rapidly growing, ethnically diverse elderly population (see Chapter 4).

BOX 1-1 Super-Centenarian Extraordinaire: Jeanne Louise Calment

Jeanne Louise Calment died in France at age 122. At that time she was believed to be the longest-lived person in the world. She outlived her husband, her daughter, her only grandson, and her lawyer. Her husband died in 1942, just four years before their 50th anniversary. Her daughter died in 1936 and her grandson in 1963. She was four when the Eiffel tower was built and reportedly once sold art supplies to Vincent Van Gogh. Not only did she live a long life, but did so with vigor. Madame Calment took up fencing at 85 and was still riding a bike at 107. She smoked until she was 117 and ate a lifelong diet rich in olive oil. Her longevity remains a mystery to experts and researchers.

From Dollemore D: *Aging under the microscope: a biological quest,* Bethesda, MD, 2006, National Institute of Aging, National Institutes of Health, Publication #02-2756.

Global Aging

Before the year 2050, the number of persons 60 years of age and older worldwide is likely to exceed those younger than 15 years for the first time in recorded history, most notably in developing or low-income countries (National Institute on Aging, National Institutes of Health, 2007) (Figure 1-2). This occurred in Europe in 1995 but will not occur in North America until 2015. Those older than 60 years of age will not surpass children until 2040 in Asia, Latin American, and the Caribbean (United Nations [UN], 2007a). However in 2007, Japan already had the highest percentage of persons 60 years of age and older at 27.9% (UN, 2007b). These changes pose major challenges in meeting the needs of the aging global community as the number of younger adults providing care and financial support diminishes. Although the number of the very old remains small, the relative number of centenarians in the world's population is growing dramatically in the United States alone (Figure 1-3). The U.N. estimates that a worldwide population of 270,000 centenarians will grow to 2.3 million by the year 2050 (Kinsella & He, 2009, p. 28).

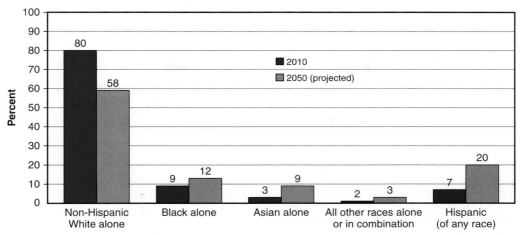

FIGURE 1-1 Population 65 years of age and over, by race and Hispanic origin: 2010 and projected 2050. (Redrawn from Federal Interagency Forum on Aging-Related Statistics: *Older Americans 2012: key indicators of well-being*, Washington DC, 2012, U.S. Government Printing Office.)

BOX 1-2   Use of Select Clinical Preventive Services by Race and Ethnicity

American Indian/Alaskan Native Adults
40% need influenza vaccination
35% need pneumococcal vaccination

Asian/Pacific Islander Adults
49% need colorectal cancer screening
47% need diabetes screening

Black American Adults
47% need pneumococcal vaccination
44% need influenza vaccination

Hispanic Adults
51% need pneumococcal vaccination
47% need colorectal screening

White Adults
34% need colorectal cancer screening
31% need diabetes screening

From Centers for Disease Control and Prevention, Administration on Aging, Agency for Healthcare Research and Quality and Centers for Medicare and Medicaid Services: *Enhancing use of clinical preventive services among older adults*, Washington, D.C., AARP, 2011. Available at www.cdc/gov/aging.

Among centenarians, women are between four and five times more numerous than men (UN, 2007b, p. xxviii) (Figure 1-4).

Africa stands out as the only major region where the population is still relatively young and the number of elderly, although increasing, will still be far below the number of those 0 to 59 years of age in 2050. Those between 15 and 59 years of age in Africa is projected to rise from half a billion in 2005 to more than 1.2 billion in 2050 (UN, 2007a), while those older than 60 will only increase from 0.05 billion to 0.2 billion in the same period.

Moving Toward Healthy Aging

The definitions of health vary greatly and are influenced by both culture and where one is on the life span. The strong emergence of the holistic health movement has resulted in even broader definitions of wellness and changes in Medicare (see Chapter 23) to support preventive care have promoted healthier aging (Table 1-1). Wellness involves one's whole being—physical, emotional, mental, and spiritual—all of which are vital components (Figure 1-5). In a classic work, Dunn (1961) defined the holistic approach to health as "an integrated method of functioning which is oriented toward maximizing the potential of which the individual is capable within the environment where he [or she] is functioning." Wellness involves achieving a balance between one's internal and external environment and one's emotional, spiritual, social, cultural, and physical processes.

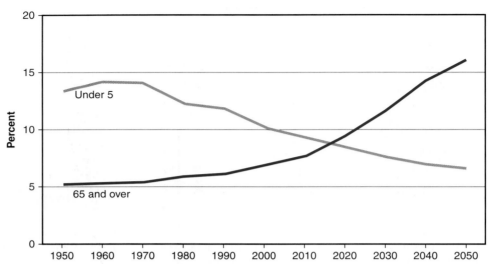

FIGURE 1-2 Average annual percent growth of older population in developed and developing countries: 1950 to 2050. (From Kinsella K, Wan H: U.S. Census Bureau, International Population Reports, P95/09-1, *An aging world: 2008*, Washington DC, 2009, U.S. Government Printing Office.)

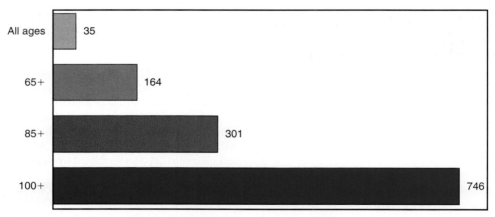

FIGURE 1-3 Percent change in world population by age, 2005 to 2040. (From U.N. Department of Economic and Social Affairs, 2007. Available at www.un.org/esa/population/publications/WPA2007/wpp2007.htm.)

Wellness is a state of being and feeling that one strives to achieve through effective health practices. An individual must work hard to achieve wellness. In working toward wellness, an individual may reach plateaus in his or her ascension to higher-level wellness. The person may also regress because of an illness or acute event or crisis, but these events can be a potential stimulus for growth and a return to moving along the wellness continuum (Figure 1-6).

Consistent with Dunn (1961), health in later life is often thought of in terms of functional ability (i.e., the ability to do what is important to a given person) rather than the absence of disease. This may mean the person's ability to live independently or the ability to enjoy great-grandchildren when they visit at the nursing home, but it is always individually determined. Well-being for those older than 60 years of age is strongly related to functional status but is affected also by socioeconomic factors, degree of social interaction, marital status, and aspects of one's living situation and environment.

In a push toward wellness, the health goals of the United States were recently updated in the document *Healthy People 2020* (U.S. Department of Health and

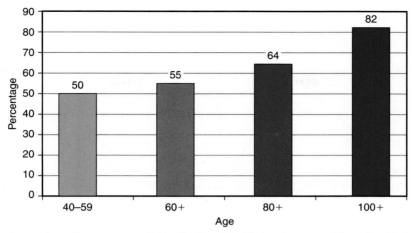

FIGURE 1-4 Proportion of women in specific age groups, worldwide, 2009. (From United Nations, Department of Economic and Social Affairs: *World population ageing 2009*, New York, 2009, United Nations. Available at www.un.org/esa/population/publications/WPA2009/WPA2009_WorkingPaper.pdf.)

TABLE 1-1	Intervention to Promote Wellness
Preventive Service	**Wellness and Person-Oriented Intervention**
Promoting influenza[†] and pneumococcal vaccination*	Consider new approaches to community outreach, such as home visits, neighbor-to-neighbor campaigns. Develop effective reminder systems.
Breast Cancer Screening Mammogram and Clinical Breast Exam*	Develop effective reminder systems. One-to-one education and counseling. Reduce structural barriers, such as transportation difficulties.
Colorectal Screening	Coverage depends on type of test used. Develop effective reminder systems. Reduce structural barriers, such as transportation difficulties.
Abdominal Aortic Aneurysm Screening*	For those persons at risk on physician referral. Inform the public.
Bone Mass Measurement*	Once every 24 months. May be covered 100%. Nurse can participate in community screening efforts.
Cervical and Vaginal Screening*	Covered at least every 24 months, depending on circumstances. Help person determine eligibility and appropriateness.
Diabetes Screenings*	Covered at least two times a year based on risk factors. Help identify persons at risk
Diabetes Self-Management Training*	For those with diabetes. Encourage participation.
Glaucoma Tests[‡]	Once a year for those at high risk. Help identify persons at risk.
Hearing and Balance Exams[‡]	For those with identified potential problems. Identify those with impairments and work with them to obtain care.
Hepatitis B Immunizations*	Identify those at risk. Nurse usually administers the vaccine.
HIV Screening[†]	Once every 12 months for persons at risk. Participate in campaigns to inform persons about who is at risk and how to reduce their risk.
Prostate Screenings (PSA and digital rectal exam (DRE))	Covered for the PSA, 20% co-pay for the DRE. Stay informed about current status and recommendations about this screening.
Tobacco Use Cessation[‡]	Coverage depends on circumstances. Co-pay and deductible may apply.
Welcome to Medicare and Annual "Wellness" Visits*	Thorough exam including a Health Risk Appraisal and wellness counseling. Inform persons of this health care benefit and help them make the best of the visit.

*This is of no cost if the provider "accepts assignment" or that amount that Medicare has approved. No co-pays are required.
[†]No cost
[‡]In most cases a 20% co-pay and deductible apply
From Centers for Medicare and Medicaid Services: *Medicare & you*. Publication #10050-27, August 2011. Baltimore, MD. See also http://www.healthcare.gov/news/factsheets/2010/07/preventive-services-list.html#CoveredPreventiveServicesforWomenIncludingPregnantWomen.

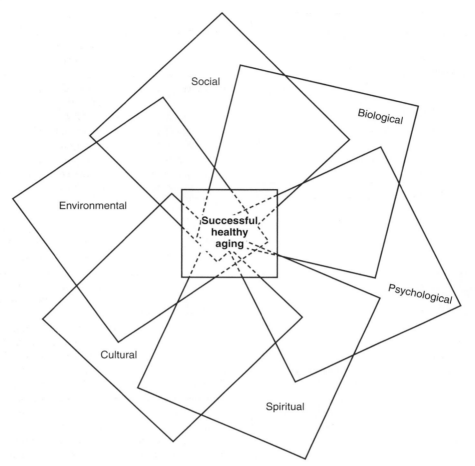

FIGURE 1-5 Healthy aging. (Developed by Patricia Hess.)

Human Services [USDHHS], 2012; see the Healthy People boxes). For the first time, older adults are identified as a priority group, with the specific goal to improve their health, function, and quality of life (USDHHS, 2012). The importance of this is triggered by the recognition of the growth of the population and the number of chronic conditions they are or will be facing as well as an emphasis on the use of clinical preventive services (USDHHS, 2012).

Approaching aging from a viewpoint of health even if the person has an illness emphasizes strengths, resilience, resources, and capabilities rather than focusing on existing pathological conditions. A wellness perspective is based on the belief that every person has an optimal level of health independent of his or her situation or functional ability or ability to manage day-to-day activities. Movement toward higher wellness is possible if the emphasis of care is placed

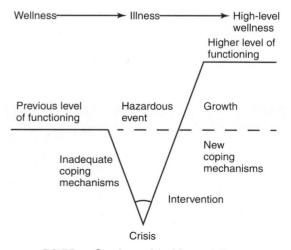

FIGURE 1-6 Growth potential: crisis as a challenge.

HEALTHY PEOPLE 2020

Overarching Goals
- Attain high-quality, longer lives free of preventable disease, disability, injury, and premature death.
- Achieve health equity, eliminate disparities, and improve the health of all groups.
- Create social and physical environments that promote good health for all.
- Promote quality of life, healthy development, and healthy behaviors across all life stages.

From U.S. Department of Health and Human Services, Office of Disease Prevention and Health Promotion: *Introducing healthy people 2020* (2012). Available at http://www.healthypeople.gov/2020.

 HEALTHY PEOPLE 2020

Emerging Issues in the Health of Older Adults
- Coordinate care.
- Help older adults manage their own care.
- Establish quality measures.
- Identify minimum levels of training for people who care for older adults.
- Research and analyze appropriate training to equip providers with the tools they need to meet the needs of older adults.

From U.S. Department of Health and Human Services: *Healthy people 2020.* Topics and objectives: older adults (2012). Available at http://www.healthypeople.gov/2020.

on the promotion of well-being in the least restrictive environment, with support and encouragement for the person to find meaning in the situation, whatever it is.

Maslow's Hierarchy of Human Needs

Maslow's theory of the hierarchy of human needs provide an organizing framework for this text and for understanding individuals and their concerns at any particular time or situation (Figure 1-7). It also can serve as a guide for prioritizing nursing interventions to promote healthy aging and as a framework for this text. The hierarchy ranks needs from the most basic, related to the maintenance of biological integrity, to the most complex, associated with self-actualization.

According to this theory, the needs of higher levels cannot be met without first meeting those of lower levels at least to some extent. In other words, moving toward healthy aging is an evolving and developing process. As basic-level needs are met, the satisfaction of higher-level needs is possible, with ever deepening richness to life, regardless of one's age. The nurse prioritizes care from the most essential to those things thought of as quality of life.

As far back as Hippocrates and Galen, the necessities of all living people were recognized as the need for air, fluids, nutrition, hygiene, elimination, activity, and skin integrity. In 1990, nurse theorist Dorothea Orem described basic human needs of Maslow's model as *self-care requirements* (Box 1-3). Along with those listed in the box is the need for comfort or relief from suffering. The gerontological nurse works to ensure that these needs are met for older adults and realizes that as this is accomplished, higher levels of wellness are possible. The person with dementia may begin to wander or become agitated because of the need to find a toilet and not knowing where to look. Until toileting needs are met, the nurse's attempt to comfort may be ineffective. As people's basic needs are met they will feel safe and secure (Maslow's second level). They will likely sleep better and feel more comfortable interacting with others. While interacting with others, people often begin to meet their needs of belonging (Maslow's third level). Participation in church, synagogue, or mosque activities; civic or social organizations; and the maintenance of ties to family and friends all are ways people fulfill belonging needs. After retirement a member of a work organization may instead become involved in special interest groups. Involvement is an opportunity to form new alliances and associations and to create environments in which relationships and activities can remain a part of life and contribute to bring life meaning (fourth level) regardless of the setting.

According to Maslow's model, a person whose basic needs are met, who feels safe and secure, and who has a sense of belonging will also develop self-esteem and a belief in self-efficacy (fourth level). In other words, people will accept and honor who they are and feel that they have some personal power and self-confidence; they will know that they are important as people and that they inherently have value. Self-esteem is not something that can be given. It is, however, something that others can negatively influence through ageist attitudes and behavior. For example, a nurse who assumes that a patient cannot do something based solely on the person's age is being ageist and is actually belittling the individual. Unfortunately this is common, but it can be challenged by the knowledgeable and sensitive gerontological nurse.

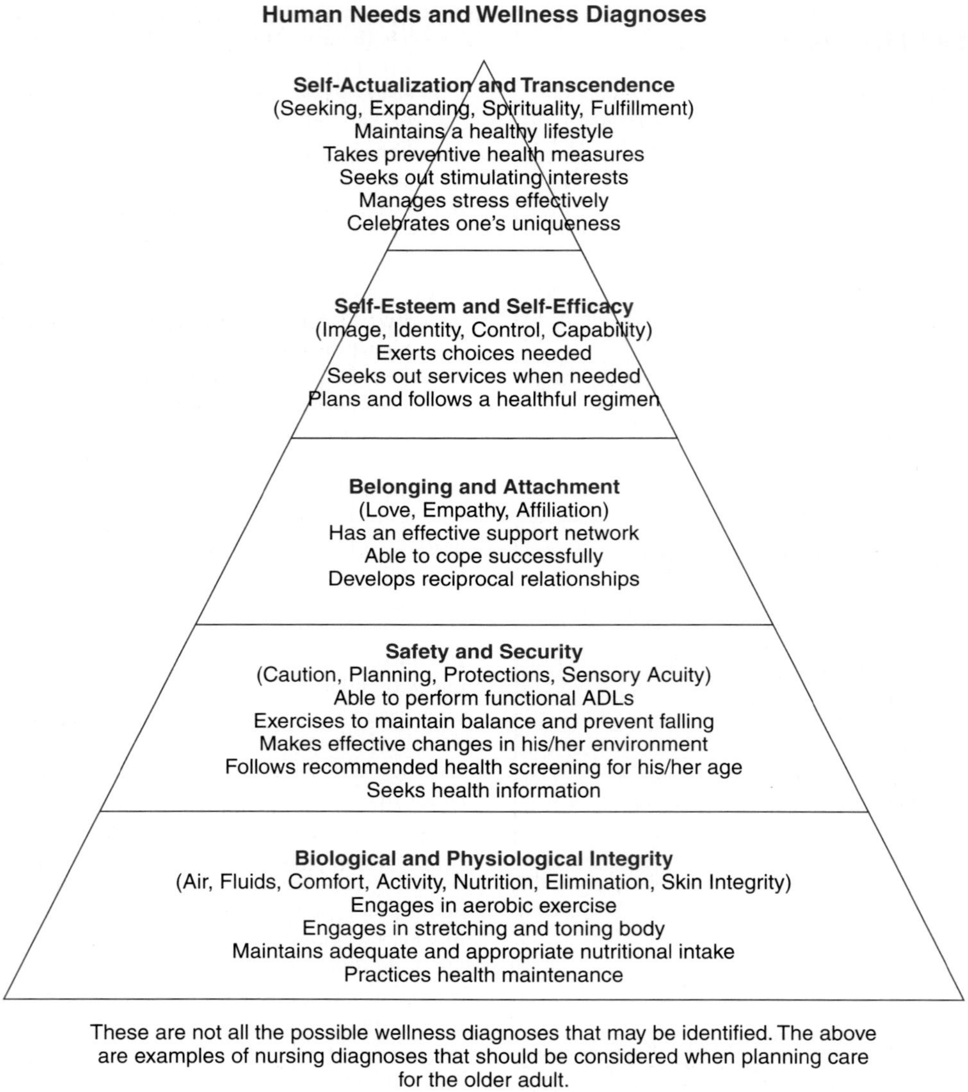

Human Needs and Wellness Diagnoses

Self-Actualization and Transcendence
(Seeking, Expanding, Spirituality, Fulfillment)
Maintains a healthy lifestyle
Takes preventive health measures
Seeks out stimulating interests
Manages stress effectively
Celebrates one's uniqueness

Self-Esteem and Self-Efficacy
(Image, Identity, Control, Capability)
Exerts choices needed
Seeks out services when needed
Plans and follows a healthful regimen

Belonging and Attachment
(Love, Empathy, Affiliation)
Has an effective support network
Able to cope successfully
Develops reciprocal relationships

Safety and Security
(Caution, Planning, Protections, Sensory Acuity)
Able to perform functional ADLs
Exercises to maintain balance and prevent falling
Makes effective changes in his/her environment
Follows recommended health screening for his/her age
Seeks health information

Biological and Physiological Integrity
(Air, Fluids, Comfort, Activity, Nutrition, Elimination, Skin Integrity)
Engages in aerobic exercise
Engages in stretching and toning body
Maintains adequate and appropriate nutritional intake
Practices health maintenance

These are not all the possible wellness diagnoses that may be identified. The above
are examples of nursing diagnoses that should be considered when planning care
for the older adult.

FIGURE 1-7 Human needs and wellness diagnoses using Maslow's Hierarchy framework. *ADLs,* Activities of daily living.

Finally, some people reach Maslow's highest level of wellness, that of self-actualization. Self-actualization is seen as people reaching out beyond themselves and finding meaning and a sense of fulfillment. This may not seem possible for all, but the nurse can foster this in unique and important ways. The author was asked to speak to a group in a nursing home about death and dying. To her surprise the room was not filled with staff, as she had expected, but with the frailest of elders in wheelchairs. Instead of the usual lecture, she spoke of legacies and asked the silent audience, "What do you want people to remember about you? What made your life worthwhile?" Without exception each member of the audience had something to say, from "I had a beautiful garden" to "I was a good mother" to "I helped design a bridge." Meaning can be found for life everywhere—you just have to ask.

BOX 1-3   Orem's Universal Self-Care Requirements

1. Maintaining sufficient intake of air, water, food
   a. Taking in the quantity required for normal functioning
   b. Preserving the integrity of associated anatomic structures and physiologic processes
2. Maintaining satisfactory elimination function
   a. Preserving the integrity of associated anatomic structures and physiologic processes
   b. Providing hygienic care of body surfaces and parts to the extent necessary to prevent injury or exposure to infection
   c. Maintaining adequate and sanitary disposal systems
3. Maintaining a balance between activity and rest
   a. Selecting activities that stimulate, engage, and keep in balance physical movement and rest adequate for health

   b. Responding to manifestations of needs for rest and activity
   c. Using personal capabilities, interests, and values as well as culturally prescribed norms as bases for development of a rest-activity pattern
4. Maintaining a balance between solitude and social interaction
   a. Maintaining the ability and interest necessary for the development of personal autonomy and enduring social relations
   b. Fostering bonds of affection, love, and friendship
   c. Participating in situations of social warmth and closeness
   d. Pursuing opportunities for satisfying group interactions

Based on the work of Dorothea Orem. See Hartweg, D: *Dorothea Orem: self-care deficit theory*, Newbury Park, CA, 1991, SAGE.

Implications for Gerontological Nursing and Healthy Aging

It is the responsibility of the nurse to assist elders to achieve the highest level of wellness in relation to whatever situation exists. The nurse can, through knowledge and affirmation, empower, enhance, and support the person's movement toward the highest level of wellness and quality of life possible. The nurse assesses and helps explore the underlying situation that may be interfering with the achievement of wellness, and work with the person and significant others to develop affirming and appropriate plans of care. The nurse can utilize the resources available, such as *Healthy People 2020* and the *Clinical Preventive Services Guidelines* to maximize the potential for health (see Table 1-1). The nurse and the elder collaboratively implement interventions to achieve individual goals and evaluate their effectiveness. The goals of the nurse are to care and comfort always, to cure sometimes, and to prevent that which can be prevented.

KEY CONCEPTS
- Gerontological nursing is an opportunity to make a significant difference in the lives of older adults.
- The meaning of aging is influenced by many factors.
- Nurses have a responsibility to contribute to the nation's goals of increasing the quality of life lived and to reduce health disparities.

- Health, history, and gender are among the major factors influencing the aging experience.
- Each age cohort is distinctly different from others in some ways.
- Individual persons become more unique the longer they live. Thus one must be cautious in attributing any specific characteristics of older adults to "old age."
- All persons, regardless of age or life and/or health situation, can be helped to achieve a higher level of wellness, which is uniquely and personally defined.
- Maslow's Hierarchy of Needs can be used as an organizing framework for health promotion, regardless of age or situation.
- Gerontological nurses have key roles in the provision of the highest quality of care to older adults in a wide range of settings and situations.
- Ageist attitudes and behaviors undermine not only the self-esteem of the individual but society's acknowledgment of the value of the contributions of older adults.

ACTIVITIES AND DISCUSSION QUESTIONS
1. Discuss the ways in which elders contribute to society today.
2. Activity: Interview an older person, and ask what has changed since he or she was 25 years of age. Compare your findings with others in your class.
3. Discuss health and wellness with your peers. Develop a definition of aging.

4. Consider Maslow's Hierarchy of Needs and discuss the level you feel is the most important. Explain your choice.
5. Explain wellness in the context of chronic illness.
6. Discuss how you seek wellness in your own life.
7. Discuss what you can do to enhance the wellness and quality of life for the persons to whom you provide care.
8. Activity: Draw a picture of yourself at 80 years of age. Compare your drawing to those of others who have done the same and discuss the implications of the representation.
9. Discuss how older adults are portrayed in popular TV shows, commercials, and movies.

REFERENCES

Administration on Aging [AOA]: *Aging statistics* (2011). Available at http://www.aoa.gov/AoARoot/Aging_Statistics/index.aspx.

Centers for Medicare and Medicaid Services: *Enhancing use of clinical services among older adults*, Washington, DC, 2011, AARP.

Dunn HL: *High-level wellness*, Arlington, VA, 1961, Beatty.

Kinsella K, He W: *An aging world* (2009). Available at http://www.census.gov/prod/2009pubs/p95-09-1.pdf.

National Institute on Aging, National Institutes of Health: *Why population aging matters: a global perspective* (2007). Available at http://www.nia.nih.gov/sites/default/files/WPAM.pdf.

United Nations [UN], Department of Economic and Social Affairs, Population Division: *Fact sheet, Series A* (2007a). Available at http://www.un.org/esa/population/publications/wpp2006/FS_aging.pdf.

United Nations [UN]: *World population aging* (2007b). Available at http://www.un.org/esa/population/publications/WPA2007/wpp2007.htm.

U.S. Department of Health and Human Services [USDHHS], Office of Disease Prevention and Health Promotion: *Healthy people 2020* (2012). Available at http://www.healthypeople.gov/2020.

Willcox BJ, Willcox DC, Ferrucci L: Secrets of healthy aging and longevity from exceptional survivors around the globe: Lessons from octogenarians to supercentenarians, *J Gerontol A Biol Sci Med Sci* 63(11):1201–1208, 2008.

Gerontological Nursing History, Education, and Roles

Theris A. Touhy

evolve evolve.elsevier.com/Ebersole/gerontological

LEARNING OBJECTIVES

Upon completion of this chapter, the reader will be able to:
- Discuss the implications of a growing older adult population on nursing education, practice, and research.
- Identify several factors that have influenced the development of gerontological nursing as a specialty practice.
- Examine the American Nurses Association Scope and Standards of Gerontological Nursing Practice and the recommended competencies for gerontological nursing practice.
- Recognize and discuss the importance of certification.
- Compare various gerontological nursing roles and requirements.
- Discuss formal gerontological organizations and their significance to the gerontological nurse.

THE LIVED EXPERIENCE

I don't think I will work in gerontological nursing; it seems depressing. I don't know many older people, but they are all sick without much hope to get better. I'll probably go into labor and delivery or the emergency room where I can really make a difference.

Student nurse, age 24

To know that I have made them feel they are human, that they're loved...that someone still cares about them. I believe that lots of times they feel ignored and as if they have no value. It's very important to me that they feel valued and they know that they still contribute not only to society but to the personal growth of everyone who comes into interaction with them.

Gerontological nurse, age 35, working in a nursing home

Care of Older Adults: A Nursing Imperative

The world population is aging. By 2050, one in five Americans will be over 65 years of age, with those over 85 showing the greatest increase in numbers. The number of people living to 100 years of age is projected to grow at more than 20 times the rate of the total population by 2050. Older people today are healthier, better educated, and expect a much higher quality of life as they age than did their elders. Healthy aging is now an achievable goal for many and it is essential that we have the knowledge and skills to help people of all ages, races, and cultures achieve this goal.

11

The developmental period of elderhood is an essential part of a healthy society and as important as childhood or adulthood (Thomas, 2004). We can expect to spend 40 or more years as older adults and our preparation for this time in our lives certainly demands attention as well as expert care from nurses. How does one maximize the experience of aging and enrich the years of elderhood despite the physical and psychological changes that may occur?

Most nurses care for older people during the course of their careers. In addition, the public looks to nurses to have knowledge and skills to assist people to age in health. Every older person should expect to receive care provided by nurses with competence in gerontological nursing. Gerontological nursing is not only for a specialty group of nurses. Knowledge of aging and gerontological nursing is core knowledge for the profession of nursing (Young, 2003).

Eldercare is projected to be the fastest growing employment sector in the health care industry. Older adults are the core consumers of health care, with higher rates of outpatient provider visits, hospitalizations, home care, and long-term care service use than other age groups. Despite demand, the number of health care workers who are interested in and prepared to care for older people remains low. America's eldercare workforce is dangerously understaffed and unprepared to care for the growing numbers of older adults (Institute of Medicine, 2008). Less than 1% of registered nurses (RNs) and only 3% of advanced practice registered nurses (APRNs) are certified in gerontology (Institute of Medicine, 2008; Stierle et al., 2006).

Geriatric medicine faces similar challenges with just 7,128 geriatricians, one for every 2,546 older Americans. By 2030, it is estimated that this number will increase to only 7,750, one for every 4,254 older Americans, far short of the predicted need for 36,000 geriatricians (Institute of Medicine, 2008). Other professions such as social work have similar shortages. These issues are critical not only in the United States but across the globe. "If these issues remain unresolved, the cumulative impact for our aging population and our overall health care system will be significant. Projected consequences include, but are not limited to extremely high nurse-patient ratios; proliferation of high-tech, low-touch care systems; and a decline in public trust for nursing" (American Nurses Association, 2010, p. 23). *Healthy People 2020* includes goals related to geriatric education (see the Healthy People box).

Enhancing interest, recruitment, and preparation of students and practicing nurses in care of older adults across the continuum is essential. Positive role models, a deep commitment to caring, and an appreciation of the significant contribution of a nursing model of care to the well-being of older people, are often the motivating factors that draw nurses to the specialty. Box 2-1 presents the views of some of the geriatric nursing pioneers, as well as current leaders, on the practice of gerontological nursing and what draws them to care of older adults.

BOX **2-1**   **Reflections on Gerontological Nursing from Gerontological Nursing Pioneers and Current Leaders in the Field**

Doris Schwartz, Gerontological Nursing Pioneer

"We need to remind ourselves constantly that the purpose of gerontic nursing is to prevent untimely death and needless suffering, always with the focus of doing *with* as well as doing *for,* and in every instance to attempt to preserve personhood as long as life continues." (From interview data collected by Priscilla Ebersole between 1990 and 2001.)

Mary Opal Wolanin, Gerontological Nursing Pioneer

"I believe that one of the most valuable lessons I have learned from those who are older is that I must start with looking inside at my own thinking. I was very guilty of ageism. I believed every myth in the book, was sure that I would never live past my seventieth birthday, and made no plan for my seventies. Probably the most productive years of my career have been since that dreaded birthday and I now realize that it is very difficult, if not impossible, to think of our own aging." (From interview data collected by Priscilla Ebersole between 1990 and 2001.)

Terry Fulmer, Dean, College of Nursing, New York University and Co-Director, John A. Hartford Institute for Geriatric Nursing

"I soon realized that in the arena of caring for the aged, I could have an autonomous nursing practice that would make a real difference in medical outcomes. I could practice the full scope of nursing. It gave me a sense of freedom and accomplishment. With older patients, the most important component of care, by far, is nursing care. It's very motivating." (From Ebersole P, Touhy T: *Geriatric nursing: growth of a specialty,* New York, 2006, Springer, p. 129.)

BOX 2-1   **Reflections on Gerontological Nursing from Gerontological Nursing Pioneers and Current Leaders in the Field—cont'd**

Neville Strumpf, Edith Clement Chair in Gerontological Nursing, University of Pennsylvania, Director of the Hartford Center of Geriatric Nursing Excellence and Center for Gerontological Nursing Science

"My philosophy remains deeply rooted in individual choice, comfort, and dignity, especially for frail, older adults. I fervently hope that the future will be characterized by a health care system capable of supporting these values throughout a person's life, and that we shall someday see the routine application of evidence based practice to the care of all older adults, whether they are in the community, a hospital, or the nursing home. We have not yet achieved that dream." (From Ebersole P, Touhy T: *Geriatric nursing: growth of a specialty*, New York, 2006, Springer, p. 145.)

Mathy Mezey, Professor Emeritus and Associate Director, The Hartford Institute for Geriatric Nursing, New York University College of Nursing

"Because geriatric nursing especially offers nurses the unique opportunity to dramatically impact people's lives for the better and for the worst, it demands the best that you have to offer. I am very optimistic about the future of geriatric nursing. Increasing numbers of older adults are interested in marching into old age as healthy and involved. Geriatric nursing offers a unique opportunity to help older adults meet these aspirations while at the same time maintaining a commitment to the oldest and

frailest in our society." (From Ebersole P, Touhy T: *Geriatric nursing: growth of a specialty*, New York, 2006, Springer, p. 142.)

Jennifer Lingler, PhD, FNP

"When I was in high school, a nurse I knew helped me find a nursing assistant position at the residential care facility where she worked. That experience sparked my interest in older adults that continues today. I realized that caring for frail elders could be incredibly gratifying, and I felt privileged to play a role, however small, in people's lives. At the same time, I became increasingly curious about what it means to age successfully. I questioned why some people seemed to age so gracefully, while others succumbed to physical illness, mental decline, or both. As a Building Academic Geriatric Nursing Capacity (BAGNC) alumnus, I now divide my time serving as a nurse practitioner at a memory disorders clinic, teaching an ethics course in a gerontology program, and conducting research on family caregiving. I am encouraged by the realization that as current students contemplate the array of opportunities before them, seek counsel from trusted mentors, and gain exposure to various clinical populations, the next generation of geriatric nurses will emerge. And, I am confident that in doing so, they will set their own course for affecting change in the lives of society's most vulnerable members." (Jennifer Lingler as cited in Fagin C, Franklin P: Why choose geriatric nursing? Six nursing scholars tell their stories, *Imprint*, September/October, 2005, p. 74.)

 HEALTHY PEOPLE 2020

Older Adults

- Increase the proportion of the health care workforce with geriatric certification (physicians, geriatric psychiatrists, registered nurses, dentists, physical therapists, dietitians)

From U.S. Department of Health and Human Services, Office of Disease Prevention and Health Promotion: *Healthy people 2020* (2012). Available at http://www.healthypeople.gov/2020.

History of Gerontological Nursing

Historically, nurses have always been in the frontlines of caring for older people. They have provided hands-on care, supervision, administration, program development, teaching, and research and are, to a great extent, responsible for

the rapid advance of gerontology as a profession. Nurses have been, and continue to be, the mainstay of care of older adults (Mezey & Fulmer, 2002). Gerontological nurses have made substantial contributions to the body of knowledge guiding best practice in care of older people. In examining the history of gerontological nursing, one must marvel at the advocacy and perseverance of nurses who have remained deeply committed to the care of older adults despite struggling against insurmountable odds over the years. We are proud to be the standard-bearers of excellence in care of older people. Table 2-1 presents a timeline of significant accomplishments in the history of gerontological nursing.

Early History

The origins of gerontological nursing are rooted in England and began with Florence Nightingale as she accepted a position in the Institution for the Care of Sick Gentlewomen in

TABLE 2-1	Professionalization of Gerontological Nursing
1906	First article is published in *American Journal of Nursing* (AJN) on care of the elderly.
1925	AJN considers geriatric nursing as a possible specialty in nursing.
1950	Newton and Anderson publish first geriatric nursing textbook. Geriatrics becomes a specialization in nursing.
1962	American Nurses Association (ANA) forms a national geriatric nursing group.
1966	ANA creates the Division of Geriatric Nursing. First master's program for clinical nurse specialists in geriatric nursing developed by Virginia Stone at Duke University.
1970	ANA establishes Standards of Practice for Geriatric Nursing.
1974	Certification in geriatric nursing practice offered through ANA; process implemented by Laurie Gunter and Virginia Stone.
1975	*Journal of Gerontological Nursing* published by Slack; first editor, Edna Stilwell.
1976	ANA renames Geriatric Division "Gerontological" to reflect a health promotion emphasis. ANA publishes Standards for Gerontological Nursing Practice; committee chaired by Barbara Allen Davis. ANA begins certifying geriatric nurse practitioners. *Nursing and the Aged* edited by Burnside and published by McGraw-Hill.
1977	First gerontological nursing track funded by Division of Nursing and established by Sr. Rose Therese Bahr at University of Kansas School of Nursing.
1979	Education for Gerontic Nursing written by Gunter and Estes; suggested curricula for all levels of nursing education.
1980	*Geriatric Nursing* first published by AJN; Cynthia Kelly, editor.
1983	Florence Cellar Endowed Gerontological Nursing Chair established at Case Western Reserve University, first in the nation; Doreen Norton, first scholar to occupy chair. National Conference of Gerontological Nurse Practitioners is established.
1984	National Gerontological Nurses Association is established. Division of Gerontological Nursing Practice becomes Council on Gerontological Nursing (councils established for all practice specialties).
1989	ANA certifies gerontological clinical nurse specialists.
1992	John A. Hartford Foundation funds a major initiative to improve care of hospitalized older patients: Nurses Improving Care for Healthsystem Elders (NICHE).
1996	John A. Hartford Foundation establishes the Institute for Geriatric Nursing at New York University under the direction of Mathy Mezey.
2000	Recommended baccalaureate competencies and curricular guidelines for geriatric nursing care published by the American Association of Colleges of Nursing and the John A. Hartford Foundation Institute for Geriatric Nursing. The American Academy of Nursing established Building Academic Geriatric Nursing Capacity (BAGNC) in 2000 with support from the John A. Hartford Foundation.
2001	Hartford Coalition of Geriatric Nursing Associations formed.
2002	Nurse Competence in Aging (funded by the Atlantic Philanthropies Inc.) initiative to improve the quality of health care to older adults by enhancing the geriatric competence of nurses who are members of specialty nursing.
2004	Nurse Practitioner and Clinical Nurse Specialist Competencies for Older Adult Care published by the American Association of Colleges of Nursing and the Hartford Institute for Geriatric Nursing. Atlantic Philanthropies committed its resources to postdoctoral fellowships in gerontology nursing.
2007	Atlantic Philanthropies provides a grant to the American Academy of Nursing of $500,000 to improve care of older adults in nursing homes by improving the clinical skills of professional nurses. American Association for Long-Term Care Nurses formed.

TABLE 2-1	**Professionalization of Gerontological Nursing—cont'd**
2008	Four new Centers of Geriatric Nursing Excellence (CGNE) are funded by the John A. Hartford Foundation bringing the total number of Centers to nine. Existing Centers are at the University of Iowa, University of California San Francisco, Oregon Health Sciences University, University of Arkansas, University of Pennsylvania, Arizona State University, Pennsylvania State University, University of Minnesota, and University of Utah. *Research in Gerontological Nursing* launched by Slack Inc; Dr. Kitty Buckwalter, Editor. Geriatric Nursing Leadership Academy established by Sigma Theta Tau International with funding from the John A. Hartford Foundation. John A. Hartford Foundation funds the Geropsychiatric Nursing Collaborative (Universities of Iowa, Arkansas, Pennsylvania, American Academy of Nursing) Institute of Medicine publishes *Retooling for an aging America: building the health care workforce* report.
2009	*National Consensus Model for APRN Regulation, Licensure, Accreditation, Certification and Education* designates adult-gerontology as one of 6 population foci for APRNs. John A. Hartford Foundation funds Phase 2 of the Fostering Geriatrics in Pre-Licensure Nursing Education, a partnership between the Community College of Philadelphia and the National League for Nursing.
2010	Adult-gerontology primary care nurse practitioner competencies published by the John A. Hartford Foundation Institute for Geriatric Nursing, the AACN, and NONPF. Sigma Theta Tau's Center for Nursing Excellence established. ANCC Pathways to Excellence – Long-Term Care Program.
2012	The Gerontological Society of America is now home to the Coordinating Center for the National Hartford Centers of Gerontological Nursing Excellence (HCGNE), also known as the Building Academic Geriatric Nursing Capacity Initiative. U.S. Department of Health and Human Services provides funding to five designated medical center hospitals for clinical training to newly enrolled APRNs to deliver primary care, preventive care, transitional care, chronic case management, and other services appropriate for Medicare recipients.
2013	Adult-Gerontology Acute Care Nurse Practitioner and Adult-Gerontology Primary Care Nurse Practitioner certifications through ANCC begin.

For a complete listing of John A. Hartford Foundation funding for geriatric nursing, see http://www.hgni.org/091008%20HGNI%20Project%20Descriptions.pdf.

Distressed Circumstances. Nightingale's concern for the frail and sick elderly was continued by Agnes Jones, a wealthy Nightingale-trained nurse, who in 1864 was sent to Liverpool Infirmary, a large Poor Law institution. The care in the institution was poor, the diet meager, and the nurses often drunk. But Miss Jones, under the tutelage of Nightingale, improved the care dramatically, as well as reduced the costs.

In the United States, almshouses were the destination of destitute older people and were insufferable places with "deplorable conditions, neglect, preventable suffering, contagion, and death from lack of proper medical and nursing care" (Crane, 1907, p. 873). As early as 1906, Lavinia Dock and other early leaders in nursing addressed, in the *American Journal of Nursing* (AJN), the needs of the elderly chronically ill in almshouses. Dock and her colleagues cited the immediate need for trained nurses and pupil education in almshouses, "so that these evils, all of which lie strictly in the sphere of housekeeping and nursing,—two spheres which have always been lauded as women's own—might not occur" (Dock, 1908, p. 523). In 1912 the American Nurses Association (ANA) Board of Directors appointed an Almshouse Committee to continue to oversee nursing in these institutions. World War I

distracted them from attention to these needs. But in 1925, the ANA advanced the idea of a specialty in the nursing care of the aged.

With the passage of the Social Security Act of 1935, federal monies were provided for old-age insurance and public assistance for needy older people not covered by insurance. To combat the fear of almshouse placement, Congress stipulated that the Social Security funds could not be used to pay for care in almshouses or other public institutions. This move is thought to have been the genesis of commercial nursing homes. During the next 10 years, many almshouses closed and the number of private boarding homes providing care to elders increased. Because retired and widowed nurses often converted their homes into such living quarters and gave care when their boarders became ill, they can be considered the first geriatric nurses and their homes the first nursing homes.

Two nursing journals in the 1940s described centers of excellence for geriatric care: the Cuyahoga County Nursing Home in Ohio and the Hebrew Home for the Aged in New York. An article in the AJN by Sarah Gelbach (1943) recommended that nurses should have not only an aptitude for working with the elderly but also specific geriatric education. The first textbook on nursing care of the elderly was published by Newton and Anderson in 1950, and the first published nursing research on chronic disease and the elderly (Mack, 1952) appeared in the premier issue of *Nursing Research* in 1952.

In 1962 a focus group was formed to discuss geriatric nursing, and in 1966 a geriatric practice group was convened. However, it was not until 1966 that the ANA formed a Division of Geriatric Nursing. The first geriatric standards were published by the ANA in 1968, and soon after, geriatric nursing certification was offered. Geriatric nursing was the first specialty to establish standards of practice within the ANA. In 1976 the Division of Geriatric Nursing changed its name to the Gerontological Nursing Division to reflect the broad role nurses play in the care of older people. In the mid 1970s, certificate and master's programs to prepare gerontological nurse practitioners were begun with funding from the Department of Health, Education, and Welfare. Whereas most specialties in nursing practice developed from those identified in medicine, this was not the case with the specialty of gerontological nursing since health care of older adults was traditionally considered to fall within the domain of nursing (Davis, 1984).

In 1984 the Council on Gerontological Nursing was formed and certification for geriatric nurse practitioners (GNPs) and gerontological clinical nurse specialists (GCNSs) became available. Nursing was the first of the professions to develop standards of gerontological care and the first to provide a certification mechanism to ensure specific professional expertise through credentialing (Ebersole & Touhy, 2006). The most recent edition of *Scope and Standards of Gerontological Nursing Practice* (ANA, 2010) provides a comprehensive overview of the scope of gerontological nursing and identifies levels of gerontological nursing practice (basic and advanced) and standards of clinical gerontological nursing care and gerontological nursing performance.

Current Initiatives

The most significant influence in enhancing gerontological nursing has been the work of the Hartford Institute for Geriatric Nursing, funded by the John A. Hartford Foundation. Mathy Mezey, EdD, RN, FAAN, directed the institute, located in the College of Nursing at New York University, from its inception in 1996 until 2010 and now serves as an Associate Director. It is the only nurse-led organization in the country seeking to shape the quality of the nation's health care for older Americans by promoting geriatric nursing excellence to both the nursing profession and the larger health care community. Initiatives in nursing education, nursing practice, nursing research, and nursing policy include enhancing geriatrics in nursing education programs through curricular reform and faculty development; the development of nine Centers of Geriatric Nursing Excellence; predoctoral and postdoctoral scholarships for study and research in geriatric nursing; and clinical practice improvement projects to enhance care for older adults (Mackin et al., 2006; Miller et al., 2006; Souder et al., 2006) (see www.hartfordign.org).

Another significant influence on improving care for older adults was the Nurse Competence in Aging (NCA) project, a five-year initiative created in 2002 through an alliance of the ANA, the American Nurses Credentialing Center (ANCC), and the Hartford Institute for Geriatric Nursing. Funded by Atlantic Philanthropies, through the American Nurses Foundation, the initiative addressed the need to ensure competence in geriatrics among nursing specialty organizations. The initiative provided grant and technical assistance to more than 50 specialty nursing organizations; developed a free web-based comprehensive gerontological nursing resource center (http://consultgerirn. org) where nurses can access evidence-based information on topics related to the care of older adults; and conducted a national gerontological nursing certification outreach (Stierle et al., 2006). An extension of this work, the Resourcefully Enhancing Aging in Specialty Nursing (REASN) project, will focuses on building intensive collaborations with 13 hospital-based specialty associations to create geriatric educational products and resources to ensure the geriatric competencies of their members (see http://hartfordign.org/practice/reasn/).

In 2008 a $1.6 million grant from the John A. Hartford Foundation was awarded to Sigma Theta Tau International (STTI) to establish the Geriatric Nursing Leadership Academy (GNLA). Working with the Hartford Centers of Geriatric Nursing Excellence, the purpose of the GNLA is to develop the leadership skills of geriatric nurses in positions of influence in a variety of health care settings and to improve the quality of health care for older adults and their families (www.nursingsociety.org/LeadershipInstitute/GeriatricAcademy/Pages/introduction.aspx).

Gerontological Nursing Education

According to the ANA Scope and Standards of Gerontological Nursing Practice (2010), "Nurses require the knowledge and skills to assist older adults in a broad range of nursing care issues, from maintaining health and preventing illnesses, to managing complex, overlapping chronic conditions and progressive/protracted frailty in physical and mental functions, to palliative care" (p. 12-13). Basic competence is critical to ensure the best possible care for diverse populations of older adults. All nursing education programs, from entry-level to advanced practice, should be "gerontologized" to ensure that graduates are competent to meet the needs of an aging population.

Essential educational competencies and academic standards for care of older adults have been developed by national organizations such as the American Association of Colleges of Nursing (AACN) for both basic and advanced nursing education (ANA, 2010). *The Essentials of Baccalaureate Education for Professional Nursing Practice* (AACN, 2008) specifically address the importance of geriatric content and structured clinical experiences with older adults across the continuum in the education of students. In 2010, AACN and the Hartford Institute for Geriatric Nursing, New York University, published the *Recommended Baccalaureate Competencies and Curricular Guidelines for the Nursing Care of Older Adults,* a supplement to The Essentials document. In addition, gerontological nursing competencies for advanced practice graduate programs have also been developed. All of these documents can be accessed from http://www.aacn.nche.edu/education-resources/competencies-older-adults.

"Despite these lists of competencies, however, there remains a lack of consistency among nursing schools in helping students gain needed gerontological nursing information and skills" (ANA, 2010, p.12). Those in the field of nursing education must seriously consider specific minimal requirements in the care of older adults at each level of education to fulfill the responsibility of nurses to the public and the profession and to meet accreditation criteria. However, schools of nursing have only begun to include gerontological nursing content in their curricula and most still do not have freestanding courses in the specialty similar to courses in maternal/child or psychiatric nursing. When content is integrated throughout the curriculum, less than 25% of the content is devoted to geriatric care (Berman et al., 2005). "Gerontological nursing content needs to be integrated throughout the curriculum, in addition to a stand-alone course, so that gerontology is valued and viewed as an integral part of nursing care" (Miller et al., 2009, p. 198).

It is important to provide students with nursing practice experiences caring for elders across the continuum of care. For clinical practice sites, one is not limited to the acute care setting or the nursing home. Experiences with well elders in the community and opportunities to focus on health promotion should be the first experience for students. This will assist them to develop more positive attitudes toward older people, understand the full scope of nursing practice with older adults, and learn nursing responses to enhance health and wellness. Rehabilitation centers, subacute and skilled nursing facilities, and hospice settings provide opportunities for leadership experience, nursing management of complex problems, interprofessional teamwork, and research application for more advanced students.

Faculty with expertise in gerontological nursing are scarce; less than 30% of baccalaureate programs have at least one full-time faculty member certified in gerontological nursing (Berman et al., 2005; Mackin et al., 2006). Important resources for faculty education in gerontological nursing include the Geriatric Nursing Education Consortium (GNEC), the Advancing Care Excellence for Seniors (ACES), the Hartford Geriatric Nursing Initiative (HGNI), and the Building Academic Geriatric Nursing Capacity (BAGNC).

The purpose of the GNEC, a national initiative of the American Association of Colleges of Nursing (AACN) with funding from the John A. Hartford Foundation, is to enhance geriatric content in senior-level undergraduate courses. The GNEC educational curriculum and evidence-based modules reflecting the state-of-the-science approach to care for older adults are available electronically and via webinars (see http://www.aacn.nche.edu/gnec.htm).

Advancing Care Excellence for Seniors (ACES), a three-year grant funded by the John A. Hartford Foundation to foster gerontological nursing education in prelicensure programs, is a collaborative effort between the National League for Nursing (NLN) and the Community College of Philadelphia. ACES provides faculty with development materials, teaching tools and strategies, curricular guidelines, and essential nursing actions (see www.nln.org/ACES).

The BAGNC initiative includes the Building Geriatric Nursing Capacity Scholars and Fellows Awards Program and the nine Hartford Centers of Geriatric Nursing Excellence. This program, coordinated by the American Academy of Nursing, has stimulated increasing interest in academic geriatric nursing through scholarships and fellowships for research, faculty, and leadership development (see http://www.geriatricnursing.org/about/about.asp).

The Patient Protection and Affordable Care Act, signed into law in March 2010, provides many initiatives that will have a direct impact on gerontological nursing with regard to workforce, education, and practice. It is anticipated that there will be additional federal funding to support advanced education in gerontological nursing, education of faculty, and advanced training for direct care workers employed in long-term care settings.

Gerontological Nursing Research

Nursing research has significantly affected the quality of life of older people and gains more prominence each decade. Nurses have generated significant research over the past 20 years in the management of common conditions of older adults and settings of care. A solid foundation has been established for the practice of gerontological nursing. Some of the most important nursing studies have investigated interventions for improving the care for individuals with dementia, reducing falls, the use of restraints, pain management, delirium, care transitions, and end-of-life care. More research is needed on community and home-care resources for older adults, family caregiving issues (particularly minority elders), research on diverse older populations, and health in aging. Translational research and continued attention to interdisciplinary studies are increasingly important. Gerontological nurse scholars and researchers May Wykle and Ruth Tappen have identified areas in most need of research (Box 2-2).

Research with older adults receives considerable funding from the National Institute of Nursing Research (NINR). Their website (www.nih.gov/ninr) provides information about results of studies as well as funding opportunities. Gerontological nurse researchers publish in many of the journals devoted to gerontology. Although nursing research has contributed significantly to knowledge about care of older adults, "aging has become a public health issue requiring new approaches to care. More nurse scientists are needed to provide the evidence for interventions and healthcare policy to improve the quality and quantity of life for older adults" (ANA, 2010, p. 23).

Roles in Gerontological Nursing

Gerontological nursing roles encompass every imaginable venue and circumstance. The opportunities are expanding rapidly because we are a rapidly aging society. "Nurses have the potential to improve elder care across settings through effective screening and comprehensive assessment, facilitating access to programs and services, educating and empowering older adults and their families to improve their health and manage chronic conditions, leading and coordinating the efforts of members of the health care team, conducting and applying research, and influencing policy" (Young, 2003, p. 9).

A gerontological nurse may be a generalist or a specialist. The generalist functions in a variety of settings (primary care, acute care, home care, subacute and long-term care facilities, the community) providing nursing

---

BOX 2-2   Future Directions for Gerontological Nursing Research as Suggested by Wykle and Tappen

- Staffing patterns and the most appropriate mix to improve care outcomes in long-term care settings
- The influence of culture, diversity, and ethnicity on aging
- Health disparities and health literacy
- Factors contributing to successful aging, health promotion, and wellness in the Baby Boomer generation
- Retirement decisions of the Baby Boomers: how they are made and how they are changing
- Dementia as a chronic illness and staying well in the presence of the disease
- Caregiving, particularly intergenerational
- Values and attitudes of the current generation toward aging and expectations of its members
- Interventions to assist with the increasing prevalence of drug and alcohol abuse and other mental health problems of the current and future generations of older adults
- Integration of current best practice protocols into settings across the continuum in cost-effective and care-efficient models
- Models of acute care designed to prevent negative outcomes in elders
- Strategies to increase preparation in gerontological nursing and increased recruitment of the brightest and best into gerontological nursing
- Models of interdisciplinary practice
- Health promotion and illness management interventions in the assisted living setting; role of professional nurses and advanced-practice nurses in this setting; aging in place
- Development of models for end-of-life care in home and nursing home

From Ebersole P, Touhy T: *Geriatric nursing: growth of a specialty,* New York, 2006, Springer.

---

care to individuals and their families. The gerontological nursing specialist has advanced preparation at the master's level and performs all of the functions of a generalist but has developed advanced clinical expertise, as well as an understanding of health and social policy and proficiency in planning, implementing, and evaluating health programs. With shortages in nursing faculty prepared in gerontological nursing, there is a critical need for nurses who have master's and doctoral preparation and expertise in care of older adults to assume faculty roles.

Certifications in gerontological nursing are available at the generalist and specialist level and should be encouraged as a way of enhancing and recognizing the needed knowledge and skills to care for this rapidly growing population (see www.nursecredentialing.org). The majority of nurses practicing today and in the future will be caring for older adult patients and the public will expect nurses to have this specialized knowledge.

Specialist Roles

Under the Consensus Model for APRN Regulation: Licensure, Accreditation, Certification, and Education (2008), APRNs must be educated, certified, and licensed to practice in a role and a population. APRNs may specialize but they may not be licensed solely within a specialty area. APRNs are educated in one of four roles; one of which is the adult-gerontology nurse practitioner. This population focus encompasses the young adult to the older adult, including the frail elder. Titles of APRNs educated and certified across both areas of practice will include the following: Adult-Gerontology Acute Care Nurse Practitioner (2013), Adult-Gerontology Primary Care Nurse Practitioner (2013), and Adult-Gerontology Clinical Nurse Specialist (2014) (http://www.nursecredentialing. org/Certification/APRNCorner/APRN-FAQ.aspx#10). Because the number of APRNs with gerontological certification and interest in the specialty practice is low, this new focus in role and population, combining ANP and GNP specialty education, will assist in meeting the critical need for APRNs well prepared to care for the growing numbers of older people.

Advanced practice nurses have demonstrated their skill in improving health outcomes and cost-effectiveness. Advanced practice nurses with certification in adult-gerontology will find a full range of opportunities for collaborative and independent practice both now and in the future. Practice sites include geriatric and family practice clinics, long-term care, acute and subacute care, home health care agencies, continuing care retirement communities, assisted living facilities, hospice, managed care organizations, specialty care clinics (e.g., Alzheimer's, heart failure, diabetes), Area Agencies on Aging, public health departments, care management, elder care consulting, schools of nursing, and private practice (see www. gapna.org). One of the most important advanced practice nursing roles that emerged over the last 30 years is that of the gerontological nurse practitioner (GNP) and the gerontological clinical nurse specialist (GCNS) in skilled nursing facilities. The education and training programs arose from evident need, particularly in the long-term care setting.

Many of these advanced practice nurses have nursing facility practices managing complex care of frail older adults in collaboration with interprofessional teams. This role is well established and positive outcomes include increased patient and family satisfaction, decreased costs, less frequent hospitalizations and emergency room visits, and improved quality of care (Bakerjian, 2008; Kane et al., 2004; Kappas-Larson, 2008). The Evercare Care Model, a federally funded Medicare demonstration project, originally designed by two nurse practitioners, is a very successful innovative model with a long history of positive outcomes. This model utilizes APRNs either certified in gerontology or specially trained by Evercare, for care of long-term nursing home residents and individuals with severe or disabling conditions (Kappas-Larson, 2008) (see www.innovativecaremodels.com).

Generalist Roles

Acute Care

Even though most nurses working in acute care are caring for older patients, many have not had gerontological nursing content in their basic nursing education programs and few are certified in the specialty. Only a small number of the country's 6000 hospitals have institutional practice guidelines, educational resources, and administrative practices that support best practice care of older adults" (Boltz et al., 2008, p. 176). Kagan (2008) reminds us that "older adults are the work of hospitals but most nurses practicing in hospitals do not say they specialize in geriatrics . . . We, as a profession and a force in an aging society, must make the transformation to understanding care of older adults is acute care nursing . . . Care of older adults would be the rule instead of the exception" (2008, p. 103). Kagan goes on to suggest that such a transformation would mean that acute care nurses would proudly describe themselves as geriatric nurses with subspecialties (geriatric vascular nurses, geriatric radiology nurses) and, along with geriatric nurse generalists, would populate hospital nursing services across the country.

Nurses caring for older adults in hospitals may function in the direct care provider role, as care managers, discharge planners, transitional care coordinators, as well as in leadership and management positions. The Nurses Improving Care for Health System Elders (NICHE), a program developed by the Hartford Geriatric Nursing Institute in 1992 to prevent iatrogenesis and improve outcomes for hospitalized older adults, offers many opportunities for new roles for acute care nurses. "NICHE is built on the premise that the bedside nurse plays a pivotal role in influencing the older adult's hospital experience and outcomes, through direct nursing care, as well as coordination of interdisciplinary activities" (Resnick, 2009, p. 81). More than 300 hospitals in more than 40 states, as well as parts of Canada, are involved in NICHE projects. NICHE units of various types have been developed, including the geriatric resource nurse (GRN) model and the acute care of the elderly (ACE) unit (www. nicheprogram.org).

Community- and Home-Based Care

Nurses will care for older adults in hospitals and long-term care facilities, but the majority of older adults live in the community. Community-based care settings include home care, independent senior housing, retirement communities, residential care facilities, adult day health programs, primary care clinics, and public health departments. The growth in home- and community-based health care is expected to continue because older people prefer to age in place. Other factors influencing the growth of home and community-based care include rapidly escalating health care costs.

The Independence at Home Act, part of the Affordable Care Act, supports home-based primary care teams, including physicians and nurse practitioners, to deliver primary care services to high-risk patients. This three-year demonstration project will receive mandatory appropriations of $5 million per year. After the project ends, the Department of Health and Human Services will evaluate the program and report to Congress. See the Centers for Medicare and Medicaid Services Innovations at http://www.cms.gov/ and http://www.aoa.gov/AoARoot/Aging_Statistics/docs/AoA_Affordable_Care.pdf for more information.

Advances in technology for remote monitoring of health status and safety, and point-of-care testing devices show promise in improving outcomes for elders who want to age in place (see Chapter 13). These technologies present exciting opportunities for nurses in the management and evaluation of care and call for increased education and practice experiences for nursing students in home-based care.

Nurses in the home setting provide comprehensive assessments and care management. They may provide and supervise care for elders with a variety of care needs including chronic wounds, intravenous therapy, tube feedings, unstable medical conditions, and complex medication regimens, and for those receiving rehabilitation and palliative and hospice services. Gerontological nurses will find opportunities to create practices in community-based settings with a focus not only on care for those who are ill, but also on health promotion.

Skilled Nursing Facilities/Nursing Homes

Nursing homes are the settings for the delivery of around-the-clock skilled care for those needing specialized care that cannot be provided elsewhere. Nursing homes have evolved into a significant location where health care is provided across the continuum. Nursing homes today are complex health care settings that are a mix of hospital, rehabilitation facility, hospice, and dementia-specific units, and are for many elders a final home. The settings called nursing homes or nursing facilities most often include up to two levels of care: a *skilled nursing care* (also called *subacute care*) facility is required to have licensed professionals with a focus on the management of complex medical needs; and a *chronic care* (also called *long-term* or *custodial*) facility is required to have 24-hour personal assistance that is supervised and augmented by professional and licensed nurses. Often, both kinds of services are provided in one facility. Most nursing homes offer subacute units that function much like the general medical-surgical hospital units of the past.

Subacute care is more intensive than traditional nursing home care and several times more costly, but far less costly than care in an acute-care hospital. The expectation is that the patient will be discharged home or to a less intensive setting. In addition to skilled nursing care, rehabilitation services are an essential component of subacute units. Length of stay is usually less than 1 month and is largely reimbursed by Medicare. Patients in subacute units are usually younger and less likely to be cognitively impaired than those in traditional nursing home care. Generally, higher levels of professional staffing are found in the subacute setting than those in the traditional nursing home setting because of the acuity of the patient's condition.

Nursing homes also care for patients who may not need the intense care provided in subacute units but still need ongoing 24-hour care. This may include individuals with severe strokes, dementia, or Parkinson's disease, and those receiving hospice care. More than 50% of residents in nursing homes are cognitively impaired, and nursing homes are increasingly caring for people at the end of life. In the United States, one in four persons die in a nursing home, and by 2020 nearly one in two will die in this setting (Federal Interagency Forum on Aging-Related Statistics, 2012; Teno, 2004). Nursing home residents represent the most frail of all older adults. Their need for 24-hour care could not be met in the home or residential care setting, or may have exceeded what the family was able to provide.

Roles for professional nursing may include nursing administrator, manager, supervisor, charge nurse, educator, infection control nurse, Minimum Data Set (MDS) coordinator, case manager, quality improvement coordinator, and direct care provider. The American Health Care Association (2010) predicts a 41% increase in the need for RNs in long-term care between 2000 and 2020.

Professional nurses in nursing facilities must be highly skilled in the complex care concerns of older people, ranging from subacute care to end-of-life care. Excellent assessment skills; ability to work with interprofessional teams in partnership with residents and families; skills in acute, rehabilitative, and palliative care; and leadership, management, supervision, and delegation skills are essential. Practice in this setting calls for independent decision making and is guided by a nursing model of care because there are fewer physicians and other professionals on site at all times. In addition, stringent federal regulations governing care practices and greater use of licensed practical nurses and nursing assistants influence the role of professional nursing in this setting. Many new graduates will be entering this setting upon graduation so it is essential to provide education and practice experiences to prepare them to function competently in this setting, particularly leadership and management skills.

Nurses accustomed to practicing in an acute care hospital will find many differences in subacute and skilled nursing facilities. Differences in focus of care and goals between acute and long-term care are presented in Boxes 2-3 and 2-4. For many nurses at both the generalist and specialist levels, nursing in long-term care settings (home, skilled nursing facilities) offers the opportunity to practice the full scope of nursing, establish long-term relationships with patients and families, and make a significant difference in patient outcomes. Although medical management is important, the need for expert nursing care is the most essential service provided. The American Association for Long Term Care Nursing offers a certification program for long-term care nurses (www.LTCNursing.org).

Professional nurse staffing ratios continue to be a critical concern in this setting, especially with the increasing acuity of patients. Current federal standards require only one RN in the nursing home for 8 hours a day—a figure quite shocking considering the ratio of RNs to patients in acute care. More RN direct-care per resident time in nursing homes is associated with fewer pressure ulcers, hospitalizations, urinary tract infections, catheterizations, and with less weight loss,

---

BOX 2-3 Focus of Acute and Long-Term Care

Acute Care Orientation
- Illness
- High technology
- Short term
- Episodic
- One-dimensional
- Professional
- Medical model
- Cure

Long-Term Care Orientation
- Function
- High touch
- Extended
- Interdisciplinary model
- Ongoing
- Multidimensional
- Paraprofessional and family
- Care

Adapted from Ouslander J, Osterweil D, Morley J: *Medical care in the nursing home*, New York, 1997, McGraw-Hill.

BOX 2-4 Goals of Long-Term Care

1. Provide a safe and supportive environment for chronically ill and functionally dependent people.
2. Restore and maintain highest practicable level of functional independence.
3. Preserve individual autonomy.
4. Maximize quality of life, well-being, and satisfaction with care.
5. Provide comfort and dignity at the end of life for residents and their families.
6. Provide coordinated interdisciplinary care to subacutely ill residents who plan to return to home or a less restrictive level of care.
7. Stabilize and delay progression, when possible, of chronic medical conditions.
8. Prevent acute medical and iatrogenic illnesses and identify and treat them rapidly when they do occur.
9. Create a homelike environment that respects dignity of each resident.

Adapted from Ouslander J, Osterweil D, Morley J: *Medical care in the nursing home*, New York, 1997, McGraw-Hill.

less deterioration in the ability to perform activities of daily living, and fewer quality of care deficiencies (Harrington et al., 2010; Horn et al., 2005; Kim et al., 2009). Many groups dealing with issues of the aging, as well as the American Nurses Association, have supported the critical need for adequate staffing in nursing homes, but to date, the federal government has not acted to mandate increases in minimum staffing requirements nor provided funding to support increases.

There are several new initiatives nurses can be involved with that are aimed at improving professional nursing practice and quality outcomes in long-term care, including Sigma Theta Tau's new Center for Nursing Excellence in Long Term Care, and the Advancing Excellence in America's Nursing Homes (www.nhqualitycampaign.org). The culture change movement (see Chapter 3) is an exciting opportunity that is transforming our vision of traditional nursing homes from an institutional model to a person-centered culture. Continued research on new models of care delivery and the appropriate mix of all levels of nursing staff in subacute and long-term care units is needed to improve outcomes.

Certified Nursing Assistants and Nurse Aides

Although it is important to promote professional nursing care for all elders, certified nursing assistants (CNAs) provide the majority of direct care in nursing homes and significantly contribute to the quality of life for nursing home residents. Critical shortages of CNAs exist now in both skilled care and home care, and these shortages will worsen in the future. Difficulty recruiting and retaining these long-term care workers continues to plague nursing homes, as turnover rates approach 100%" (Carpenter & Thompson, 2008). Several recent studies have investigated the relationship of factors such as turnover, work satisfaction, staffing, and power relations to quality of care and positive outcomes in nursing homes. Results support the importance of developing a culture of respect in which the work of CNAs is understood and valued at all levels of the organization. Research findings also indicate that the most influential factor in turnover among CNAs was the perception that they were not appreciated or valued by the organization (Bowers et al., 2003).

Results of several studies confirm the deep committment and passion that nursing assistants bring to their jobs as they "struggle to find and maintain a balance between the task-oriented needs of residents (e.g. bathing, toileting, feeding) and developing relationships and building community" (Carpenter & Thompson, 2008, p. 31). The significance and importance of close personal relationships between nursing assistants and residents, often described as "like family," is emerging as a central dimension of quality of care and

postive outcomes (Bowers et al., 2000, 2003; Carpenter & Thompson, 2008; Ersek et al., 2000; Fisher & Wallhagen, 2008; Sikma, 2006; Touhy et al., 2005). The commitment and dedication of nursing home staff must be honored and supported. They have much to teach us about aging, nursing, and caring.

One of the most important components of the culture change movement is the creation of models of care that value and honor the important work of nursing assistants. Culture change (see Chapter 3) must be equally concerned about the needs of residents and the well-being of staff (Thomas & Johnson, 2003). "An organization that learns to give love, respect, dignity, tenderness, and tolerance to all members of the staff will soon find these same virtues being practiced by the staff" (Thomas & Johnson, 2003, p. 3). Until health care professionals and society make a real commitment to providing adequate wages, individual supports (e.g., health insurance, education, career ladders), and an appreciation of their significant contribution to quality of nursing home care, these neglected workers cannot be expected to have the energy or incentive to extend themselves to the elders in their care (Kash et al., 2007).

Gerontological Nursing and Gerontology Organizations

The Gerontological Society of America (GSA) demonstrates the need for interdisciplinary collaboration in research and practice. The divisions of Biological Sciences, Health Sciences, Behavioral and Social Sciences, Social Research, and Policy and Practice include individuals from myriad backgrounds and disciplines who affiliate with a section based on their particular function rather than their educational or professional credentials. Nurses can be found in all sections and occupy important positions as officers and committee chairs in the GSA.

This mingling of the disciplines based on practice interests is also characteristic of the American Society on Aging (ASA). Other interdisciplinary organizations have joined forces to strengthen the field. The Association for Gerontology in Higher Education (AGHE) has partnered with the GSA, and the National Council on Aging (NCOA) is affiliated with the ASA. These organizations and others have encouraged the blending of ideas and functions, furthering our understanding of aging and of the integration necessary for optimal care. International gerontology associations, such as the International Federation on Aging and the International Association of Gerontology and Geriatrics, also have interdisciplinary membership and offer the opportunity to study aging internationally.

Organizations specific to gerontological nursing include the National Gerontological Nursing Association (NGNA), the Gerontological Advanced Practice Nurses Association (GAPNA), the National Association Directors of Nursing Administration in Long Term Care (NADONA/LTC) (also LPNs/LVNs as associate members), the American Association for Long-term Care Nursing (AALTCN), the American Assisted Living Nurses Association (AALNA), and the Canadian Gerontological Nursing Association (CGNA). The CGNA, founded in 1985, addresses the health needs of older Canadians and the nurses who care for them. In 2003, the CGNA formed an alliance with the NGNA to exchange information and share mutual goals and opportunities for the advancement of both groups (Mantle, 2005). In 2001, the Coalition of Geriatric Nursing Organizations (CGNO) was established to improve the health care of older adults across care settings. The CGNO represents more than 28,700 geriatric nurses from eight national organizations and is supported by the Hartford Institute for Geriatric Nursing and located at New York University College of Nursing (New York, NY).

An important organization for nursing assistants in nursing homes is the National Association of Geriatric Nursing Assistants (NAGNA). NAGNA was established in 1995 as a professional association of CNAs. The purpose of NAGNA is to ensure that the highest quality of care is provided to elders living in nursing homes, achieved by elevating the professional standing and performance of the caregivers. With a membership of more than 30,000 CNAs representing more than 500 nursing homes, the organization provides recognition for outstanding achievements, development training for CNAs, mentoring programs to reduce CNA turnover, and advocacy for issues important to long-term care and CNAs.

Another organization, the National Clearinghouse on the Direct Care Workforce, supports efforts to improve the quality of jobs for frontline workers who assist people who are elderly and/or living with disabilities. This organization provides information and resources needed to effect change in industry practice, public policy, and public opinion. The clearinghouse is also working with the Paraprofessional Healthcare Institute to improve understanding for the direct care workforce crisis through research and analysis funded by the U.S. Department of Health and Human Services and the Centers for Medicare and Medicaid Services.

Implications for Gerontological Nursing and Healthy Aging

Nursing is a vital aspect of the health care of older people, and the practice of gerontological nursing provides a unique vantage point from which to make an impact on it.

Nurses attracted to this specialized field recognize that expertise in caring for older adults can make a significant difference in the quality of life of the persons served. In times of illness and rehabilitation and end-of-life care, outcomes for the older person most often depend on the nursing care received. Through research, gerontological nurses have made substantial contributions to the body of knowledge of best practices in the care of elders, and they are recognized as leaders in aging care.

Gerontological nurses have opportunities to provide care across the continuum of aging services, caring for everyone from the most ill and frail elders to those who are active and independent. As phrased by Mezey and Fulmer (2002), the commitment of gerontological nurses to "tackle difficult but exceptionally meaningful issues that impact profoundly on the health and quality of life for older adults, the opportunities for decision making, independent action, innovation, and the significant contribution of geriatric nursing research to improved patient outcomes and health policy position the specialty for continued growth, recognition, contribution and value to society" (Mezey & Fulmer, 2002, p. 440). Gerontological nursing may be the most needed specialty in nursing, both now and in the future (Ebersole & Touhy, 2006).

KEY CONCEPTS

- Certification assures the public of nurses' commitment to specialized education and qualification for the care of older adults.
- All students graduating from nursing programs and all practicing nurses working with older adults should have competency in gerontological nursing.
- The major changes in health care delivery and the increasing numbers of older adults have resulted in numerous revised, refined, and emergent roles for nurses in the field of gerontological nursing. There is a critical shortage of competent and compassionate gerontological nurses.
- Advanced practice registered nurses may have either nurse practitioner qualifications or clinical nurse specialist education or a combination of both.
- Advanced practice role opportunities for nurses are numerous, offer more independence, are cost-effective, and facilitate more holistic health care and improved outcomes for patients.

ACTIVITIES AND DISCUSSION QUESTIONS

1. Identify factors that have influenced the progress of gerontological nursing as a specialty practice.
2. Consider and discuss with classmates the various gerontological nursing roles that you find most interesting and stimulating.

3. Discuss the gerontological organizations of today and their significance to the practicing nurse.

4. Why do you think more students do not choose gerontological nursing as a specialty? What would increase interest in this area of nursing?

5. What do you think are the most important issues in gerontological nursing education at this time?

6. Discuss your clinical education experiences and reflect on how they have influenced your views about care of older people and gerontological nursing?

REFERENCES

American Association of Colleges of Nursing (AACN): *The essentials of baccalaureate education for professional nursing practice* (2008). Available at http://www.aacn.nche.edu/education-resources/baccessentials08.pdf.

American Health Care Association: *U.S. long term care workforce at a glance* (2010). Available at http://www.ahcancal.org/research_data/staffing/Documents/WorkforceAtAGlance.pdf.

American Nurses Association: *Scope and standards of gerontological nursing practice*, Silver Springs, MD, 2010, Nursesbooks.org.

Consensus model for APRN regulation: licensure, accreditation, certification and education. Completed through the work of the APRN Consensus Work Group and the National Council of State Boards of Nursing APRN Advisory Committee, July 7, 2008. Available at http://www.aacn.nche.edu/education-resources/APRNReport.pdf.

Bakerjian D: Care of nursing home residents by advanced practice nurses: a review of the literature, *Res Gerontol Nurs* 1:177, 2008.

Berman A, Mezey M, Kobayashi M, et al: Gerontological nursing content in baccalaureate programs: comparison of findings from 1997 and 2003, *J Prof Nurs* 21:268, 2005.

Boltz M, Capezuti E, Bower-Ferres S, et al: Changes in the geriatric care environment associated with NICHE (Nurses Improving Care for Health System Elders), *Geriatr Nurs* 29(3):176–185, 2008.

Bowers B, Esmond S, Jacobson N: The relationship between staffing and quality in long-term care facilities: exploring the views of nurses aides, *J Nurs Care Qual* 14(4):55–64, 2000.

Bowers B, Esmond S, Jacobson N: Turnover reinterpreted: CNAs talk about why they leave, *J Gerontol Nurs* 29(3):36–43, 2003.

Carpenter J, Thompson SA: CNAs' experience in the nursing home: "it's in my soul," *J Gerontol Nurs* 34(9):25–32, 2008.

Crane C: Almshouse nursing: the human need, *Am J Nurs* 7:872, 1907.

Davis B: Nursing care of the aged: historical evolution, *Bull Am Assoc Hist Nurs* 47, 1985.

Dock L: The crusade for almshouse nursing, *Am J Nurs* 8(7):520, 1908.

Ebersole P, Touhy T: *Geriatric nursing: growth of a specialty*, New York, 2006, Springer.

Ersek M, Kraybill B, Hansberry J: Educational needs and concerns of nursing home staff, *J Gerontol Nurs* 26(10):91–99, 2000.

Federal Interagency Forum on Aging-Related Statistics: *Older Americans 2012: key indicators of well-being* (2012). Available at http://www.agingstats.gov/agingstatsdotnet/main_site/default.aspx.

Fisher L, Wallhagen M: Day-to-day care: the interplay of CNAs' views of residents and nursing home environments, *J Gerontol Nurs* 34:26, 2008 .

Geldbach S: Nursing care of the aged, *Am J Nurs* 43(12):1113, 1943.

Harrington C, Carrillo H, Blank B, et al: *Nursing facilities, staffing, residents and deficiencies by state, 2001-2007* (2010). Available at www.theconsumervoice.org/node/444.

Horn S, Buerhaus P, Bergstrom N, et al: RN staffing time and outcomes of long-stay nursing home residents, *Am J Nurs* 105(11):58–70, 2005.

Institute of Medicine, National Academies: *Retooling for an aging America: building the health care workforce* (2008). Available at http://www.iom.edu/Reports/2008/Retooling-for-an-Aging-America-Building-the-Health-Care-Workforce.aspx.

Kagan S: Moving from achievement to transformation, *Geriatr Nurs* 203:102–104, 2008.

Kane R, Flood S, Bershadsky B, Keckhafer F: Effect of an innovative Medicare managed care program on the quality of care for nursing home residents, *Gerontologist* 44(1):95–103, 2004.

Kappas-Larson P: The Evercare story: reshaping the health care model, revolutionizing long-term care, *Nurs Pract* 4(2):132–136, 2008.

Kash B, Castle N, Phillips C: Nursing home spending, staffing and turnover, *Health Care Manage Rev* 32(3):253–262, 2007.

Kim H, Kovner C, Harrington C, et al: A panel data analysis of the relationships of nursing home staffing levels and standards of regulatory deficiencies, *J Gerontol B Psychol Sci Soc Sci* 64B:269, 2009 .

Mack M: Personal adjustment of chronically ill old people under home care, *Nurs Res* 1:9, 1952.

Mackin L, Kayser-Jones J, Franklin P, et al: Successful recruiting into geriatric nursing: the experience of the Hartford Centers of Geriatric Nursing Excellence, *Nurs Outlook* 54:197, 2006.

Mantle JH: Personal communication, March 2, 2005.

Mezey M, Harrington C, Kluger M: NPs in nursing homes: an issue of quality, *Am J Nurs* 104(9):71, 2004.

Miller J, Coke L, Moss A, et al: Reluctant gerontologists: integrating gerontological nursing content into a prelicensure program, *Nurse Educ* 34(5):198–203, 2009.

Miller L, Beck C, Dowling G, et al: Building gerontological nursing research capacity: research initiatives of the John A. Hartford Foundation Centers of Geriatric Nursing Excellence, *Nurs Outlook* 54:189-196, 2006.

Newton K, Anderson H: *Geriatric nursing*, St. Louis, 1950, Mosby.

Resnick G: A big welcome to our NICHE hospitals, *Geriatr Nurs* 3:81, 2009.

Sikma S: Staff perceptions of caring: the importance of a supportive environment, *J Gerontol Nurs* 32(6):22–29, 2006.

Souder E, Kagan S, Hansen L, et al: Innovations in geriatric nursing curricula: experiences from the John A. Hartford Centers of Geriatric Nursing Excellence, *Nurs Outlook* 54:219, 2006.

Stierle L, Mezez M, Schumann M, et al: Professional development: the nurse competence in aging initiative: encouraging expertise in the care of older adults, *Am J Nurs* 106(9):93–96, 2006.

Teno J: Now is the time to embrace nursing homes as a place of care for dying persons, *J Palliat Med* 6(2):293–296, 2004.

Thomas W: *What are old people for? how elders will save the world.* St. Louis, 2004, Vanderwyk & Burnham.

Thomas W, Johnson C: Elderhood in eden, *Top Geriatr Rehabil* 19(4):282–289, 2003.

Touhy T, Strews W, Brown C: Staff perceptions of caring as lived by nursing home staff, residents and families, *Int J Hum Caring* 9(3):31–36, 2005.

Young H: Challenges and solutions for care of frail older adults, *Online J Issues Nurs* 8(2):1–13, 2003.

CHAPTER 3

Care Across the Continuum

Theris A. Touhy

⊖volve   evolve.elsevier.com/Ebersole/gerontological

LEARNING OBJECTIVES
Upon completion of this chapter, the reader will be able to:
- Compare the major features, advantages, and disadvantages of several residential options available to the older adult.
- Identify interventions to improve care for older adults in acute and long-term care settings.
- Describe factors influencing the provision of long-term care including the culture change movement.
- Discuss interventions to improve transitions of care and outcomes for older adults moving between health care settings.
- Discuss strategies to assist an older adult and their family in making an informed choice when relocation to a more protected setting becomes necessary.

GLOSSARY
Hospital-acquired events (HACs) Target conditions that are high cost or high volume, resulting in a higher payment when present as a secondary diagnosis in hospitalized patients, are not present on admission, and could have reasonably been prevented through use of evidence-based guidelines (e.g. catheter-associated urinary tract infections, pressure ulcers, falls).

Orthotist A person specially trained to measure, design, fabricate, fit, or service orthoses, and/or assists in the formulation of orthoses. An orthosis is a device that is intended to be fitted to a person to correct a disability, or to support the person who has a disability

Physiatrist Medical doctors who have completed training in the medical specialty of physical medicine and rehabilitation

Prosthetist A health care professional who is skilled in making and fitting artificial parts (prosthetics) for the human body

Transitional care The broad range of services and environments designed to promote the safe and timely passage of patients between levels of care and across care settings (Naylor & Keating, 2008, p. 65).

THE LIVED EXPERIENCE
"This is my home. We are all like a family, and I will die here. The girls that help me during the day, we treat one another like family members. We have some days when we are grumpy, some days we are happy, and we don't hold our feelings back, like you would do with your own family at home."

An 85-year-old resident of a skilled nursing facility

"We are their family now, and that is how we have to treat them. I think we do a pretty good job here because a lot of patients say when they leave and come back, 'Oh, I am so glad to be home.' Our philosophy here is that we don't work at this facility, we are guests in these people's home."

A 50-year-old director of nursing in a skilled nursing facility

A mobile, youth-oriented society may find it difficult to fully comprehend the insecurity that elders feel when moving from one site to another in their later years. In addition to the stress of relocation and the initial anxiety of adapting to a new setting, elders typically move to ever more restrictive environments, often in times of crisis. This chapter discusses residential care options across the continuum and transitions between health care settings with related implications for nursing practice. Professional nursing roles in settings across the continuum where care is provided to older adults are discussed in Chapter 2.

Elder-Friendly Communities

"Home" provides basic shelter, is a place to establish security, and is the place where one "belongs." It should provide the highest possible level of independence, function, safety, and comfort. Most older people prefer to remain in their own homes and "age-in-place," rather than relocate to more protected settings, especially institutional living. Future generations of older people will be much more likely to want to remain living independently and seek opportunities to adapt homes and communities to meet their needs. The ability to age-in-place depends on appropriate support for changing needs so the older person can stay where he or she wants. Developing elder-friendly communities and increasing opportunities to age-in-place can enhance the health and well-being of older people. Enabling the community to become the good neighbor to older citizens provides mutual benefits to all who are involved.

Components of an elder-friendly community include the following: (1) addresses basic needs; (2) optimizes physical health and well-being; (3) maximizes independence for the frail and disabled; and (4) provides social and civic engagement. Figure 3-1 presents elements of an elder-friendly community. Many state and local governments are assessing the community and designing interventions to enhance the ability of older people to remain in their homes and familiar environments. These interventions range from adequate transportation systems to home modifications and universal design standards for barrier-free housing. Home design features such as 36-inch-wide doorways and hallways, a bathroom on the first floor, an entry with no steps, outlets at wheelchair level, and reinforced walls in bathrooms to support grab bars will become standard nationwide in the next 50 years (Robinson & Reinhard, 2009).

Advancements in all types of technology hold promise for improving quality of life, decreasing the need for personal care, and enhancing the ability to live safely at home and age-in-place (Daniel et al., 2009). Some emerging technologies to enhance safety and independent living for older adults are discussed in Chapter 13.

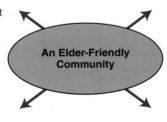

Addresses Basic Needs

- Provides appropriate and affordable housing
- Promotes safety at home and in the neighborhood
- Ensures no one goes hungry
- Provides useful information about available services

Optimizes Physical and Mental Health and Well-Being

- Promotes healthy behaviors
- Supports community activities that enhance well-being
- Provides ready access to preventive health services
- Provides access to medical, social, and palliative services

Promotes Social and Civic Engagement

- Fosters meaningful connections with family, neighbors, and friends
- Promotes active engagement in community life
- Provides opportunities for meaningful paid and voluntary work
- Makes aging issues a community-wide priority

Maximizes Independence for Frail and Disabled

- Mobilizes resources to facilitate "living at home"
- Provides accessible transportation
- Supports family and other caregivers

An Elder-Friendly Community

FIGURE 3-1 Essential elements of an elder-friendly community. (From Advantage Initiative, Center for Home Care Policy and Research, Visiting Nurse Service of New York. Available at www.vnsny.org/advantage/.)

Residential Options In Later Life

Some older people, by choice or by need, move from one type of residence to another. A number of options exist, especially for those with the financial resources that allow them to have a choice. Residential options range along a continuum from remaining in one's own home; to senior retirement communities; to shared housing with family members, friends, or others; to residential care communities such as assisted living settings; to nursing facilities for those with the most needs (Figure 3-2). There are many different models of senior housing, and older people may seek assistance from nurses in choosing what kind of living situation will be best for them. It is important to be aware of the various options available in your local community as well as the advantages, disadvantages, cost, and services provided in each option. When discharging older people from the hospital or long-term care facility, knowledge of where they live or the type of setting to which they are being discharged will assist in providing appropriate resources and teaching so that outcomes can be enhanced for both the individual and his or her family.

Shared Housing

Shared housing among adult children and their older relatives has become a choice for many because of cultural preferences or need. The sharing may relieve the economic burdens of maintaining a home after widowhood or retirement on a fixed income. Historically, strong cultural influences predict the frequency of multigenerational residences.

Among Asians, South Americans, and African Americans, it is often an expectation. Growth of multigenerational households has accelerated during the economic downturn among all cultures and races and this trend is expected to continue (Hooyman & Kiyak, 2011). Relocating from one's own home to the home of an adult child can have many benefits for both, but without adequate preparation it can also be stressful. Box 3-1 presents some factors to consider when planning to add an older person to the household.

A variation of multigenerational housing has long existed in what has become known as "granny flats." These may be apartments added to existing homes or the construction of small housing units on family property with privacy as well as sharing of time and resources. Such arrangements allow families to be close enough to be of assistance if needed but to remain separate. They are practical and economical, and their production has continually expanded, particularly in Australia. In the United States, use of this model is minimal, but existing "mother-in-law" cottages and apartments have served a similar purpose for many families for years.

Another model of shared housing is that of opening one's personal home to others. Older people often live in houses that were purchased in their young adult years and find that, as they age, much of the space may be underused. Sharing a house can be easily implemented by locating, screening, and matching older people looking for houses to share with those who have them. The National Shared Housing Resource Center (NSHRC) (http://www.nationalsharedhousing.org/) has established subgroups to assist individuals interested in home sharing. Those who have done so report feeling safer and less lonely.

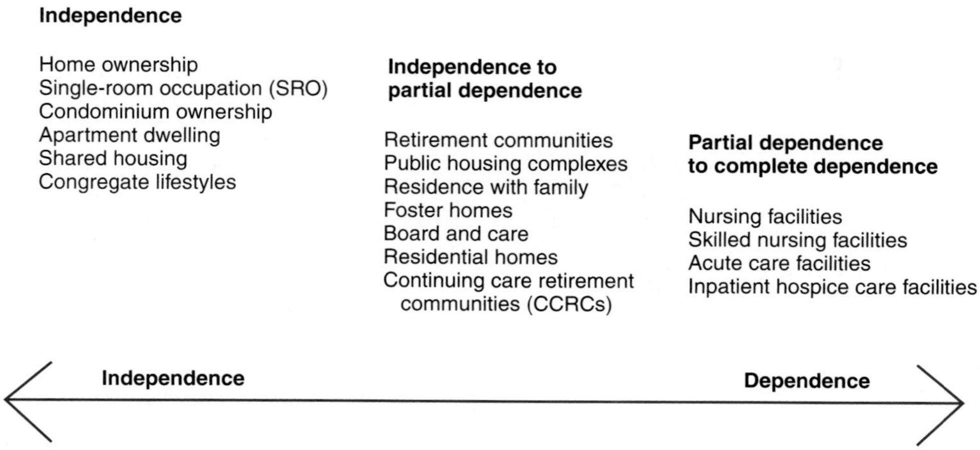

Independence

Home ownership
Single-room occupation (SRO)
Condominium ownership
Apartment dwelling
Shared housing
Congregate lifestyles

Independence to partial dependence

Retirement communities
Public housing complexes
Residence with family
Foster homes
Board and care
Residential homes
Continuing care retirement communities (CCRCs)

Partial dependence to complete dependence

Nursing facilities
Skilled nursing facilities
Acute care facilities
Inpatient hospice care facilities

Independence ⟵   ⟶ **Dependence**

FIGURE 3-2 Continuum of residential options based on level of assistance needed.

BOX 3-1 Planning to Add an Older Person to the Household

Questions You Should Ask:
- What are the needs of the new member and of the family?
- Where will space be allotted for the new member?
- How will this new member be included in existing family patterns?
- How will responsibilities be shared?
- What resources in the community will assist in the adjustment phase?
- Is the environment safe for this new member?
- How will family life change with the added member, and how does the family feel about it?
- What are the differences in socialization and sleeping patterns?
- What are the older person's strong needs and expectations?
- What are the older person's skills and talents?

Modifications You Have to Make:
- Arrange semiprivate living quarters if possible.
- Regularly schedule visits to other relatives to give each family respite and privacy.
- Arrange adult day health programs and senior activities for the older person to help keep contact with members of his or her own generation. Consider how the older person will feel about giving up familiar surroundings and friends.

Discuss Potential Areas of Conflict:
- Space: especially if someone has given up his or her space to the older relative.
- Possessions: older people may want to move possessions into the house; others may not find them

attractive or may insist on replacing them with new things.
- Entertaining: times when old and young feel the need or desire to exclude the other from social events.
- Responsibilities and chores: the older person may feel useless if he or she does nothing and may feel in the way if he or she does something; the young may feel that their position is usurped or may be angry if they are expected to wait on the parent.
- Expenses: increased cost of home maintenance, food, clothing, and recreation may not be shared appropriately.
- Vacations: whether to go together or alone; the young may feel uneasy not taking the older person out and resentful if they must.
- Child rearing: disagreement over child-rearing policies.
- Child care: grandparental babysitting may be welcomed by family and resented by the older person; or if not allowed, the older person may feel a lack of trust in capability.

Decrease Areas of Conflict by the Following:
- Respecting privacy.
- Discussing space allocations.
- Discussing the elder person's furnishings before move.
- Making it clear in advance when social events include everyone or exclude someone.
- Clearing decisions about household tasks—all should have responsibility geared to ability.
- Paying a share of expenses and maintaining a separate phone reduces strain and increases feelings of independence.

Population-Specific Communities

As the number of senior communities expands, older adults will have more options of moving somewhere that they find especially welcoming. These options include communities that emphasize a particular sport, like tennis or golf. Groups of people can also come together to form intentional communities, buying a cluster of home tracts and building in such a way to support their particular lifestyles or needs or personalities. Still others provide unique additional services, such as those in communities that specialize in providing residences for persons with, for example, a mental illness, alcoholism, or developmental disabilities.

Lesbian, gay, bisexual, and transgender (LGBT) seniors face several problems in housing in their older years. They

may have little family support and may face discrimination in housing options. Many LGBT seniors say they do not feel welcome at traditional residential options. Those who want to live together are discouraged from doing so by some organizations. Residential facilities and communities designed specifically for LGBT seniors are increasing in number across the country. Nurses should be aware of this heretofore invisible group of older adults who need access to welcoming resources. Chapter 24 discusses issues specific to LGBT seniors in more depth.

Senior Retirement Communities

Communities designed for elders are proliferating. Numerous combinations of single-family homes, apartments, activities, optional services, meals in the home, cafeterias, restaurants, housekeeping, and security are available. In some cases, emergency services and health clinics are adjacent. These are all designed to make independent living feasible with the least effort on the part of the elder. Some senior communities are luxurious and have a wide range of physical and cultural amenities; others are simpler, providing only the basic necessities. Prices are consistent with the level of luxury provided and the range of services available.

Although the costs of the majority of senior communities are borne by the consumers, for elders with limited incomes, federally subsidized rental options are available in some areas of the country. Older adults benefiting from this option are assisted through rental housing subsidized by the U.S. Department of Housing and Urban Development (HUD). Although not all HUD housing is designated for senior living, Section 202 of the Housing Act, U.S. Department of Housing and Urban Development, approved the construction of low-rent units especially for older people. These units may also have provisions for health care, recreation, and transportation.

Community and Home Care

Nurses will care for older adults in hospitals and long-term care, but the majority of older adults live in the community. Community-based care settings include home care services, independent senior housing, retirement communities, residential care facilities, adult day health programs, primary care clinics, and public health departments. The growth in home and community health care is expected to continue because older people prefer to age in place. Other factors influencing the growth of home-based care include rapidly escalating health care costs. Chapter 2 discusses roles for nurses in home and community care.

An innovative long standing community-based program is Program for All-Inclusive Care for the Elderly (PACE). PACE is an alternative to nursing home care for frail older people who want to live independently in the community with a high quality of life. It provides a comprehensive continuum of primary care, acute care, home care, nursing home care, and specialty care by an interdisciplinary team. PACE is a capitated system in which the team is provided with a monthly sum to provide all care to the enrollees, including medications, eyeglasses, and transportation to care as well as urgent and preventive care. Participants must meet the criteria for nursing home admission, prefer to remain in the community, and be eligible for Medicare and Medicaid. Adult day services are also provided.

PACE is now recognized as a permanent provider under Medicare and a state option under Medicaid. PACE has been approved by the U.S. Department of Health and Human Services (USDHHS) as an evidence-based model of care. Models such as PACE are innovative care delivery models, and continued development of such models are important as the population ages. More information about PACE models and outcomes of care can be found at http://www.npaonline.org/website/article.asp?id=12.

Adult Day Services

Adult day services (ADS) are community-based group programs designed to provide social and some health services to adults who need supervised care in a safe setting during the day. They also offer caregivers respite from the responsibilities of caregiving, and most provide educational programs for caregivers and support groups. The most recent nationwide survey of adult day centers confirmed that there are over 4600 adult day services centers in the United States providing care for 150,000 care recipients each day—a 35% increase since 2002. Adult day centers are serving populations with higher levels of physical disability and chronic disease, and the number of older people receiving adult day services has increased 63% over the last 8 years (National Adult Day Services Association, Ohio State University College of Social Work, MetLife Mature Market Institute, 2010).

Adult day services are an important part of the long-term care continuum and a cost-effective alternative or supplement to home care or institutional care. ADS are increasingly being utilized to provide community-based care for conditions like Alzheimer's disease and for transitional care and short-term rehabilitation following hospitalization. Local Area Agencies on Aging are good sources of information about adult day services and other community-based options.

Residential Care Facilities

Residential care facility (RCF) is the broad term for a range of nonmedical, community-based residential settings that house two or more unrelated adults and provide services such as meals, medication supervision or reminders, activities, transportation, or assistance with activities of daily living (ADLs). RCFs are known by more than 30 different names across the country, including *adult congregate facilities, foster care homes, personal care homes, homes for the elderly, domiciliary care homes, board and care homes, rest homes, family care homes, retirement homes,* and *assisted living facilities.*

RCFs are the fastest growing housing option available for older adults in the United States. This kind of facility is viewed as more cost effective than nursing homes while providing more privacy and a homelike environment. Medicare does not cover the cost of care in these types of facilities. In some states, costs may be covered by private and long-term care insurance and some other types of assistance programs. Residential care payment is primarily private pay, although 41 states currently have a Medicaid Waiver/Medicaid State Plan for a limited amount of eligible individuals. The use of Medicaid financing for services in RCFs has gradually increased in recent years. The rates charged and what services those rates include vary considerably, as do regulations and licensing.

Assisted Living

A popular type of residential care can be found in assisted living facilities (ALFs), also called *board and care homes* or *adult congregate living facilities* (ACLFs). Assisted living is a residential long-term care choice for older adults who need more than an independent living environment but do not need the 24 hours/day skilled nursing care and the constant monitoring of a skilled nursing facility. The typical ALF resident is an 86-year-old woman who is mobile but needs assistance with two ADLs (Box 3-2). Assisted living settings may be a shared room or a single-occupancy unit with a private bath, kitchenette, and communal meals. They all provide some support services.

Assisted living is more expensive than independent living and less costly than skilled nursing home care, but it is not inexpensive. There are 31,110 ALFs in the United States and most are private, for-profit facilities. Costs vary by geographical region, size of the unit, and relative luxury. The national average base rate for an ALF (single room and board and limited other services) is $3300 monthly (AssistedLivingFacilities.org, 2012). Most ALFs offer two or three meals per day, light weekly housekeeping, and laundry services, as well as optional social activities. Each added service increases the cost of the setting but allows for individuals with resources to remain in the setting longer, as functional abilities decline.

Many seniors and their families prefer ALFs to nursing homes because they cost less, are more homelike, and offer more opportunities for control, independence, and privacy. However, many residents of ALFs have chronic care needs and over time may require more care than the facility is able to provide. Services (e.g., home health, hospice, homemakers) can be brought into the facility, but some question whether this adequately substitutes for 24-hour supervision by registered nurses (RNs). Not every ALF has an RN or licensed practical–vocational nurse (LPN/LVN), and, in most states, any skilled nursing provided by the staff other than nurse-delegated assistance with self-administered medication is prohibited. In the ALF, there is no organized team of providers such as that found in nursing homes (i.e., nurses, social workers, rehabilitation therapists, pharmacists).

With the growing number of older adults with dementia residing in ALFs, many are establishing dementia-specific units. It is important to investigate services available as well as staff training when making decisions as to the most appropriate placement for older adults with dementia. Continued research is needed on best care practices as well as outcomes of care for people with dementia in both ALFs and nursing homes. The Alzheimer's Association has issued a set of dementia care practices for ALFs and nursing homes (Alzheimer's Association, 2009)

BOX 3-2   Profile of a Resident in an Assisted Living Facility

- 86.9 years old
- Female (74%)
- 70% moved to the ALF from a private home or apartment
- Needs help with at least two activities of daily living (ADLs)
  - Bathing: 64%
  - Dressing: 39%
  - Toileting: 26%
  - Transferring: 19%
  - Eating: 12%
- Needs help with instrumental activities of daily living (IADLs)
  - Meal preparation: 87%
  - Medications: 81%
- 42% have Alzheimer's disease or other dementia types of diagnosis
- Length of stay: 28.3 months
  - 59% move to a nursing facility
  - 33% die while a resident

Data from National Center for Assisted Living: *Resident profile* (2010). Available at http://www.ahcancal.org/ncal/resources/Pages/ResidentProfile.aspx.

and an evidence-based guideline, *Dementia Care Practice Recommendations for Assisted Living Residences and Nursing Homes* is also available (Tilly & Reed, 2006) (see also www.guideline.gov).

The Joint Commission and the Commission for Accreditation of Rehabilitation Facilities have published standards for accreditation of ALFs, but many are advocating for more comprehensive federal and state standards and regulations. Appropriate standards of care must be developed and care outcomes monitored to ensure that residents are receiving quality care in this setting, which is almost devoid of professional nursing. Further research is needed on care outcomes of residents in ALFs and the role of unlicensed assistive personnel, as well as RNs, in these facilities.

The American Assisted Living Nurses Association has established a certification mechanism for nurses working in these facilities and has also developed a *Scope and Standards of Assisted Living Nursing Practice for Registered Nurses* (www.alnursing.org). Advanced practice gerontological nurses are well suited to the role of primary care provider in ALFs, and many have assumed this role. Consumers are advised to inquire as to exactly what services will be provided and by whom if an ALF resident becomes more frail and needs more intensive care. The Assisted Living Federation of America provides a consumer guide for choosing an assisted living residence (http://www.alfa.org/images/alfa/PDFs/getfile.cfm_product_id=94&file=ALFAchecklist.pdf).

Continuing Care Retirement Communities

Continuing care retirement communities (CCRCs), also known as life care communities, provide the full range of residential options, from single-family homes to skilled nursing facilities all in one location. Most of these communities provide access to these levels of care for a community member's entire remaining lifetime, and for the right price, the range of services may be guaranteed. Having all levels of care in one location allows community members to make the transition between levels without life-disrupting moves. For married couples in which one spouse needs more care than the other, life care communities allow them to live nearby in a different part of the same community. This industry is maturing, and there are 1900 CCRCs in the United States, housing more than 745,000 older adults (Leading Age, 2011).

Most CCRCs are managed by not-for-profit organizations. They usually charge an entry fee ranging from $60,000 to $120,000 that covers and reflects the cost of the residence in which the member will live, the possible future care needed, and the quality and quantity of the community services. The average monthly cost of living in a not-for-profit CCRC is $2,672. Important to remember about these types of communities is that the residence purchased usually belongs to the community after the death of the owner.

Acute Care

Older adults often enter the health care system with admissions to acute care settings. Older adults comprise 60% of medical-surgical patients and 46% of critical care patients (Mezey et al., 2007). Acutely ill older adults frequently have multiple chronic conditions and comorbidities and present many care challenges. Hospitals are dangerous places for elders: 34% experience functional decline, and iatrogenic complications occur in as many as 29% to 38%, a rate three to five times higher than in younger patients (Inouye et al., 2000; Kleinpell, 2007). Common iatrogenic complications include functional decline, pneumonia, delirium, new-onset incontinence, urinary tract infections (UTIs), malnutrition, pressure ulcers, medication reactions, and falls—many of the geriatric syndromes. Geriatric syndromes are groups of specific signs and symptoms that occur more often in older adults and can impact morbidity and mortality. Normal aging changes, multiple comorbidities, and adverse effects of therapeutic interventions contribute to the development of geriatric syndromes. These syndromes are discussed in Chapters 7, 9 to 13, and 21. Nursing roles in acute care and model programs to improve care are discussed in Chapter 2.

Recognizing the impact of iatrogenesis, both on patient outcomes and cost of care, the Centers for Medicare and Medicaid Services (CMS) has instituted changes to the inpatient prospective payment system that will reduce payment to hospitals relative to poor care. The changes target conditions (hospital-acquired events (HACs) that are high cost or high volume, result in a higher payment when present as a secondary diagnosis, are not present on admission, and could have reasonably been prevented through the use of evidence-based guidelines. Targeted conditions include catheter-associated UTIs, pressure ulcers, and falls. Use of evidence-based nursing protocols, particularly for these geriatric syndromes, thorough assessment, prevention, and monitoring of treatment responses, and accurate documentation is essential.

Nursing Homes (Long-Term Care Facilities)

There are approximately 16,100 certified nursing homes in the United States, and more than 1.4 million older adults reside in nursing homes. The majority of nursing homes are for-profit organizations (67%), and nursing home chains own 54% of all nursing homes (Leading Age, 2011). The number of nursing home beds is decreasing in the United States and the number of Medicaid-only beds has decreased by half since 1995 (Gleckman, 2009). This is most likely a result of the increased use of RCFs and more reimbursement by Medicaid programs for community-based care alternatives.

However, skilled nursing facilities are the most frequent site of postacute care in the United States, treating 50% of all Medicare beneficiaries requiring postacute care following hospitalization (Alliance for Quality Nursing Home Care and the American Health Care Association, 2011). With the increasing number of older people, projections are that there will be a threefold increase in the number who will need care in this setting by 2030. Although the percentage of older people living long-term in nursing homes at any given time is low (4% to 5%), people who reach age 65 will likely have a 40% chance of entering a nursing home and those who live to age 85 will have a 1 in 2 chance of spending some time in this setting (Medicare.gov, 2012). This could be for subacute care, ongoing long-term care, or end-of-life care. Chapter 2 discusses the changing nature of skilled nursing facilities and roles for professional nurses in more depth.

People who are cared for in subacute units, as well as long-term units of nursing facilities, require access to rehabilitation and restorative care services that maintain or improve their function and prevent excess disability. These services are required under federal and state regulations and are integral to quality indicators in nursing facilities. Restorative nursing programs for ADLs (e.g., toileting, range of motion, ambulation, and feeding) contribute to restoration and maintenance of function for nursing facility residents who may have been discharged from skilled therapy services or who are not eligible for Medicare

reimbursement for rehabilitation services by physical, occupational, or speech therapists. Both rehabilitation and restorative programs require comprehensive multidisciplinary assessment and involvement of the patient and family in development of a plan of care with short and long-term goals (Box 3-3). Rehabilitation and restorative care is increasingly important in light of shortened hospital stays that may occur before conditions are stabilized and the older adult is not ready to function independently.

Costs of Care

Costs for nursing homes vary by geographical location, ownership, and amenities, but the average annual cost for a semiprivate room is $215 per day or $78,475 annually. Nursing home rates have increased more than 10% since 2008 and nearly 50% since 2004. The majority of the cost of care in nursing homes is borne by Medicaid (42%), followed by Medicare (25%), out of pocket (22%), and private insurance and other sources (11%) (Prudential Insurance Company of America, 2010). Medicare covers 100% of the costs for the first 20 days if the individual requires skilled care services. Beginning on day 21 of the nursing home stay, there is a significant co-payment. This co-payment may be covered by a Medigap policy. After 100 days, the individual is responsible for all costs. For a nursing home stay to be covered by Medicare, you must enter a Medicare-approved "skilled nursing facility" or nursing home within 30 days of a hospital stay that lasted at least 3 days (Medicare.gov, 2012). Complex medical treatments (e.g., feeding tube, tracheostomy, intravenous [IV] therapy) and rehabilitation services such as occupational therapy (OT), physical therapy (PT), or speech therapy (ST), are considered skilled care.

Medicare does not cover the costs of care in chronic, custodial, and long-term units. If the older person was admitted to the nursing home because of a dementia diagnosis

---

BOX 3-3   Members of the Rehabilitation Care Team

- Rehabilitation nurse specialist
- Physical therapist
- Occupational therapist
- Speech therapist
- Social worker
- Discharge planner
- Psychologist
- Prosthetist and orthotist

- Physiatrist
- Chaplain
- Dietitian
- Audiologist
- Physician, nurse practitioner
- Vocational rehabilitation specialist
- Person in rehabilitation
- Person's significant others

and the need for assistance with ADLs and maintenance of safety, Medicare would not cover the cost of care unless there was some skilled need. Medicare does provide coverage for hospice care services in nursing homes with some exceptions (room charges) provided eligibility requirements are met.

Concern is growing nationwide about the financing of long-term care and the ability of the states and the federal government to continue to support costs through the Medicaid programs. The reimbursement levels of both Medicare and Medicaid do not cover actual costs, and there is fear that if further cuts are made, quality of care will be more drastically compromised. The increasing burden on Medicaid is unsustainable. The purchase of long-term care insurance is an option, but it is expensive and pays for less than 5% of long-term care costs. Health care coverage for people with long-term care needs is a major national issue that demands attention.

Quality of Care

Nursing homes are one of the most highly regulated industries in the United States. The Omnibus Reconciliation Act (OBRA) of 1987, and the frequent revisions and updates, are designed to improve the quality of resident care and have had a positive impact. Some of the requirements of OBRA and subsequent legislation include the following: comprehensive resident assessments (Minimum Data Set [MDS]), increased training requirements for nursing assistants, elimination of the use of medications and restraints for the purpose of discipline or convenience, higher staffing requirements for nursing and social work staff, standards for nursing home administrators, and quality assurance activities.

Both the federal and state governments describe the standards that nursing facilities must meet to comply with the law and qualify for reimbursement. Quality trends are monitored and available to the public (https://www.cms.gov/MDSPubQIandResRep/01_Overview.asp#TopOfPage). Nursing homes were the first to publish online quality information, which is now available for hospitals and other health care organizations. Findings from the recent report on care quality in nursing and rehabilitation facilities reported that since 2009, nursing facilities have made measurable improvements in 9 out of 10 quality measures (Leading Age, 2011).

Although nursing homes recognize the need to ensure quality and have responded to improvement initiatives, the lack of additional funding for legislated initiatives has left many nursing homes struggling to maintain quality and meet standards with few resources. Care of the frail elderly and seriously ill persons is labor-intensive, costly, and requires specialized knowledge. Reasonable workloads, enhanced education and training, and adequate reimbursement are essential. Oversight has too often been conducted in a punitive fashion rather than a collaborative effort to enhance outcomes similar to that which is seen in other health care institutions.

The Five-Star Quality Rating system for nursing homes, established by the CMS, was created to help consumers, their families, and caregivers to compare nursing homes (www.medicare.gov/NHCompare). This rating system is based on the nursing home's most recent health inspection, staffing, and quality measures. The CMS advises consumers to use additional sources of information because the Five Star rating system should not substitute for visiting nursing homes since it is a "snap shot" of the care in individual nursing homes.

The most appropriate method of choosing a nursing home is to personally visit the facility, meet with the director of nursing, observe care routines, discuss the potential resident's needs, and use a format such as the one presented in Box 3-4 to ask questions. The CMS provides a nursing home checklist on their website, and the National Citizens' Coalition for Nursing Home Reform also provides resources for choosing a nursing home (http://www.theconsumervoice.org/resident/nursinghomes/fact-sheets). Nurse researchers Marilyn Rantz and Mary Zywgart-Stauffacher published a book, *How to Find the Best Eldercare*, based on their research.

Regulations have also been created to protect the rights of the residents of nursing homes. Residents in long-term care facilities have rights under both federal and state law. The staff of the facility must inform residents of these rights and protect and promote their rights. The rights to which the residents are entitled should be conspicuously posted in the facility (Box 3-5). Also, the Long-Term Care Ombudsman Program is a nationwide effort to support the rights of both the residents and the facilities. In most states, the program provides trained volunteers to investigate rights and quality complaints or conflicts. All reporting is anonymous. Each facility is required to post the name and contact information of the ombudsman assigned to the facility.

The Culture Change Movement

Across the United States, the movement to transform nursing homes from the typical medical model into "homes" that nurture quality of life for older people and support and empower frontline caregivers is changing the face of long-term care. Begun by the Pioneer Network, a national not-for-profit organization that serves the culture change movement,

BOX 3-4 Selecting a Nursing Home

Central Focus
- Residents and families are the central focus of the facility

Interaction
- Staff members are attentive and caring
- Staff members listen to what residents say
- Staff members and residents smile at one another
- Prompt response to resident and family needs
- Meaningful activities provided on all shifts to meet individual preferences
- Residents engage in activities with enjoyment
- Staff members talk to cognitively impaired residents; cognitively impaired residents involved in activities designed to meet their needs
- Staff members do not talk down to residents, talk as if they are not present, ignore yelling or calling out
- Families are involved in care decisions and daily life in facility

Milieu
- Calm, active, friendly
- Presence of community, volunteers, children, plants, animals

Environment
- No odor, clean and well maintained
- Rooms personalized
- Private areas

- Protected outside areas
- Equipment in good repair

Individualized Care
- Restorative programs for ambulation, ADLs
- Residents well dressed and groomed
- Resident and family councils
- Pleasant mealtimes, good food, residents have choices
- Adequate staff to serve meals and assist residents
- Flexible meal schedules, food available 24 hours per day
- Ethnic food preferences

Staff
- Well trained, have high level of professional skill
- Professional in appearance and demeanor
- RNs involved in care decisions and care delivery
- Active staff development programs
- Physicians and advanced practice nurses involved in care planning and staff training
- Adequate staff (more than the minimum required) on each shift
- Low staff turnover

Safety
- Safe walking areas indoors and outdoors
- Monitoring of residents at risk for injury
- Restraint-appropriate care, adequate safety equipment and training on its use

ADLs, Activities of daily living; *RNs,* registered nurses.
Adapted from Rantz MJ, Mehr DR, Popejoy L, et al: Nursing home care quality: a multidimensional theoretical model, *J Nurs Care Qual* 12(3):30-46, 1998.

BOX 3-5 Bill of Rights for Long-Term Care Residents

- The right to voice grievances and have them remedied
- The right to information about health conditions and treatments and to participate in one's own care to the extent possible
- The right to choose one's own health care providers and to speak privately with one's health care providers
- The right to consent to or refuse all aspects of care and treatments
- The right to manage one's own finances if capable, or to choose one's own financial advisor
- The right to be transferred or discharged only for appropriate reasons

- The right to be free from all forms of abuse
- The right to be free from all forms of restraint to the extent compatible with safety
- The right to privacy and confidentiality concerning one's person, personal information, and medical information
- The right to be treated with dignity, consideration, and respect in keeping with one's individuality
- The right to immediate visitation and access at any time for family, health care providers, and legal advisors; the right to reasonable visitation and access for others

NOTE: This list of rights is a sampling of federal and several states' lists of rights of residents or participants in long-term care. Nurses should check the rules of their own state for specific rights in law for that state.

many facilities are changing from a rigid institutional approach to one that is person-centered (http://www.pioneernetwork.net/). "Culture change is the process of moving from a traditional nursing home model—characterized as a system unintentionally designed to foster dependence by keeping residents, as one observer put it, 'well cared for, safe, and powerless'—to a regenerative model that increases residents' autonomy and sense of control" (Brawley, 2007, p. 9).

Older people in need of long-term care want to live in a homelike setting that does not look and function like a hospital. They want a setting that allows them to make decisions they are used to making for themselves, such as when to get up, take a bath, eat, or go to bed. They want caregivers who know them and understand and respect their individuality and their preferences. "No matter how old, how sick, how disabled, how forgetful we are, each of us deserves to have a home—not an institution" (Baker, 2007; Baker as cited by Haglund, 2008, p. 8). Box 3-6 presents some of the differences between an institution-centered culture and a person-centered culture.

Although further research is needed, some results suggest that person-centered care is associated with improved organizational performance, including higher resident and staff satisfaction, better workforce performance, and higher occupancy rates. Examples of philosophies and programs of culture change are the Eden Alternative (www.edenalt.com) founded by Dr. Bill Thomas, the Green House Project (www.thegreenhouseproject.org), and the Wellspring Model developed by Wellspring Innovative Solutions in Seymour, Wisconsin (http://www.innovations.ahrq.gov/content.aspx?id=259).

The Eden Alternative is best known for the addition of animals, plants, and children to nursing homes. However, cats and dogs are not the heart of culture change. Truly transforming a nursing home starts at the top and requires involvement of all levels of staff and changes in values, attitudes, structures, and management practices. Some of the principles of culture change activities are as follows:

- Staff empowerment
- Resident involvement in decision making
- Individualized rather than routine task-oriented care
- Relationship building
- A sense of community and belonging
- Meaningful activities
- A homelike environment
- Increased attention to respect of staff and the value of caring

Culture change has moved from a grassroots movement to one supported by policy makers, providers, national and state associations, and CMS. The CMS has endorsed culture change and has also released a self-study tool for nursing homes to assess their own progress toward culture change. The Affordable Care Act includes a national demonstration project on culture change to develop best practices and the development of resources and funding to

---

BOX 3-6 Changing the Culture in Nursing Homes

Institution-Centered Culture
- Schedules and routines are designed by the institution and staff, and residents must comply.
- Focus is on tasks to be accomplished.
- Rotation of staff from unit to unit occurs.
- Decision making is centralized with little involvement of staff or residents and familes.
- There is a hospital environment.
- Structured activities are provided to all residents.
- There is little opportunity for socialization.
- Organization exists for employees rather than residents.
- There is little respect for privacy or individual routines.

Person-Centered Culture
- Emphasis is on relationships between staff and residents.
- Individualized plans of care are based on residents' needs, usual patterns, and desires.
- Staff members have consistent assignments and know the residents' preferences and uniqueness.
- Decision making is as close to the resident as possible.
- Staff members are involved in decisions and plans of care.
- Environment is homelike.
- Meaningful activities and opportunities for socialization are available around the clock.
- There is a sense of community and belonging— "like family."
- There is involvement of the community—children, pets, plants, outings.

From The Pioneer Network. Available at www.pioneernetwork.net.

undertake culture change. The culture change movement is growing rapidly, and ongoing research is needed to demonstrate costs, benefits, and outcomes (Rahman & Schnelle, 2008; White-Chu et al., 2009).

Improving Transitions Across the Continuum of Care

Care transition refers to the movement of patients from one health care practitioner or setting to another as their condition and care needs change. Older people have complex health care needs and often require care in multiple settings across the continuum. An older person may be treated by a family practitioner in the community, hospitalized and treated by a hospitalist, discharged to a nursing home and followed by another practitioner, and then discharged home or to a less care-intensive setting (e.g., ALF) where the primary care provider may or may not continue to follow him or her. Most health care providers practice in only one setting and are not familiar with the specific requirements of other settings. "Many factors contribute to gaps in care during critical transitions including poor communication, incomplete transfer of information, inadequate education of older adults and their family members, medication errors, limited access to essential services, and the absence of a single point person to ensure continuity of care" (Naylor & Keating, 2008, p. 65). Language and health literacy issues and cultural differences exacerbate the problem (Corbett et al., 2010).

Transitions happen often, and there is increasing evidence that serious deficiencies exist for older patients undergoing transitions across sites of care. Approximately one fifth of Medicare beneficiaries discharged from a hospital were rehospitalized within 30 days, and 34% were rehospitalized within 90 days of hospital discharge. Of these rehospitalizations, about 10% were planned. Estimated costs to Medicare for unplanned hospitalizations is $17.4 billion (Jencks et al., 2009). Additionally, 1 in 4 Medicare patients admitted to skilled nursing facilities from hospitals is readmitted to the hospital within 30 days. Up to two thirds of hospital transfers are rated as potentially avoidable by expert long-term care health professionals (see http://interact2.net/). These rehospitalizations are costly, potentially harmful, and often preventable.

Transitions during the course of hospitalization can also be problematic for older patients. Minimizing the number of transfers from unit to unit during a single hospitalization is associated with more consistent nursing care, fewer adverse incidents (e.g., nosocomial infections, falls, delirium, medication errors), shorter hospital stays, and lower overall costs (Kanak et al., 2008).

Individuals at high risk for transitional care problems include older people with multiple medical conditions or depression or other mental health disorders, isolated elders without family or friends, non-English speakers, recent immigrants, and low-income individuals (Graham et al., 2009). Compared to other groups of older adults, ethnically and racially diverse elders have slower rates of recovery after hospitalization and increased incidence of potentially preventable rehospitalizations (Graham et al., 2009). Heart failure is the most frequent reason for rehospitalization, and patients with heart failure experience a 27% rate of readmission within 30 days of a hospital discharge (Hines et al., 2010).

Improving Transitional Care

Transitional care "encompasses a broad range of services and environments designed to promote the safe and timely passage of patients between levels of care and across care settings" (Naylor & Keating, 2008, p. 65). National attention to improving patient safety during transfers is increasing, and a growing body of evidence-based research provides data for design of care to improve transition outcomes. Nurses play a very important role in ensuring the adequacy of transitional care, and many of the successful models involve the use of advanced practice nurses and registered nurses in roles such as transition coaches and care managers (Coleman et al., 2006; Chalmers & Coleman, 2008; Naylor et al., 2009).

Nurse researcher Mary Naylor has significantly contributed to knowledge in the area of transitional care. The Transitional Care Model (TCM): Hospital Discharge Screening Criteria for High Risk Older Adults (Bixby & Naylor, 2009) can be found at http://consultgerirn.org/uploads/File/trythis/try_this_26.pdf. In a study by Hain et al. (2012), skilled nursing facilities had the highest rehospitalization rates followed by home with home health care, areas in which nursing had a strong presence. "Nurses

---

 SAFETY ALERT

Medication discrepancies are the most prevalent adverse event following hospital discharge and the most challenging component of a successful hospital-to-home transition. Nurses' attention to an accurate prehospital medication list, medication reconciliation during hospitalization and at discharge, identification of high-risk medications, and patient and family education about medications is required to enhance safety.

play an important role in the development of interventions aimed at reducing rehospitalization" (p. 32). In addition to roles as care managers and transition coaches, nurses play a key role in many of the elements of successful transitional care models, such as medication management, family caregiver education, comprehensive discharge planning, and adequate and timely communication between providers and sites of service (Box 3-7).

Further research is needed to evaluate what transitional care models are most effective in various settings and for which group of patients. Particularly important is research on transitions from nursing home to hospital, racial and cultural disparities in transitional care, and ways to improve family caregiver preparation and involvement during transitions. The Family Caregiver Alliance provides a hospital discharge planning guide for families and caregivers (www.caregiver.org). Other transitional care resources can be found at http://interact2.net/care.html, http://www.caretransitions.org/, and www.ahrq.gov/qual/pips.

The CMS and The Joint Commission (TJC) have also increased efforts to promote better outcomes, patient safety, and effective care by requiring hospitals to collect data on the core measures and other quality indicators. The CMS posts 30-day, all cause, risk-adjusted readmission rates on its website for heart failure, acute myocardial infarction, and pneumonia. Participating hospitals are classified as better than U.S. national rate; no different than U.S. national rate; or worse than U.S. national rate (see www.hospitalcompare.gov). Medicare is also implementing initiatives to reduce the amount of improper payments to providers as a result of medically unnecessary care (Hines et al., 2010).

A major goal of the Patient Protection and Affordable Care Act (PPACA) is improving care coordination and outcomes for individuals with multiple comorbid conditions who require high-cost care. The health care reform law creates several programs based on promising models that include the following: the Medicare Community-Based Care Transitions Program; the Medicare Independence at Home demonstration; bonus payments for Medicare Advantage plans with care management programs; Medical (Health) Home models in Medicare and Medicaid; and Community Health Teams to support the Medical (Health) Homes. Many of these new initiatives include nurse practitioners and offer opportunities for new roles for registered nurses with preparation in care of older adults as well. The American Nurses Association provides information on key provisions related to nursing in health care reform (http://www.nursingworld.org/MainMenuCategories/Policy-Advocacy/HealthSystemReform).

Relocation

For many older adults, relocation is a major stressor and often a crisis for the older person and his or her family. Relocation to a long-term care facility is identified as one of the most stressful and one that many older people fear. With each move, if the adaptation is to be satisfying, one must begin to claim personal space by somehow placing

---

BOX 3-7 Suggested Elements of Transitional Care Models

- Utilize interdisciplinary teams guided by evidence-based protocols
- Comprehensive geriatric assessments
- Performance measures and evaluation
- Use information systems such as electronic medical records that span traditional settings
- Target high-risk patients
- Improve communication between patients, family caregivers, and providers
- Improve communication between sending and receiving clinicians
- Well-designed and structured patient transfer records
- Simplify posthospital medication regimen; identifying high-risk medications
- Reconcile patients' prehospitalization and posthospitalization medication lists

- Improve patient/family knowledge of medications prior to discharge
- Educational materials adapted for language and health literacy
- Schedule follow-up care appointments prior to discharge
- Discuss warning signs that require reporting and medical evaluation
- Follow up discharge with home visits/telephone calls
- Care coordination by advanced nurse practitioners
- Assessment of informal support
- Involvement, education, and support of family caregivers
- Knowledge of community resources and appropriate referrals to resources and financial assistance
- Enhance discussions of palliative and end-of-life care and communication of advance directives

one's stamp of individuality on the new surroundings. Because the older adult is particularly likely to move or be moved, the subject of relocation is significant. Nurses in hospitals, the community, and long-term care institutions frequently care for elders experiencing relocation.

The first issue to address in any move is whether it is necessary and whether it will provide the least restrictive lifestyle appropriate for the individual. Questions that must be asked to assess the impact on the individual after a move are presented in Box 3-8. Nurses' concerns are with assessing the impact of relocation and determining methods to mitigate any negative reactions.

Relocation stress syndrome is a nursing diagnosis describing the confusion resulting from a move to a new environment. Characteristics of relocation stress syndrome include anxiety, insecurity, altered mental status, depression, insecurity, loss of control, and physical problems. An abrupt and poorly prepared transfer actually increases illness and disorientation. Research suggests that individuals are better able to meet the challenges of relocation if they have a sense of control over the circumstances and the confidence to carry out the needed activities associated with a move.

To avoid some of the effects of relocation stress syndrome, the individual must have some control over the environment, preparation regarding the new situation, and maintenance of familiar situations to the greatest degree possible. Nurses must carefully assess and monitor older people for relocation stress syndrome effects. Working with families to help them plan relocations, understanding the effects of relocation, and implementing effective approaches are also necessary. It is important that some

familiar and some treasured items accompany the transfer. Too often, elders arrive at long-term care institutions via ambulance stretcher from the hospital with nothing but a hospital gown. Everything familiar and necessary in their lives remains at the home they have left when they became ill.

Even more distressing is when families or responsible parties sell the home to finance long-term care stays without the input of the elder. It is no wonder so many residents with dementia in nursing homes wander the hallways looking for home and for something familiar and comforting. Family members will need considerable support when an elder is moved into an institution. No matter what the circumstances, the family invariably feels that they have in some way failed the elder (see Chapter 24). A summary of relocation stress syndrome and nursing actions to prevent relocation stress during transition to long-term care are presented in Box 3-9.

Implications for Gerontological Nursing and Healthy Aging

Nurses in all practice settings play a key role in improving care for older people across the continuum. New roles for nursing are emerging in the era of health care reform and heightened attention to improved patient outcomes. Most nurses work in only one setting and are not familiar with the requirements of other settings or the needs of patients in those settings. As a result, there are often significant misunderstandings and criticisms of care in the different settings across the continuum. As Barbara Resnick pointed out: "We can stop the finger pointing and start working

---

BOX 3-8   Assessment of Relocation

- Are significant persons as accessible in the new location as they were before the move?
- Is the individual developing new and reciprocal relationships in the new setting?
- Is the individual functioning as well, better, or not as well in the new location? This determination cannot be made immediately, but this assessment must be done within at most 6 weeks of the move.
- Was the individual given options before the move?
- Was the individual given the opportunity to assess the new environment before making a decision to move?
- Has the individual been able to move important items of furniture and memorabilia to the new setting?

- Has a particular individual who is familiar with the environment been available to assist with orientation?
- Was the decision to move made hastily or with inadequate information?
- Does the new situation provide adequately for basic needs (food, shelter, physical maintenance)?
- Are individual idiosyncratic needs recognized, and is there an opportunity to actualize them?
- Does the new situation decrease the possibility of privacy and autonomy?
- Is the new living situation an improvement over the previous situation, similar in quality, or worse?

BOX 3-9   Relocation Stress Syndrome

Relocation stress syndrome is a physiological and/or psychosocial disturbance as a result of transfer from one environment to another.

Defining Characteristics
Major
Change in environment or location
Anxiety
Apprehension
Increased confusion
Depression
Loneliness

Minor
Verbalization of unwillingness to relocate
Sleep disturbance
Change in eating habits
Dependency
Gastrointestinal disturbances
Increased verbalization of needs
Insecurity
Lack of trust
Restlessness
Sad affect
Unfavorable comparison of posttransfer and pretransfer staff
Verbalization of being concerned or upset about transfer
Vigilance
Weight change
Withdrawal

Related Factors
Past, concurrent, and recent losses
Losses involved with the decision to move
Feeling of powerlessness
Lack of adequate support system
Little or no preparation for the impending move
Moderate to high degree of environmental change
History and types of previous transfers
Impaired psychosocial health status
Decreased physical health status

Sample Diagnostic Statement
Relocation stress syndrome related to admission to
   long-term care setting as evidenced by anxiety,
   insecurity, and disorientation

Expected Outcomes
1. The resident will socialize with family members, staff,
   and/or other residents.
2. Preadmission weight, appetite, and sleep patterns will
   remain stable. If previous patterns were dysfunctional,
   more appropriate health patterns will develop.
3. The resident will verbalize feelings, expectations, and
   disappointments openly with members of the staff and/
   or family.
4. Inappropriate behaviors (e.g., "acting out," refusing to
   take medicines) will not occur.

Expected Short-Term Goals
1. The resident will become independent in moving to
   and from areas within the facility during the next
   3 months.
2. The resident will react in a positive manner to staff
   effort to assist in adjusting to nursing home placement
   in the next 3 months.
3. The resident will express his or her thoughts or concerns
   about placement when encouraged to do so during
   individual contacts in the next 3 months.
4. During the next 3 months, the resident will not develop
   physical or psychosocial disturbances indicative of translocation
   syndrome as a result of the change in living
   environment.

Expected Long-Term Goals
1. The resident will verbalize acceptance of nursing home
   placement within the next 6 months.
2. The resident will indicate acceptance of nursing home
   placement through positive body language within the
   next 6 months.

Specific Nursing Interventions
1. Identify previous coping patterns during admission
   assessment. Clearly document these, and share the
   information with other staff members.
2. Include the resident in assessing problems and developing
   the care plan on admission.
3. Adjust for limitations in sensory-perceptual disturbances
   when planning care for residents. Visual disturbances
   necessitate special intervention to assist residents in
   finding their way around.
4. Staff members will introduce themselves when entering
   the resident's room, indicating the nature of their
   relationship with the resident. Example: "Hello, Mr. S.
   My name is Nancy. I'll be your nurse attendant today,
   helping you with your meals and your bath."
5. Each staff member providing care for the resident should
   make it a point to spend at least 5 minutes each day
   with new admissions to "just visit."

BOX 3-9 Relocation Stress Syndrome—cont'd

6. Allow the resident as many opportunities to make independent choices as possible.
7. Identify previous routines for activities of daily living (ADLs). Try to maintain as much continuity with the resident's previous schedule as possible. Example: If Mr. S. has taken a bath before bed all of his life, adjust his schedule to continue that practice.
8. Familiarize the resident with unit schedules.
9. Encourage family participation through frequent visits, phone calls, and activity sessions. Be sure to let the family know schedules.
10. Establish familiar landmarks for the resident when leaving his or her room so that he or she can recognize areas more quickly.

11. Encourage family members to bring familiar belongings from home for the resident's room decorations.
12. Provide reorientation cues frequently. Example: "You are in the dining room. Your room is down the hall three doors just past the window."
13. Encourage the resident to talk about expectations, anger, and/or disappointments and the recent life changes that he or she has experienced.
14. Review the patient's medication list with the physician to verify the need for medications that might promote disorientation.
15. Provide for constructive activities. Initiate activity therapy consultation.

together through the common transitions patients endure in our health care system. This will be a win-win situation for patients and providers alike" (2008, p. 154).

It is essential that educational programs prepare students for competent care of older adults in a variety of health care settings, including acute, long-term, home, and community-based care. Nurses in all settings need to increase awareness of the roles and responsibilities of nursing practice across the continuum and work collaboratively to improve care outcomes, particularly during times of transition. We can no longer work in our individual "silos" and not be concerned with what happens after the patient is out of our particular unit or institution. Nurses are well positioned "to create services and environments that embrace values that are at the core of this profession—patient/caregiver centered care, communication and collaboration, and continuity (Naylor, 2002, p. 140).

KEY CONCEPTS

- A familiar and comfortable environment allows an elder to function at his or her highest capacity.
- Nurses must be knowledgeable about the range of residential options for older people so they can assist the elder and the family to make appropriate decisions.
- Nursing homes are an integral part of the long-term care system, providing both skilled (subacute) care and chronic, long-term, and palliative care. Projections are that this setting will provide increasing amounts of care to the growing numbers of older adults.
- Culture change in nursing homes is a growing movement to develop models of person-centered care and improve care outcomes and quality of life.

- Nurses play a key role in insuring optimal outcomes during transitions of care.
- Relocation has variable effects, depending on the individual's personality, health, cognitive capacities, sense of control, opportunities for choice, self-esteem, and preferred lifestyle.

ACTIVITIES AND DISCUSSION QUESTIONS

1. Identify three objects in your living space that are important to you, and explain why these are significant. Will you take these with you whenever you relocate?
2. Ask an older relative about the items or conditions in his or her home that make him or her feel secure and comfortable.
3. Discuss with this elder various moves he or she has made and how he or she felt about them.
4. How might the care needs of an older adult in assisted living, subacute care, and a nursing home differ? What is the role of the professional nurse in each of these settings?
5. Select three places listed in your phone book as retirement communities, and make inquiries regarding possible placement of an older adult parent. What questions did you ask? What is the cost? What are the provisions for health care? What types of activities and assistance are available? Which would you select for your grandmother and why?
6. In your experience in the acute care setting, what improvements would you suggest to improve transitions to other care settings? Discuss any experience you or your friends or family may have had with transitions after hospital discharge.

7. If you were the director of nursing, what would your nursing home be like (design, staffing, quality of care, training)?

REFERENCES

Alliance for Quality Nursing Home Care and the American Health Care Association: *Annual quality report: a comprehensive report on the quality of care in America's nursing homes and rehabilitation facilities* (2011). Available at http://www.aqnhc.org/www/file/AHCA_Alliance_2011_Quality_Report_v2.pdf.

Alzheimer's Association: *Dementia care practice: recommendations for assisted living residences and nursing homes* (2009). Available at http://www.alz.org/national/documents/brochure_DCPRphases1n2.pdf.

AssistedLivingFacilities.org: *Assisted living costs* (2012). Available at http://www.assistedlivingfacilities.org/articles/assisted-living-costs.php.

Baker B: *Old age in a new age: the promise of transformative nursing homes*, Nashville, TN, 2007, Vanderbilt University Press.

Baker B, as cited in Haglund K: Closing keynote speaker found hope in changes benefiting residents and staff, *Caring Ages* 9(6):8, 2008.

Bixby M, Naylor M: *The Transitional Care Model (TCM): hospital discharge screening criteria for high risk older adults* (2009). Available at http://consultgerirn.org/uploads/File/try this/try_this_26.pdf.

Brawley E: What culture change is and why an aging nation cares, *Aging Today* 28:9–10, 2007.

Chalmers S, Coleman E: Transitional care. In Capezuti E, Swicker D, Mezey M, et al, editors: *The encyclopedia of elder care*, ed 2, New York, 2008, Springer.

Coleman EA, Parry C, Chalmers S, et al: The Care Transitions Intervention: results of a randomized controlled trial, *Arch Intern Med* 166(17):1822–1928, 2006.

Corbett C, Setter S, Daratha K, et al: Nurse identified hospital to home medication discrepancies: implications for improving transitional care, *Geriatr Nurs* 31:188, 2010.

Daniel K, Carson C, Ferrell S: Emerging technologies to enhance safety of older people in their homes, *Geriatr Nurs* 30(6): 384–389, 2009.

Gleckman H: *The death of nursing homes* (2009). Available at http://www.kaiserhealthnews.org/Columns/2009/September/092809Gleckman.aspx.

Graham C, Ivey S, Neuhauser L: From hospital to home: assessing the transitional care needs of vulnerable seniors, *Gerontologist* 49:23, 2009.

Hain D, Tappen R, Diaz S, Ouslander J: Characteristics of older adults rehospitalized within 7 and 30 days of discharge: implications for nursing practice, *J Gerontol Nurs* 38(8):32–44, 2012.

Hines P, Yu K, Randall M: Preventing heart failure readmissions: is your organization prepared? *Nurs Econ* 28:74, 2010.

Hooyman N, Kiyak A: *Social gerontology*. Boston, 2011, Pearson.

Inouye S, Baker DI, Leo-Summers L: The hospital elder life progress: a model of care to prevent cognitive and functional decline in older hospitalized patients, *J Am Geriatr Soc* 48(12):1657–1706, 2000.

Jencks SF, Williams MV, Coleman EA: Rehospitalizations among patients in the Medicare fee-for-service program, *N Engl J Med* 360(14):1418–1428, 2009.

Kanak MF, Titler M, Shever L, et al: The effect of hospitalization on multiple units, *Appl Nurs Res* 21(1):15–22, 2008.

Kleinpell R: Supporting independence in hospitalized elders in acute care, *Crit Care Nurs Clin N Am* 19:242–252, 2007.

Leading Age: *Choosing a provider* (2011). Available at http://www.leadingage.org/Choosing_A_Provider.aspx.

Medicare.gov: *What is Medicare?* (2012). Available at http://www.medicare.gov/navigation/medicare-basics/medicare-basics-overview.aspx.

Mezey M, Stierle L, Huba G, et al: Ensuring competence of specialty nurses in care of older adults, *Geriatr Nurs* 28(6S): 9–13, 2007.

National Adult Day Services Association, Ohio State University College of Social Work, MetLife Mature Market Institute: *The MetLife National Study of Adult Day Services: providing support to individuals and their family caregivers* (2010). Available at http://www.metlife.com/assets/cao/mmi/publications/studies/2010/mmi-adult-day-services.pdf.

Naylor M: Transitional care of older adults. In Archbold P, Fitzpatrick J, Stewart B, editors: *Annual review of nursing research*. New York, 2002, Springer, pp. 127–147.

Naylor M, Keating S: Transitional care: moving patients from one care setting to another, *Am J Nurs* 108(9 Suppl):58, 2008.

Naylor M, Kurtzman E, Pauly M: Transitions of elders between long-term care and hospitals, *Policy Polit Nurse Pract* 10:187, 2009.

Omnibus Budget Reconciliation Act (OBRA) of 1987 (Public Law No. 100-203): *Amendments 1990, 1991, 1992, 1993, and 1994*, Rockville, MD, U.S. Department of Health and Human Services, Health Care Financing Administration.

Prudential Insurance Company of America: *Prudential research report: long-term care cost study* (2010). Available at http://www.prudential.com/media/managed/LTCCostStudy.pdf.

Rahman A, Schnelle J: The nursing home culture change movement: recent past, present, and future directions for research, *Gerontologist* 48(2):142–148, 2008.

Resnick B: Hospitalization of older adults: are we doing a good job? *Geriatr Nurs* 29(3):153–154, 2008.

Robinson K, Reinhard S: Looking ahead in long-term care: the next 50 years, *Nurs Clin North Am* 44(2): 253–262, 2009.

Tilly J, Reed P, editors: *Dementia care practice recommendations for assisted living residences and nursing homes*, Washington, DC, 2008, Alzheimer's Association.

White-Chu E, Graves W, Godfrey S, et al: Beyond the medical model: The culture change revolution in long-term care, *J Am Med Direct Assoc* 6:370, 2009.

CHAPTER 4

Culture and Aging

Kathleen F. Jett

evolve evolve.elsevier.com/Ebersole/gerontological

LEARNING OBJECTIVES

Upon completion of this chapter, the reader will be able to:

- Identify factors contributing to the nurse's cultural sensitivity.
- Discuss approaches that facilitate an appreciation of diverse cultural and ethnic experiences.
- Explain the prominent health care belief systems.
- Identify nursing care interventions appropriate for ethnically diverse elders.
- Formulate a plan of care incorporating ethnically sensitive interventions.

GLOSSARY

Culture Beliefs, customs, and values that are shared by a group and passed on from one generation to the next.

Ethnicity Identifying with or deriving from the cultural, racial, religious, or linguistic traditions of a people or country.

Ethnocentrism The belief in the inherent superiority of one's ethnic group, accompanied by devaluation of other groups.

Folk medicine Healing methods originating among the people of a given culture and primarily transmitted from person to person.

Interpreter A person who transmits the meaning of what is spoken in one language to another spoken language.

Stereotype Belief applied to a group of persons based on assumed knowledge of an individual member of the group.

Translator A person who converts written materials from one language to another.

THE LIVED EXPERIENCE

I feel so out of place here. If my children weren't so busy, I suppose I could live with them, but they seemed so relieved when this retirement home would accept me. I wonder if they knew I was the only Chinese person in this place. A sweet young Chinese student tried to talk with me, but she only spoke Mandarin and I speak Cantonese. She had never lived in China. I want so much to talk to someone my age who lived in China and speaks my language.

Shin, a 75-year-old woman

Interest in and attention to culture and health care are increasing. In the field of gerontology, this interest is stimulated to a great extent by two major issues: the realization of a "gerontological explosion" and the recognition of the significant health disparities and inequities in the Unites States. The *gerontological explosion* refers both to the rapid increases in the total numbers of older adults, especially those over 85 years of age, and to the relative proportion of older adults in most countries across the globe (see Chapter 1). *Health disparities* refers to the differences in the state of health and health outcomes between people.

Health disparities adversely affect groups of people who have systematically experienced greater obstacles to health based on racial or ethnic group; religion; socioeconomic status; gender; age; mental health; cognitive, sensory or physical disability; sexual orientation or gender identity; geographic location; or other characteristics historically linked to discrimination or exclusion (U.S. Department of Health and Human Services [USDHHS], 2012).

Health inequities refers to the excess burden of illness or the difference between an expected incidence and prevalence and that which actually occurs in excess in a comparison population group. The inequities are often the result of both historical and contemporary injustices. Those found to be especially vulnerable to health disparities and inequities are older adults from ethnically distinct groups (Table 4-1).

Today's nurse is expected to provide competent care to persons with different life experiences, cultural perspectives, values, styles of communication and ages than their own. The nurse may need to effectively communicate with people regardless of the languages and manner being spoken. In doing so, the nurse may have to depend on limited verbal exchanges and attention to more facial expressions, postures, and gestures. However, these forms

TABLE 4-1	Blacks Compared with Whites on Measures of Quality and Access: Specific Measures, 2009*	
Topic	**Better than Whites**	**Worse than Whites**
Cancer		Colorectal cancer diagnosed at advanced stage
		Adults 50 years of age and over who report they ever received a colonoscopy, sigmoidoscopy, proctoscopy, or fecal occult blood test
		Colorectal cancer deaths per 100,000 population
		Breast cancer diagnosed at advanced stage
		Cancer deaths per 100,000 female population due to breast cancer
Heart disease	Deaths per 1000 admissions with acute myocardial infarction as principal diagnosis, 18 years of age and over	
	Hospital patients who received recommended care for heart failure	
HIV and AIDS		New AIDS cases per 100,000 population 13 years of age and over
Respiratory diseases		Adults 65 years of age and over who ever received pneumococcal vaccination
		Hospital patients with pneumonia who received recommended care
Functional status preservation and rehabilitation		Female Medicare beneficiaries 65 years of age and over who reported ever being screened for osteoporosis
Supportive and palliative care	Long-stay nursing home residents who were physically restrained	High-risk long-stay nursing home residents with pressure sores
		Short-stay nursing home residents with pressure sores
		Home health care patients who were admitted to the hospital
Timeliness		Emergency department visits in which patients left without being seen
Access	People without a usual source of care due to a financial or insurance reason	People who have a usual primary care provider

From The National Healthcare Quality Report, 2009; Chapter 4. Priority Populations. Available at http://www.ahrq.gov/qual/nhdr09/Chap4.htm.
*Modified for those most relevant to older adults.

of communication are heavily influenced by age, culture and ethnicity and easily may be misunderstood. To skillfully assess and intervene, nurses must first develop sensitivity through awareness of their own ethnocentrism and ageist attitudes. Effective nurses develop competence and the ability to work sensitively with older adults through new knowledge about aging, ethnicity, culture, language, and health belief systems, and develop the skills needed to optimize communication.

Knowing how to provide competent care is especially important in gerontological nursing because many older adults are just now immigrating to the United States. Many others have spent their lives in self-contained, homogeneous communities and may not have become acculturated to a Western model of care. This situation is likely to result in cultural conflict in the health care setting.

This chapter provides an overview of culture and aging, as well as strategies that gerontological nurses can use to best respond to the changing face of aging and in doing so, help reduce health inequities. These strategies include increasing sensitivity, knowledge and skills, decreasing ageism and working with diverse groups of older adults.

The Gerontological Explosion

The population of the United States is rapidly becoming more diverse. Persons of color, who have long been classified as those from "minority groups," will represent about 50% of the population in the next 50 years. The greatest increase in the number of ethnically diverse elders in the United States will be those who identify themselves as African American, followed by Hispanic, followed by Asian and Pacific Islanders (Table 4-2). Those who report "white alone" will decrease from 87% to 77%; African American alone will increase from 9% to 12% between 2010 and 2050 (Vincent & Velkoff, 2010). The effect of the overall growth in the numbers of elders currently in all groups is being

seen in all aspects of nursing (Administration on Aging [AOA], 2010). For example, it would not be unusual for nurses working in states with the greatest number of immigrant elders (especially California, Nevada, Florida, Texas, New Jersey, and Illinois) to care for persons from a variety of backgrounds in the same day (Gelfand, 2003). It must be noted, however, that these and many of the figures available today are drawn from the U.S. Census, in which persons of color are often underrepresented and those who reside illegally are not included at all. In reality, the numbers of elders from diverse backgrounds residing in the United States may be and may become substantially higher.

Health Disparities

In 2003 the Institute of Medicine (IOM) prepared the landmark analysis of health disparities. It began with the acknowledgement that persons of color had difficulty accessing the same care as their white counterparts. The study showed that even among those who had the same access, health care treatment in the United States in and of itself was unequal (Smedley et al., 2003) (Box 4-1). The barriers to quality care were found to be wide and were consistently found across the spectrum of disease areas and clinical services. Although there has been some improvement, significant problems remain (Centers for Disease Control and Prevention, 2009; National Institute on Aging, 2010). The goals published in *Healthy People 2020* are to work to achieve health equity, eliminate disparities and improve the health of all groups (USDHHS, 2012).

TABLE 4-2	Percentage of Persons 65 Years of Age and Older in the United States from Minority Groups in 2009
African American	8.3
Asian/Pacific Islander	3.4
American Indian/ Native Alaskan	<1
More than one race	0.6
Hispanic (any race)	7.0

Data from *A profile of older Americans* (2010). Available at www.aoa.gov/AoARoot/Aging_Statistics/Profile/2010/7.aspx.

BOX 4-1	Examples of Health Disparities Relevant to Older Adults

African Americans
- Although African American adults are 40% more likely to have hypertension , they are 10% less likely than their non-Hispanic white counterparts to have their blood pressures controlled.
- In 2009 African American men were 30% more likely than non-Hispanic white men to die of heart disease.
- African American women are 1.6 times more likely to have hypertension than their non-Hispanic white counterparts.

From CDC Office of Minority Health Disparities: Heart disease and African Americans. From: *Summary statistics for U.S. adults: 2010.* Available at http://minorityhealth.hhs.gov/templates/content.aspx?lvl=2&lvlID=51&ID=3018.

Reducing Health Disparities

The IOM study also provided a number of recommendations for reducing health disparities. However, before change can occur, health care providers must become more culturally competent. The objective is not just to become competent but to become culturally proficient, that is, able to move smoothly between the world of the nurse and the world of the patient (in this case, the world of the elder). Moving toward proficient gerontological nursing care is one of the major strategies to improve the health of all persons regardless of age or ethnicity.

Increasing Cultural Competence

As nurses move toward gerontological cultural proficiency, they increase their awareness, knowledge, and skills. Nurses can learn of their personal biases, prejudices, attitudes, and behaviors toward persons different from themselves in race, ethnicity, age, gender, sexual orientation, social class, economic situations, and many other factors. Through increased knowledge, nurses can better assess the strengths and weaknesses of the older adult within the context of their lives and know when and how to effectively intervene to support rather than hinder long-held patterns that enhance wellness and coping. Competence means having the skills to put cultural knowledge to use in assessment, communication, negotiation, and intervention.

Awareness

Increased awareness calls for openness and self-reflection. It is a conscious effort to recognize the bias we express in our interactions with others, especially those who are different than we are (Stone & Moskowitz, 2011). If the nurse is white, especially those who are younger, it is realizing that this means special privilege and freedoms in a predominantly white and youth-oriented society. Those who are especially affected are older adults of color who may not have had the same advantages or experiences as the nurse (McIntosh, 1989). For example, in many regions of the United States, especially in the rural South, the current cohort of African Americans was limited to a fourth-grade education, with far-reaching implications. African Americans who are elders today lived during the time of Jim Crow laws which legalized discrimination and segregation and significantly restricted their lives. Events of the time included numerous murders by lynching (see www.jimcrowhistory.org and Box 4-2). These elders are also aware of the Tuskegee Experiment, in which black men with syphilis were purposely deceived and not treated

---

BOX 4-2   Racism in the Boston Naming Test*

During a study to evaluate the cultural applicability of several standard psychological tools sometimes administered by nurses, an 82-year-old African American woman reluctantly agreed to take what is called the Boston Naming Test. This measure of verbal fluency used in the diagnosis of dementia comprises a packet of pictures. The patient is asked to name the pictures. After doing so the volunteer shared, "Did you know that one of the pictures is a hangman's noose? Do you have any idea what that means to a black person to look at that picture!" Indeed, none of the white researchers had noticed this.

*Personal experience of Kathleen Jett.

---

so scientists could study its effect over time (see www.cdc.gov/tuskegee/timeline.html). For some, this has left a continuing distrust of the health care system and a reluctance to become involved in research.

Cultural awareness means recognizing the presence of the "isms" such as the racism just described. It is imperative to understand how these affect not only the pursuit and receipt of health care, but also the quality of life for older adults (Smedley et al., 2003). Moreover, as older adults they also may have faced sexism, classism, ageism, and so on.

Ageism is a term coined in 1968 by Robert Butler, the first director of the National Institute on Aging, to describe the discrimination and negative stereotypes that are based solely on age. Cole (1997) examined the historic roots of ageism in America. At one time, power in the United States was held almost exclusively by older white males. With the shift to urban industrialism and a growing emphasis on productivity and the ability to withstand the rigors of factory work, power and influence shifted from older to younger white men. With a near cultural obsession with youth today, it is easy to see that ageism is alive and well. Gift shops and department stores are replete with products such as "antiaging" products and graphic portrayals mocking the abilities of those formerly known as elders (Associated Press, 2011). In 2004, Americans spent $45.5 billion on antiaging products, and spending is expected to reach $72 billion by 2009 (International Longevity Center, 2006, p. 28). We often think in personal terms when negative stereotypes are applied to the person due to his or her age, but ageism may also be institutional, such as in mandatory retirement policies or the absence of older adults in research clinical trials. Ageism may be intentional, such as when older workers are targeted in financial scams, but

BOX 4-3   **Unintentional Ageism in Language and Its Effects**

- Use of general labeling terms: sweet old lady, little old lady, geezer.
- Use of terms applied in the health care setting: fossil, bed blocker (debilitated person in the hospital awaiting a bed in a nursing home), GOMER (get out of my emergency room).
- When speaking: exaggerated pitch, demeaning emotional tone, lower quality of speech.
- Consequences of ageism in language: reduced sense of self, lowered self-esteem, lowered sense of self-competence, decreased memory performance.

From International Longevity Center: *Ageism in America* (2006). Available at http://www.graypanthersmetrodetroit.org/Ageism_In_Amerca_-_ILC_Book_2006.pdf.

more often in nursing it is unintentional, but nonetheless present and hurtful (Box 4-3). Some health care professionals demonstrate ageism, undoubtedly in part because providers tend to see many frail older persons and fewer of those who are healthy and active. The impact of these perceptions has largely been ignored but almost certainly negatively affects health outcomes.

We now know that ageism is not universal but is most often reflective of the Euro-American culture. In many other cultures, elders are treated with special respect and honor. For example, for the most part, African American elders are respected. They may provide wisdom and insight to younger members of the family. Owing to a number of factors, African American grandparents are increasingly assuming the role of parent, for grandchildren and other teenage and younger relatives (Caminha-Bacote, 2008) (see Chapter 24).

Before the nurse provides quality care to elders, it is useful to self-reflect and consider whether one holds any personal beliefs about such persons and whether these beliefs are negative or positive, how they affect care delivery, and if they are based on facts rather than anecdotal experiences resulting in stereotypes.

Knowledge

Cultural knowledge is both what the nurse brings to the caring situation and what the nurse learns about older adults, their families, their communities, their behaviors, and their expectations. Essential knowledge includes the elder's way of life (ways of thinking, believing, and acting).

This knowledge is obtained formally and informally through the individual's professional experience of nursing.

Some nurses prefer to use what can be called an "encyclopedic" approach to details of a particular culture or ethnic group, such as proper name usage, touch, greeting, eye contact, gender roles, foods, and beliefs about relevant topics such as health promoting practices, pain expression, death rituals, or caregiving. This information is available in many compendiums of cross-cultural information (see the Evolve website for this book). The work of the Stanford Geriatric Education Center is especially helpful in this area (http://sgec.stanford.edu/training). When working with elders from a specific culture, knowledge about attitudes toward caregiving, decision making, and death rituals are especially important and may be particularly sensitive.

Although cultural knowledge is helpful and essential, caution must be used with regard to the potential for stereotyping. Stereotyping is the application of limited knowledge about one person with specific characteristics to other persons with the same characteristics; negative characteristics are especially prone to this treatment. Stereotyping limits the recognition of the heterogeneity of the group. At the same time, relying on knowledge of a positive stereotype can be useful as a starting point in understanding, but it too can be used to limit understanding of the uniqueness of the individual and impose unrealistic expectations. For example, a common stereotype of the African American culture is to assume that the church is a source of support. The nurse's assumption can easily have a negative outcome, such as fewer referrals for formal services support (e.g., home-delivered meals). This stereotype can also be used to shortcut conversation about discharge planning. In discussing discharge plans with an African American elder, the non–African American nurse may say, "I understand that the church is often a source of support in the African American community. Is this one of the resources you will be able to depend on when you return home?"

Persons from a specific ethnic group may share a common geographical origin, migratory status, race, language or dialect, or religion. Traditions, symbols, literature, folklore, food preferences, and dress are expressions of ethnicity. These may be particularly seen in older adults who have had no need to leave their culture-specific neighborhoods such as Chinatowns in the major cities, or the barrios of the Southwest. Persons who identify with the same ethnic group may or may not share a common race. For example, persons who consider themselves Hispanic are members of the most diverse ethnic group in the United States and may be from any race and from any one of a number of countries.

However, they usually have the Catholic religion and the Spanish language in common.

Health beliefs and practices are usually a mixed expression of life experience and cultural knowledge. In most cultures, older adults are likely to treat themselves for familiar or chronic conditions in ways they have found successful in the past, practices that are referred to as domestic medicine, folk medicine, or folk healing. The basis for much folk medicine was, and remains, to make the most of whatever is available. When self-treatment fails, a person will consult others known to be knowledgeable or experienced with the problem, such as a community or indigenous healer, often an elder known to the community. Only when this too fails do people seek help within the formal health care system.

The culture of nursing and health care in the United States is one that advocates what is called the Western or biomedical system with its own set of beliefs about the cause of illness, the choice of treatments, and so on. In most settings this belief system is considered superior to all others, an ethnocentric viewpoint. However, many of the world's people have different beliefs, such as those of the personalistic (magicoreligious) system or the naturalistic (holistic) system. Each system is complete with beliefs about disease causation and recommendations for prevention and treatment. It is not uncommon for ethnic elders to adhere to belief systems other than the biomedical system or a combination of systems. Nurses who are familiar with the range of health beliefs and realize their importance will be able to provide more sensitive and appropriate care. In the absence of understanding there is great potential for conflict. This is especially important to remember when working with those who have lived in culturally homogeneous communities.

Western or Biomedical System

In the Western or biomedical belief system, disease is thought to be the result of abnormalities in the structure and function of body organs and systems, often caused by an invasion of germs or genetic mutation. The terms *disease* and *illness* are subjective; they are used by care providers and not always understood by others. In the biomedical system, assessment and diagnosis are directed at identifying the pathogen or the process causing the abnormality by using laboratory and other procedures. Treatment is based on removing or destroying the invading organism or repairing, modifying, or removing the affected body part. Prevention involves the avoidance of pathogens, chemicals, activities, and dietary agents known to cause abnormalities. Health is often considered the absence of disease (see Chapter 1).

Personalistic or Magicoreligious System

Those who follow the personalistic or magicoreligious system believe that illness is caused by the actions of the supernatural, such as gods, deities, or nonhuman beings, such as ghosts, ancestors, or spirits. Health is viewed as a blessing or reward of God and illness as a punishment for a breach of rules, breaking a taboo, or displeasing or failing to please the source of power. Beliefs about illness and disease being caused by the wrath of God are prevalent among members of the Holiness, Pentecostal, and Fundamentalist Baptist churches. Examples of magical causes that illness can be attributed to are voodoo, especially among persons from the Caribbean; root work among southern African Americans; hexing or spells among Mexican Americans and African Americans; and Gaba among Filipino Americans. Knowledge about hexing became popularized in the *Harry Potter* series. Treatments may include religious practices, such as praying, meditating, fasting, wearing amulets, burning candles, and establishing family altars. Making sure that social networks with their fellow humans are in good working order is viewed as the essence of prevention. It is therefore important to avoid angering family, friends, neighbors, ancestors, and gods. This belief system can be traced back to the ancient Egyptians, thousands of years before the common era, and persists in its entirety or in parts in many groups. Current practices that would be included in this group include rituals such as "laying of the hands" and prayer circles. It is not uncommon to hear an older adult pray for a cure or lament, "What did I do to cause this?"

Naturalistic or Holistic Health System

The naturalistic or holistic health belief system is based on the concept of balance and stems from the ancient civilizations of China, India, and Greece (Wang & Paulanka, 2008). Many people throughout the world view health as a sign of balance—of the right amount of exercise, food, sleep, evacuation, interpersonal relationships, or the geophysical and metaphysical forces in the universe, such as *chi*. Disturbances in this balance result in disharmony and subsequent illness. Diagnosis calls for the determination of the type and extent of imbalance. The appropriate intervention, therefore, is to restore balance and harmony.

Traditional Chinese medicine is based on this belief, on the balance between *yin* and *yang*, darkness and light. Older adults who were raised in one of the countries on the Pacific Rim (especially in Asia and the Pacific Islands) or in a traditional American Indian community frequently rely on this system. The naturalistic system practiced in India and some of its neighboring countries is known as *ayurvedic* medicine.

Another variation is seen in those who follow the hot-cold beliefs, apart from traditional Chinese medicine. Held by many of Hispanic backgrounds, illness is believed to be the result of an excess of heat or cold that has entered the body and caused an imbalance. Hot and cold are generally metaphoric, although at times actual temperature is considered. Various foods, medicines, environmental conditions, emotions, and body conditions, such as menopause, may possess the characteristics of either hot or cold (Spector, 2008). Selecting an appropriate treatment requires the identification of disease type, either hot or cold; treatments are likewise divided. They are focused on using the opposite element; if the disease is the result of excess heat, treatment will be with something that has cold properties, and vice versa. The treatments include teas, herbs, food, dietary restrictions, techniques, or medications from Western medicine that have hot and cold properties.

Naturalistic healers can also be advanced practice nurses, physicians, or herbalists who specialize in symptomatic treatment and know which medicines will restore the body's equilibrium. In the American Indian culture, the healer is referred to as a medicine man or woman who combines naturalistic and magicoreligious systems. Prevention is directed at protecting oneself from imbalance.

Skills

Skillful nursing requires mutual respect between the nurse and the elder. It is working "with" the person rather than "on" the person. Providing the highest quality of care for diverse elders and enhancing healthy aging calls for a new or refined set of skills. These skills include listening carefully to the person, especially for his or her perception of the situation, and attending not just to the words but to the nonverbal communication and the meaning behind the words. It is a skill to be able to listen to the elder's perception of the situation, desired goals, and ideas for treatment. Cultural skills include the ability to explain your (the nurse's) perceptions clearly and without judgment, acknowledging that there are both similarities and differences between your perceptions and goals and those of the elder. Finally, cross-cultural skills include the ability to develop a plan of action that takes both perspectives into account and negotiate an outcome that is mutually acceptable (Berlin & Fowkes, 1983).

Working with Interpreters

Caring for persons cross-culturally often includes working with an *interpreter*. Interpreting is the process of rendering oral expressions made in one language into another in a manner that preserves the meaning and tone of the original

without adding or deleting anything. The job of the interpreter is to work with two different linguistic codes in a way that will produce equivalent messages. The interpreter tells the elder what the nurse has said and the nurse what the elder has said without adding meaning or opinion but in a way in which communication is as accurate as possible. This is often confused with translation (when interpreters are called "translators"), which instead deals with the written word.

Respectful communication is called for at all times; it is essential, however, with older adults from cultures in which this is the expectation and for those with limited or no English proficiency. Respectful communication includes addressing the person in the appropriate manner (surname unless otherwise instructed by the elder) and using acceptable body language. For example in most cultures other than those of northern Europe (including Euro-Americans) direct eye contact is considered disrespectful. To press eye contact with an elder may be particularly rude.

An interpreter is needed any time the nurse and the elder speak different languages, when the elder has limited English proficiency, or when cultural tradition prevents the elder from speaking directly to the nurse, for example as a result of the nurse's being a man or woman. The more complex the decision that must be made, the more important the skills of the interpreter are, such as when determining the elder's wishes regarding life-prolonging measures or the family's plan for caregiving.

It is ideal to engage persons who are trained medical interpreters who are of the same age, sex, and social status as the elder whenever possible. Unfortunately it is usually necessary to call upon younger interpreters; the effectiveness of the exchange may be hampered by the presence of intergenerational boundaries. Children and grandchildren are often called on to act as interpreters. In such a situation the nurse should realize that the child or the elder is "editing" comments because of cultural restrictions about the sharing of certain information (i.e., what is or is not considered appropriate to speak of to an elder or a child).

When working with an interpreter, the nurse first introduces herself or himself to the client and the interpreter and sets guidelines for the interview. Sentences should be short, employ the active voice, and avoid metaphors because they may be impossible to convert from one language to another. The nurse asks the interpreter to articulate exactly what is being said, and all conversation is addressed directly to the client (Enslein et al., 2002). Most guides will have the interpreter sit to the side and slightly behind the person. However, due to age-related hearing loss the interpreter may need to sit aside the nurse so the speaker can be seen for optimal communication (Box 4-4).

BOX 4-4   Working with Interpreters

- Before an interview or session with a client, meet with the interpreter to explain the purpose of the session.
- Encourage the interpreter to meet with the client before the session to identify the client's educational level and attitudes toward health and health care and to determine the depth and type of information and explanation needed.
- Look and speak directly to the client, not the interpreter.
- Be patient. Interpreted interviews take more time because long, explanatory phrases are often needed.
- Use short units of speech. Long, involved sentences or complex discussions create confusion.
- Use simple language. Avoid technical terms, professional jargon, slang, abbreviations, abstractions, metaphors, or idiomatic expressions.

- Encourage interpretation of the client's own words rather than paraphrased professional jargon to get a better sense of the client's ideas and emotional state.
- Request that the interpreter avoid inserting his or her own ideas and to avoid omitting information.
- Listen to the client and watch nonverbal communication (facial expression, voice intonation, body movement) to learn about emotions regarding a specific topic even when words are not understood.
- Clarify the client's understanding and the accuracy of the interpretation by asking the client to tell you in his or her own words what he or she understands, facilitated by the interpreter.

From Enslein J, Tripp-Reimer T, Kelley LS, et al: Evidence-based protocol: interpreter facilitation for individuals with limited English proficiency, *J Gerontol Nurs* 28(7):5-13, 2002.

Implications for Gerontological Nursing and Healthy Aging

The contact between elders and gerontological nurses often begins with assessment. During that process, each has an opportunity to know the other. Listening is the key; the nurse tries to understand the meaning of the person's perceptions. A thorough assessment includes a cultural assessment. A comprehensive assessment takes time. It is clear that this cannot be done in all situations, but even if it must be done bit by bit over time, it will give the caregiver a better understanding of how to work with and within the culture of the client.

Several tools or instruments can assist the nurse in the conduct of sensitive assessments. Although Leininger's Sunrise Model (Shen, 2004; Schim et al., 2007) is often recommended, alternative models may be more useful in the fast-paced health care situations of today. The explanatory model developed by Kleinman and associates (1978) has become a classic and has helped nurses and other health care professionals obtain the basic information needed in a culturally sensitive manner (Box 4-5). An adaptation of this assessment, LEARN, appears in Box 4-6. The LEARN Model (Berlin & Fowkes, 1983) serves as a guide in the clinical setting and can be used easily to increase the effectiveness of nursing interventions. Through it, the nurse will increase his or her cultural sensitivity and in doing so will be instrumental in providing more proficient care, thus helping reduce health disparities.

With an understanding of the basics, the nurse can negotiate a clear understanding of problems and solutions with the person or with the identified support figure in his or her life. When an understanding is reached, the nurse may need to include consultation or collaboration with traditional or alternative healers if the patient believes this is important. Priests, monks, rabbis, ministers, or indigenous healers may provide expert consultation, support, and interventions of their own. A sense of caring is conveyed in giving support to the elder's traditional beliefs and practices. Unbiased caring can surmount cultural and age differences.

Also critical to the cultural assessment is to determine the person's system of health beliefs. Most people (nurses and patients alike) subscribe to more than one system, combining Western biomedical approaches with those that may be considered more traditional. People choose among the health belief systems or include aspects of several of them in their attempt to make sense of health, illness, and treatments. To optimize the healthy aging of the person who depends on the nurse for intervention and caring, the nurse must be sensitive to the possibility that the person may hold one or more of these beliefs.

When a patient refuses biomedical treatments because the health problem is viewed as God's will or destiny, this is often particularly difficult for the nurse and other health

---

BOX 4-5   The Explanatory Model for Culturally Sensitive Assessment

1. How would you describe the problem that has brought you here? (*What do you call your problem; does it have a name?*)
   a. Who is involved in your decision making about health concerns?
2. How long have you had this problem?
   a. When do you think it started?
   b. What do you think started it?
   c. Do you know anyone else with it?
   d. Tell me what happened to that person when dealing with this problem.
3. What do you think is wrong with you?
   a. How severe is it?
   b. How long do you think it will last?
4. Why do you think this happened to you?
   a. Why has it happened to the involved part?
   b. What do you fear most about your sickness?
5. What are the chief problems your sickness has caused you?
6. What do you think will help clear up this problem? (*What treatment should you receive; what are the most important results you hope to receive?*)
   a. If specific tests and/or medications are listed, ask what they are and do.
7. Apart from me, who else do you think can make you feel better?
   a. Are there therapies that make you feel better that I do not know? (*Maybe in another discipline?*)

Modified from Kleinman A: *Patient and healers in the context of culture: an exploration of the borderland between anthropology, medicine, and psychiatry,* Berkeley, 1980, University of California Press; Pfeifferling JH: A cultural prescription for mediocentrism. In Eisenberg L, Kleinman A, editors: *The relevance of social science for medicine,* Boston, 1981, Reidel.

---

care providers. Finding out more about the person's beliefs about disease causation and the type of treatments he or she believes are appropriate in the given circumstances can enable the nurse to navigate the cultures of the medical establishment and that of the patient and work to promote better health.

Nurses should not attempt to change the person's belief system. It is difficult, if not impossible, and usually counterproductive. This is particularly so when working with older adults who carry a lifetime of beliefs and illness experiences. However, negotiating health, treatment, or prevention options may be possible. The nurse attempts to preserve helpful beliefs and practices, accommodate beliefs that are neither helpful nor harmful, and help clients to modify beliefs or practices that have been shown to be harmful. While it was not about aging, the book *The Spirit Catches You and You Fall Down* (Anne Fadiman), describes the hardships caused by a lack of sensitivity and the benefits when attempts to understand are made. For the nurse who has little or no knowledge of a belief or practice, it will be necessary to study and evaluate it to determine its helpfulness or its potential harm. In this way beliefs and practices can be preserved whenever possible. Respectfully explaining concern about potentially harmful practices with the offer of possible alternatives may show the person that the nurse is considering the person's preferences.

When care is provided in the home, nurses must adapt home care strategies to the beliefs and culture of the individual and the family if they hope to promote healthy aging and wellness. Special attention should be given to caregivers who are torn between their acculturated beliefs such as those related to nursing home stays, work versus caregiver demands, and expectations of the role of the child. The fictionalized accounts portrayed in Amy Tan's *The Bonesetter's Daughter* and Julia Alvarez' *Yo!* present some of the dilemmas and conflicts between the traditional elder and the acculturated children. Nurses work with the family to attempt to find a solution to potential cross-cultural and intergenerational conflicts in the caregiving and health

---

BOX 4-6   The LEARN Model

L Listen carefully to what the elder is saying. Attend to not just the words but to the nonverbal communication and the meaning behind the stories. Listen to the elder's perception of the situation, the desired goals, and the ideas for treatment.

E Explain your perception of the situation and the problems.

A Acknowledge and discuss both the similarities and the differences between your perceptions and goals and those of the elder.

R Recommend a plan of action that takes both perspectives into account.

N Negotiate a plan that is mutually acceptable.

From Berlin EA, Fowkes WC: A teaching framework for cross-cultural health care: application in family practice, *West J Med* 139(6):934-938, 1983.

care settings. The nurse also focuses on the elder's overall health and assists the elder and the family in gaining access to needed services. This is done by ascertaining the following: affordability, efficacy, accessibility, and availability of information; satisfaction; illness perspective; and informal support systems. Maintaining respect for clients' health beliefs is always paramount.

Cross-Cultural Caring and Long-Term Care

The term *long-term care* refers to ongoing assistance provided to persons who are physically or mentally fragile and unable to independently meet their basic needs (see Chapter 3). In many cultures outside the United States and in subcultures in the United States, families are expected to take care of their older members; institutional long-term care is less often used than in families of European descent (Jett, 2006) (see Table 4-2). Long-term care takes place in family homes, group homes, assisted living, skilled nursing facilities, and hospices. The preference for where care is received is culturally determined but often economically influenced. Senior centers also provide a type of ongoing long-term care, most of it social in nature. Only rarely do they provide service or a setting that is welcoming to other groups, such as new immigrants (McCaffrey, 2008) (Box 4-7).

The On Lok Project in San Francisco is the ultimate model for the provision of long-term care services to diverse elders. Originally designed to meet the home care needs of Chinese and Italian immigrants, it now has the capacity to provide every level of short- and long-term care as well as senior housing to the diverse populations of San Francisco. Services are provided in the language of the elder and in the manner that optimizes each person's wellness and cultural heritage (Kornblatt et al., 2003). Nurses can learn from the work of On Lok and other programs to enhance the care and encourage the health of ethnically diverse elders (AOA, n.d.).

Modifications to existing long-term care services that On Lok and others have found to enhance the well-being of ethnically diverse elders includes:

1. Ensuring that the resident has access to professional interpreter services if needed
2. Developing programs that reflect the diversity of the residents and the staff
3. Considering monocultural facilities or units, where population demographics warrant
4. Attempting to employ staff that reflects the diversity of the residents or participants

The study of the uniqueness and individuality of each elder is one of the most complex and intriguing opportunities of our day. Realistically it is almost impossible to become familiar with the whole range of clinically relevant cultural differences of older adults one may encounter. Caring for elders holistically and sensitively is the most challenging and potentially satisfying opportunity.

Culture, Nursing, and Maslow's Hierarchy of Needs

Promoting healthy aging in the care of diverse elders frequently provides the gerontological nurse with new challenges and necessitates a slightly different conceptualization of Maslow's Hierarchy. Unfortunately, poverty is very common in many older adult households especially those elders of color, and meeting basic needs (level one) may be difficult. The nurse can be sensitive to this possibility without making assumptions. The nurse can assess the components of biological integrity and, if necessary, facilitate the elder or the family in obtaining whatever supports (e.g., food stamps, home-delivered meals) are possible and appropriate.

Although some elders born outside of the United States did not experience trauma during their move to the United States, there are many others who suffered horrifically in their home country prior to the move or during their immigration process and for whom safety and security (level two) may have special meaning. The staff of a nursing home for Jewish residents complained that it was particularly difficult getting some of the residents with

---

BOX 4-7   Providing Culturally Welcoming Services

Dr. Ruth McCaffrey and colleagues received a grant in 2006 and "integrated" Haitian elders into a senior center in the very diverse community of Belle Glade, Florida. The center's staff and usual participants were introduced to culturally oriented ideas, music, art, and language. They were given an opportunity to ask questions of the local Haitian priest. The Haitian elders were similarly oriented. On a prearranged date, transportation was provided to the Haitian elders and a "welcoming" party was held; the event was facilitated by a bilingual native speaker-advocate-helper. The project was a success; both the long-term participants of the center and the newer participants expressed a new appreciation of each other and of the center.

Summarized from McCaffrey RG: Integrating Haitian older adults into a senior center in Florida: understanding cultural barriers for immigrant older adults, *J Gerontol Nurs* 33(12):13-18, 2007.

dementia to shower. Some were Holocaust survivors. It was some time before the staff realized that as the residents' dementia progressed, they were no longer able to distinguish the difference between a shower for hygiene and the fear of "going to the showers" (i.e., to the gas chamber) in the concentration camps of their youth (Weissman, 2004).

Cultural identity may be one of the major elements of self-concept and a key to self-esteem—increasingly so as a person becomes more mentally or physically frail. Often elders of a distinct ethnic background are closely tied to family and community. Estrangement from their country of origin may be ameliorated if they live in homogeneous communities and exacerbated if they live in social isolation or away from persons with similar backgrounds (Averill, 2005). The ethnic community (e.g., barrios, Nihonmachi, Chinatown) serves as a buffer and a means of strengthening social cohesiveness for elders and others of various cultural groups (Chiang-Hanisko, 2005). Within the community, members are protected from discrimination and the language and customs of the society outside.

Family, religion, community, and history are important reference points for self-worth and identity for persons from any ethnic group. Familial supports vary among groups, social classes, and subcultures, yet the nuclear or extended family is the chief avenue of transmitting cultural values, beliefs, customs, and practices. In some groups, elders are considered repositories of cultural knowledge. The elder and extended family provides orientation, stability, and often, sanctuary. In gross generalizations, we must consider the possibility that persons of Asian descent value familial piety; Hispanics, the extended family; African Americans, extended or fictive kin (family "members" due to emotional bond) supports; Native Americans, a system of kinship and line of descent; and persons of northern European descent, the desire for independence and autonomy above all other things (Purnell & Paulanka, 2008).

Changes are threatening the historical role of the older adult in the traditional family (see Chapter 24). Economic independence and mobility of the younger members of the family are chipping away at the insulation afforded by the community (Jett, 2006). Intergenerational discontinuities created by assimilation produce a communication gap between the young and the old. This may cause isolation and estrangement between the oldest and youngest generations. Members of ethnic minorities are extremely vulnerable in old age. They may be devalued by the majority culture because of both age and ethnicity or any of the "isms." Nurses can take an active role in facilitating self-actualization by facilitating expression of the uniqueness of the individual, by attending to the elder's spiritual and cultural needs, and

by taking the lead in optimizing the health and abilities of those who seek our care.

KEY CONCEPTS

- Population diversity will continue to increase rapidly for many years. This suggests that nurses will be caring for a greater number of persons from a broad range of ethnicities and ages than in the past.
- Recent research has revealed significant and persistent inequities in the outcomes of health for persons from minority groups, with the members of these groups bearing the burden of morbidity and mortality in most areas.
- Nurses can contribute to the reduction of health disparities and inequities through increasing their own awareness, knowledge, and skills.
- Negative stereotyping is never appropriate.
- Cultural awareness, knowledge, and skills are necessary to increase cultural competence.
- Nurses caring for diverse elders must let go of their own ethnocentrism before they can give effective care.
- Many elders hold health beliefs that are different from those of the biomedical or Western medicine used by most health care professionals in the United States.
- Lack of awareness of the elder's health belief system has the potential to produce conflict in the nursing situation.
- The more complex the communication or decision-making needs in a given situation, the greater the need for skilled interpreter services for persons with limited English proficiency.
- Programs staffed by persons who reflect the ethnic background of the participants and speak their language may be preferred by the elderly.
- Kleinman's explanatory model and the LEARN Model provide a useful framework for working with elders of any ethnicity or background.

ACTIVITIES AND DISCUSSION QUESTIONS

1. Discuss your personal beliefs regarding health and illness and how they fit into the three major classifications of health systems. How can this affect culturally competent care for ethnically diverse elders?
2. Explain the types of questions that would be helpful in assessing an elder's health problem or problems in a way that is respectful of the person and his or her cultural background and ethnic identity.
3. Propose strategies that would be helpful in planning care for elders from different ethnic backgrounds.
4. Activity: Discuss your familial and culturally determined views of aging after speaking to older family members.

REFERENCES

Administration on Aging [AOA]: *A profile of older Americans: 2010*. Available at http://www.aoa.gov/AoARoot/Aging_Statistics/Profile/2010/7.aspx.

Administration on Aging [AOA]: *A toolkit for serving diverse communities* (n.d). Available at http://www.aoa.gov/AoARoot/AoA_Programs/Tools_Resources/DOCS/AoA_Diversity Toolkit_full.pdf.

Associated Press: *Ageism in America: as boomers age, bias against the elderly becomes a hot topic* (2011). Available at http://www.msnbc.msn.com/id/5868712/ns/health-aging/t/ageism-america.

Averill JB: Studies of rural elderly individuals: merging critical ethnography with community-based action research, *J Gerontol Nurs* 31(2):11–18, 2005.

Berlin EA, Fowkes WC: A teaching framework for cross-cultural health care: application in family practice, *West J Med* 139(6):934–938, 1983.

Caminha-Bacote J: People of African American heritage. In Purnell L, Paulanka BJ, editors: *Transcultural health care: a culturally competent approach*, Philadelphia, 2008, Davis.

Centers for Disease Control and Prevention [CDC]. *The state of aging and health in America* (2009). Available at http://www.cdc.gov/aging/data/stateofaging.htm.

Chiang-Hanisko L: Transnational perspective: ethnic identity and older adult immigrant's health care decision making, *Geriatr Nurs* 26(6):349, 2005.

Cole T: *The journey of life: cultural history of aging in America*, Cambridge, England, 1997, Cambridge University Press.

Enslein J, Tripp-Reimer T, Kelley LS, et al: Evidence-based protocol: interpreter facilitation for individuals with limited English proficiency, *J Gerontol Nurs* 28(7):5–13, 2002.

Gelfand D: *Aging and ethnicity: knowledge and service*, ed 2, New York, 2003, Springer.

International Longevity Center. *Ageism in America* (2006). Available at http://www.graypanthersmetrodetroit.org/Ageism_In_America_-_ILC_Book_2006.pdf. See also http://www.mssm.edu/research/programs/international-longevity-center.

Jett K: Mind-loss in the African American community: a normal part of aging, *J Aging Stud* 20(1):1–10, 2006.

Kleinman A, Eisenberg L, Good B: Culture, illness, and care: clinical lessons from anthropologic and cross-cultural research, *Ann Intern Med* 88(2):251–258, 1978.

Kornblatt S, Eng C, Hansen JC: Cultural awareness in health and social services: the experience of On Lok, *Generations* 26(3):46–53, 2003.

McCaffrey R: The lived experience of integrating Haitian elders into a senior center, *J Transcult Nurs* 19(1):33–39, 2008.

McIntosh P: *White privilege: unpacking the invisible knapsack* (1989). Available at http://www.library.wisc.edu/EDVRC/docs/public/pdfs/LIReadings/InvisibleKnapsack.pdf.

National Institute on Aging [NIA]: *Review of minority aging research at the NIA* (2010). Available at http://www.nia.nih.gov/AboutNIA/MinorityAgingResearch.htm.

Purnell L, Paulanka BJ: *Transcultural health care: a culturally competent approach*, Philadelphia, 2008, Davis.

Schim SN, Doorenbos A, Benkert R, et al: Culturally congruent care: putting the pieces together, *J Transcult Nurs* 18(2):57–62, 2007.

Shen Z: Cultural competence models in nursing: a selected annotated bibliography, *J Transcult Nurs* 15(4):317–322, 2004.

Smedley B, Stith A, Nelson A, editors: *Unequal treatment: confronting racial and ethnic disparities in health care*, Washington, DC, 2003, National Academy Press. Available at http://www.nap.edu/catalog.php?record_id=12875.

Spector RE: *Cultural diversity in health and illness*, ed 7, Uppar Saddle River, NJ, 2008, Prentice-Hall Health.

Stone J, Moskowitz GB: Non-conscious bias in medical decision making: what can be done to reduce it? *Medical Education* 45(8):768–776, 2011.

U.S. Department of Health and Human Services [USDHHS], Office of Disease Prevention and Health Promotion: *Disparities* (2012). Available at http://www.healthypeople.gov/2020/about/DisparitiesAbout.aspx.

Vincent GK, Velkoff VA: *Current Population Reports: The next four decades: the older population in the United States, 2010 to 2050*, U.S. Department of Commerce (2010). Available at http://www.census.gov/prod/2010pubs/p25-1138.pdf.

Wang Y, Paulanka BJ: People of Chinese culture. In Purnell L, Paulanka BJ, editors: *Transcultural health care: a culturally competent approach*, Philadelphia, 2008, Davis, pp. 129–144.

Weissman G: Personal communication, April 10, 2004.

CHAPTER 5

Theories of Aging and Physical Changes

Kathleen F. Jett

evolve.elsevier.com/Ebersole/gerontological

LEARNING OBJECTIVES

Upon completion of this chapter, the reader will be able to:

- Identify the physical changes that are associated with normal aging.
- Begin to differentiate normal age-related changes from those that are potentially pathological.
- Describe at least one age-related change for each body system.
- Develop a plan of care for the older adult that targets prevention and health promotion.

GLOSSARY

Glomerular filtration rate (GFR) The rate at which the kidneys filter blood.

Kyphosis C-shaped curvature of the cervical vertebrae.

Presbycusis Progressive, bilaterally and symmetrical age-related hearing loss.

Presbyopia Reduced near vision occurring normally with age, usually resulting in improved distance vision.

Xerostomia Excessive mouth dryness.

THE LIVED EXPERIENCE

Strange how these things creep up on you. I really was surprised and upset when I first realized it was not the headlights on my car that were dim but only my aging night vision. Then I remembered other bits of awareness that forced me to recognize that I, that 16-year-old inside me, was experiencing changes that go along with getting older.

Sally, age 60

Aging comprises a series of complex changes and occurs in all living organisms. Most of these changes are intrinsic, coming from within; others are a result of extrinsic, environmental factors, such as exposure to smoke or other pollutants. Some changes are beneficial (e.g., learned experiences, resistance to some infections), others are to one's disadvantage (e.g., slowed reaction time) and others are neutral (e.g., graying of hair). Just why the changes occur has been of interest to scientists for decades as they have unceasingly searched for the mythical "fountain of youth," yet it is now well accepted that the maximum possible age in the human is about 120 years (Walston, 2010). It is known that the triggers of aging are greatly influenced by genetics and by injury to or abuse of the body earlier in life.

Later life is a time of challenge and opportunity. Among the challenges are physical changes which occur to many or most persons as they accumulate years. Other challenges are the result of pathological conditions, many of which are the manifestations of lifestyle choices made at younger ages, such as smoking and obesity. Some indications of pathological conditions are mistakenly considered an expected part of the aging process.

In this chapter the prominent biological theories of aging and some of the major physical changes associated with normal aging are discussed. For a more thorough discussion see *Toward Healthy Aging* (Jett, 2011). With this knowledge the nurse can begin to differentiate normal aging from health problems that necessitate treatment and help facilitate prompt intervention, which in turn promotes healthy aging. When health is optimized the person can more easily move toward self-actualization (see Chapter 1).

Biological Theories of Aging

A theory is an explanation of some phenomenon that makes sense to us. Theories remain reasonable explanations until someone finds them to be incorrect. Most theories can neither be proved nor disproved, but they are useful as points of reference. Each theory in its own right provides a clue to the aging process. However, many unanswered questions remain.

The biological theories of aging today have evolved from the early study of changes over the life span of the organism. Two related theoretical views form the foundation of biological theories: error (stochastic) theories and predetermined aging (nonstochastic) theories. Although they differ, both viewpoints agree that, in the end, the cells in the body become disorganized or chaotic and are no longer able to replicate, and cells die. When enough cells die, so does the organism. In recent years, research on the biological theories of aging has emphasized the cells, the genes, and other components within the cell. The physical traits that identify one as older (e.g., gray hair, wrinkled skin) are referred to as the aging phenotype, that is, an outward expression of one's individual genetic makeup (Carnes, Staats, Sonntag, 2008). A short description of emerging theories can be found in Box 5-1.

Error (Stochastic) Theories

Error theories explain aging as the result of an accumulation of errors in the synthesis of cellular DNA and RNA, the basic building blocks of the cell (Short et al., 2005). With each replication, more errors occur, until the cell is no longer able to function. The visible signs of aging, such as gray hair, are thought to be the result of the accumulation

---

BOX 5-1 Emerging Biological Theories of Aging

Neuroendocrine Control or Pacemaker Theory
The neuroendocrine system regulates many essential activities related to an organism's growth and development. The neuroendocrine (or pacemaker) theory focuses on the changes in these systems over time. It may be that common neurons in the higher brain centers act as pacemakers that regulate the biological clock during development and aging, and slow down and eventually "shut off" at the predetermined time. Much of the current research in this area is on the examination of the influence of hormones on neuroendocrine functioning over time, especially dehydroepiandrosterone (DHEA) and melatonin.

Genetic Research
As the human genome is being mapped, scientists continue to examine the roles that genetics, and RNA in particular, has in both random and programmed aging and may eventually be able to explain senescence. Among the findings are that telomeres, which serve to cap the ends of the chromosomes, shorten with each cellular reproduction until a time when the telomere disappears and the cell can no longer reproduce and dies. Abnormal cells such as cancer cells produce an enzyme called *telomerase*, which actually lengthens the telomeres, enabling the cells to continue to reproduce. Learning to manipulate telomerase may have significant implications for controlling both cellular reproduction and aging.

Progerin and Telomers
Some of the latest research in this field has found an association between telomeres which cap either end of chromosomes and a toxic protein call progerin. As long as a telomere is securely bound to the chromosome, the cell is able to replicate and in essence live forever. However, the telomeres actually wear away with aging at the same time the cell produces more and more progerin. The progerin, a mutated version of normal cell protein, interferes with the stability of the telomeres and ultimately the length of the cell's life. (From Cao K, Faddah DA, Kieckhaefer JE, et al: Progerin and telomere dysfunction collaborate to trigger cellular senescence in normal fibroblasts, *J Clin Invest* 121(7): 2833–2844, 2011.)

of these cellular errors. Three of the most common theories of error are wear-and-tear, cross-linkage, and free radical.

Wear-and-Tear Theory

One of the earliest theories of aging is known as "wear-and-tear." According to this theory, cell errors are the result of "wearing out" over time because of continued use and trauma. Internal and external stressors increase the numbers of errors and the speed with which they occur (e.g., in shoulder joints of pitchers or knees of runners). These errors may cause a progressive decline in cellular function.

Cross-Link Theory

Cross-link theory explains aging in terms of the accumulation of errors by cross-linking, or the stiffening of proteins in the cell. Proteins link with glucose and other sugars in the presence of oxygen and become stiff and thick (Marin-Garcia, 2008). Because collagens are the most plentiful proteins in the body, this is where the cross-linking is most easily seen. Skin that was once smooth, silky, firm, and soft becomes drier and less elastic with age. Collagen is also a key component of the lungs, the arteries, and the tendons, and similar changes can be seen there, such as in stiffened joints.

Oxidative Stress Theory (Free Radical Theory)

The oxidative stress theory, otherwise known as the free radical theory of aging, is among those most understood and accepted (Jang & Van Remmen, 2009). Free radicals are natural by-products of cellular activity and are always present to some extent. It is believed that cellular errors are the result of random damage from molecules in the cells called free radicals.

It is known that exposure to environmental pollutants increases the production of free radicals and increases the rate of damage. The best-known pollutants include smog and ozone, pesticides, and radiation (Abdollahi et al., 2004; Lodovici & Bigagli, 2011). Other environmental sources thought to cause increases in free radicals are gasoline, by-products from the plastic industry, and drying linseed oil paints. There is also new evidence that chronic exposure to racial discrimination increases evidence of oxidative stress. This may provide some explanation for a number of the disparities in incidence and prevalence of several diseases that are associated with free radicals, such as heart disease (Pashkow, 2011). In youth, naturally occurring vitamins, hormones, enzymes, and antioxidants neutralize the free radicals as needed (Valko et al., 2005). However, with aging, the damage caused by free radicals occurs faster than the cells can repair themselves, and cell death occurs (Hornsby, 2009; Marin-Garcia, 2008).

Programmed Aging (Nonstochastic Theories)

The nonstochastic theories attribute the changes of aging to a process that is thought to be predetermined or "programmed" at the cellular level. This means that each cell has a natural life expectancy. As more and more cells cease to replicate, the signs of aging appear, and ultimately the person dies at a "predetermined" age. These theories evolved from the groundbreaking work of Hayflick and Moorehead (1981). They referred to this process as the inner *biological clock*. In other words, each cell is "born" with a limited number of replications and then it dies.

Neuroendocrine-Immunological Theory

Closely tied to both programmed and free radical theory is the immunity theory of aging. It is based on changes in the integrated neuorendocrine and immune systems. In this case, the emphasis is on the programmed deaths of the immune cells from damage caused by the increase of free radicals as aging progresses (Effros et al., 2005; Marin-Garcia, 2008). The immune system in the human body is a complex network of cells, tissues, and organs that function separately and together to protect the body from substances from the outside, such as bacteria. It is highly dependent on the release of hormones. In the simplest terms, the specialized B lymphocytes (humoral) and the T lymphocytes (cellular) protect the body against invasion by infection or other matter that is considered foreign, such as tissue or organ transplants. The results of animal studies have demonstrated that the cells of the immune system become progressively more diversified with age and in a somewhat predictable fashion lose some of their ability to self-regulate. The T lymphocytes show more signs of "aging" than do the B lymphocytes. The reduced T cells are thought to be responsible for hastening the age-related changes caused by autoimmune reactions as the body battles itself; healthy cells are mistaken for foreign substances and are attacked.

It is important for the nurse to understand that the exact cause of aging is unknown; there is considerable variation in the aging process. Not only is there variation between persons but also between the systems of any one person. Aging is a wholly unique and individual experience.

Physical Changes that Accompany Aging

Integumentary

The skin is composed of the epidermis, the dermis, and the hypodermis. As the largest, most visible organ of the body, the various layers of the skin mold and model the individual to give much of his or her personal and sexual identity. The skin and hair provide clues to heredity, race, and physical and emotional health.

Many age-related changes in the skin are functionally inconsequential, but others have implications for organs throughout the body and have more far-reaching impact. Skin changes occur due to both genetic (intrinsic) factors and environmental (extrinsic) factors such as wind, sun, and pollution, to which skin is especially sensitive. Cigarette smoking causes coarse wrinkles, and the photo-damage of the sun is evidenced by rough, leathery texture, itching, and mottled pigmentation, among other signs. Changes that may be genetic, environmental, or both include dryness, thinning, decreased elasticity, and the development of prominent small blood vessels. Skin tears, purpura (large purple spots), and xerosis (excessive dryness) are common but not normal aspects of physical aging. Visible changes of the skin—quality of color, firmness, elasticity, and texture—affirm that one is aging.

Epidermis

The epidermis is the outer layer of skin and is composed primarily of tough keratinocytes and squamous cells. Melanocytes produce melanin, which gives the skin color. With age, the epidermis thins, making blood vessels and bruises much more visible. T-cell function declines, and there may be a reactivation of latent conditions such as herpes zoster (shingles) or herpes simplex, making a shingles immunization particularly important for persons who had "chicken pox" or varicella when younger.

Cell renewal time increases by up to one third after 50 years of age; 30 or more days may be necessary for new epithelial replacement (Gosain & DiPietro, 2004). This change significantly affects wound healing. In a younger adult, if the skin is injured (e.g., a cut or scrape), the surrounding tissue becomes red (erythematous) almost immediately. This inflammatory response is the first step in the natural healing process. In an older adult, this inflammation may not begin to occur for 48 to 72 hours. A laceration that becomes pink several days after the event may be misinterpreted by the nurse as having become "infected," when in reality, the healing process has only just started. Evidence of true skin infection in older adults is no different than in younger adults, namely, *increasing* redness and purulent drainage.

The number of melanocytes in the epidermis decreases. Fewer melanocytes means a lightening of the overall skin tone, regardless of original skin color, and a decrease in the amount of protection from ultraviolet rays; the importance of sunscreen is thus significantly increased (see Chapter 12).

However, in some body areas, melanin synthesis is increased. Pigment spots (freckles and nevi) enlarge and can become more numerous with increased exposure to natural and artificial light. Lentigines appear, commonly referred to as "age spots" or "liver spots." They are frequently found on the backs of the hands and the wrists, and on the faces of light-skinned persons older than 50 years of age. Thick, brown, raised lesions with a "stuck on" appearance (seborrheic keratoses) are more common in men and are of no clinical significance but can become cosmetically disfiguring if severe.

Dermis

The dermis, lying beneath the epidermis, is a supportive layer of connective tissue composed of a combination of yellow elastic fibers that provide stretch and recoil and white fibrous collagen fibers that provide strength. It also supports hair follicles, sweat glands, sebaceous glands, nerve fibers, muscle cells, and blood vessels, which provide nourishment to the epidermis. Sun exposure accelerates skin tissue changes by hastening changes in collagen fiber.

Many of the visible signs of aging skin are reflections of changes in the dermis. The dermis loses about 20% of its thickness (Friedman, 2011). This thinness causes older skin to look more transparent and fragile. Dermal blood vessels are reduced, which accounts for resultant skin pallor and cooler skin temperature. Collagen synthesis decreases, causing the skin to "give" less under stress and tear more easily. Elastin fibers thicken and fragment, leading to loss of stretch and resilience and a "sagging" appearance. Loss of elasticity accentuates jowls and elongated ears and contributes to the formation of a "double" chin. Breasts that were full and firm begin to sag. As will be seen, the impact of the change in elastin has implications for a number of other systems as well.

Hypodermis: Subcutaneous Layer

The hypodermis is the innermost layer of the skin, and it contains connective tissues, blood vessels, and nerves, but the major component is subcutaneous fat (adipose tissue). The primary purposes of the adipose tissue are to store calories and provide temperature regulation. It also provides shape and form to the body and acts as a shock absorber against trauma. With age, some areas of the hypodermis thin. As the natural insulation of fat decreases, a person becomes more sensitive to the cold.

Changes in the hypodermis also increase the chance for the person to become overheated (hyperthermia) as a result of the reduced efficiency of the eccrine (sweat) glands. Sweat glands are located all over the body and respond to thermostimulation and neurostimulation in response to internal changes (e.g., fever, menopausal "hot flashes") or increases in environmental temperatures. The usual body response to heat is to produce moisture or sweat from these glands and thus cool the skin by evaporation. With aging, the glands become fibrotic, and surrounding connective tissue becomes avascular, leading to a decline in the efficiency of the body to cool down. It is not uncommon for persons to complain of being either too hot or too cold in environments that are comfortable to others.

Sebaceous (oil) glands also atrophy. Sebum, produced by the gland, protects the skin by preventing the evaporation of water from the epidermis; it possesses bactericidal properties and contains a precursor of vitamin D. When the skin is exposed to sunlight, vitamin D is produced and absorbed into the skin. Continuing to produce Vitamin D is especially important because of the high incidence of osteoporosis (see "Structure, Posture, and Body Composition" later in this chapter and Chapter 18). All people need some sunshine and probably vitamin D supplementation every day, especially those living in residential care facilities who have fewer opportunities to be outside.

Older adults are at significant risk for both hyperthermia and hypothermia. When caring for frail older adults, gerontological nurses can promote healthy aging by helping their patients avoid extremes of temperature, prevent drying, and prevent exposure to toxic products (see Chapter 13).

Hair and Nails

Hair, as part of the integument, has biological, psychological, and cosmetic value. Hair is composed of tightly fused horny cells that arise from the dermal layer of the skin and are colored by melanocytes. Genetics, race, sex, and hormones influence hair color and distribution in both men and women.

Men and women in all racial groups have less hair as they grow older. Hair on the head thins. Scalp hair loss is prominent in men, beginning as early as the twenties. The hair in the ears, the nose, and the eyebrows of older men increases and stiffens. Women have less pronounced scalp hair loss (Luggen, 2005). For some, the accustomed hair color remains, but for most, there is a gradual loss of pigmentation (melanin) and it becomes dryer and coarser. Older women develop chin and facial hair because of the decreased estrogen to testosterone ratio. Leg, axillary, and pubic hair lessens and in some instances disappears in postmenopausal women. The absence of leg hair can be misinterpreted as a sign of peripheral vascular disease in the older adult, whereas it is a normal change of aging.

The various races have distinctive hair characteristics, which should be kept in mind when caring for or assessing the person. Almost all Asians have sparse facial and body hair that is dark, silky, and most often straight. African Americans have slightly more head and body hair than Asians; however, the hair texture varies widely. It is always fragile, and it ranges from straight to spiraled, and thin to thick. Whites have the most head and body hair, with an intermediate texture and form ranging from straight to curly, fine to coarse, and thick to thin.

The nail becomes harder and thicker, and more brittle, dull, and opaque. It changes shape, becoming at times flat or concave instead of convex. Vertical ridges appear because of decreasing water, calcium, and lipid content. The blood supply, as well as the rate of nail growth, decreases. The half moon (lunule) of the fingernail may entirely disappear; the color of the nails may vary from yellow to gray, although with the widespread use of acrylics on the nails, long-term effects are not yet known. The development of a fungal infection of the nails (onychomycosis) is not the result of aging but is quite common. Fungus invades the space between the layers of the nails, leaving a thick and unsightly appearance. The slowness of growth and the reduced circulation in the older nail make it very difficult to treat.

For suggestions of nursing interventions that promote healthy skin during aging see Box 5-2.

Musculoskeletal

A functioning musculoskeletal system is necessary for the body's movement in space, for gross responses to environmental forces, and for the maintenance of posture. This complex system comprises bones, joints, tendons, ligaments, and muscles.

Although none of the age-related changes to the musculoskeletal system are life-threatening, any of them could affect one's ability to function and therefore one's quality of life. Some of the changes are visible to others and have the potential to affect the individual's self-esteem. As seen with the skin, changes in the musculoskeletal system are influenced by many factors, such as age, sex, race, and environment; signs begin to become obvious in the forties.

BOX 5-2 **Promoting Healthy Skin While Aging**
• Avoid excessive exposure to ultraviolet light. • Keep skin moisturized. • Avoid use of drying soaps. • Always use sunscreens. • Keep well hydrated.

The musculoskeletal changes that have the most effect on function are related to the ligaments, tendons, and joints; over time these become dry, hardened, and less flexible. In joints that had been subjected to trauma earlier in life (injuries or repetitive movement), these changes can be seen earlier and are more severe. If joint space is reduced, arthritis is diagnosed.

Muscle mass can continue to build until the person is in his or her fifties. However, between 30% and 40% of the skeletal muscle mass of a 30-year-old may be lost by the time the person is in his or her nineties (Crowther-Radulewicz, 2010). Disuse of the muscles accelerates the loss of strength. Age-related changes to muscles are known as *sarcopenia* and are seen almost exclusively in the skeletal muscle. Muscle tissue mass decreases (atrophies) whereas adipose tissue increases in key areas. The replacement of lean muscle by adipose tissue is most noticeable in men in the area of the waist and in women between the umbilicus and the symphysis pubis. The nurse can encourage older adults to exercise, especially through weight-bearing exercises, to help maintain healthy bones and muscles and flexibility (Box 5-3). See Chapter 11 for discussion on exercise.

Structure, Posture, and Body Composition

Changes in stature and posture are two of the more obvious signs of aging and are associated with multiple factors involving skeletal, muscular, subcutaneous, and fat tissue. Vertebral disks become thin as a result of dehydration, causing a shortening of the trunk. These changes may begin to be seen as early as the fifties (Crowther-Radulewicz, 2010). The trunk shortens as a result of gravity and dehydration of the vertebral disks. The person may have a stooped appearance from kyphosis, a curvature of the cervical vertebrae arising from reduced bone mineral density (BMD). Some loss of BMD in women is associated with the reduction of estrogen levels after menopause. With the shortened appearance, the bones of the arms and the legs may appear disproportionate in size. If a person's bone mineral density is very low, it is diagnosed as osteoporosis and a loss of 2 to 3 inches in height is not uncommon (see Chapter 18).

Alteration in body shape and weight occurs as lean body mass declines and body water is lost: 54% to 60% in men; 46% to 52% in women (Kee et al., 2009). Fat tissue increases until 60 years of age; therefore body density is higher in youth because of the density of muscle compared to the lightness of fat. From 25 to 75 years of age, fat content of the body increases by 16%. Cellular solids and bone mass decline; extracellular water, however, remains relatively constant. The water loss has significant implications for the dramatically increased risk for dehydration (Figure 5-1).

Cardiovascular

The cardiovascular system is responsible for the transport of oxygen and nutrient-rich blood to the organs and the transport of metabolic waste products to the kidneys and the bowels. The most relevant age-related changes in this system are myocardial and blood vessel stiffening and decreased responsiveness to sudden changes in demand (Brashers & McCance, 2010). Changes in the cardiovascular (CV) system are progressive and cumulative.

Cardiac

The age-related changes of the heart (presbycardia) are structural, electrical, and functional. The size of the heart remains relatively unchanged in healthy adults. However, the left ventricle wall thickens by as much as 50% by 80 years of age, and the left atrium increases in size slightly—an adaptation that enhances ventricular filling (Taffet & Lakatta, 2003). Maximum coronary artery blood flow, stroke volume, and cardiac output are decreased. In health, the changes have little or no effect on the heart's ability to function in day-to-day life. The changes only become significant when there are environmental, physical, or psychological stresses. With sudden demands for more oxygen the heart may not be able to respond adequately (Marin-Garcia, 2008). It takes longer for the heart to accelerate and then return to a resting state.

For the gerontological nurse, this means that the increased heart rate one might expect to see when the person is in pain, anxious, febrile, or hemorrhaging may not be present or will be delayed. Similarly, the older heart may not be able to respond to other calls for increased cardiac demand such as infection, anemia, pneumonia, cardiac dysrhythmias, surgery, diarrhea, hypoglycemia, malnutrition, and drug-induced and noncardiac illnesses such as

---

BOX 5-3 Promoting Healthy Bones and Muscles

- Ensure regular and adequate intake of vitamin D and calcium.
- Engage in regular weight-bearing exercise, for example, T'ai Chi.
- Engage in regular flexibility and balance exercises, for example, yoga.
- For women: consider preventive pharmacotherapeutics.

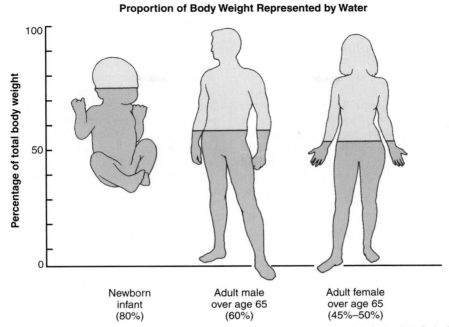

Proportion of Body Weight Represented by Water

FIGURE 5-1 Changes in body water distribution. (From Thibodeau GA, Patton KT: *Structure and function of the body,* ed 12, St. Louis, 2004, Mosby.)

renal disease and prostatic obstruction. Instead, the nurse must depend on other signs of distress in the older patient and be diligently alert to signs of rapid decompensation of both the previously well elder and one who is already medically fragile, such as those in nursing homes.

Heart disease is the number one cause of nonaccidental death in developed nations. Often the changes associated with disease are thought to be "normal," but they are not. The nurse promotes healthy aging with recommendations for heart-healthy life choices and urging the elder to seek and receive excellent health care.

Blood Vessels

Several of the same age-related changes seen in the skin and muscles affect the lining (intima) of the blood vessels, especially the arteries. As in the skin, the most significant change is decreased elasticity which allows some blood to circulate. The blood supply to various organs decreases, and resistance in the blood vessels increases. Change in flow to the coronary arteries and the brain is minimal, but decreased blood flow to other organs, especially the liver and kidneys, has potentially serious implications for medication use (see Chapter 8). When a person already has or develops arteriosclerosis or hypertension, the age-related changes can have serious consequences.

Less dramatic changes are found in the veins; although they do stretch somewhat, the valves which keep the blood from flowing backward become less efficient. This means that lower extremity edema develops more quickly and that the older adult is more at risk for deep vein thrombosis (blood clots) because of the increased sluggishness of the venous circulation. The normal changes, when combined with long-standing but unknown weakness of the vessels, may become visible in varicose veins and explain the increased rate of stroke and aneurysms in older adults. However, the promotion of a healthier cardiovascular system is always possible (Box 5-4).

BOX 5-4   Promoting a Healthy Heart

- Engage in regular exercise.
- Eat a low-fat, low-cholesterol, balanced diet.
- Maintain tight control of diabetes.
- Do not smoke, and avoid exposure to smoke.
- Avoid environmental pollutants.
- Practice stress management.
- Minimize sodium intake.
- Maintain ideal body weight.

Respiratory

The respiratory system is the vehicle for ventilation and gas exchange, particularly the transfer of oxygen into and the release of carbon dioxide from the blood. The respiratory structures depend on the musculoskeletal and nervous systems to function fully. The respiratory system matures by the age of 20 and then begins to decline even in healthy individuals. Although subtle changes occur in the lungs, the thoracic cage, the respiratory muscles, and the respiratory centers in the central nervous system, the changes are small and, for the most part, insignificant. The specific changes include loss of elasticity resulting in stiffening of the chest wall, inefficiency in gas exchange, and increased resistance to air flow (Figure 5-2). Respiratory problems are common but almost always the result of exposure to environmental toxins (e.g., pollution, cigarette smoke) rather than the aging process (Sheahan & Musialowski, 2001).

Like the cardiovascular system, the biggest change is in the efficiency, in this case, of gas exchange. Under usual conditions, this has little or no effect on the performance of customary life activities. However, when an individual is confronted with a sudden demand for increased oxygen, a respiratory deficit may occur. The body is not as sensitive to low oxygen levels or elevated carbon dioxide levels, each

indicating the need to increase the rate of breathing. The changes that occur in the anatomical structures of the chest and altered muscle strength can significantly affect one's ability to cough forcefully enough to quickly expel materials that accumulate in or obstruct airways. In addition, the respiratory cilia, small fibers in the respiratory system, are less effective. Together these place the person at high risk of potentially life-threatening infections and aspiration. In the presence of impairment, such as difficulty swallowing or decreased movement in the esophagus, the risk is significantly increased; this is often the case after a person has had a stroke. All of these make the promotion of health through the prevention of respiratory illnesses of the highest importance (Box 5-5).

Renal

The renal system is responsible for regulating water and salts in the body and maintaining the acid/base balance in the blood. The glomerulus is the key structure in the kidney that controls the rate of filtering (glomerular filtration rate [GFR]). With each beat of the heart the blood passes through the smallest tubes (nephrons) in the kidneys for filtering. This filtering is the mechanism wherein waste products are removed by the production of urine and needed products like water and salts are held back. Among the many changes to the kidneys are those of blood flow, GFR, and the ability to regulate body fluids. Blood flow through the kidneys decreases by about 10% per decade, from about 1200 mL/min in young adults to about 600 mL/min by 80 years of age, as a result of vascular and fixed anatomical and structural changes (Macias-Nunez & Cameron, 2008; Wiggins & Patel, 2009). Yet the kidneys lose as many as 50% of the nephrons with little change in the body's ability to regulate body fluids and maintain adequate day-to-day fluid homeostasis. The age-related decrease in size and function

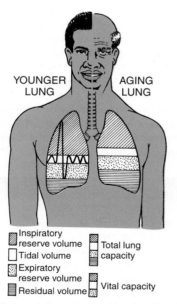

YOUNGER LUNG   AGING LUNG

▨ Inspiratory reserve volume
☐ Tidal volume
▦ Expiratory reserve volume
▤ Residual volume
☐ Total lung capacity
▨ Vital capacity

FIGURE 5-2 Changes in lung volumes with aging. (From McCance KL, Huether SE, editors: *Pathophysiology: the biologic basis for disease in adults and children*, ed 5, St. Louis, 2006, Mosby.)

BOX 5-5   **Promoting Healthy Lungs**

- Obtain pneumonia immunization.
- Obtain annual influenza immunization.
- Avoid exposure to smoke and pollutants.
- Do not smoke.
- Avoid persons with respiratory illnesses.
- Seek prompt treatment of respiratory infections.
- Wash hands frequently.
- Eat meals in relaxed atmosphere.
- Practice regular oral hygiene.

occurs primarily in the kidney cortex, the top of the kidney, begins in the thirties, and becomes significant by the seventies. There is no significant variation by sex or race (Macias-Nunez & Cameron, 2008). Like the other organs, renal reserve is lost and/or the ability to quickly respond to the stress of either a salt or water excess or loss is decreased even in a healthy elder (Choudhury & Levi, 2011). Kidney function is measured through the calculation of the creatinine clearance rate (CrCl) (see Chapter 8).

Creatinine is the end product of the breakdown in muslces as they are used. Whereas creatinine in the plasma is constant throughout life, urine creatinine shows a decline because of normal age-related loss of lean muscle mass. The urine creatinine clearance is an important indicator for appropriate drug therapy, reflecting the ability to handle medications passing through and metabolized by the kidneys (see Chapter 8). Persons with a reduced creatinine clearance usually need a reduction in the dosages of their medications to prevent potential toxicity, and caution must be used in the administration of intravenous fluids.

Age-related changes in the renal system are significant due to resultant heightened susceptibility to fluid and electrolyte imbalance and structural damage from medications and contrast media of diagnostic tests. Under normal circumstances, renal function is sufficient to meet the regulation and excretion demands of the body (Macias-Nunez & Cameron, 2008). However, with the stress of disease, surgery, or fever, the kidneys have reduced capacity to respond and are therefore at greater risk for damage or even acute failure.

Endocrine

The endocrine system, working along with the neurological system, helps regulate and control the activities within the body so that they work together. This is done through the secretion and distribution of hormones from glands found throughout the body. As the body ages, most glands atrophy and decrease their rate of secretion. However, other than a dramatic decrease in estrogen, which causes menopause, the impact of the changes is not clear.

Pancreas

The endocrine pancreas secretes insulin, glucagon, somatostatin, and pancreatic polypeptides. The secretion of these substances does not appear to decrease to any level of clinical significance. However, for reasons unknown, the tissues of the body often develop decreased sensitivity to insulin. When combined with increased needs for insulin in the presence of obesity, the result is often the development of type 2 diabetes (see Chapter 17). Older adults have the highest rate of type 2 diabetes of any age group, with significant variation by ethnicity and region. When the pancreas is stressed with sudden concentrations of glucose, such as a high carbohydrate meal, blood levels are higher for longer. These temporary levels of increased blood glucose sometimes make the diagnosis of true diabetes difficult.

Thyroid

Slight changes occur in the structure and function of the thyroid gland, which may explain the slight, but nonetheless important, increased incidence of hypothyroidism, or lowered function, in older adults (Brashers & Jones, 2010). Some atrophy, fibrosis, and inflammation occurs. Although other evidence of change is inconclusive at this time, diminished secretion of thyroid-stimulating hormone (TSH) and thyroxine (T_4) and decreased plasma triiodothyronine (T_3) appear to be age related. Serum T_3 decreases with age, perhaps as a result of decreased secretion of TSH by the pituitary gland. When thyroid replacement is needed, lower doses are usually effective and higher doses contraindicated. In addition, the therapeutic dose of medication may change over time and monitoring is required (see Chapter 17).

Collective signs, such as a slowed basal metabolic rate, thinning of the hair, and dry skin, are characteristic of hypothyroidism in the young but are normal manifestations in the aged who have no history of thyroid deficiencies, making the recognition of thyroid disturbances difficult.

Reproductive

The reproductive systems in men and women serve the same physiological purpose—human procreation and also control the phyenotypes (external appearance) that we recognize as male and female. Although both aging men and women undergo age-related changes, the changes affect women significantly more than men. Women lose the ability to procreate after the cessation of ovulation (menopause), whereas men remain fertile their entire lives. Regardless of the physical changes, the need for sexual expression remains (see Chapter 24).

Female Reproductive System

As menopause signals the end of the reproductive phase in a woman's life, several other age-related changes occur, particularly in breast tissue and urogenital structures. Older breasts are smaller, pendulous, and less firm. Outwardly, the labia majora and minora become less prominent and pubic hair thins. The ovaries, cervix, and uterus slowly atrophy. The vagina shortens, narrows, and loses some of its elasticity, typical of aging muscle and skin. Vaginal walls also lose their ability to lubricate quickly, especially if the woman is not sexually active. More stimulation is needed to achieve orgasm. The vaginal epithelium changes considerably; the pH rises from 4.0 to 6.0 before menopause to 6.5 to 8.0 afterward (Deneris & Huether, 2010). The vaginal changes result in the potential for dyspareunia (painful intercourse), trauma during intercourse, and increased susceptibility to infection.

Male Reproductive System

Although men have the ability to produce sperm throughout their lives, they also experience changes in the functioning of the reproductive and the urogenital organs in late life. The changes are usually more subtle and noticed only as they accumulate, beginning when men are in their 50s. The testes atrophy and soften. The seminiferous tubules where semen is produced thicken, and obstruction caused by sclerosis and fibrosis can occur. Although sperm count does not decrease, fertility may be reduced because of the higher number of sperm lacking motility or because of the structural abnormalities just noted. Erectile changes are also seen: more stimulation is needed to achieve a full erection, ejaculation is slower and less forceful, and the period between the ability to have an erection increases (Deneris & Huether, 2010). As with women, alterations in hormone balances may play a part in the age-related changes in men. Testosterone level is reduced in all men but only rarely to the level at which it would be considered a true deficiency.

By 80 years of age, up to 80% of men have some degree of prostatic enlargement (Kamel & Dornbrand, 2004). The condition known as *benign prostatic hyperplasia* (BPH) is so common that some are beginning to call it a normal part of aging. The only time it is considered a problem is when the enlargement is such that it causes compression of the urethra and urinary retention. BPH is most often the cause of repeated urinary tract infections. Intervention is pursued only when the symptoms of BPH interfere with the man's quality of life (Kamel & Dornbrand, 2004).

Digestive

The digestive system includes the gastrointestinal (GI) tract and the accessory organs that aid in digestion. Like the endocrine system, few true age-related changes affect function. However, a number of common health problems can have a great effect on the digestive system. Changes in other systems can also affect GI structure and function; with these changes seen as early as the fifties (Huether, 2010).

Mouth

Age-related changes affect both the teeth and the mouth. With the wear and tear of years of use, the teeth eventually lose enamel and dentin and then become more vulnerable to decay (caries). The roots become more brittle and break more easily. For unknown reasons, the gums are also more susceptible to periodontal disease. Without care, teeth may be lost. Taste buds decline in number, and salivary secretion lessens. A very dry mouth (xerostomia) is common. It is still common to care for persons over 80 or 90 years of age who have had all of their teeth removed (edentulous) and who may or may not wear dentures. It is important that the nurse ensure the fit and cleanliness of the dentures or the appropriate choice of diet. Even in health, these changes combine to create the potential for decreased pleasure and comfort in eating, which in turn can lead to loss of appetite (anorexia) and weight loss. A number of medications taken for common health problems can quickly exacerbate potential problems, especially xerostomia. When the gerontological nurse administers medications to an older adult or conducts medication education, he or she needs to know if these effects apply and should warn persons about this potential and work with the person to manage this problem (see Chapter 8).

Esophagus

In youth, food passes quickly through the esophagus to the stomach because of the strong and coordinated contractions of the surrounding muscles. In aging, the contractions increase in frequency but are more disordered, and therefore movement forward is less effective. This is referred to as *presbyesophagus*. The sluggish emptying of the esophagus may cause the lower end to dilate, creating greater stress in this area and possibly causing digestive discomfort. Pathological processes that are increasingly seen as adults become older include gastroesophageal reflux disease (GERD) and hiatal hernias.

Stomach

There are several age-related changes in the stomach. These include decreased gastric motility and volume and reductions in the secretion of bicarbonate and gastric mucus. The reductions are caused by gastric atrophy and result in hypochlorhydria (insufficient hydrochloric acid). Decreased production of something called "intrinsic factor" can lead to pernicious anemia if the stomach is not able to utilize an adequate amount of ingested vitamin B_{12}, needed for the production of red blood cells. The protective alkaline viscous mucus of the stomach is lost because of the increase in stomach pH. This makes the stomach more susceptible to peptic ulcer disease, particularly with the use of nonsteroidal antiinflammatory drugs such as aspirin and ibuprofen. Loss of smooth muscle in the stomach delays emptying time, which may lead to anorexia or weight loss as a result of distention, or the sensation of being overfull after a meal (Price & Wilson, 2002).

Intestines

The age-related changes of the small intestine include those noted earlier that involve smooth muscles and those related to the gastric villi, the anatomical structures in the intestinal walls where nutrients are absorbed from ingested food. The villi become broader and shorter and less functional. Nutrient absorption is affected; proteins, fats, minerals (including calcium), vitamins (especially B_{12}), and carbohydrates (especially lactose) are absorbed more slowly and in lesser amounts (Huether, 2010b). Changes in motility, epithelial membranes, vascular perfusion, and gastrointestinal membrane transport may affect absorption of lipids, amino acids, glucose, calcium, and iron.

Peristalsis (surrounding muscular contraction) is slowed with aging and there is blunted response to rectal filling; the extent of the change should not be such to cause problems with defecation. In other words, constipation, which is often thought of as a normal part of aging, is not. Instead, constipation is more often a side effect of medications, life habits, immobility, inadequate fluid intake, and lack of attention to the gastrocolic reflex, the urge to defecate following a meal. The role of the gerontological nurse and elimination needs are presented in Chapter 9 and suggestions on promoting healthy digestion are found in Box 5-6.

Accessory Organs

The accessory organs of the digestive system are the liver and the gallbladder. The liver continues to function

---

throughout life despite a decrease in volume and weight (mass) and a concomitant decrease in liver blood flow of 30% to 40% by the late nineties (Hall, 2009); this carries implications for impaired drug metabolism and is associated with an increased half-life of fat-soluble medications (see Chapter 8). While slow, liver regeneration is not greatly impaired, and liver function tests remain unaltered with age.

There does not seem to be a specific change in the gallbladder; however, the incidence of gallstones increases (Hall, 2009). This is possibly caused by the increased lipogenic composition of bile from biliary cholesterol. The decrease in bile salt synthesis increases the incidence of gallstones (Hall, 2009). In addition, the decrease in bile acid synthesis causes a reduction in the ability of the body to rid itself of unnecessary cholesterol. This, in conjunction with a decrease in hepatic extraction of low-density lipoprotein (LDL) cholesterol from the blood, increases the level of serum cholesterol in the older adult. For women, the increase in cholesterol begins to be seen following menopause.

Neurological

Contrary to popular belief, the older nervous system, including the brain, is remarkably resilient and other than very slight disturbances in recent memory, changes in cognitive functioning are not a normal part of aging. Neither the elder nor the nurse should accept an assessment of "confusion" without making sure the cause is identified and treated if at all possible. Although many neurophysiological changes occur in some older adults, they do not occur in all and do not affect everyone the same way, therefore cannot be attributed to normal aging. For example, the presence of neurofibrillary tangles is a classic sign of dementia and is found in the brains of all persons with Alzheimer's disease, but they are found also in the brains of persons without dementia. Although it is very difficult to show a true cause and effect of age-related changes in the nervous system, several changes appear to be consistent.

Central Nervous System (CNS)

The major changes in the aging nervous system are found in the CNS. With aging, the number of neurons (cells in the nervous system) decreases and the dendrites which extend from the neurons appear to be "wearing out," and correlate with a decrease in brain weight and size (Figure 5-3). This change in size is seen primarily in the frontal lobe and appears as "atrophy" on computed tomography (CT) scans or magnetic resonance imaging (MRI) While its meaning is controversial (Snowdon, 2002), it is usually considered clinically

---

> **BOX 5-6   Promoting Healthy Digestion**
>
> - Practice good oral hygiene.
> - Wear properly fitting dentures.
> - Seek prompt treatment of dental caries and periodontal disease.
> - Eat meals in relaxed atmosphere.
> - Maintain adequate intake of fluids.
> - Provide time for response to gastrocolic reflex.
> - Respond promptly to urge to defecate.
> - Eat a balanced diet.
> - Avoid prolonged periods of immobility.
> - Avoid tobacco products.

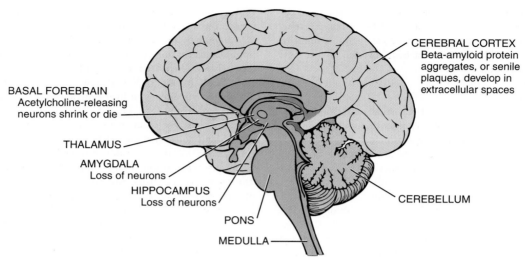

FIGURE 5-3 Changes in the brain with aging. (Courtesy Carole Donner, Tucson, Ariz.)

insignificant. Decreased adherence of the brain matter to the skull, and other changes increase the potential damage if a traumatic brain injury should occur such as a result of a fall (Sugarman, 2010).

Sleep disturbances may also be a normal part of aging as a result of changes in the part of the nervous system called the reticular formation (RF). The RF is a set of neurons that extend from the spinal cord through the brainstem and into the cerebral cortex. With aging, a loss of deep sleep (stages 3 and 4) may be seen. Elders spend more time in bed to get the same amount of "sleep" since the time in light sleep increases in proportion to that spent in deep sleep (Huether, 2010a). However, excessive daytime drowsiness is not expected and, if it occurs, a thorough assessment of potential causes should be done, especially for the side effects of medication or depression.

Subtle changes in cognitive (thinking) and motor functioning (movement) occur in the very old. Mild memory impairments and difficulties with balance may be seen as normal age-related changes in neurodegeneration and neurochemistry (see Chapter 20). Intellectual performance of the older adult without brain dysfunction remains constant; however, the performance of tasks may take longer, which is an indication that central processing is slowed. There are also decreasing levels of the neurotransmitters (chemicals in the brain) choline acetylase, serotonin, and catecholamines. Reduced levels of circulating serotonin probably increase the elder's risk for endogenous depression. Enzymes such as monoamine oxidase (MAO) increase. The fact that there are many brain cells which seem to do the same thing may

blunt the effects of these changes, but the exact number of cells required for certain functions is unknown.

Peripheral Nervous System

The most important effect of the normal changes in the aging peripheral nervous system is the increased risk for injury. Vibratory sense in the lower extremities may be nonexistent. Somesthetics, or tactile sensitivity, decreases in connection with the loss of nerve endings in the skin. This is most notable in the fingertips, the palms of the hands, and the lower extremities. This decreased sensitivity is translated into delayed reactions to things such as hot surfaces, significantly increasing the risk for burns and the extent of burns should they occur. The presence of a functioning smoke detector is particularly important for healthy and safer aging (see Chapter 13 for a further discussion of safety).

Kinesthetic sense, or proprioception (awareness of one's position in space), is altered because of changes in both the peripheral and central nervous systems. If one is less aware of body position and has less tactile awareness, the risk for falling is dramatically increased. The person may be walking on a flat surface when it suddenly becomes uneven. With reduced proprioception, it takes a little longer to realize the surface is uneven and a little longer still to realize that one has tripped (changed position in space). Where a younger person would be able to immediately right herself or himself and prevent a fall, this slight delay may result in a fall in an older adult. Conditions such as arthritis, stroke, some cardiac disorders, or damage to the structures of the inner ear may also affect peripheral and central mechanisms of mobility and exacerbate the problem.

Sensory

A number of changes occur in the sensory organs as a result of a combination of internal and external factors. As we age, we cannot totally escape some changes in our senses, especially vision and hearing. Creative gerontological nurses can make a big difference in the quality of life for the person with sensory changes (Boxes 5-7 and 5-8).

Eye and Vision

Changes in vision and eyes begin very early and are both functional and structural. All the changes affect visual acuity and accommodation, or the ability for the vision to adjust to changes in environmental light.

Presbyopia is an age-related decrease in near vision that begins to become noticeable in midlife. Nearly 95% of adults older than 65 years of age wear glasses for close vision (Burke & Laramie, 2000), and 18% also use a magnifying glass for reading and close work. Although presbyopia is first seen between 45 and 55 years of age, 80% of those older than 65 years of age have fair to adequate far vision past 90 years of age.

BOX 5-7	**Promoting Healthy Eyes**

- Protect eyes from ultraviolet light.
- Avoid eye strain; use a bright light when needed.
- See health care provider promptly if there are changes in vision.
- Have yearly dilated eye examination.

BOX 5-8	**Promoting Healthy Hearing**

- Avoid exposure to excessively loud noises.
- Avoid injury with cotton-tipped applicators and other cleaning materials.
- Use assistive devices as appropriate, for example, hearing aids.
- See health care provider promptly if there are sudden changes in hearing.
- Do not insert foreign objects into the ears, such as q-tips.

Extraocular. Like the skin elsewhere, age-related changes affect both form and function of the extraocular structures. The eyelids lose elasticity, and drooping (senile ptosis) results. In most cases, this only affects appearance. In extreme cases the lids sag far enough to block vision. Spasms of the muscle of the lower lid may cause it to turn inward. If it stays this way, it is called *entropion.* The lower lashes can irritate and scratch the cornea. Surgery may be needed to prevent permanent damage. Decreases in the muscle strength of the lower lid may result in *ectropion,* or an out-turning. Without the integrity of the trough of the lower lid, tears run down the cheek instead of bathing the cornea. This and an inability to close the lid completely lead to excessively dry eyes and the need for artificial tears. The person may need to tape the eyes shut during sleep. To make this problem worse, the number of goblet cells that provide mucin (essential for eye lubrication and movement) decreases. A severe deficiency of lubrication is known as *dry eye syndrome.*

Ocular. The cornea is the avascular transparent outer surface of the eye that refracts (bends) light rays entering the eye through the pupil. With aging, the cornea becomes flatter, less smooth, thicker, and duller in appearance. The result is increased far-sightedness (hyperopia). For the person who was myopic (near-sighted) earlier in life, this change may actually improve vision. Arcus senilis, a gray-white to silver ring or partial ring, may be observed at the juncture of the iris and cornea; it is composed of deposits of calcium and cholesterol salts. It does not appear to have any clinical significance.

The anterior chamber is the space between the cornea and the lens. The edges of the chamber include canals that control the volume and movement of aqueous fluid within the space. With aging, the chamber decreases slightly in size and capacity because of thickening of the lens. Resorption of the intraocular fluid becomes less efficient. If the decrease is significant, it can lead to increased intraocular pressure and glaucoma (Huether, 2010a). Any acute changes in vision or eye pain should be considered medical emergencies and responded to accordingly.

The ability to adjust to changes in light and the need for greater levels of lighting are the result of reduced responsiveness of the pupils and changes in the lens. The lens, a small, flexible, biconvex, crystal-like structure just behind the iris (the colored part of the eye), is most responsible for visual acuity; it adjusts the light entering the pupil and focuses it on the retina. Age-related changes in the lens are probably universal and begin in the forties. The origins of these changes are not fully understood, although ultraviolet rays of the sun contribute to the problem, with cross-linkage of collagen creating a more rigid and thickened lens structure. Promoting healthy aging means encouraging the use of protective lenses, such as sunglasses, whenever the person is exposed to ultraviolet light.

Light scattering increases, and color perception decreases. As a result, glare is a problem, not only that created by sunlight outdoors, but also the reflection of light on any shiny object, such as light striking polished floors and surfaces found in many care facilities (Meisami et al., 2007). Eventually people require 3 times as much light to see things as they did when they were in their twenties. It is more effective to place high-intensity light on the object or surface to be observed rather than increasing the intensity of the light in the entire room. For example, it would be more effective to focus a light directly on the newspaper a person was reading than to increase the lighting overhead which produces glare.

Intraocular. The retina, which lines the inside of the eye, has less distinct margins and is duller in appearance than in younger adults. Color clarity diminishes by 25% in the sixth decade and by 59% in the eighth decade, especially that of the blues, the violets, and the greens of the spectrum; light colors such as reds, oranges, and yellows are more easily seen. Some of this difficulty is linked to the yellowing of the lens and impaired transmission of light to the retina. Finally, the number of rods and associated nerves at the periphery of the retina is reduced, resulting in peripheral vision that is not as clear or is absent (Meisami et al., 2007). If the person has cardiovascular disease the arteries in back of the eye may show atherosclerosis and slight narrowing. Veins may show indentations (nicking) as they pass over the arteries if the person has a long history of hypertension. As long as these changes are not accompanied by distortion of objects or a significant decrease in vision, they are not clinically significant.

Ear and Hearing

Like the eye, age-related changes affect both the structure and the function of the ear. Some hearing loss affects about one third of all adults between 65 and 74 years of age and about one half of those aged 75 to 79 years.

The appearance of the ear changes, especially in men. The auricle loses flexibility and becomes longer and wider as a result of diminished elasticity. The tragus enlarges. The lobe sags, elongates, and wrinkles. Together, these changes make the ear appear larger. Coarse, wiry, stiff hairs grow at the periphery of the auricle.

The auditory canal narrows and the hairs that line it become stiffer and coarser. Cerumen glands atrophy, causing the wax to become thicker and dryer and more difficult to remove. Ear wax blocking the canal can cause temporary and reversible obstructive hearing loss. The gerontological nurse should be sensitive to this possibility and be skilled at safe cerumen removal.

A major and irreversible type of hearing loss is known as presbycusis. This is the loss in the ability to hear high-frequency sounds and sensorineural in origin, affecting more than 10 million people (Meisami et al., 2007).

Structurally, the bones in the inner ear become calcified and the auditory nerve becomes "frayed" resulting in a reduction in the amount and change in the type of sounds transmitted to the brain.

Presbycusis is primarily the loss of the ability to hear high-frequency sounds such as consonants, the chirping of birds, and the rustling of leaves. The phrase "The Cat in the Hat" may be heard as "e at in e at." Although the person may be able to decipher what is said if it is within context, this processing takes longer than usual or language is processed incorrectly. It is important to note that with normal age-related hearing loss the person can still hear but may not be able to make sense of the partially heard words especially in places where there is a great deal of environmental noise such as restaurants. Inaccurate responses too often lead to the incorrect suspicion of dementia or confusion when in fact it is a hearing loss.

Immunological

The function of the immune system is to protect the body from invasions from foreign substances and organisms, and in doing so reduce infections. To do this, it must be able to differentiate the self from the non-self (Shames & Kishiyama, 2009). The immune system includes elements of many of the systems already discussed, and also white blood cells, bone marrow, thymus, lymph nodes, and spleen.

A number of age-related changes increase the risk for infection in the older adult. For example, the skin is thinner and therefore less resistant to bacterial invasion. The reduced number of cilia in the lungs leads to the increased risk for pneumonia and the stiffening of the urethra increases the risk for urinary tract infections in women. But perhaps the most important of all is the reduced immunity at the cellular level, which is now understood to have a significant genetic underpinning.

Late life brings a decrease in T-cell function that results from a decrease in innate immunity, adaptive immunity, and self-tolerance. The response to foreign materials (antigens) decreases, but antibodies, or the materials needed for the body to protect itself, increase. As a result, the body may actually see itself as a foreign material, creating what is referred to as an *autoimmune response* (Michel & Proust, 2000). Being alert for signs and symptoms of autoimmune changes is especially important to gerontological nursing, as is the responsibility to promote disease prevention and protection from infection for the older adult. Goals for healthy aging related to the reduction of potentially preventable infections are provided in the document *Healthy People 2020* (see the Healthy People boxes).

HEALTHY PEOPLE 2020

Goals to Reduce Potentially Preventable Infections

Objective IID-4.2 Reduce new invasive pneumococcal infections among persons 65 years of age and older

Baseline: 40.4 confirmed new cases per 10,000 persons 65 years of age and older (2008)

Target: 31 new cases per 10,000 persons 65 years of age and older

Objective IID-4.4: Reduce new cases of penicillin-resistant invasive pneumococcal infections among persons 65 years of age and older

Baseline: 2.6 confirmed new cases per 10,000 persons 65 years of age and older (2008)

Target: 2 new cases per 10,000 persons 65 years of age and older

Data from U.S. Department of Health and Human Services, Office of Disease Prevention and Health Promotion: *Healthy people 2020.* Immunizations and infectious disease: objectives (2012). Available at http://healthypeople.gov/2020/topicsobjectives2020/objectiveslist.aspx?topicId=23.

 HEALTHY PEOPLE 2020

Goals for Immunizations

Objective IID-12.7: Increase percentage of persons who receive a seasonal influenza immunization—65 years of age and older living in the community

Baseline: 67% (2008)

Target: 90%

Objective IID-12.8: Increase percentage of persons who receive a seasonal influenza immunization—18 years of age and older living in long-term or nursing home settings

Baseline: 62% (2006)

Target: 90%

Objective IID-13.1: Increase percentage of persons who are vaccinated against pneumococcal disease—65 years of age and older and living in the community

Baseline: 60% (2008)

Target: 90%

Objective IID-13.3: Increase percentage of persons who are vaccinated against pneumococcal disease—18 years of age and older living in certified long-term or nursing home settings

Baseline: 66% (2006)

Target: 90%

Objective IID-14: Increase percentage of persons who are vaccinated against herpes zoste—60 years of age and older

Baseline: 7% (2008)

Target: 30%

Data from U.S. Department of Health and Human Services, Office of Disease Prevention and Health Promotion: *Healthy people 2020.* Immunizations and infectious disease: objectives (2012). Available at http://healthypeople.gov/2020/topicsobjectives2020/objectiveslist.aspx?topicId=23.

The changes in immune function affect the older person's response to illness as well. Early studies by Stengel (1983) found oral temperature norms in well elders significantly lower. In women older than 80 years of age, the temperature was lower than in younger women; older men consistently had an even lower temperature than women of comparable age. This means that a febrile response suggestive of infection is no longer restricted to a temperature above 98.6° or 99° F. Instead, an older adult may have a core temperature elevation at much lower numbers. The old-old may have an average normal temperature of 96° F, with an average range of 95° to 97° F (Hogstel, 1994). These findings emphasize the need to carefully evaluate the basal temperature of older adults and recognize that even low-grade fevers (98.6° F) in later life may signify serious illness. When this is combined with the age-related delay in the increase in the white blood cell count compared to younger adults, early detection of serious illness is difficult in many cases. *A lack of fever (temperature greater than 98.6° F) or a normal white blood cell count cannot be used to rule out an infection.* Instead, the nurse must consider the person as a whole—mood, level of consciousness, or other signs such as a recent fall or change in level of cognitive abilities.

Concluding Statement

Based on the current biological theories of aging, with support of clinical evidence, it can be concluded that com-plex functions of the body decline before simple body processes; that coordinated activity, which relies on interacting systems such as nerves, muscles, and glands, has a greater decremental loss than single-system activity; and that a uniform and predictable loss of cell function occurs in all vital organs. Yet many older adults are able to function effectively within the physical dictates of their body and continue to live to a healthy old age, capable of wisdom, judgment, and satisfaction.

Application of Maslow's Hierarchy

The normal physical changes with aging have the potential to affect the person at all levels of Maslow's Hierarchy. For example, the most basic need for air can be compromised by the combination of decreased pulmonary ciliary movement, cough reflex, and immunity. The need for safety may be compromised by reduced sensory function, such as the reduced ability to hear a smoke detector and escape a fire emergency in time. Meeting belonging needs can be compromised when decreased response time restricts the ability to drive safely and social opportunities are missed. Self-esteem may be threatened by changes in appearance, especially in skin and hair color. Finally, the overall changes with aging require a readjustment in how one looks at transcendence—what is most important in later life will probably be very different from what was most important in earlier periods of life.

The physical changes that accompany aging affect every body system, and the theories of why they occur are many. Although there are numerous ways nurses can promote healthy aging in the presence of these changes, when nurses are able to begin to differentiate these normal changes from signs and symptoms of potential health problems, the positive effect of the nurse's interventions is multiplied.

KEY CONCEPTS

- There are many physical changes that accompany aging; however, a number of these are relatively insignificant in the absence of disease or unusual stress.
- Physiological aging begins at birth and is universal, progressive, and intrinsic.
- There are enormous individual variations in the rate of aging of body systems and functions.
- Many of the normal changes with aging may be misinterpreted as being pathological, and some pathological conditions may be mistaken for normal changes of aging.
- Careful assessment of individual aging changes, lifestyle, and desires is fundamental to caring and the promotion of health in later life.
- The nurse cannot rely on the "typical" signs of infection in the older adult but must use a more holistic approach.

ACTIVITIES AND DISCUSSION QUESTIONS

1. Identify at least two normal changes that accompany aging for each body system.
2. Activity: Discuss the changes of aging you do or would find most difficult to accept.

REFERENCES

Abdollahi M, Ranjbar A, Shadnia S, et al: Pesticides and oxidative stress: a review, *Med Sci Monit* 10(6):RA141–147, 2004.

Brashers VL, Jones RE: Mechanism of hormonal regulation. In McCance KL, Huether SE, Brashers VL, et al., editors: *Pathophysiology: the biological basis for disease in adults and children*, ed 6, St. Louis, 2010, Mosby, pp. 696-726.

Brashers VL, McCance KL: Structure and function of the cardiovascular and lymphatic systems. In McCance KL, Huether SE, Brashers VL, et al, editors: *Pathophysiology: the biologic basis for disease in adults and children*, St. Louis, 2010, Mosby, pp. 1091–1141.

Burke M, Laramie JA: *Primary care of the older adult: a multidisciplinary approach*, ed 2, St. Louis, 2003, Mosby.

Carnes BA, Staats DO, Sonntag WE: Does senescence give rise to disease? *Mech Ageing Dev* 129(12): 693–699, 2008. [Epub.]

Choudhury D, Levi M: Kidney aging—inevitable or preventable? *Nat Rev Nephrol* 7(12):706–17, 2011.

Crowther-Radulewicz CL: Structure and function of the musculoskeletal system. In McCance KL, Huether SE, Brashers VL, et al, editors: *Pathophysiology: the biologic basis for disease in adults and children*, St. Louis, 2010, Mosby, pp. 1540–1567.

Deneris A, Huether SE: Structure and function of the reproductive systems. In McCance KL, Huether SE, Brashers VL, et al, editors: *Pathophysiology: the biologic basis for disease in adults and children*, ed 6, St. Louis, 2010, Mosby, pp. 781–815.

Effros RB, Dagarag M, Spaulding C, et al: The role of CD8 T-cell replicative senescence in human aging, *Immunol Rev* 205:147–157, 2005.

Friedman S: Integumentary function. In Meiner SE, editor: *Gerontologic nursing*, St. Louis, 2011, Mosby, pp. 596–627.

Gosain A, DiPietro LA: Aging and wound healing, *World J Surg* 28(3):321–326, 2004.

Hall KE: Effect of aging on gastrointestinal function. In Halter B, Ouslander J, Tinetti M, et al, editors: *Hazzard's principles of geriatric medicine and gerontology*, New York, 2009, McGraw-Hill, pp. 1059–1064.

Hayflick L, Moorehead PS: The serial cultivation of human diploid cell strains, *Exp Cell Res* 25:585, 1981.

Hogstel MO: Vital signs are really vital the old-old. *Geriatr Nurs* 15(5): 253, 1994.

Hornsby PJ: Senescence and the life span, *Eur J Physiol* 459: 291–299, 2009.

Huether SE: Pain, temperature regulation, sleep, and sensory function. In McCance KL, Huether SE, Brashers VL, et al, editors: *Pathophysiology: the biologic basis for disease in adults and children*, St. Louis, 2010a, Mosby, pp. 481–524.

Huether SE: Structure and function of the digestive system. In McCance KL, Huether SE, Brashers VL, et al, editors: *Pathophysiology: the biologic basis for disease in adults and children*, St. Louis, 2010b, Mosby, pp. 1420–1451.

Jang Y, Van Remmen H: The mitochondrial theory of aging: insight from transgenic and knockout mouse models, *Exp Gerontol* 44: 256–260, 2009.

Jett K: Physiological changes with aging. In Touhy T, Jett K, editors: *Ebersole and Hess' toward healthy aging*, St. Louis, 2011, Mosby, pp. 44–61.

Kamel H, Dornbrand L: Health issues of the aging male. In Landefeld CS, Palmer R, Johnson MA, et al, editors: *Current geriatric diagnosis and treatment*, New York, 2004, McGraw-Hill, pp. 368–375.

Kee JL, Paulanka BJ, Polek C: Fluids and their influence on the body. In Kee JL, Paulanka BJ, Polek C: *Handbook of fluids, electrolytes and acid-base imbalances,* Albany, NY, 2009, Delmar, pp. 1–48.

Lodovici M, Bigagli E: Oxidative stress and air pollution exposure, *J Toxicol,* 13 Aug 2011. [Epub.]

Luggen AS: Rapunzel no more: hair loss in older women, *Adv Nurse Pract* 13(10):28–33, 2005.

Macias-Nunez JF, Cameron JS: The ageing kidney. In Davison AM, et al, editors: *Oxford textbook of clinical nephrology,* New York, 2008, Oxford University Press, pp. 33–87.

Marin-Garcia J: *Aging and the heart: a post genomic view,* ed 1, New York, 2008, Springer.

Meisami E, Brown CM, Emerle HF: Sensory systems: normal aging, disorders, and treatments of vision and hearing in humans. In Timiras PS, editor: *Physiological basis of aging and geriatrics,* New York, 2007, CRC Press, pp. 109–137.

Michel J, Proust J: Aging and the immune system. In Beers MH, Berkow R, editors: *The Merck manual of geriatrics,* Whitehouse Station, NJ, 2000, Merck Research Laboratories, pp. 1351–1382.

Pashkow FJ: Oxidative stress and inflammation in heart disease: do antioxidants have a role in treatment and/or prevention? *Int J Inflam,* 11 Aug 2011. [Epub.]

Price S, Wilson L: *Pathophysiology: clinical concepts of disease processes,* ed 6, St. Louis, 2002, Mosby.

Shames RS, Kishiyama JL: Disorders of the immune system. In McPhee SJ, Hammer GD, editors: *Pathophysiology of disease: an introduction to clinical medicine,* ed 6, 2009, McGraw-Hill Medical, pp. 28–49.

Sheahan SL, Musialowski R: Clinical implications of respiratory system changes in aging, *J Gerontol Nurs* 27(5):26, 2001.

Short KR, Bigelow ML, Kahl J, et al: Decline in skeletal muscle mitochondrial function with aging in humans, *Proc Natl Acad Sci USA* 102(15):5618–5623, 2005.

Snowdon D: *Aging with grace: what the nun study teaches us about leading longer, healthier and more meaningful lives,* New York, 2002, Bantam Books.

Stengel GB: Oral temperature in the elderly, *Gerontologist* 23(special issue):306, 1983.

Sugarman RA: Structure and function of the neurologic system. In McCance KL, Huether SE, Brashers VL, et al, editors: *Pathophysiology: the biologic basis for disease in adults and children,* St. Louis, 2010, Mosby, pp. 442–480.

Taffet GE, Lakatta EG: Aging of the cardiovascular system. In Hazzard WR, Blass J, Halter B, et al., editors: *Principles of geriatric medicine and gerontology,* ed 5, New York, 2003, McGraw-Hill, pp. 403–422.

Valko M, Morris H, Cronin M, et al: Metals, toxicity and oxidative stress, *Curr Med Chem* 12(10):1161–1208, 2005.

Walston J: Aging. In Durson SC, Bowker LK, Price JD, Smith SC, editors: *Oxford American handbook of geriatric medicine,* New York, 2010, Oxford University Press, pp. 1–12.

Wiggins J, Patel S: Changes in kidney function. In Halter B, Ouslander J, Tinetti M, et al, editors: *Hazzard's principles of geriatric medicine and gerontology,* New York, 2009, McGraw-Hill, pp. 1009–1016.

CHAPTER 6

Social, Psychological, Spiritual, and Cognitive Aspects of Aging

Theris A. Touhy

evolve elsevier.com/Ebersole/gerontological

LEARNING OBJECTIVES

Upon completion of this chapter, the reader will be able to:
- Explain the major psychological and sociological theories of aging.
- Discuss the influence of culture and cohort on psychological and social adaptation.
- Discuss the importance of spirituality to healthy aging.
- Explain cognitive changes with age and strategies to enhance cognitive health.
- Discuss factors influencing learning in late life, including health literacy, and appropriate teaching and learning strategies.

GLOSSARY

Cognition The mental process characterized by knowing, thinking, learning, and judging.

Cross-sectional A study design in which data are collected at one point in time on several variables such as gender, income, education, and health status.

Eurocentric The practice of viewing the world from a European perspective, with an implied belief, either consciously or subconsciously, in the preeminence of European (and more generally, of Western) culture, concerns, and values at the expense of non-Europeans.

Geragogy The application of the principles of adult learning theory to teaching for older adults.

Health literacy The degree to which individuals have the ability to obtain, process, and understand basic health information and services needed to make appropriate health decisions.

Longitudinal research A study design that studies a group of subjects over time, assessing their experiences at predetermined stages. The Harvard Nurses' Study is an example of this in that a large group of nurses have been assessed every few years since 1976.

THE LIVED EXPERIENCE

If I Had My Life to Live Over

I'd dare to make more mistakes next time, I'd relax, I would limber up. I would be sillier than I've been this trip. I would take fewer things seriously. I would take more chances. I would climb more mountains and swim more rivers. I would eat more ice cream and less beans. I would perhaps have more actual troubles, but I'd have fewer imaginary ones.

You see, I'm one of those people who live sensibly and sanely hour after hour, day after day. Oh, I've had my moments, and if I had to do it over again, I'd have more of them. In fact, I'd try to have nothing else. Just moments, one after another, instead of living so many years ahead of each day. I've been one of those persons who never goes anywhere without a thermostat, a hot water bottle, a raincoat, and a parachute. If I had it to do again, I would travel lighter than I have.

If I had my life to live over, I would start barefoot earlier in the spring and stay that way later in the fall. I would go to more dances. I would ride more merry-go-rounds. I would pick more daisies.

Nadine Stair (1992)

Social, Psychological, Spiritual, and Cognitive Aspects of Aging

There are normal biological, psychological, social, and cognitive changes in the process of aging. The biological changes are discussed in Chapter 5. This chapter is meant to provide the reader with information on the psychological, social, cognitive, and spiritual aspects of aging. Factors influencing learning in late life, appropriate teaching and learning strategies, and health literacy are also discussed.

Each individual has unique life experiences and because of this must be seen holistically, through the lens of his or her time, place, culture, gender, and personal history. The close relationship among biological, social, and psychological development that exists through childhood and adolescence varies more in adulthood because of the greater variations in life experiences and demands as one matures.

Life Span Development Approach

Human development goes on throughout life and is a lifelong process of adaptation. Life span development refers to an individual's progress through time and an expected pattern of change: biological, sociological, and psychological. A summary of the key principles of the life span developmental approach, provided by Papalia and colleagues (2002), is based on the work of Paul Baltes and colleagues (Baltes, 1987; Baltes et al., 1998). Principles include the following:

- Development is lifelong. Each part of the life span is influenced by the past and will affect the future. Each period of the life span has unique characteristics and value; none is more important than any other.
- Development depends on history and context. Each person develops within a certain set of circumstances or conditions defined by time and place. Humans are influenced by historical, social, and cultural context.
- Development is multidimensional and multidirectional and involves a balance of growth and decline. Whereas children usually grow consistently in size and abilities, in adulthood, the balance gradually shifts. Some abilities, such as vocabulary, continue to increase, whereas others,

such as speed of information retrieval, may decrease. New abilities, such as wisdom and expertise, may emerge as one ages.
- Development is plastic rather than rigid. Function and performance can improve throughout the life span with training and practice. However, there are limits on how much a person can improve at any age.

Types of Aging

People age in a number of ways. Aging can be viewed in terms of *chronological age, biological age, psychological age,* and *social age.* These ages may or may not be the same. Chronological age is measured by the number of years lived. Biological age is predicted by the person's physical condition and how well vital organ systems are functioning. Psychological age is expressed through a person's ability and control of memory, learning capacity, skills, emotions, and judgment. Maturity and capacity will direct the manner in which one is able to adapt psychologically over time to the requirements of the physical and social environment. Social age may be quite different from chronological age and is measured by age-graded behaviors that conform to an expected status and role within a particular culture or society. A person may be chronologically 80 years of age but biologically 60 years of age because he or she has remained fit with a healthy lifestyle. Or, a person with a chronic illness may be biologically 80 years of age but psychologically is much younger because he or she has remained active and involved in life.

There are several psychological and sociological theories of aging. In contrast to biological theories of aging, the psychological and sociological theories are not always based on empirical evidence because of methodological and measurement-related problems. The majority of these theories were developed from a Eurocentric perspective and may be less useful to describe aging within other cultures, especially those that are collective rather than individualistic (see Chapter 4). The importance of opportunity, ethnicity, gender, and social status is largely ignored. In addition, the theories have little to do with personal meaning and motivation; however, they may be useful as a guide in helping us understand the world around us and move toward healthy aging. As current generations of elders move through this period of life development, many of the ideas we have about this period of life are being, and will continue to be, redefined.

Sociological Theories of Aging

Sociological theories of aging attempt to explain and predict the changes in roles and relationships in middle and late life, with an emphasis on adjustment. Many of the basic theories were developed in the 1960s and 1970s and must be viewed within the context of the historical period from which they emerged. Some of the theories continue to generate interest and thought, such as modernization and social exchange theories, and others, such as disengagement theory, are no longer considered relevant.

Disengagement Theory

The disengagement theory states that "aging is an inevitable, mutual withdrawal or disengagement, resulting in decreased interaction between the aging person and others in the social system he belongs to" (Cummimg & Henry, 1961, p. 2). This means that withdrawal from one's society and community is natural and acceptable for the older adult and his or her society. The measures of disengagement are based on age, work, and decreased interest or investment in societal concerns. The theory is seen as universal and applicable to older people in all cultures, although there are expected variations in timing and style.

Activity Theory

The activity theory is based on the belief that remaining as active as possible in the pursuits of middle age is the ideal in later life. Because of improved general health and wealth, this is more possible than it was 40 years ago when Maddox (1963) proposed this theory. The activity theory may make sense when individuals live in a stable society, have access to positive influences and significant others, and have opportunities to participate meaningfully in the broader society if they continue to desire to do so. Attempts at clarifying activity theory as a general concept of satisfactory aging have not been supported.

Continuity Theory

The continuity theory, proposed by Havighurst and co-workers (1968), explains that life satisfaction with engagement or disengagement depends on personality traits. Three ideas about personality (Neugarten et al., 1968) are important to understanding continuity theory:

- In the normal progression of aging, personality traits remain quite stable.
- Personality influences role activity and one's level of interest in particular roles.
- Personality influences life satisfaction regardless of role activity.

Age-Stratification Theory

Age-stratification theory is a newer approach to understanding the role, the reactions, and the adaptations of older adults. Like continuity theory, it specifically challenges activity theory and disengagement theory. Age-stratification theory goes beyond the individual to the age structure of society (Marshall, 1996). The structuring of different ages can take a number of different forms, including the conceptualization of "young," "middle-aged," and "old." With the increasing life expectancy and compressed morbidity, age categories are changing. Readers have probably heard that "60 is the new 40." In the future, 60 to 80 years of age may be considered "young-old," 80 to 100 years of age "middle-old," and 100 years of age and over, "oldest-old."

Historical context is a key component of age-stratification theory. Elders can be understood as members of cohorts along with others who have shared similar historical periods in their lives, with age-graded systems of expectations and rewards. They have been exposed to similar events and conditions and common global, environmental, and political circumstances (e.g., World Wars, Great Depression, Viet Nam, civil rights movement) (Riley et al., 1972). Hooks (2000) reminds us that race must be considered when understanding cohort effects.

This theory may be particularly useful to examine aging within a global context. The definitions of age strata usually encompass social and cultural expressions of aging as well as who is placed in a given stratum and when. The cohort effect can be used as a powerful tool for understanding the potential life experiences of people from not only different cultures, but also different parts of the world.

Social Exchange Theory

Challenging both activity theory and disengagement theory, social exchange theory is based on the consideration of the cost-benefit model of social participation (Dowd, 1980). It explains that withdrawal or social isolation is the result of an imbalance in the exchanges between older persons and younger members of society and that the balance is what determines one's personal satisfaction and social support at any point in time.

Older adults are often viewed as unequal partners in the exchange and may need to depend on metaphorical reserves of contributions to the pool of reciprocity. This may be seen in the expectation of elderly African Americans for care as "pay-back" for their providing care to others earlier in their lives (Jett, 2006). Other elders care for younger grandchildren so that their adult children can work. For this they may receive total support (i.e., room, board, income). Although this exchange may appear uneven, it can also be viewed from the more holistic perspective of a lifetime of exchanges and contributions. Hooyman and Kiyak (2011) noted that "although older individuals may have fewer economic and material resources, they often have nonmaterial resources such as respect, approval, love, wisdom, and time for civic engagement and giving back to society" (p. 323). Intergenerational programs are an example of the value of social exchange between generations.

Modernization Theory

Modernization theory attempts to explain the social changes that have resulted in the devaluing of both the contributions of elders and the elders themselves. Historically (before about 1900 in the United States), materials and political resources were controlled by the older members of society (Achenbaum, 1978). The resources included not only their time, as shown in the examples just described, but also their knowledge, traditional skills, and experience. According to this theory, the status, and therefore the value, of elders is lost when their labors are no longer considered useful. Kinship networks are dispersed, the information they hold is no longer useful to the society in which they live, and the culture in which they live no longer reveres them. It is proposed that these changes are the result of advancing technology, urbanization, and mass education.

Treatment of the elderly in modern Japan was long considered evidence of the inaccuracy of the theory. Historically, Japanese elders were given the highest status and held the greatest power. This did not seem to change with the industrialized advances after World War II. However, today Japan not only is a highly modern country from an industrial point but also is showing signs of "modernization" in social relations with elders. Other researchers have also found support of the modernization theory in other societies such as India and Taiwan (Dandekar, 1996; Silverman et al., 2000).

Symbolic Interaction Theories

Symbolic interaction theories focus on the interaction between the older adult and their social world. The interactions between older adults and their environment significantly affect their experience of the aging process and of themselves. "People reflect on their lives and design ways of understanding their position in the social system. When confronted with change, whether in the process of relocating to a long-term care facility or learning to use a computer, elders are expected to try to master the new situation while extracting from the larger environment what they need to retain a positive self-concept" (Hooyman & Kiyak, 2011, p. 320). With this perspective, one has to examine how the individual's resources and activities, as well as the environmental demands and supports, can be altered to enhance satisfaction and self-concept.

Implications for Gerontological Nursing and Healthy Aging

The sociological theories of aging provide the gerontological nurse with useful information and a background for enhancing healthy aging and adaptation (Box 6-1). Although these theories have neither been proved nor disproved, many of the ideas they discuss have withstood the test of time. The theories have been adapted and applied to contemporary approaches to aging in many ways, from the concept of senior centers (activity theory) to nursing assessments of social support (social exchange theory). And, unfortunately, the disengagement theory is still applied any time one incorrectly assumes depression and isolation to be a "normal" part of aging. Further research is needed to explore how culture, ethnicity, and gender influence aging and adaptation. This is particularly important in light of the expected growth of a very diverse aging population.

Psychological Theories of Aging

Psychological theories presuppose that aging is one of many developmental processes experienced between birth and death. Life, then, is a dynamic process. Although these are widely accepted because of their face validity, like the sociological theories, they are not well suited to testing or measurement and do not address the influence of culture, gender, and ethnicity.

Jung's Theories of Personality

Psychologist Carl Jung (1971), a contemporary of Freud, proposed a theory of the development of a personality throughout life, from childhood to old age. He was one of the

> **BOX 6-1   Areas of Potential Nursing Assessment and Education Consistent with the Sociological Theories of Aging**
>
> - Current level of activity and satisfaction with such (*Activity*)
> - Effect of changes in health on usual roles and activities (*Activity*)
> - Cultural beliefs and expectations related to roles, activity, and both engagement and disengagement related to these (*Activity, Disengagement*)
> - Usual life patterns and personality and attention to any change in these as an indication of a potential problem (*Continuity*)
>
> - Knowledge of the historical context of the individual and its potential influence on perception and responses (*Age-Stratification*)
> - Complexity of social support and network (*Social/Exchange*)
> - Opportunities for contributions of knowledge to society (*Modernization*)
> - Sense of self and self-worth (*Modernization*)

first psychologists to define the last half of life as having a purpose of its own, quite apart from species survival. The last half of life is often a time of inner discovery, quite different from the biological and social issues that demand a great deal of outward attention during the first half of life. The last half of life, ideally, is less intensely demanding and allows more time for inner growth, self-awareness, and reflective activity.

According to this theory, a personality is either extroverted and oriented toward the external world or introverted and oriented toward the subjective inner world of the individual. Jung suggested that aging results in the movement from extraversion to introversion. Beginning perhaps at midlife, individuals begin to question their own dreams, values, and priorities. The potentially resulting crisis or emotional upheaval is a step in the process of personality development. With chronological age and personality development, Jung proposed that the person is able to move from a focus on outward achievement to one of acceptance of the self and to the awareness that both the accomplishments and challenges of a lifetime can be found within oneself. The development of the psyche and the inner person is accomplished by a search for personal meaning and the spiritual self. This personality of late life can easily be compared to Erikson's ego integrity, Maslow's self-actualization (see Chapter 1), and Tornstam's gerotranscendence, described in the following sections.

Developmental Theories

Psychologist Eric Erikson is well known for articulating the developmental stages and tasks of life, from early childhood to later "elderhood." Most students have studied Erikson's eight-stage or task model. Erikson (1963) theorized a predetermined order of development and specific tasks that

were associated with specific periods in one's life course. He proposed that one needed to successfully accomplish one task before complete mastery of the next was possible and originally articulated these in "either/or" language. He proposed that all persons would return again and again to a task that had been poorly resolved in the past.

Erikson's task of middle age is generativity. If successful in this task, one establishes oneself and contributes in meaningful ways for the future and future generations. Failure to accomplish this task results in stagnation. Erikson saw the last stage of life as a vantage point from which one could look back with ego integrity or despair on one's life. Ego integrity implies a sense of completeness and cohesion of the self. In achieving this final task, individuals can look back over their lives, at the joys and the sorrows, the mistakes and the successes, and feel satisfied with the way they lived.

In later years, as octogenarians, Erikson and his wife, Joan, reconsidered his earlier work from the perspective of their own aging. They modified their "either/or" stance of the developmental tasks to the recognition of the balance of each of the tasks. Thus ego integrity is tinged with some regrets, wisdom is balanced with frivolity, and letting go is balanced with hanging on (Erikson et al., 1986).

Robert Peck (1968) expanded on the original work of Erikson with the identification of specific tasks of old age that must be addressed to establish ego integrity. Peck's tasks represent the process or movement toward Erikson's final stage. Peck's tasks are as follows:

- *Ego differentiation* versus *work role preoccupation*. The individual is no longer defined by his or her work.
- *Body transcendence* versus *body preoccupation*. The body is cared for but does not consume the interest and attention of the individual.

- *Ego transcendence* versus *ego preoccupation*. The self becomes less central, and one feels a part of the mass of humanity, sharing their struggles and their destiny.

To achieve ego integrity, according to Peck's theoretical model, one must develop the ability to redefine the self, to let go of occupational identity, to rise above bodily discomforts, and to establish meanings that go beyond the scope of self-centeredness. Although these are admirable and idealistic goals, they place a considerable burden on the older person. Not everyone may have the courage or the energy to laugh in the face of adversity or surmount all of the assaults of old age. The wisdom of old age involves a crisis of understanding in which the ordinary structures are shaken and the meaning of life is reexamined. It may or may not include the wisdom of questioning assumptions in the search for meaning in the last stage of life.

Robert Havighurst (1971) is another developmental theorist who has proposed specific tasks to be accomplished in middle age and later maturity. Havighurst's developmental tasks are presented in Box 6-2.

BOX 6-2   Havighurst's Developmental Tasks

Middle Age
- Assisting teenage children to become responsible and happy adults
- Achieving adult social and civic responsibility
- Reaching and maintaining satisfactory performance in one's occupational career
- Developing adult leisure-time activities
- Relating to one's spouse as a person
- Accepting and adjusting to the physiological changes of middle age
- Adjusting to aging parents

Later Maturity
- Adjusting to decreasing physical strength and health
- Adjusting to retirement and reduced income
- Adjusting to death of a spouse
- Establishing an explicit affiliation with one's age group
- Adopting and adapting social roles in a flexible way
- Establishing satisfactory living arrangements

From Havighurst R: *Developmental tasks and education*, ed 3, New York, 1971, Longman.

BOX 6-3   Characteristics of Gerotranscendence

- A high degree of life satisfaction
- Midlife patterns and ideals are no longer prime motivators
- Complex and active coping patterns
- A greater need for solitary philosophizing, meditation, and solitude
- Social activities are not essential to well-being
- Satisfaction with self-selected social activities
- Less concern with body image and material possessions
- Decreased fear of death
- Affinity with past and future generations
- Decreased self-centeredness and increased altruism

Theory of Gerotranscendence

Lars Tornstam (1994, 1996, 2005), a Swedish sociologist, proposed the theory of gerotranscendence. According to Tornstam, human aging brings about a general potential for what he terms *gerotranscendence*, a shift in perspective from the material world to the cosmic and, concurrent with that, an increasing life satisfaction. Gerotranscendence is thought to be a gradual and ongoing shift that is generated by the normal processes of living, sometimes hastened by serious personal disruptions. An understanding of transcendence and the unique characteristics of this transformation in older people is important to the continued growth and development of older people. It is associated with wisdom and spiritual growth, similar to Erikson's concept of integrity and Maslow's self-actualization. Characteristics of gerotranscendence are presented in Box 6-3.

Spirituality and Aging

Spirituality has been defined as a "quality of a person derived from the social and cultural environment that involves faith, a search for meaning, a sense of connection with others, and a transcendence of self, resulting in a sense of inner peace and well-being" (Delgado, 2007, p. 230). The spiritual aspect of people's lives transcends the physical and psychosocial to reach the deepest individual capacity for love, hope, and meaning. Erickson's concept of ego integrity and Maslow's concept of self-actualization seem closely related to development of a spiritual self.

Aging as a biological process has been studied extensively. Less attention has been paid to the study of aging as a spiritual process. As people age and move closer to death, spirituality may become more important. Declining physical health, loss of loved ones, and a realization that life's end may be near often challenge older people to reflect on the meaning of their lives. Spiritual belief and practices often play a central role in helping older adults cope with life challenges and are a strength in the lives of older adults (Hodge et al., 2010).

Distinguishing between religion and spirituality is a concern for many health professionals. Religious beliefs and participation in religious obligations and rites are often the avenues of spiritual expression, but they are not necessarily interchangeable. "Religion can be described as a social institution that unites people in a faith in God, a higher power, and in common rituals and worshipful acts. A god, divinity, and/or soul is always included in the concept" (Strang & Strang, 2002, p. 858). Each religion involves a particular set of beliefs.

Spirituality is a broader concept than religion and encompasses a person's values or beliefs, search for meaning, relationships with a higher power, with nature, and with other people. The concept of spirituality is found in all cultures and societies. For some people, particularly older people, formalized religion helps them feel fulfilled. The majority of older adults describe themselves as both spiritual and religious (Hodge et al., 2010).

Spirituality is also a significant factor in understanding healthy aging. Rowe and Kahn's (1998) model of successful aging includes active engagement in life, minimal risk and disability, and high cognitive and physical function. Crowther and colleagues (2002) maintain that spirituality must be the fourth element of the model and is interrelated with all of the others. The ultimate goal for promoting spirituality is to support and enhance quality of life.

Spiritual well-being may be considered the ability to experience and integrate meaning and purpose in life through connectedness with self, others, art, music, literature, nature, or a power greater than oneself (Gaskamp et al., 2006). Spirituality may be particularly important to healthy aging in "historically disadvantaged populations who display remarkable strengths despite adversities in their lives (Hooyman & Kiyak, 2005, p. 213).

Spirituality and Nursing

An emphasis on spirituality in nursing is not new; nursing has encompassed the spiritual from its origin. The science of nursing was not seen as separate from the art and spirit of the discipline. Florence Nightingale's view of nursing was derived from her spiritual philosophy, and she considered nursing a spiritual experience, "intrinsic to human nature, our deepest and most potent resource for healing" (Macrae, 1995, p. 8). Many nursing theories address spirituality, including those of Neuman, Parse, and Watson (Martsolf & Mickley, 1998). Nursing and medicine are beginning to reclaim some of the essential healing values from their roots.

A nursing evidence-based guideline for promoting spirituality in the older adult (Gaskamp et al., 2006) provides a framework for spiritual assessment and interventions. The guideline identifies older adults who may be at risk for spiritual distress and who might be most likely to benefit from use of the guideline (Box 6-4). Spiritual distress or spiritual pain is "an individual's perception of hurt or suffering associated with that part of his or her person that seeks to transcend the realm of the material. Spiritual distress is manifested by a deep sense of hurt stemming from feelings of loss or separation from one's God or deity, a sense of personal inadequacy or sinfulness before God and man, or a pervasive condition of loneliness" (Gaskamp et al., 2006, p. 9). The person experiencing spiritual distress is unable to experience the meaning of hope, connectedness, and transcendence. Spiritual distress may be manifested by anger, guilt, blame, hatred, expressions of alienation, turning away from family and friends, inability to enjoy, and inability to participate in religious activities that have previously provided comfort.

BOX 6-4 Identifying Elders at Risk for Spiritual Distress

- Individuals experiencing events or conditions that affect the ability to participate in spiritual rituals
- Diagnosis and treatment of a life-threatening, chronic, or terminal illness
- Expressions of interpersonal or emotional suffering, loss of hope, lack of meaning, need to find meaning in suffering
- Evidence of depression
- Cognitive impairment
- Verbalized questioning or loss of faith
- Loss of interpersonal support

Data from Gaskamp C, Sutter R, Meraviglia M, et al: Evidence-based guideline: promoting spirituality in the older adult, *J Gerontol Nurs* 32(11): 8-11, 2006.

Implications for Gerontological Nursing and Healthy Aging

Assessment

Patients welcome a discussion of spiritual matters and want health professionals to consider their spiritual needs. The older person may have a pressing need to talk about philosophy and spiritual development. Private time for prayer, meditation, and reflection may be needed. Nurses may neglect to explore this issue with elders because religion and spirituality may not seem a high priority. The client should be assured that religious longings and rituals are important and that opportunities will be made available as desired. Nurses need to be knowledgeable and respectful about the rites and rituals of varying religions, cultural beliefs, and values (see Chapter 4). Religious and spiritual resources, such as pastoral visits, should be available in all settings where older people reside. It is important to avoid imposing one's own beliefs and to respect the person's privacy on matters of spirituality and religion (Touhy & Zerwekh, 2006).

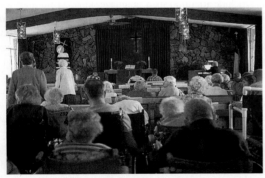

Residents attend a religious service at a nursing center. (From Sorrentino SA, Gorek B: *Mosby's textbook for long-term care assistants, ed 5,* St. Louis, 2007, Mosby.)

A spiritual history opens the door to a conversation about the role of spirituality and religion in a person's life. People often need permission to talk about these issues. Without a signal from the nurse, patients may feel that such topics are not welcome or appropriate. There are formal spiritual assessments, but open-ended questions can also be used to begin dialogue about spiritual concerns (Box 6-5). Simply listening to patients as they express their fears, hopes, and beliefs is important. Spiritual assessments

---

BOX 6-5   Questions to Begin Dialogue About Spiritual Concerns

- Tell me more about your life.
- What has been most meaningful in your life?
- To whom do you turn when you need help?
- What brings you joy and comfort?
- What are you most proud of?
- How have you found strength throughout your life?
- What are you hopeful about?
- Is spiritual peace important to you? What would help you achieve it?
- Is your religion or God significant in your life? Can you describe how?
- Is prayer or meditation helpful?
- What spiritual or religious practices bring you comfort?
- Are there religious books or materials that you want nearby?
- What are you afraid of right now?
- What do you wish you could still do?
- What are your concerns at this time for the future?
- What matters most to you right now?

Adapted from Touhy T, Zerwekh J: Spiritual caring. In Zerwekh J: *Nursing care at the end of life: palliative care for patients and families,* Philadelphia, 2006, Davis; Hospice of the Florida Suncoast, 2001; Blues A, Zerwekh J: *Hospice and palliative care nursing,* Orlando, 1984, Grune & Stratton.

are intended to elicit information about the core spiritual needs and how the nurse and other members of the health care team can respond to them. A spiritual assessment (FICA Spiritual History Tool) can be found at http://consultgerirn.org/uploads/File/trythis/try_this_sp5.pdf.

The Joint Commission requires spiritual assessments in hospitals, nursing homes, home care organizations, and many other health care settings providing services to older adults. The process of spiritual assessment is more complex than completing a standardized form and must be done within the context of the nurse-patient relationship.

Interventions

The caring relationship between nurses and persons nursed is the heart of nursing that touches and supports the spirit. Knowing persons in their complexity, responding to that which matters most to them, identifying and nurturing connections, listening with one's being, using presence and silence, and fostering connections to that which is held

BOX 6-6 Spiritual Nursing Responses

- Relief of physical discomfort, which permits focus on the spiritual
- Creating a peaceful environment
- Comforting touch, which fosters nurse-patient connection
- Authentic presence
- Attentive listening
- Knowing the patient as a person
- Listening to life stories
- Sharing fears and listening to self-doubts or guilt
- Fostering forgiveness and reconciliation
- Validating the person's life and assuring them they will be remembered
- Sharing caring words and love
- Encouraging family support and presence
- Fostering connections to that which is held sacred by the person
- Praying with and for the patient
- Respecting religious traditions and providing for access to religious objects and rituals
- Referring the person to a spiritual counselor

From Gaskamp C, Sutter R, Meraviglia M, et al: Evidence-based practice guideline: promoting spirituality in the older adult, *J Gerontol Nurs* 32(11):8-11, 2006; Touhy T, Brown C, Smith C: Spiritual caring: end of life in a nursing home, *J Gerontol Nurs* 31(9):27-35, 2004; Touhy T, Zerwekh H: Spiritual caring. In Zerwekh J: *Nursing care at the end of life: palliative care for patients and families*, Philadelphia, 2006, FA Davis.

sacred by the person are spiritual nursing responses that arise from within the caring, connected relationship (Touhy, 2001). Suggestions for spiritual care interventions are presented in Box 6-6.

Nurturing the Spirit of the Nurse

"Because spiritual care occurs over time and within the context of relationship, probably the most effective tool at the nurse's disposal is the use of self" (Soeken & Carson, 1987, p. 607). Thinking about what gives your own life meaning and value helps in developing your spiritual self and assists you in being able to offer spiritual support to patients. Examples of activities include finding quiet time for meditation and reflection; keeping your own faith traditions; being with nature; appreciating the arts; spending time with those you love; and journaling (Touhy & Zerwekh, 2006). Find ways to nourish your own spirit.

Nurses often do not take the time to do so and become dispirited. This is especially true for nurses who work with dying patients and experience grief and loss repeatedly. Having someone to talk to about feelings is important. Practicing compassion for oneself is essential to authentic practice of compassion for others (Touhy & Zerwekh, 2006) (Box 6-7).

Cognition and Aging

Cognition is both a biological and a psychological factor that must be considered in caring for the older adult. Processes of normal cognition and learning in late life and cognitive health are discussed in this chapter. Assessment of cognition and care of older adults with impairment of cognition is discussed in Chapter 21.

Cognition is the process of acquiring, storing, sharing, and using information. Components of cognitive function include language, thought, memory, executive function, judgment, attention, and perception (Desai et al., 2010). The determination of intellectual capacity and performance has been the focus of a major portion of gerontological research. Cognitive functions may remain stable, or decline with increasing age. The cognitive functions that remain stable include attention span, language skills, communication skills, comprehension and discourse, and visual perception. The cognitive skills that decline are verbal fluency, logical analysis, selective attention, object naming, and complex visuospatial skills.

Early studies about cognition and aging were cross-sectional rather than longitudinal and were often conducted with older adults who were institutionalized or had coexisting illnesses. It has been generally believed that

BOX 6-7 Personal Questions on Spirituality for Reflection by Nurses

- What do I believe in?
- How do I find purpose and meaning in my life?
- How do I take care of my physical, emotional, and spiritual needs?
- What are my hopes and dreams?
- Who do I love, and who loves me?
- How am I with others?
- What would I change about my relationships?
- Am I willing to heal relationships that trouble me?

From Touhy T, Zerwekh J: Spiritual caring. In Zerwekh J: *Nursing care at the end of life: palliative care for patients and families*, Philadelphia, 2006, Davis.

cognitive function declines in old age because of a decreased number of neurons, decreased brain size, and diminished brain weight. Although these losses are features of aging, they are not consistent with deteriorating mental function, nor do they interfere with everyday routines. Neuron loss occurs mainly in the brain and spinal cord and is most pronounced in the cerebral cortex. The neuronal dendrites atrophy with aging, resulting in impairment of the synapses and changes in the transmission of the chemical neurotransmitters dopamine, serotonin, and acetylcholine. This causes a slowing of many neural processes. However, overall cognitive abilities remain intact. If brain function becomes impaired in old age, it is the result of disease, not aging (Crowley, 1996).

The aging brain maintains resiliency or the ability to compensate for age-related changes. The old adage "use it or lose it" applies to cognitive as well as physical health. Stimulating the brain increases brain tissue formation, enhances synaptic regulation of messages, and enhances the development of cognitive reserve (CR). CR is based on the concept of neuroplasticity, which is the capacity of the brain to change in response to various stimuli, such as daily stressors and activities. Neuroplasticity was once thought to decrease with age, but current literature suggests that cognitive performance can be enhanced with mental stimulation. Maximizing the potential benefits of brain plasticity and CR requires engaging in challenging cognitive, sensory, and motor activities, as well as meaningful social interactions, on a regular basis throughout life.

High CR may allow the individual to continue to learn and adapt to changing stimuli, despite the presence of age-related changes. CR is probably set early in the first two to three decades of life, and stimulating environments, education, and healthy lifestyles throughout life appear to enhance cognitive reserve. CR affects the ability of the adult brain to sustain normal function in the face of significant disease or injury. Brain diseases and injuries may be less apparent in those with greater CR because they are able to tolerate lost neurons and synapses (Desai et al., 2010; Yevchak et al., 2008). For example, individuals who attained more years of education may have high levels of Alzheimer's disease pathology, but few, if any, clinical symptoms.

There are many myths about aging and the brain that may be believed by both health professionals and older adults. It is important to understand cognition and memory in late life and dispel the myths that can have a negative effect on wellness and may, in fact, contribute to unnecessary cognitive decline (Box 6-8). Many skills improve with age but are not identified on standard cognitive screens, and certain testing conditions have exaggerated age-related declines in performance. The bulk of research has focused

---

BOX 6-8   Myths About Aging and the Brain

MYTH: People lose brain cells every day and eventually just run out.
FACT: Most areas of the brain do not lose brain cells. Although you may lose some nerve connections, it can be part of the reshaping of the brain that comes with experience.
MYTH: You can't change your brain.
FACT: The brain is constantly changing in response to experiences and learning, and it retains this "plasticity" well into aging. Changing our way or thinking causes corresponding changes in the brain systems involved, that is, your brain believes what you tell it.
MYTH: The brain doesn't make new brain cells.
FACT: Certain areas of the brain, including the hippocampus (where new memories are created) and the olfactory bulb (scent-processing center), regularly generate new brain cells.

MYTH: Memory decline is inevitable as we age.
FACT: Many people reach old age and have no memory problems. Participation in physical exercise, stimulating mental activity, socialization, healthy diet, and stress management helps maintain brain health. The incidence of dementia does increase with age, but when there are changes in memory, older people need to be evaluated for possible causes and receive treatment.
MYTH: There is no point in trying to teach older adults anything because "you can't teach an old dog new tricks."
FACT: Basic intelligence remains unchanged with age, and older adults should be provided with opportunities for continued learning. Minimizing barriers to learning such as hearing and vision loss and applying principles of geragogy enhance learning ability.

Modified from American Association of Retired Persons: *Myths about aging and the brain* (2007). Available at www.aarp.org/health/brain/aging/myths_about_aging_and_the_brain.html.

on cognitive declines and strategies to help older people find ways to overcome cognitive failings rather than on cognitive capacities (Helmuth, 2003).

Late adulthood is no longer seen as a period when growth has ceased and cognitive development halted; rather it is seen as a life stage programmed for plasticity and the development of unique capacities. Over the last two decades, there has been renewed interest in the concept of wisdom and the ability of the aging brain to develop unique capacities (Ardelt, 2004; Baltes & Smith, 2008). Moving beyond Piaget's formal operational stage of cognitive development, adult development theories propose a more advanced cognitive stage, the postformal operational stage. In this stage, individuals develop the skills to view problems from multiple perspectives, utilize reflection, and communicate thoughtfully in complex and emotionally challenging situations (Parisi et al., 2009).

Recent neuroimaging research has suggested that changes in the brain, once seen only as compensation for declining skills, are now thought to indicate the development of new capacities. These changes include using both hemispheres more equally than younger adults, greater density of synapses, and more use of the frontal lobes, which are thought to be important in abstract reasoning, problem solving, and concept formation (Hooyman & Kiyak, 2011; Grossman et al., 2010). The renewed emphasis on the development of cognitive capabilities that can develop with age provides a view of aging that reflects the history of many cultures and provides a much more hopeful view of both aging and human development.

Fluid and Crystallized Intelligence

Fluid intelligence (often called native intelligence) consists of skills that are biologically determined, independent of experience or learning. It is associated with flexibility in thinking, inductive reasoning, abstract thinking, and integration; it assists people to identify and draw conclusions about complex relationships. Crystallized intelligence is composed of knowledge and abilities that the person acquires through education and life. Measures of crystallized intelligence include verbal meaning, word association, social judgment, and number skills. Older people perform more poorly on performance scales (fluid intelligence), but scores on verbal scales (crystallized intelligence) remain stable. This is known as the classic aging pattern (Hooyman & Kiyak, 2011). The tendency to do poorly on performance tasks may be related to age-related changes in sensory and perceptual abilities as well as psychomotor skills. Speed of cognitive processing and slower reaction time also affect performance.

Memory

Memory is defined as the ability to retain or store information and retrieve it when needed. Memory is a complex set of processes and storage systems. Three components characterize memory: immediate recall; short-term memory (which may range from minutes to days); and remote or long-term memory. Biological, functional, environmental, and psychosocial influences affect memory development throughout adulthood. Recall of newly encountered information seems to decrease with age, and memory declines are noted in connection with complex tasks and strategies. Even though some older adults show decrements in the ability to process information, reaction time, perception, and capacity for attentional tasks, the majority of functioning remains intact and sufficient.

Familiarity, previous learning, and life experience compensate for the minor loss of efficiency in the basic neurological processes. In unfamiliar, stressful, or demanding situations, however, these changes may be more marked. Healthy older adults may complain of memory problems, but their symptoms do not meet the criteria for mild cognitive impairment (MCI) or dementia (see Chapter 21). The term *age-associated memory impairment (AAMI)* has been used to describe memory loss that is considered normal in light of a person's age and educational level. This may include a general slowness in processing, storing, and recalling new information, and difficulty remembering names and words. However, these concerns can cause great anxiety in older adults who may fear dementia. Many medical or psychiatric difficulties (delirium, depression) also influence memory abilities, and it is important for older adults with memory complaints to have a comprehensive evaluation.

Implications for Gerontological Nursing and Healthy Aging

Interventions to Promote Cognitive Health

Knowledge about cognition and memory in older adults is still developing. However, accumulating evidence suggests that there are many strategies to maintain and enhance cognitive health and vitality throughout life. At present, there is not enough evidence to identify which factors or interventions may increase or decrease the risk of developing Alzheimer's disease or other cognitive declines, but attention to brain health remains an important part of overall health promotion activities and should be encouraged (Agency for Healthcare Research and Quality, 2010). "Modification of risk factors remains a cornerstone for dementia prevention until disease-modifying agents prove efficacious" (Desai et al., 2010, p. 1).

Cognitive health is defined as "the development and preservation of the multidimensional cognitive structure that allows the older adult to maintain social connectedness, an ongoing sense of purpose, and the abilities to function independently, to permit functional recovery from illness or injury, and to cope with residual functional deficits" (Hendrie et al., 2006, p. 12). This view of healthy cognitive aging (healthy brain aging) is comprehensive and proactive; it implies that cognitive health is much more than simply a lack of decline with aging (Desai et al., 2010).

Nurses need to educate people of all ages about effective strategies to enhance cognitive health and vitality and to promote cognitive reserve and brain plasticity. Suggested strategies include prevention and management of chronic conditions, maintaining a healthy weight, avoiding excess caloric intake, limiting sodium and fat intake, increasing antioxidant defense by consuming fresh fruits and vegetables, physical activity, participation in mentally stimulating activity, and social engagement (Yevchak et al., 2008; Desai et al., 2010). *The Healthy Brain Initiative: A National Public Health Road Map to Maintaining Cognitive Health* (http://www.cdc.gov/aging/healthybrain/roadmap.htm) and the *Cognitive and Emotional Health Project: The Healthy Brain* (http://trans.nih.gov/cehp/index.htm) are examples of national efforts to promote cognitive health.

Learning in Late Life

Basic intelligence remains unchanged with increasing years, and older adults should be provided with opportunities for continued learning. Adapting communication and teaching to enhance understanding requires knowledge of learning in late life and effective teaching-learning strategies with older adults. *Geragogy* is the application of the principles of adult learning theory to teaching interventions for older adults.

The older adult demands that teaching situations be relevant; new learning must relate to what the person already knows and should emphasize concrete and practical information. Aging may present barriers to learning, such as hearing and vision losses and cognitive impairment. Moreover, the process of aging may accentuate other challenges that had already been factors in a person's life, such as cultural and cohort variations and education. Many older adults may have special learning needs based on educational deprivation in their early years and consequent anxiety about formalized learning.

Attention to literacy level and cultural variations is important to enhance learning and the usefulness of what is learned. Mood is extremely important in terms of what

individuals (young and old) will recall. In other words, when we attempt to measure recall of events that may have occurred in a crisis situation or an anxiety state, recall will be impaired. This is significant for health care professionals who give information to older adults who are ill or upset, particularly at times of crisis such as hospital discharge. They are not likely to remember the information provided, which contributes to problematic transitions (see Chapter 3). Box 6-9 presents strategies to enhance the learning of older adults.

Opportunities for older adults to learn are available in many formal and informal modes: self-teaching, college attendance, participation in seminars and conferences, public television programs, CDs, internet courses, and countless others. In most universities, older people are taking classes of all types. Fees are usually lower for individuals older than 60 years of age, and elders may choose to work toward a degree or audit classes for enrichment and enjoyment. The Elderhostel program is an example of a program designed for older people that combines continued learning with travel (www.elderhostel.org).

Older adults comprise the fastest growing population using computers and the Internet. According to data from the Pew Research Center's Internet and American Life Project, 92% of adults aged 50 to 64 years of age and 89% of those 65 years of age and over send and receive emails (Pew Research Center, 2010). Older adults also comprise the fastest growing group using social-networking sites such as Facebook. More than any other age group, older adults perceive the Internet as a valuable resource to help them connect to loved ones and more easily obtain information.

AARP and other organizations such as CyberSeniors provide basic computer and Internet training for older people. Although there has been little research on the use of computers among nursing home residents or among those with dementia, the technology has great potential to meet psychosocial needs for family contact, enjoyment, and stimulation (Tak et al., 2007).

Health Literacy

Health literacy is defined as the degree to which individuals have the capacity to obtain, process, and understand basic health information and services needed to make appropriate health decisions (Kobylarz et al., 2010). Limited health literacy has been linked to increased health disparities, poor health outcomes, inadequate preventive care, increased use of health care services, higher risk of mortality for older adults, and several health care safety issues, including medical and medication errors. Improving health literacy for

BOX 6-9   Guiding Older Adult Learners

- Make sure the client is ready to learn before trying to teach. Watch for cues that would indicate that the client is preoccupied or too anxious to comprehend the material.
- Be sensitive to cultural, language, and other differences among the older adults you serve. Some suggestions may not be appropriate for everyone.
- Provide adequate time for learning, and use self-pacing techniques
- Create a shame-free environment where older adults feel free to ask questions and stay informed.
- Provide regular positive feedback.
- Avoid distractions, and present one idea at a time.
- Present pertinent, specific, practical and individualized information. Emphasize concrete rather than abstract material.
- Use past experience; connect new learning to what has already been learned.
- Use written material to supplement verbal instruction. Use a list format, a low-literacy level, and large readable font (e.g., Arial, 14 to 16 points).

- Use high contrast on visuals and handout materials (e.g., black print on white paper).
- Consider using Braille and audio-taped information whenever necessary.
- Pay attention to reading ability; use tools other than printed material such as drawings, pictures, and discussion.
- Use bullets or lists to highlight pertinent information.
- Sit facing the client so he or she can watch your lip movements and facial expressions.
- Speak slowly.
- Keep the pitch of your voice low; older people can hear low sounds better than high-frequency sounds.
- Encourage the learner to develop various mediators or mnemonic devices (e.g., visual images, rhymes, acronyms, self designed coding schemes).
- Use shorter, more frequent sessions with appropriate breaks; pay attention to fatigue and physical discomfort.

Modified from: *Bridging principles of older adult learning: reconnaissance phase final report,* Washington, DC, 1999, SPRY Foundation; and Hayes K: Designing written medication instructions: effective ways to help older adults self-medicate, *J Gerontol Nurs 32(5):5-10, 2005; From Arozullah A, Yarnold P, Bennett C, et al: Development and validation of a short-form rapid estimate of adult literacy in medicine, Med Care* 45(11):1026-1033, 2007; Hayes K: Designing written medication instructions: effective ways to help older adults self-medicate, *J Gerontol Nurs* 31(5):5-10, 2005; Hayes K: Literacy for health information of adult patients and caregivers in the rural emergency department, *Clinical Excellence for Nurse Practitioners,* 4(1):35-40, 2000. *Quick guide to health literacy, fact sheet.* Available at www.health.gov/communication/literacy/quickguide/factsliteracy.htm.

all Americans has been identified as one of the 20 necessary actions to improve health care quality on a national scale (Agency for Healthcare Research and Quality, 2011: Centers for Disease Control and Prevention [CDC], 2009.)

Health literacy is more than the basic reading and writing skills. It includes the ability to understand instructions on prescription drug bottles, appointment slips, medical education brochures, provider instructions, and consent forms; to interact with health professionals in health care settings; and to negotiate complex health care systems (National Network of Libraries of Medicine, 2011). Health literacy is "approximately five grade levels lower than the last school year completed" (Hayes, 2000, p. 7). Many health education materials, as well as information on the Internet, are written at reading levels above the recommended fifth-grade reading level.

Being health literate "involves a multitude of cognitive processes that are challenging for any one at any age"

(Speros, 2009). Nearly 9 of 10 adults do not have the level of proficiency in health literacy skills necessary to successfully navigate the health care system. Older adults are disproportionately affected by inadequate health literacy. Chronic illness and sensory impairments further contribute to challenges related to communication and understanding. Among adult age groups, those 65 years of age and older have the smallest proportion of persons with proficient health literacy skills. This group also has the highest proportion of persons with health literacy defined as "below basic." More than half of individuals over 65 years of age are at the below-basic level (CDC, 2009; Kobylarz et al., 2010).

Older adults are a heterogeneous group in their characteristics and literacy skills, and therefore strategies to enhance their understanding of health information need to be individualized. Individuals residing in urban areas, those with poor education or low income, and people for whom

English is a second language are more likely to perform at lower levels of literacy. Other factors influencing health literacy include the person's basic literacy skills and situations encountered in the health care system as well as the cultural competence and communication skills of health professionals. *Improving Health Literacy for Older Adults* (CDC, 2009) and *Quick Guide to Health Literacy* (http://www.health.gov/communication/literacy/quickguide/) provide health professionals with information related to health literacy and strategies for communicating effectively.

Implications for Gerontological Nursing and Healthy Aging

Knowledge about the process of life span development and the various ways people experience aging assists nurses in understanding the meaning of healthy aging for each individual and provides the foundation for nursing interventions that enhance lifelong growth, development, health, and well-being. A rich and stimulating environment should be available to all older adults in all settings so that they can thrive, not merely survive, in old age.

Future generations of older adults will redefine what we now consider the "norms" for aging. People can expect to spend 30 or more years in "late life," and there are still many important tasks to be accomplished during this period. Concerns of the young are to become established as adults; middle-aged persons are overwhelmed with the requirements of success and survival. Focusing on the reason for being and the meaning of life is the concern of elders.

Application of Maslow's Hierarchy

Nurses can provide the opening for elders to discuss the process of aging and its psychological and social effects. In our highly biomedicalized approach to aging, it is imperative that we seek to know individuals beyond the problem that brings them to the attention of the health care team. Care addressing only biological needs robs older people of the opportunity to grow toward self-actualization—a major task of late life. Ask elders, "How has aging affected your inner life and outlook?" "What gives your life meaning and purpose?" Listen to the answers, and learn. We are all aging, and those whom we serve are our best teachers.

KEY CONCEPTS

- Normal aging involves a gradual process of biopsychosocial change over the course of time.
- Life span development theorists tend to study the total life course of cohort groups to determine the influence of major historical events on their development.

- The impact of gender, culture, and cohort must always be considered when discussing the validity of biopsychosocial theories.
- Spirituality must be considered a significant factor in understanding healthy aging.
- Late adulthood is no longer seen as a period of when growth ceases and cognitive development halts; rather it is seen as a life stage programmed for plasticity and the development of unique capacities.
- Cognitive stimulation and attention to brain health is just as important as attention to physical health.
- Learning in late life can be enhanced by utilizing principles of geragogy and adapting teaching strategies to minimize barriers such as hearing and vision impairment and low literacy.

ACTIVITIES AND DISCUSSION QUESTIONS

1. Identify and discuss the major flaws in the sociological theories of aging.
2. How well do the psychological and sociological theories of aging "fit" within your own cultural perspective?
3. Discuss the variables that must constantly be considered when assessing the psychosocial aspects of the aging experience. Identify and discuss those that seem most significant.
4. Discuss some of the problems of adequately testing the cognitive function of elders.
5. How would you respond to the following myth of aging: "You can't teach an old dog new tricks"?
6. Discuss some ways that nurses can respond to the spiritual needs and concerns of older adults.

REFERENCES

Achenbaum WA: *Old age in a new land*, Baltimore, 1978, Johns Hopkins Press.

Agency for Healthcare Research and Quality: *Health literacy interventions and outcomes: an updated systematic review* (2011). Available at http://www.ahrq.gov/clinic/epcsums/lituptsum.pdf.

Agency for Healthcare Research and Quality, U.S. Department of Health and Human Services: *Preventing Alzheimer's disease and cognitive decline* (2010). Available at http://www.ahrq.gov/downloads/pub/evidence/pdf/alzheimers/alzcog.pdf.

Ardelt M: Wisdom as expert knowledge system: a critical review of a contemporary operationalization of an ancient concept, *Human Development* 47:257–285, 2004.

Arozullah A, Yarnold P, Bennett C, et al: Development and validation of a short-form rapid estimate of adult literacy in medicine, *Med Care* 45(11):1026–1033, 2007.

Baltes PB: Theoretical propositions on life-span developmental theory: on the dynamics between growth and decline, *Dev Psychol* 23(5):611–626, 1987.

Baltes PB, Lindenberger U, Staudinger U: Life-span theory in developmental psychology. In Lerner R, editor: *Handbook of child psychology, vol 1. theoretical models of human development,* New York, 1998, Wiley.

Baltes P, Smith J: The fascination of wisdom: it's nature, ontogeny, and function, *Perspectives on Psychological Science* 3:56–62, 2008.

Centers for Disease Control and Prevention [CDC]. *Improving health literacy for older adults: expert panel report 2009,* Atlanta, 2009, U.S. Department of Health and Human Services.

Crowley SL: Aging brain's staying power, *AARP Bulletin 37:1,* 1996.

Crowther M, Parker M, Achenbaum W, et al: Rowe and Kahn's model of successful aging revisited: positive spirituality—the forgotten factor, *Gerontologist* 42(5):613, 2002.

Cumming E, Henry W: *Growing old,* New York, 1961, Basic Books.

Dandekar K: *The elderly in India,* Thousand Oaks, CA, 1996, Sage.

Delgado C: Sense of coherence, spirituality, stress and quality of life in chronic illness, *J Nurs Scholarsh* 39(3):229–234, 2007.

Desai A, Grossberg G, Chibnall J: Healthy brain aging: a road map, *Clinics in Geriatric Medicine* 26:1, 2010.

Dowd JJ: *Stratification among the aged,* Monterey, CA, 1980, Brooks Cole.

Erikson EH: *Childhood and society,* ed 2, New York, 1963, WW Norton.

Erikson EH, Erikson JM, Kivnick HQ: *Vital involvement in old age: the experience of old age in our time,* New York, 1986, WW Norton.

Gaskamp C, Sutter R, Meraviglia M, et al: Evidence-based guideline: promoting spirituality in the older adult, *J Gerontol Nurs* 32(11):8–11, 2006.

Havighurst R, Neugarten B, Tobin S: Disengagement and patterns of aging. In Neugarten BL, editor: *Middle age and aging,* Chicago, 1968, University of Chicago Press.

Havighurst R: *Developmental tasks and education,* ed 3, New York, 1971, Longman.

Hayes K: Literacy for health information of adult patients and caregivers in the rural emergency department, *Clin Excel Nurse Pract* 4(1):35–40, 2000.

Helmuth L: The wisdom of the wizened, *Science* 299:1300–1302, 2003.

Hendrie H, Albert M, Butters M, et al: The NIH Cognitive and Emotional Health Project: report of the Critical Evaluation Study Committee, *Alzheimers Dement* 2:12, 2006.

Hodge D, Bonifas R, Chou R: Spirituality and older adults: ethical guidelines to enhance service provision, *Adv Soc Work* 11:1, 2010.

Hooks B: *Feminist theory: from margin to center,* Cambridge, MA, 2000, South End Press.

Hooyman N, Kiyak H: *Social gerontology,* ed 7, Boston, 2005, Pearson.

Hooyman N, Kiyak H: *Social gerontology,* ed 9, Boston, 2011, Pearson.

Jett KR: Mind loss in the African-American community: a normal part of aging, *J Aging Stud* 20(1):1, 2006.

Jung C: The stages of life. In Campbell J, editor: *The portable Jung* (RFC Hull, translator), New York, 1971, Viking Press.

Kobylarz F, Pomidor A, Pleasant A: Health literacy as a tool to improve the public understanding of Alzheimer's disease, *Ann Longterm Care* 18:34, 2010.

Macrae J: Nightingale's spiritual philosophy and its significance for modern nursing, *Image J Nurs Scholarsh* 27:8, 1995.

Maddox G: Activity and morale: a longitudinal study of selected older adult subjects, *Soc Forces* 42(2):195, 1963.

Marshall V: The state of theory in aging and the social sciences. In Binstock RH, Geroge LK, editors: *Handbook of aging and the social sciences,* San Diego, 1996, Academic Press.

Martsolf D, Mickley J: The concept of spirituality in nursing theories: differing world views and extent of focus, *J Adv Nurs* 27:294, 1998.

National Network of Libraries of Medicine: *Health literacy* (2012). Available at http://nnlm.gov/outreach/consumer/hlthlit.html.

Neugarten BL, Havighurst R, Tobin SS: Personality and patterns of aging. In Neugarten B, editor: *Middle age and aging,* Chicago, 1968, University of Chicago Press.

Papalia D, Sterns H, Feldman R, et al: *Adult development and aging,* Boston, 2002, McGraw-Hill.

Parisi J, Rebok G, Carlson M, et al: Can the wisdom of aging be activated and make a difference socially? *Educ Gerontol* 35:867–879, 2009.

Peck R: Psychological developments in the second half of life. In Neugarten B, editor: *Middle age and aging,* Chicago, 1968, University of Chicago Press.

Pew Research Center: *Older adults and social media* (2010). Available at http://www.pewinternet.org/Reports/2010/Older-Adults-and-Social-Media.aspx.

Riley M, Johnson M, Forner A: *Aging and society: a sociology of age stratification, vol. 3,* New York, 1972, Russell Sage Foundation.

Rowe JW, Kahn RL: *Successful aging,* New York, 1998, Pantheon-Random House.

Stair N: If I had my life to live over. In Martz S, editor: *If I had my life to live over I would pick more daisies,* Watsonville, CA, 1992, Papier Mache Press.

Silverman P, Hecht L, McMillin J: Modeling life satisfaction among the aged: a comparison of Chinese and Americans, *J Cross Cult Gerontol* 15(4):289, 2000.

Soeken K, Carson V: Responding to the spiritual needs of the chronically ill, *Nurs Clin North Am* 22:604, 1987.

Speros C: More than words: promoting health literacy in older adults, *Online J Issues Nurs* 14(3), 2009.

Strang S, Strang P: Questions posed to hospital chaplains by palliative care patients, *J Palliat Med* 5:857, 2002.

Tak S, Beck C, McMahon E: Computer and Internet access for long-term care residents, *J Gerontol Nurs* 33:32, 2007.

Tornstam L: Gerotranscendence: a theoretical and empirical exploration. In Thomas LE, Eisenhandler SA, editors: *Aging and the religious dimension,* Westport, CT, 1994, Greenwood Publishing Group.

Tornstam L: Gerotranscendence: a theory about maturing into old age, *J Aging Ident* 1(1):37, 1996.

Tornstam L: *Gerotranscendence: a developmental theory of positive aging,* New York, 2005, Springer.

Touhy T: Touching the spirit of elders in nursing homes: ordinary yet extraordinary care, *Int J Human Caring* 6(1):12–17, 2001.

Touhy T, Zerwekh J: Spiritual caring. In Zerwekh J: *Nursing care at the end of life: palliative care for patients and families,* Philadelphia, 2006, FA Davis.

Yevchak A, Loeb S, Fick D: Promoting cognitive health and vitality: a review of clinical implications, *Geriatr Nurs,* 29(5): 302–330, 2008.

CHAPTER 7

Assessment and Documentation for Optimal Care

Kathleen F. Jett

evolve evolve.elsevier.com/Ebersole/gerontological

LEARNING OBJECTIVES

Upon completion of this chapter, the reader will be able to:

- Identify key differences in assessing older adults and younger adults.
- Describe the range of tools that may be used in the comprehensive gerontological assessment.
- Discuss the advantages and disadvantages of the use of standardized assessment tools in gerontological nursing.
- Begin to develop the skills needed to select an evidence-based and appropriate tool for a specific situation and use it correctly.
- Discuss the impact of common normal changes with aging on the assessment.
- Describe the reasons for accurate and thorough documentation in gerontological nursing.
- Identify potential problems in documentation.
- Identify ways in which errors in documentation and communication are especially dangerous when caring for older adults.
- Compare the major documentation methods used in acute, long-term, and home care.

GLOSSARY

ADLs, Activities of daily living Those tasks necessary to maintain one's health and basic personal needs.

IADLs, Instrumental activities of daily living Those tasks necessary to maintain one's home and independent living.

Health fluency The ability to understand and interpret language and wording used in the health care setting.

HIPAA Health Insurance Portability and Accountability Act of 1996, which legislated the handling of confidential patient information.

Report-by-proxy One person (the proxy) answering questions or providing information for a second person, based on the first person's knowledge of the second person.

THE LIVED EXPERIENCE

I was so happy to be able to make a big difference in Mrs. Jones's life. She was 97 and had grown slowly confused over the years. She was also profoundly hard of hearing. She spent the majority of time calling for "Mary," her deceased sister. We really could not communicate effectively with her; we could only show her we cared and keep her safe. Eventually she became acutely ill, and a decision had to be made about CPR (cardiopulmonary resuscitation). When we tried to find out what her wishes were, we could not immediately find any record of them, and she had no living relatives or friends, just an attorney. I searched and searched and finally found documentation about her wishes. We were able to provide her the comfort she wanted because of a nurse's careful documentation years before.

Kathleen, GNP, age 45

Assessment Tools in Gerontological Nursing

Gerontological nurses conduct skilled and detailed assessments of and with the persons who entrust themselves to their care. While many of the skills used in the physical assessment of younger and older adults are the same, the overall process of working with persons later in life is strikingly different if for no reason other than their medical, psychological, and social complexity. Older adults vary greatly in their health and function, from active and independent to medically fragile and dependent. The comprehensive assessment is more complex, more detailed, and takes much longer to complete. More often, partial or problem-oriented assessments are done. If a more thorough assessment is needed, this is usually performed by a nurse-led interdisciplinary health care team. The assessment is not complete until it is documented. Nursing documentation is an age-old practice of making a permanent record of the conditions of our patients, our actions, and the patients' responses to our actions or those of others. There is probably not a nurse alive who does not know the mantra, "If you didn't document it—you didn't do it!"

In this chapter the basic concepts of the general assessment process as it applies to working with elders are reviewed as well as discussions of commonly used instruments that are available for the collection of assessment data. The chapter further provides the reader with basic information about documenting the assessment and other pertinent data in the health record in the various settings in which older adults are cared for by nurses. References are provided throughout for more information about specialized assessments and documents both in other parts of this text and in other sources. (See Appendix 7-1 at the end of this chapter for a list of chapters in which assessment topics are addressed.)

The health assessment is composed of a number of parts; the collection of physical data as well as integration of biological, psychosocial, and functional information. It also may include cultural and spiritual assessments and occurs at all levels of Maslow's Hierarchy. Additional assessment areas include cognitive abilities, psychological well-being; caregiver stress or burden; and patterns of health and health care. Areas or problems frequently not addressed by the care provider or mentioned by the elder but that should be addressed are sexual function, depression, alcoholism, hearing loss, oral health, and environmental safety. Part of a safety assessment usually includes consideration of gait and balance (see Chapter 13). Although not usually conducted by a nurse, a driving assessment may be recommended any time there is a question of ability. Questions regarding genetic background in this age group, especially for those in the younger range, have most relevance as they relate to Alzheimer's disease, stroke, diabetes, and several types of cancer. The assessment is also an opportunity to review the elder's preferences for advanced care planning. Finally a comprehensive assessment includes consideration of the somewhat vague conditions referred to as *geriatric syndromes*. These most often include delirium, falls, dizziness, syncope, and urinary incontinence (see Fulmer's SPICE tool later in this chapter).

Assessment of the older adult requires special abilities: to listen patiently, to allow for pauses, to ask questions that are not often asked and to obtain data from all available sources, and to understand that not all positive findings will require interventions. The nurse must be able to recognize normal changes of aging (see Chapter 5) and atypical presentations (see Section 3) in order to appropriately and effectively conduct the assessment and interpret the findings. The assessment must be paced according to the stamina of both the person and the nurse. If the elder is physically frail, cognitively impaired, is unable to speak or does not speak the same language as the nurse, the health assessment becomes particularly difficult but even more important. The quality and speed of the assessment are a reflection of experience. Novice nurses should neither be expected to nor expect themselves to do this proficiently but should expect to see their skills, the amount of information obtained, and the speed at which it is obtained, increase over time. According to Benner (1984), assessment is a task for the expert. However, an expert is not always available. By following some basic guidelines and learning how to use the wide range of assessment tools and resources now available, the quality of data collected by all nurses can be improved.

Collecting Assessment Data

Conducting assessment data begins with establishing rapport. It is never appropriate to address the patient by the first name unless invited to do so. The assumption of familiarity in the use of the first name in addressing an elder can easily be perceived as condescending especially when the nurse is younger than the patient or of a different ethnic background.

There are three approaches used for collecting assessment data: self-report, report-by-proxy, and observation. In the self-report format, questions are either asked directly or the person is expected to respond to written questions about his or her health status. Patients tend to overestimate their own abilities and older adults in particular have been found to under-report symptoms, often due to the erroneous belief that what they are experiencing are normal parts of aging. When assessment information is obtained indirectly (report-by-proxy) the nurse asks another person, such as a staff nurse, aide, spouse, or friend, relative or caretaker to report their observations. This approach is used extensively with persons who are cognitively impaired; the elder's abilities and health are often underestimated. In the observational approach the nurse collects and records the data as she or he has measured and observed using what are believed to be objective parameters.

The usual physical examination, such as the measurement of a blood pressure, and performance-based functional assessments, such as having the person walk a certain distance, are examples of observational measures. Observation and the use of previously developed tools are probably the most accurate but are limited in that they only represent a snapshot in time.

Certain guidelines should be followed regardless of the approach used in the data collection:

- Whenever possible, conduct the assessment at a time when the patient is at his or her best.
- If a standard tool is being used, be sure it is used correctly; training may be required.
- To avoid biasing the response, do not direct the way the question is answered.
- Explore for more information only if it is needed to complete the assessment.
- Approach questions that are more personal, such as sexual functioning, in a matter-of-fact, but nonetheless sensitive, manner.
- Record the responses accurately, using the patient's own words where possible; do not analyze at the same time the data are being collected. For example, if the patient says "I have a runny nose," this is not recorded as "Patient has a cold" until analysis of the data.

Ideally, the assessment should be used to gather baseline data before the older adult has a health crisis. Periodically, the person can be reassessed to monitor health status. For example, a person who has an altered mental status as a result of an illness or medication *(delirium)* should be reassessed later when the underlying problem has been resolved.

The appropriate and accurate use of assessment and documentation instruments will increase the likelihood of obtaining reliable, useful data; especially that which can be compared over time to monitor changes in health status and therefore health needs. This of course implies that data collection is followed by the analysis and determination of the person's needs followed by the development of nursing interventions. By accomplishing both, the nurse contributes to the nation's goal of increasing the quality of life for all Americans and the health of older adults (see Chapter 1 and http://www.healthypeople.gov/2020).

Assessment instruments exist that can broadly categorize physical health, mood, motor capacity, manual ability, self-care ability, more complex instrumental abilities, and cognitive and social function. Assessments are completed in every setting. In most settings, standardized formats of some kind are used. Which assessments are done depends both on the setting and the purpose. Sometimes these tools come directly from the gerontological literature or payer sources like Medicare, and other times they are modified to meet the particular needs of the setting.

Fortunately we have a number of excellent instruments at our disposal to help us do this. Several tools are discussed or referred to in this chapter. We ask the reader to note that those described herein serve only as examples of what is available. The *Try This:*® series available from the Hartford Institute for Geriatric Nursing is one of the sources for ever-evolving information, tools, and evidence-based protocols (http://www.hartfordign.org/practice/try_this). The *Try This:* series includes copies of commonly used and tested instruments for general assessment (e.g., the Geriatric Depression Scale [GDS]) (see the Evidence-Based Practice box) as well as those needed in specialized circumstances (e.g., measurement of the Ankle-Brachial Index [ABI]) and other instruments specific to working with the person with dementia. Although several of the tools are discussed in this chapter and elsewhere throughout the book (see Appendix 7-1), complete descriptions of the tools, how they are best used in the older population, and the instruments themselves are provided for educational, non-profit use online. Information about use is provided at the ConsultGeriRN website (http://consultgerirn.org/resources). Finally, with the current volume of materials available on the Internet, additional information about the use of and research related to any of the tools discussed throughout this text can be found easily.

EVIDENCE-BASED PRACTICE

General Geriatric Assessment Instruments in the Hartford Institute for Geriatric Nursing *Try This.*® Series

SPICES: An Overall Assessment Tool of Older Adults*

Katz Index of Independence in Activities of Daily Living (ADL)*

The Mini-Cog: Mental Status Assessment*

Geriatric Depression Scale (GDS)*

The Braden Scale: Predicting Pressure Ulcer Risk[†]

The Pittsburgh Sleep Quality Index (PSQI)[†]

The Epworth Sleepiness Scale[†]

Pain Assessment Scales: Examples[†]

The Hendrich II Fall Risk Assessment[†]

The Mini-Nutritional Assessment[†]

The PLISSIT Model: A scale for assessing sexuality[†]

Urogenital Distress Inventory Short Form (UDI-6)

Incontinence Impact Questionnaire Short Form (IIQ-7)

Brief Hearing Loss Screener[†]

Confusion Assessment Method (CAM)[†]

Modified Caregiver Strain Index (CSI)[†]

Short Michigan Alcoholism Screening Instrument – Geriatric Version (SMAST-G)[†]

The Kayser-Jones Brief Oral Health Status Examination (BOHSE)[†]

Horowitz's Impact of Event Scale: An Assessment of Post Traumatic Stress in Older Adults[†]

Lawton Instrumental Activities of Daily Living (IADL) Scale*

Hospital Admission Risk Profile (HARP)[†]

Confusion Assessment Method for the Intensive Care Unit (CAM-ICU)[†]

Transitional Care Model (TCM): Hospital Discharge Screening Criteria for High Risk Older Adults[†]

The Preparedness for Caregiving Scale[†]

The Falls Efficacy Scale-International (FES-I): Assessment of Fear of Falling[†]

The FACIT Fatigue Scale (version 4): Assessment of Fatigue in Older Adults

SOURCE: The Hartford Institute for Geriatric Nursing, New York University, College of Nursing. These and other *Try This.*® issues can be found at www.ConsultGeriRN.org.

*Content discussed in this chapter

[†]Content discussed elsewhere in this text (see Appendix 7-1)

The Health History

The initiation of the health history marks the beginning of the nurse-client relationship and the assessment process. It begins with a review of what the person reports as a problem, known as the "chief complaint." This is considered subjective data that is documented in the patient's own words. In an older adult this is much more likely to be vague and less straightforward. For example, it is not unusual for the person to say "I just don't feel well."

The health history is best collected either verbally in a face-to-face interview or using the interview to review a written history completed by the patient or patient's proxy beforehand. Although longer for the patient, written formats are usually much faster than the verbal for the nurse. The written format should never be used if the person has limited vision, questionable reading level, the person has limited health fluency or written in a language or at a level in which the patient does not have reading ability. Written histories provide reliable information only when the person is able to adequately complete the documents alone or with some assistance. If collecting the history verbally or when reviewing a previously written document, the nurse

uses techniques which optimize communication. If the elder has limited language proficiency, a trained medical interpreter is needed and the interview will generally take about twice as long (see Chapter 4). If the person has limited health fluency, special attention will need to be paid to wording of questions and answers to the patient's questions. If the person is cognitively impaired he or she should be included to the extent possible with additional information obtained from the proxy.

Any health history form or interview should include a patient profile, a past medical history, a review of systems, a medication history (see Chapter 8), nutritional history (see Chapter 9) and include any other factors which influence the person's quality of life. The nurse should be aware that in an older adult the traditional review of systems may be quite lengthy due to the number of years the person has had the opportunity to have had problems. It may be easier and more appropriate to begin with reviewing the symptoms the person is currently having and gear the system review accordingly. In the oldest older adult, family history in and of itself becomes less important as the person ages, and it is replaced with the increasing importance of the social history. The social history, an essential part of the history, includes current living arrangements, economic resources to meet current health-related or food expenses, amount of family and friend support, and community resources available if needed. Tools to adequately measure social networks have been in development for a number of years. However, the many nuances and configurations of social support networks make standardized measurements difficult.

Finally, to meet the needs of our increasingly diverse population of elders, the use of questions related to the explanatory model (Kleinman, 1980) is recommended to complement the health history (see Chapter 4 and Box 4-5). The responses will better enable the nurse to understand the elder and to plan culturally and individually appropriate and effective interventions.

Physical Assessment

Nurses learn to conduct a complete "head-to-toe" when conducting a physical assessment. While this is usually done when assessing younger persons it is rarely possible when working with an older adult, especially one who is medically complex or fragile. To do so would be excessively time-consuming and burdensome to all involved. Instead the assessment is first directed to that which is most likely associated with the presenting problem or major diagnoses and progresses from there. When performing a physical assessment the gerontological nurse must be able to quickly prioritize what is the most necessary to know (based on the chief complaint) and proceed to what would be nice to know. When the chief complaint is not known, such as in persons with moderate to advanced dementia, persons who are unable to express themselves (such as those with expressive aphasia), or in the presence of any other type of language barrier, a more thorough assessment is always necessary. When the focus is on a well check or a health care contact related to health promotion and disease prevention, the emphasis is on the major preventable health problems in later life, especially those of cardiovascular and musculoskeletal origins.

The collection of data for the physical assessment begins the moment the nurse sees the person, noting skin color and texture, presence or absence of lesions. If the person "looks ill," this should be noted in the medical record. Is the person able to ambulate alone or does he or she hold on to the walls along the way to the exam room, dining room, or bathroom? Are assistive devices used? Is the person able to follow directions when the nurse uses a normal voice volume or is an elevated one needed? If unable to follow directions at all or only with difficulty, it will be necessary to determine first whether

this is related to sensory losses or indicates cognitive impairment. It may even be from something as simple as a cerumen (ear wax) impaction (see Chapter 5).

While considering the expected findings related to normal age changes discussed in Chapter 5, the manual techniques used in the physical exam are applicable to any age group and the reader is referred to any number of excellent textbooks solely dedicated to this. However, extra time is usually needed for dressing and undressing and some positions (e.g., lying flat for an abdominal exam) may not be possible. Several modifications may be necessary due to common changes see in later life (Table 7-1). For additional information, see http://www2.kumc.edu/coa/education/AMED900/PhysiologicAging/PhysicalDiagnosisinOlderAdults.htm.

Most often the physical exam is only one part of the evaluation of one or more other aspects of the person and his or her life. Due to the complexity of life and health in later life, this elevates the responsibility of the nurse. The nurse working in the geriatric setting must have a considerable repertoire of physical assessment skills and be able to draw upon these as the circumstance arises; in some cases this may need to be done quickly. In most circumstances the quality of care the elder receives is dependent on the quality of the assessment conducted.

Comprehensive Physical Assessment of the Frail and Medically Complex Elder

FANCAPES is a model for a comprehensive yet prioritized, primarily physical assessment that is especially useful for the frail elder (Resnick & Mitty, 2009). It emphasizes the determination of very basic needs and the individual's functional ability to meet these needs independently; these are the needs that form even the most basic levels of Maslow's Hierarchy. The acronym *FANCAPES* represents *F*luids, *A*eration, *N*utrition, *C*ommunication, *A*ctivity, *P*ain, *E*limination, and *S*ocialization. It can be used in all settings, may be used in part or whole depending on the need, and is easily adaptable to functional pattern grouping if nursing diagnoses are used. The nurse obtains comprehensive information in each section, guided by the questions provided in the following text.

F—Fluids

What is the current state of hydration (see Chapter 9)? Does the person have the functional capacity to consume adequate fluids to maintain optimal health? This includes the abilities to sense thirst, mechanically obtain the needed fluids, swallow them, and excrete them.

TABLE **7-1**	**Considerations of Common Changes in Late Life During the Physical Assessment**
Height and weight	Monitor for changes in weight Weight gain: especially important if the persons has any heart disease, being alert for early signs of heart failure Weight loss: be alert for indications of malnutrition from dental problems, depression, or cancer. Check for mouth lesions from ill-fitting dentures.
Temperature	Even a low-grade fever could be an indication of a serious illness. Temperatures of as low as 100° F may indicate pending sepsis.
Blood pressure	Positional blood pressure readings should be obtained due to high occurrence of orthostatic hypotension. Both arms should be checked (at heart level) and recording of the highest one used. Isolated systolic hypertension is common.
Skin	Check for indications of solar damage, especially among persons who worked outdoors or live in sunny climates. Due to thinning, "tenting" cannot be used as a measure of hydration status.
Ears	Cerumen impactions are common. These must be removed before hearing can be adequately assessed. High-frequency hearing loss (presbycusis) is common. The person often complains that he or she can hear but not understand as some, but not all sounds are lost. The person with severe but unrecognized hearing loss may be incorrectly thought to have dementia.
Eyes	Increased glare sensitivity, decreased contrast sensitivity and need for more light to see and read. Ensure that waiting rooms, hallways, and exam rooms are adequately lit. Decreased color discrimination may affect ability to self-administer medications safely.
Mouth	Excessive dryness common and exacerbated by many medications. Cannot use mouth moisture to estimate hydration status.
Neck	Due to loss of subcutaneous fat it may appear that carotid arteries are enlarged when they are not.
Chest	Any kyphosis will alter the location of the lobes, making careful assessment more important. Risk for aspiration pneumonia increased and therefore the importance of the lateral exam.
Heart	Listen carefully for third and fourth heart sounds. Fourth heart sounds common. Determine if this has been found to be present in the past or is new.
Extremities	Dorsalis pedis and posterior tibial pulses very difficult or impossible to palpate. Must look for other indications of vascular integrity.
Abdomen	Due to deposition of fat in the abdomen, auscultation of bowel tones may be difficult.
Musculoskeletal	Osteoarthritis very common and pain often undertreated. Ask about pain and function in joints. Conduct very gentle passive range of motion if active range of motion not possible. Do not push past comfort level.
Neurological	Although there is a gradual decrease in muscle strength, it still should remain equal bilaterally. Greatly diminished or absent ankle jerk (Achilles) tendon reflex is common and normal. Decreased or absent vibratory sense of the lower extremities, testing unnecessary.

A—Aeration

Is the person's oxygen exchange adequate for full respiratory functioning (see Chapter 19)? This means the ability to maintain an oxygen saturation of at least 96% in most situations. Is supplemental oxygen required, and if so, is the person able to obtain it? What is the respiratory rate and depth at rest and during activity, talking, walking, exercising, and while performing activities of daily living? What sounds are auscultated, palpated, and percussed, and what do they suggest? For the older person, it is particularly important to carefully assess lateral and apical lung fields.

N—Nutrition

What mechanical and psychological factors affect the person's ability to obtain and benefit from adequate nutrition (see Chapter 9)? What is the type and amount of food consumed? Does the person have the abilities to bite, chew, and swallow? What is the oral health status and what is the impact of periodontal disease if present? For edentulous persons, do their dentures fit properly and are they worn? Does the person understand the need for special diets? Has this diet been designed so that it is consistent with the person's eating and cultural patterns? Can the person afford the special foods needed? If the person is at risk for aspiration, including those who are tube fed, have preventive strategies been taught, including the need for meticulous oral hygiene?

C—Communication

Is the person able to communicate his or her needs adequately? Do the persons who provide care understand the patient's form of communication? What is the person's ability to hear in various environments? Are there any environmental situations in which understanding of the spoken word is inadequate? If the person depends on lip-reading, is his or her vision adequate? Is the person able to clearly articulate words that are understandable to others? Does the person have either expressive or receptive aphasia (see Chapter 20), and if so has a speech therapist been made available to the person and significant others? What is the person's reading and comprehension levels? (Assume it is no greater than fifth grade if unknown.)

A—Activity

Is the person able to participate in the activities necessary to meet basic needs such as toileting, grooming, and meal preparation? How much assistance is needed, if any, and is someone available to provide this if needed? Is the person able to participate in activities that meet higher levels of needs such as belonging (e.g., church attendance) or finding meaning in life (see Chapter 11)? What are the person's abilities to feed, toilet, dress, and groom; to prepare meals; to dial the telephone; and to voluntarily move about with or without assistive devices? Does the person have coordination, balance, ambulatory skills, finger dexterity, grip strength, and other capacities that are necessary to participate fully in day-to-day life?

P—Pain

Is the person experiencing physical, psychological, or spiritual pain? Is the person able to express pain and the desire for relief? Are there cultural barriers between the nurse and the patient that make the assessment of or expression of pain difficult? How does the person customarily attain pain relief (see Chapter 15)?

E—Elimination

Is the person having difficulty with bladder or bowel elimination (see Chapter 10)? Is there a lack of control? Does the environment interfere with elimination and related personal hygiene; for example, are toileting facilities adequate and accessible? Are any assistive devices used, such as a high rise toilet seat or bedside commode, and if so, are they available and functioning? If there are problems, how are they affecting the person's social functioning?

S—Socialization and Social Skills

Is the person able to negotiate relationships in society, to give and receive love and friendship, and to feel self-worth (see Chapter 24)?

Mental Status Assessment

As persons enter their eighties and nineties their risk for impaired cognitive abilities increases (Snowdon, 2002). With increases in age there is an increased rate of dementing illnesses, such as Alzheimer's and Lewy body dementia. Cognitive ability is also easily threatened by any disturbance in physical health. Indeed, altered or impaired mental status may be the first sign of anything from a heart attack to a urinary tract infection. The gerontological nurse must be aware of the need to conduct an assessment of mental status, especially cognitive abilities and mood whenever there is a change in an elder's condition or safety. Several of the most commonly seen instruments are described here, with more details in Chapters 21 and 22. The nurse working in the geriatric setting is often expected to be proficient in their use. To ensure that the results are valid and reliable, they must be administered exactly as they have been created and tested.

Cognitive Measures

Mini-Mental State Examination. The *Mini-Mental State Examination (MMSE)* by Folstein and colleagues (1975) is a 30-item instrument that has been used to screen for cognitive difficulties and is one of the tools often used in the determination of a diagnosis of dementia or delirium. It tests orientation, short-term memory and attention, calculation ability, language, and construction. It cannot be given to persons who cannot see or write or who are not proficient in English. It has not been tested extensively in cultures other than those of northern European descent and so culture bias must always be considered. A score of 30 suggests no impairment, and a score below 24 suggests **potential** dementia; however, adjustments are needed for educational level (Osterweil et al., 2000). In the long-term care setting, the MMSE is administered by either the nurse or the social worker as part of a required periodic assessment. It is used in primary care but not usually in the acute care setting.

Clock Drawing Test. The *Clock Drawing Test* has been used since 1992 (Mendez et al., 1992; Tuokko et al., 1992) as a tool to help identify those with cognitive impairment and is used as a measure of severity. It requires some manual dexterity to complete. It would not be appropriate to use with individuals with any limitations in the use of their dominant hand. A person is presented with a blank piece of paper. He or she is asked to draw a circle and the face of a clock so that it says 2:40 or some other time. Scoring is based on both the position of the numbers and the position of the hands on the clock (Box 7-1). This tool does not establish criteria for dementia, but if performance on the clock drawing is impaired, it suggests the need for further investigation and analysis. It has also been found very useful for assessing delirium in the hospitalized patient (Moylan & Lin, 2004). Another evidence-based version of this measure is Royall's CLOX (Kennedy, 2007).

The Mini-Cog. The *Mini-Cog* was developed as a tool that could establish cognitive status more quickly than the MMSE and without the limitations of educational adjustments. It is the evidence-based tool now recommended (Doerflinger & Carolan, 2007). It combines one aspect of the MMSE (short-term memory recall) with the test of executive function of the Clock Drawing Test. It has been found to be highly sensitive to diagnosing dementia (Borson et al., 2000) and as a predictor of delirium in older hospitalized persons (Brodaty et al., 2006; Alagiakrishnan et al., 2007) (Box 7-2).

The Global Deterioration Scale The *Global Deterioration Scale* (Reisberg et al., 1982) is a classic measure of the levels of cognitive changes as one passes through the process of dementia. It is useful to both the nurse and the family to develop appropriate interventions to help the person to optimize his or her health and anticipate future needs and changes.

Mood Measures

Other tools are needed to assess mood, especially to determine the presence or absence of depression, a common and too often unrecognized problem in older adults. Persons with untreated depression are more functionally impaired and will have prolonged hospitalizations and nursing home stays, lowered quality of life, and shortened length of life (see Chapter 22). Persons with depression may appear as if they have dementia, and many persons with dementia are also depressed. The interconnection between the two calls for skill and sensitivity in the nurse to ensure that elders receive the assessment and care they need. The most commonly used mood measure in both middle-aged and older adults is the *Geriatric Depression Scale (GDS)*, developed by Yesavage and colleagues (1982). The GDS has been extremely successful in determining depression because it deemphasizes physical complaints, sex drive, and appetite—those things most affected by medications. It cannot be used in persons with dementia or cognitive impairment. Chapter 22 provides more detail on the assessment of mood in older adults.

BOX 7-1 Clock Drawing Test

Instructions

Ask the person to do the following on a blank piece of paper:
1. Draw a circle.
2. Place the numbers 1-12 inside the circle as for a clock.
3. Place the hands at 3:45 or a similar time.

Scoring

Draws closed circle	1 point
Places numbers in correct position	1 point
Includes all 12 correct numbers	1 point
Places hands in correct position	1 point

Interpretation

Errors such as grossly distorted contour or extraneous markings are rarely produced by cognitively intact persons. Clinical judgment must be applied, but a low score indicates the need for further evaluation.

Data from Mendez MF, Ala T, Underwood KL: Development of scoring criteria for the clock drawing task in Alzheimer's disease, *J Am Geriatr Soc* 40(11):1095-1099, 1992; Tuokko H, Hadjistaropoulost T, Miller J, et al: The clock test: a sensitive measure to differentiate normal elderly from those with Alzheimer disease, *J Am Geriatr Soc* 40(6): 579-584, 1992.

BOX 7-2 The Mini-Cog

1. Tell the person that you are going to name three objects (e.g., apple, table, coin) and ask the person to repeat the objects after you and remember them.
2. Administer the clock test (see Box 7-1).
3. Ask the person to tell you the objects.
4. Give one point for each recalled word.
   SCORE: 0 recall = indication of dementia
   1-2 recall and clock abnormal = indication of dementia
   1-2 recall and clock normal = no indication of dementia
   3 recall = no indication of dementia

Borson S. The mini-cog: a cognitive "vitals signs" measure for dementia screening in multi-lingual elderly. *Int J Geriatr Psychiatry* 15(11):1021, 2000.

Functional Assessment

A determination of functional status is part of the usual gerontological assessment. If the person is healthy and active, a simple statement documenting that effect may be all that is needed, such as "Patient is active and independent; denies functional difficulties." However, if any potential problems exist, such as for the person with Parkinson's disease or a recent fall, a more detailed functional assessment is conducted.

A thorough functional assessment will help the gerontological nurse promote healthy aging by doing the following:

- Identifying the specific areas in which help is needed or not needed
- Identifying changes in abilities from one period to another
- Assisting in the determination of the need for specific service(s)
- Providing information that may be useful in determining the safety of a particular living situation

Functional abilities have been divided between those associated with the individual's ability to perform the tasks needed for self-care (i.e., those needed to maintain one's health) that is, activities of daily living (ADLs) and those tasks needed for independent living or instrumental activities of daily living (IADLs). ADLs are most often identified as eating, toileting, ambulation, bathing, dressing, and grooming. Three of these tasks (grooming, dressing, and bathing) entail higher cognitive function than the others. The IADLs such as cleaning, yard work, shopping, and money management are considered to be more complex activities necessitating higher physical and cognitive functioning than the ADLs. For persons with dementia, the progressive loss of abilities begins with IADLs and progresses to the ADLs. The nurse must keep in mind

that the willingness and skill to perform specific ADLs and IADLs are influenced by the sociocultural factors unique to the person (Box 7-3).

Numerous tools are available that describe, screen, assess, monitor, and predict functional ability. Like the health history, functional ability is measured by observation, self-report, or proxy. Most of the tools result in an arbitrary score of some kind—a rating of the person's ability to do the task alone, with assistance, or not at all. When such an assessment is needed or conducted, the use of existing and established tools is recommended. Most tools do not break down a task into its component parts, such as picking up a spoon or cup or swallowing, when assessment of eating is done; instead, eating is seen as a total task. The tools are useful in that they serve the purposes noted earlier. However, the ratings are not usually sensitive enough to show small changes in function and are more global in nature.

Activites of Daily Living

The *Katz Index* (Katz et al., 1963) developed in 1963, has served as a basic framework for most of the measures of ADLs since that time. There are several versions of the Katz Index; one is based on a 4-point scale and allows one to score performance abilities as independent, assistive, dependent, or unable to perform. Another version of the tool assigns 1 point to each ADL that can be completed independently and a zero (0) if unable to perform these activities. Scores will range from a maximum of 6 (totally independent) to 0 (totally dependent) (Wallace & Shelkey, 2007). A score of 4 indicates moderate impairment, whereas 2 or less indicates severe impairment (Table 7-2). This scoring puts equal weight on all activities, and the determination of a cutoff score is completely subjective. Despite these limitations, the tool is useful because it

---

BOX 7-3   Functional Performance Tests: Mobility

Standing Balance
Instructions: semitandem stand. The nurse:*
a. First demonstrates the task.
   (The heel of one foot is placed to the side of the first toe of the other foot.)
b. Supports one arm of the person while he or she positions the feet as demonstrated above. The person can choose which foot to place forward.
c. Asks if the person is ready, then releases the support and begins timing.
d. Stops timing when the person moves the feet or grasps the nurse for support or when 10 seconds have elapsed.

*Start with the semitandem stand. If it cannot be done for 10 seconds, then the **side-by-side** test should be done. If the semitandem can be accomplished for the requisite 10 seconds, carry out the full tandem stand following the same instructions as above, except the **full tandem** calls for placing the heel of one foot directly in front of the toes of the other foot.

BOX 7-3   Functional Performance Tests: Mobility—cont'd

Scoring	Full tandem	Semitandem	Side-by-side
0	_____	<10 seconds or unable	<10 seconds or unable
1	_____	<10 seconds or unable	10 seconds
2	<3 seconds or unable	10 seconds	_____
3	3 to 9 seconds	10 seconds	_____
4	10 seconds	10 seconds	_____

Standing Balance score: _____

Walking Speed
Instructions: The nurse:
a. Sets up an 8-foot walking course with an additional 2 feet at both ends free of any obstacles.
b. Places an 8-foot rigid carpenter's ruler to the side of the course.
c. Instructs the older adult to "walk to the other end of the course at your normal speed, just like walking down the street to go to the store." Assistive devices should be used if needed.
d. Times two walks. **The fastest of the two is used as the score.**

Scoring

0	Unable
1	>5.6 seconds
2	4.1 to 5.6 seconds
3	3.2 to 4 seconds
4	<3.2 seconds

Walking Speed score: _____

Chair Stands
Instructions: The nurse:
a. Places a straight-backed chair next to a wall.
b. Asks the older adult to fold the arms across the chest and rise from sitting in the chair to standing 1 time. If successful, the nurse goes on to Step c.
c. Asks the older adult to stand and sit 5 times as quickly as possible.
d. Times from the initial sitting position to the final standing position at the end of the fifth stand.
Scores are for the five rise-and-sits only. If the older adult performs fewer than five repetitions, the score is 0.

Scoring

0	Unable
1	>16.6 seconds
2	13.7 to 16.5 seconds
3	11.2 to 13.6 seconds
4	<11.2 seconds

Chair Stands score: _____ **Total of all performance tests (0-12)** _____

Modified from Guralnik JM, Simonsic EM, Ferrucci L, et al: A short physical performance battery assessment of lower extremity function: association with self-reported disability and prediction of mortality and nursing home admission, *J Gerontol A Biol Sci Med Sci* 49(2):M85-M94, 1994; and Bennett JA: Activities of daily living: old-fashioned or still useful? *J Gerontol Nurs* 25(5):22-29, 1999.

TABLE 7-2	Katz Index of Independence in Activities of Daily Living	
Activities (0 or 1 Point)	**Independence (1 Point)**	**Dependence (0 Points)**
	NO supervision, direction, or personal assistance	**WITH supervision, direction, personal assistance, or total care**
BATHING Points: _____	(1 point) Bathes self completely or needs help in bathing only a single part of the body such as the back, the genital area, or disabled extremity.	(0 points) Needs help with bathing more than one part of the body, or getting in or out of the tub or shower. Requires total bathing.
DRESSING Points: _____	(1 point) Gets clothes from closets and drawers and puts on clothes and outer garments complete with fasteners. May have help tying shoes.	(0 points) Needs help with dressing self or needs to be completely dressed.
TOILETING Points: _____	(1 point) Goes to toilet, gets on and off, arranges clothes, cleans genital area without help.	(0 points) Needs help transferring to the toilet or cleaning self, or uses bedpan or commode.
TRANSFERRING Points: _____	(1 point) Moves in and out of bed or chair unassisted. Mechanical transferring aids are acceptable.	(0 points) Needs help in moving from bed to chair or requires a complete transfer.
CONTINENCE Points: _____	(1 point) Exercises complete self-control over urination and defecation.	(0 points) Is partially or totally incontinent of bowel or bladder.
FEEDING Points: _____	(1 point) Gets food from plate into mouth without help. Preparation of food may be done by another person.	(0 points) Needs partial or total help with feeding or requires parenteral feeding.
TOTAL POINTS = _____	6 = High (patient independent)	0 = Low (patient very dependent)

From Katz S, Down TD, Cash HR, et al: Progress in the development of the index of ADL, *Gerontologist* 10(1):20-30, 1970.

creates a common language about patient function for all caregivers involved in planning overall care.

The *Barthel Index* (Mahoney & Barthel, 1965) is commonly used in rehabilitation settings to measure the amount of physical assistance required when a person can no longer carry out ADLs. It has proven to be especially useful as a method of documenting improvement of a patient's ability especially for those who have suffered a stroke. The Barthel Index ranks the functional status as either independent or dependent and then allows for further classification of independent into intact or limited, and dependent into needing a helper or unable to do the activity at all. Training in the correct use and scoring of this tool is required.

The *Functional Independence Measure (FIM)* is similar to the Barthel Index in that both are used to provide as accurate a picture of the patient's functional status as possible. The FIM provides much more detail and therefore a better picture; however, in the detail is the problem of the time

and skill it takes to administer it (Granger & Hamilton, 1993). It includes measure of ADLs, mobility, cognition, and social functioning. It was developed through the work of a number of experts and has been thoroughly tested. Ordinarily the tool is completed through the joint efforts of the interdisciplinary team and used for both planning and evaluation of progress, most often in the acute rehabilitation setting.

Instrumental Activities of Daily Living

The original tool for the assessment of IADLs was developed by Lawton and Brody (1969). Both the original tool and the subsequent variations use the self-report, proxy, and observed formats with three levels of functioning (independent, assisted, and unable to perform). The pros and cons of using these are the same as the measures of ADLs. Box 7-4 gives an example of a self-rated instrument for IADLs.

BOX **7-4**   **Instrumental Activities of Daily Living**

1. Telephone:
   I: Able to look up numbers, dial, and receive and make calls without help
   A: Able to answer phone or dial operator in an emergency but needs special phone or help in getting number or dialing
   D: Unable to use telephone
2. Traveling:
   I: Able to drive own car or travel alone on bus or taxi
   A: Able to travel but not alone
   D: Unable to travel
3. Shopping:
   I: Able to take care of all shopping with transportation provided
   A: Able to shop but not alone
   D: Unable to shop
4. Preparing meals:
   I: Able to plan and cook full meals
   A: Able to prepare light foods but unable to cook full meals alone
   D: Unable to prepare any meals
5. Housework:
   I: Able to do heavy housework (e.g., scrub floors)
   A: Able to do light housework but needs help with heavy tasks
   D: Unable to do any housework
6. Medication:
   I: Able to take medications in the right dose at the right time
   A: Able to take medications but needs reminding or someone to prepare them
   D: Unable to take medications
7. Money:
   I: Able to manage buying needs, write checks, pay bills
   A: Able to manage daily buying needs but needs help managing checkbook, paying bills
   D: Unable to manage money

I, Independent; *A*, assistance needed; *D*, dependent.
From *Multidimensional Functional Assessment Questionnaire*, ed 2, 1978, by Duke University Center for the Study of Aging and Human Development with permission of Duke University.

Three performance tests related to mobility are simple and quick: the ability to stand with feet together in a side-by-side manner and in a tandem and semitandem position, a timed walk of 8 feet, and a timed rise from a chair and return to a seated position, repeated five times (see Box 7-3).

When assessing both functional status and cognitive abilities, slightly different tools are needed. The *Blessed Dementia Rating Scale* (Blessed et al., 1968) is a 22-item tool scored from 0 to 27. The higher the score, the greater the degree of dementia. This tool incorporates aspects of ADLs, IADLs, memory, recalling events, and finding one's way outdoors. The American Academy of Neurology suggests that there is some evidence that this tool may be useful for persons with early dementia. The *Clinical Dementia Rating Scale Sum of Boxes (CDR-SOB)* (Morris, 1993; O'Bryant, et al., 2010) is also used to assess both functional and cognitive abilities and to promote optimal living with dementia. By determining both the functional status and cognitive stage of the dementia, the nurse can provide considerable anticipatory teaching to both the family and other caregivers.

Integrated Assessments

In some cases an integrated approach is used rather than a collection of separate tools and assessments. The original integrated assessment tool was probably the *Older American's Resources and Service (OARS)* and later the *Multidimensional Functional Assessment Questionnaire (OMFAQ)* created by Eric Pfeiffer and his colleagues at Duke (1979). It has served as the basis of many subsequent measures. All are quite comprehensive and therefore quite lengthy. Completion of these assessments requires a collaborative and interdisciplinary approach and training. When completed, they serve as a resource for a detailed plan of care. Related instruments discussed herein are Fulmer's SPICES, the Minimum Data Set used in skilled nursing facilities, and the OASIS used in certified home care agencies.

Older American's Resources and Service

The original *OARS* instrument was designed to evaluate ability, disability, and the capacity level at which the person is able to function. It is set up in such a manner in that each of five subscales may be used separately. The five subscales include social resources, economic resources, physical health, mental health, and ability to perform ADLs. The person's functional capacity in each area is rated on a scale of 1 (excellent) to 6 (completely impaired). At the conclusion of the assessment a cumulative impairment score (CIS) is established, which can range from the most capable (6) to total disability (30). This aids in establishing the degree of need and the resources required for both daily living and quality of healthy life. Similarities between some aspects of the subscales of the OARS and Maslow's Hierarchy can be found. Information considered in each domain includes the following.

Social Resources. The social resources dimension addresses the social skills and the ability to negotiate and make friends. Is the person able to seek help from friends, family, and strangers? Is there a caregiver available if needed? Who is it, and how long is the person available? Does the individual belong to any social network or group, such as a special interest or church group? How are belonging needs met?

Economic Resources. Data about monthly income and sources (e.g., Social Security, Supplemental Security Income, pensions, income generated from capital) are needed to determine the adequacy of income compared with the cost of living and food, shelter, clothing, medications, and small luxury items. This information can provide insight into the person's relative standard of living and point out areas of need that might be alleviated by use of additional resources unknown to the elder.

Mental Health. Consideration is given to intellectual function, the presence or absence of psychiatric symptoms, and the amount of enjoyment and interaction the person gets from life.

Physical Health. Diagnoses of major and common diseases of older persons, the type of prescribed and over-the-counter medications the person is taking, and the person's perception of his or her health status are the basis of evaluation. Excellent physical health includes participation in regular vigorous activity, such as walking, dancing, or biking at least twice each week, and preferably daily. Seriously impaired physical health is determined by the presence of one or more illnesses or disabilities that are severely painful or life-threatening, or necessitate extensive care.

Activities of Daily Living. The ADLs included in the OARS are walking, getting in and out of bed, bathing, combing hair, shaving, dressing, eating, and getting to the bathroom on time by oneself. The IADLs measured include tasks such as dialing the telephone, driving a car, hanging up clothes, obtaining groceries, taking medications, and having correct knowledge of their dosages.

Fulmer SPICES

The *Fulmer SPICES* is a simple and overall assessment tool of older adults focusing on geriatric syndromes (Wallace and Fulmer, 2007) which has proved reliable and valid when used with persons later life whether in health or illness; in acute, skilled nursing, long-term care facilities; or at home. The acronym *SPICES* refers to sometimes vague but nonetheless very important problems that require nursing interventions: *S*leep disorders, *P*roblems with eating or feeding, *I*ncontinence, *C*onfusion, *E*vidence of falls, and *S*kin breakdown. Nurses are encouraged to make a 3 x 5 card with this acronym on it and carry them with them to use as a reference when caring for older adults (see www.hartfordign.org). It is a system for alerting the nurse to the most common problems that occur in the health and well-being of the older adult, particularly those who have one or more medical conditions.

Resident Assessment Instrument (RAI)

In 1986 the Institute of Medicine (IOM) completed a study indicating that although there was considerable variation, residents in skilled nursing facilities (SNFs) were receiving an unacceptably low quality of care. As a result, nursing home reform was legislated as part of the Omnibus Budget Reconciliation Act (OBRA) of 1987. The creators of OBRA recognized the challenging work of caring for sicker and sicker persons discharged from acute care settings to nursing homes and, along with this, the need for comprehensive assessment, complex decision making and documentation regarding the care that was needed, planned, implemented, and evaluated.

In 1990 a Resident Assessment Instrument (RAI) was created and mandated for use in all long-term care facilities that receive compensation from either Medicare or Medicaid (see Chapter 23) (Dellefield, 2007). Now in its third version, the RAI is composed of three parts, the 450-item Minimum Data Set (MDS 3.0), the Resident Assessment Protocols (RAPs) and associated Resource Utilization Groups or RUGs. The MDS 3.0 provides a health and functional profile throughout the resident's stay; RAPs are structured, problem-oriented frameworks for the organization and direction of the care. Finally, the information forms the basis for the Resource Utilization Group data (RUGs), used to determine the reimbursement rate. The exhaustive and thorough assessment and associated documentation requirement is an attempt to improve and standardize the quality of care provided and help long-term care residents achieve the highest level of functioning and highest quality of life possible (Centers for Medicare and Medicaid Services [CMS], 2011a; Dellefield, 2007). Intended for use to develop the plan of care, the RAI - MDS is now also used for policy applications including case-mix reimbursement and research (Mor et al., 2011). It is additionally used as a quality indicator with a high degree of reliability and validity (Hutchinson et al., 2010).

Nurses are responsible for the coordination of the RAI shortly after a person's admission, at preset intervals (see current requirements at www.cms.gov), and at any time there is a significant change in the resident's health. The RAI process is dynamic and solution-oriented. It is used to gather definitive information on the resident's functioning. As reassessments are done, the nurse and other members of the care team have the opportunity to both document and track the progress toward the resolution of identified problems and make changes to the plan of care as necessary. An identified actual or potential social, medical, or psychological problem that appears in the RAP is known as a trigger. The trigger prompts the nurse to conduct a more detailed assessment, following utilization guidelines (UGs). The care plan is modified as a result of the trigger. The type and level of documentation called for in the RAI facilitates reliable and measurable communication and, when used properly, has the potential to significantly improve outcomes for residents. The resulting picture of the resident is as clear as possible. For persons who will benefit from active rehabilitation, the outcomes include discharge to a lower level of care, such as returning home. For persons whose condition is one of progressive decline, the RAI process can lead to increased comfort and appropriate care. Although the MDS is completed jointly by all members of the interdisciplinary team, the nurse, as the MDS Coordinator, is responsible for verifying the completion of the assessment with his or her signature.

The RAI is entered into computer software for ease of analysis and communication of patient profiles to the federal Centers for Medicare and Medicaid (CMS). These data then become part of an aggregate national database used to better respond to the needs of residents in skilled nursing facilities across the country.

OASIS-C

Like the requirements for standardized documentation in the SNF setting discussed earlier, the provision of skilled care to persons at home was also affected by the Balanced Budget Act of 1997. The Outcomes and Assessment Information Set (OASIS) and the revised OASIS-C were implemented to provide the format for the documentation of a comprehensive assessment, which forms the basis for planning care and measuring patient outcomes–based quality improvement (OBQI) (CMS, 2011b). As with all other assessment and documentation systems, OASIS-C is used both to improve the quality of care and the communication about the individual and serve as a guide for reimbursement. The electronic document is completed in the person's home and later transferred to a central database. These assessments are repeated at intervals during the care period, with the results electronically transmitted to CMS and added to the national database. Nurses supplement the data collected in OASIS to include pertinent information necessary to personalize the care provided.

Documentation for Quality Care

Clinical documentation chronicles, supports, and communicates the results of the assessment. Good documentation will help the nurse identify, monitor, and evaluate treatment or interventions. The recorded assessment provides the data needed for the careful development of the individualized plan of care and the evaluation of patient outcomes. Documentation also provides the communication needed to ensure that a person continues to receive continuity of care—from one shift to another and one caregiver to another and across settings. The nurse who provides care to a patient for whom the previous nurse did not document knows well the potential errors that can be made and the added risk to the patient. At the same time, documentation is the major means for the nurse to demonstrate the quality of care he or she provides. In any setting, documentation is a means to more quickly identify iatrogenic problems and hospital-acquired conditions (HACs) that frequently complicate recovery in seriously ill patients.

Documentation also serves as the basis for the determination of reimbursement in most settings. In skilled nursing facilities this is through the analysis of the RUGs already described when Medicare is the payer. Reimbursement is similarly calculated in home care through the OASIS assessment. While initial reimbursement in acute care settings (hospitals and acute rehabilitation) is preset by diagnosis codes (DRGs), documentation of the assessment at admission, with any change in condition and at discharge have become key factors in the postdischarge responsibility if HACs are found. Since the Patient Self-Determination Act was passed in 1991, all persons entering a health care facility or who begin to receive skilled home care are asked if they have an advance directive and, if not, are provided information about them (see Chapter 23). The nursing records supplement this documentation with more details regarding a person's wishes and include who they want involved in their care, who they want to have access to their records, and their wishes related to everything from organ donation to the use of cardiopulmonary resuscitation (CPR) and the handling of their bodies after death. Patients often discuss these things with nurses during quiet moments. By noting these conversations in the clinical record we are able to both officially document this important information and share it with other members of the health care team. This will better ensure that the patient's wishes are respected.

Documentation Across Health Care Settings

Documentation begins as soon as the person enters the health care system and the assessment begins. While the format may change, the purposes do not.

Documentation in Acute Care and Acute Rehabilitation Care Settings

Documentation in the acute care setting has undergone a significant change in recent years especially with the mandates for upgrading to the Electronic Medical Record. Computers can be found at the bedside, in nurses' pockets, and in strategic locations around the unit. Nurses are given passwords that may be more important than their name tags. Bar codes and even fingerprints are scanned both for access to records, the administration of treatments and medications and the identification of patients. The use of checklists, flow sheets, and standardized tools has become the norm, as has the use of electronic format for everything from the documentation of meals eaten to vital signs to discharge planning. Care maps are used to predict and document the care provided within a preestablished trajectory and to anticipate the day of discharge.

While the use of the electronic medical record or (EMR) is near universal, in some settings, "lower-tech" approaches are still used. There, documentation is done in the form of problem-oriented notes made in the clinical record. The patient is assessed (usually with a checklist); problems are identified and care plans of interventions are developed. In some cases nursing diagnoses developed by the North American Nursing Diagnosis Association (NANDA) using the Nursing Interventions Classification (NIC) are selected from preprinted forms. This format provides a standardization of language and ease of communication between nurses.

Documentation in Long-Term Care Facilities

The term long-term care facility is applied to a number of settings, including family care homes, assisted living facilities (board and care homes), nursing facilities, SNFs, and "swing beds" in rural hospitals (beds that serve for either acute or long-term care, depending on the patient's needs) (see Chapter 3). The level of documentation required varies by setting and is prescribed by state or jurisdiction statutes. In family care homes and assisted living facilities, documentation generally occurs only if a nurse has been hired or is under contract with the facility. This service is always optional and is usually limited to administration of medications or the delegation of this act to nurse's aides.

Both nursing facilities and skilled nursing facilities are making the transition to the electronic medical record but still lag considerably behind acute care facilities. In addition to nursing observations, documentation in these facilities encompasses the recording of day-to-day care such as eating and bowel movement as well as vital signs, periodic assessment, medication and treatment administration, assessment of any unusual event or change in condition, and periodic mandated comprehensive assessments. Documentation in SNFs includes narrative progress notes, flow sheets, checklists, and the RAI as already discussed. When a resident's care is no longer covered by Medicare, narrative notes are reduced to "problem-oriented only" and are completed on an "as-needed" and weekly or monthly basis depending on the facility and licensing body. Good documentation is an expectation of both trained and licensed staff that provide professional care. The nurse is ultimately responsible for both the quality of the care provided and the completeness and accuracy of the documentation of the care and serves as a means of monitoring functional, medical conditions and promoting healthy aging.

Documentation in Home Care

The majority of the care that is provided in the home is by informal caregivers such as family members and others. They will often develop documentation systems of their own to track appointments, medication administration, and health care provider instruction. This system increases the continuity of care. Nurses may need to assist the family in developing and using effective systems.

When skilled care is provided in the home, documentation of assessment and nursing activities follows the Federal requirements, primarily through OASIS and supplemental notations (see earlier). If formal but not skilled care is provided, the documentation system is designed by the providing agency and is primarily for the purpose of coordinating care.

Implications for Gerontological Nursing and Healthy Aging

Health care documentation contains highly personal and confidential information relating to clients, patients, or residents, whether it is written or electronic. For many years the confidentiality of health and medical information was protected through professional codes of ethics. The expectation has always been that the nurse and other health care providers will only access information that relates to a specific individual on a "need to know" basis. Nursing students are taught to avoid talking about patients in hallways, elevators, and lunch rooms or with persons outside their clinical groups, such as friends and family members. The nurse who notes that a neighbor has been admitted to the unit is expected to not review the chart unless he or she is the nurse assigned to provide the care.

However, we have not been as respectful of people's privacy as we should be. This, coupled with the electronic exchange of personal health information, has significantly increased the risk for breaches of confidentiality. In 1996 the Health Insurance Portability and Accountability Act (HIPAA) was passed, legislating the strict protection of the privacy of medical records. The Department of Health and Human Services has the responsibility to ensure this protection. Patients may expect that reasonable steps are taken to ensure that their verbal communications are confidential and that they have complete control as to who has access to their information. It is expected that nursing actions to protect privacy include closing the patient's or resident's door before having health-related conversations or staff's not discussing patient or residents' needs or condition in a location where it could be overheard, for example in hallways or some nurses' stations.

Communication of both assessment information and that which is needed in day-to-day care activities through documentation has become critical to ensure patients' rights, adequate care, and the economic survival of providers. It is the responsibility of the nurse to make sure that communication and documentation are of the highest quality so as to provide error-free and appropriate care and continuity and to maximize both patient outcomes and accurate reimbursement.

Whether the nurse is working with a standardized instrument or creating a new one, the goal of the gerontological nursing assessment is to promote healthy aging. To do this it is necessary to collect data that are the most accurate and to do so in the most efficient, yet caring manner possible. The use of tools serves as a way to organize the collected data necessary for assessment and makes it possible to compare the data from time to time. As noted earlier, each tool has strengths and weaknesses. A number of factors complicate assessment of the older adult. These include the difficulty of differentiating the effects of aging from those originating from disease, the coexistence of multiple diseases, the underreporting of symptoms by older adults, atypical presentation or nonspecific presentation of illness, and the increase in iatrogenic illnesses.

Overdiagnosis or underdiagnosis occurs when the normal age changes are not considered; these include both physical changes and psychosocial changes. Underdiagnosis is far more common in gerontological nursing. Many symptoms or complaints are ascribed to normal aging rather than a health problem that may be developing. Assessing the older adult with multiple chronic conditions is also a challenge. Symptoms of one condition can exacerbate or mask symptoms of another. The gerontological nurse is challenged to provide the highest level of excellence in the care of elders. If a particular tool will facilitate the achievement of this goal, it should be used. If the tool serves little purpose and is burdensome to either the nurse or the patient, it should be avoided or replaced. And without appropriate documentation neither the tool nor the assessment can contribute to the well-being of those who entrust themselves to our care.

KEY CONCEPTS

- Assessment of the physical, cognitive, psychosocial, and environmental status is essential to meeting the specific needs of the older adult and implementing appropriate interventions.
- Whether the data for an assessment tool are collected by self-report, by report-by-proxy, or through nurse observation will affect the quality and quantity of the data.
- Knowledge of how to use a particular gerontological assessment tool is needed to accurately administer it.
- The medical and social complexity of many older adults complicates obtaining and interpreting assessment data.
- Anticipate that hearing and vision may be impaired and compensation may be necessary.
- Expect findings that are abnormal from a younger adult and anticipate the need to begin to differentiate normal age-related changes from potential pathology.
- For those with cognitive impairments, obtaining some assessment data from a proxy may be necessary but can only be done with the patient or legal representative's permission.
- Excellence in documentation sets the stage for excellence in patient care.
- Standardized instruments for patient evaluation are integral to consistent determination of the needs and health status of patients and appropriate reimbursement for care provided.
- Documenting patient status and needs accurately is a key responsibility of the licensed nurse.
- Nurses have a responsibility to protect patient confidentiality at all times, both in spoken communication and in the clinical record.

ACTIVITIES AND DISCUSSION QUESTIONS

1. What is the importance of the measurement of ADLs and IADLs in older adults?
2. What makes an assessment tool effective?
3. Discuss the origins and purpose of the development of standardized documentation systems.
4. Activity: Discuss problems you have experienced with incomplete data or poor documentation in a health facility.
5. Discuss the potential uses of the MDS 3.0, and OASIS-C.
6. Discuss ways in which patient confidentiality is breached and what the nurse can do about this.
7. Explain the reasons why documentation is critical to patient care.

REFERENCES

Alagiakrishnan K, Marrie T, Rolfson D, et al: Simple cognitive testing (mini-cog) predicts in-hospital delirium in the elderly, *J Am Geriatr Soc* 55(2), 314–316, 2007.

Benner P: *From novice to expert,* Menlo Park, CA, 1984, Addison-Wesley.

Blessed G, Tomlinson BE, Roth M: The association between qualitative measures of dementia and of senile change in the cerebral grey matter of elderly subjects, *Br J Psychiatry* 114(512):797–811, 1968.

Borson S, Scanlan J, Brush M, et al: The mini-cog: a cognitive "vital signs" measure for dementia screening in multi-lingual elderly, *Int J Geriatr Psychiatry* 15(11):1021–1027, 2000.

Brodaty H, Low L, Gibson L, et al: What is the best dementia screening instrument for general practitioners to use? *Am J Geriatr Psychiatry* 14:391–400, 2006.

Centers for Medicare and Medicaid Services [CMS]: *MDS 3.0 for nursing homes and swing bed provider.* (2011a). Available at http://www.cms.gov/NursingHomeQualityInits/25_NHQ-IMDS30.asp.

Centers for Medicare and Medicaid Services [CMS]: *OASIS: overview* (2011b). Available at http://www.cms.gov/OASIS.

Dellefield ME: Implementation of the resident assessment instrument/minimum data set in the nursing home as organization: implications for quality improvement in RN clinical assessment, *Geriatr Nurs* 28(6):377–386, 2007.

Doerflinger D, Carolan M: Mental status assessment of older adults: the mini-cog (2007). Available at http://www.hartfordign.org/Resources/Try_This_Series.

Folstein MF, Folstein SE, McHugh PR: Mini-mental state: a practical method for grading the cognitive state of patients for the clinician, *J Psychiatr Res* 12(3):189–198, 1975.

Granger CV, Hamilton BB: The uniform data system for medical rehabilitation: report of first admissions for 1991, *Am J Phys Med Rehabil* 72(1):33–38, 1993.

Hutchinson AM, Milke DL, Maisey S, et al: The resident assessment instrument-minimum data set 2.0 quality indicators: a systematic review, *BMC Health Serv Res* 16(10):166, 2010.

Institute of Medicine [IOM]: *Improving the quality of care in nursing homes: consensus report* (1986). Available at http://www.iom.edu/Reports/1986/Improving-the-Quality-of-Care-in-Nursing-Homes.aspx.

Katz S, Ford AB, Moskowitz RN, et al: Studies of illness in the aged: the index of ADL: a standardized measure of biological and psychosocial function, *JAMA* 185:914–919, 1963.

Kennedy GJ: Brief evaluation of executive dysfunction: an essential refinement in the assessment of cognitive impairment (2007). Available at http://www.hartfordign.org/Resources/Try_This_Series.

Kleinman A: *Patient and healers in the context of culture: an exploration of the borderland between anthropology, medicine, and psychiatry,* Berkeley, 1980, University of California Press.

Lawton MP, Brody EM: Assessment of older people: self-maintaining and instrumental activities of daily living, *Gerontologist* 9(3): 179–186, 1969.

Mahoney FI, Barthel DW: Functional evaluation: the Barthel index, *Md State Med J* 14:61–65, 1965.

Mendez MF, Ala T, Underwood KL: Development of scoring criteria for the Clock Drawing Task in Alzheimer's disease, *J Am Geriatr Soc* 40(11):1095–1099, 1992.

Mor V, Intrator O, Unruth MA, et al: Temporal and geographic variation in the validity and internal consistency of the nursing home resident assessment minimum data set 2.0, *BMC Health Serv Res* 11:78, 2011.

Morris JC: The clinical dementia rating (CDR): current version and scoring rules, *Neurology* 43(11):2412–2414, 1993.

Moylan KC, Lin TL: *The Washington manual: geriatrics subspecialty consult,* New York, 2004, Lippincott Williams & Wilkins.

O'Bryant SE, Lacritz LH, Hall J, et al: Validation of the new interpretive guidelines for the clinical dementia rating scale sum of boxes in the national Alzheimer's coordinating database, *Arch Neurol* 67(6):746–749, 2010.

Osterweil D, Brummel-Smith K, Beck JC: *Comprehensive geriatric assessment,* New York, 2000, McGraw-Hill.

Pfeiffer E: *Physical and mental assessment—OARS,* San Francisco, 1979, Workshop Intensive, Western Gerontological Society.

Reisberg B, Ferris S, deLeon MJ, et al: The global deterioration scale for assessment of primary progressive dementia, *Am J Psychiatry* 139(9):1136–1139, 1982.

Resnick B, Mitty E, editors: *Assisted living nursing: a manual for management and practice,* New York, 2009, Springer.

Snowdon D: *Aging with grace: what the nun study teaches us about leading longer, healthier and more meaningful lives.* New York, 2002, Bantam Books.

Tuokko H, Hadjistaropoulost T, Miller J, et al: The clock test: a sensitive measure to differentiate normal elderly from those with Alzheimer disease, *J Am Geriatr Soc* 40(6):579–584, 1992.

Wallace M, Fulmer T: Fulmer SPICES: an overall assessment tool for older adults (2007). Available at http://www.hartfordign.org/Resources/Try_This_Series.

Wallace M, Shelkey M: Katz index of independence in activities of daily living (2007). Available at http://www.hartfordign.org/Resources/Try_This_Series.

Yesavage JA, Brink TL, Rose T, et al: Development and validation of a geriatric depression screening scale: a preliminary report, *J Psychiatr Res* 17(1):37–49, 1982.

Chapters in Which Assessment Topics Are Addressed

Assessment Topic	Chapter(s)
Activities of daily living (ADLs)	7
Advance care planning	25
Caregiver stress	24
Confusion	21
Cognition	6, 7, 21
Culture	4
Depression	8, 22
Discharge planning/Transitional Care Model (TCM)	3
Functional status	7
Gait, balance, and exercise	12, 13
Hearing	16
Instrumental activities of daily living (IADLs)	7
Integrated assessments	7
Medication use	8
Mental health	7, 22
Nutritional status and hydration	9
Physical assessment	7
Pressure ulcer	12
Safety	12
Sexual function	24
Sleep	11
Social support	24
Spirituality	6
Urinary continence	10
Vision	16

CHAPTER 8

Safe Medication Use

Kathleen F. Jett

evolve evolve.elsevier.com/Ebersole/gerontological

LEARNING OBJECTIVES

Upon completion of this chapter, the reader will be able to:

- Explain age-related pharmacokinetic changes.
- Discuss potential use of chronotherapy.
- Describe drug use patterns and their implications for the older adult.
- Explain the roles of elder, caregiver, and social network in reducing medication misuse.
- List interventions that can help promote medication adherence by the elder.
- Identify diagnoses or symptoms for which psychotropic drugs are prescribed.
- Discuss issues concerning psychotropic medication management in the older population.
- Develop a nursing care plan for patients prescribed psychoactive medications.

GLOSSARY

Adverse reaction A harmful, unintended reaction to a drug.

Bioavailability The amount of drug that becomes available to effect changes in target tissues.

Biotransformation A series of chemical alterations of a drug occurring in the body.

Half-life The time it takes after administration to inactivate half of a drug.

Iatrogenic A result of something that is done or given to a person in the context of providing care.

Potentiation The strengthening of the effect of one or more substances (e.g., food or another drug) when they are used in combination.

Regimen A scheduled plan for the taking of medications, such as twice a day, with food, etc.

Side effect A consequence of a drug or procedure other than that for which it is used (e.g., dry mouth).

Target tissue Tissue or organ intended to receive the greatest concentration of a drug or to be most affected by the drug.

Therapeutic window The range of the plasma concentration of a drug within which it is safe and effective.

THE LIVED EXPERIENCE

It is so hard to keep track of my medications. I try arranging them in little cups to take with each meal, but then there are the ones that I take at odd times. Those are the easiest to forget. I get really confused and think sometimes I have taken them twice and then think I must be going crazy. I really wish I didn't have to take so many pills, but I'm not sure what would happen if I stopped any of them. I don't even know why I'm taking most of them.

Geraldo, hypertensive, diabetic, and having cardiac problems

In the United States, persons 65 years of age and older are the largest users of prescription and over-the-counter (OTC) medications; with the number of medications taken increasing with age. Making up only 13% of the population, they consume 33% of the prescribed medications or a range somewhere between 0 and 13 prescription drugs per person, and about 40% of OTC medications or other supplements such as herbs (Steinman et al., 2006; Gallagher et al., 2007; Brandt, 2010). Ninety percent of the persons at least 65 years of age take at least 1 drug a week, over 40% take at least 5, and 12% use at least 10 different drugs every week. Residents of long-term care facilities take the most medications of all, typically 7 to 8 different ones (Ruscin, 2009; Brandt, 2010). Elders accumulate prescriptions as they accumulate chronic diseases and number of health care providers (Green et al., 2007).

Unfortunately, the number of adverse drug reactions increases with the number of medications used. Adverse drug reactions (ADRs) have been found to be a notable cause for hospitalization as well as a cause of iatrogenic mortality and morbidity for those already hospitalized. This has been found to occur not only in the United States but in countries across the globe.

How elders use their prescribed medicines and other bioactive products depends on many factors related to the person's own unique characteristics, situations, beliefs, understanding about illness, functional and cognitive status, perception of the necessity of the drugs, severity of symptoms, reactions to the medications, finances, access, and alternatives, and the compatibility of such products with their lifestyle. From the perspective of Maslow's Hierarchy of Needs, drugs impinge on all levels. When used appropriately, prescription medications can afford basic survival or even enhance one's quality of life and help achieve self-actualization for those with chronic conditions and disabilities. When they are used inappropriately, they threaten even the most basic level of physiological stability. Yet, at times, even when drugs are used appropriately, they may adversely affect the elder's health and well-being.

Gerontological nurses have a responsibility to help minimize the risks and maximize the safety of medication use in the persons who receive their care. A review of the changes in pharmacokinetics, pharmacodynamics, and issues in drug use are presented in this chapter. The final section deals with the use of psychotropic agents. These are frequently prescribed to frail elders with the potential for both great benefit and significant risk and require special attention.

Pharmacokinetics

The term *pharmacokinetics* refers to the movement of a drug in the body from the point of administration as it is absorbed, distributed, metabolized, and finally, excreted. There is no conclusive evidence of an appreciable change in overall pharmacokinetics with aging; however, there are several changes with aging (see Chapter 5) that may have an effect (Figure 8-1). This chapter is not intended to replace a pharmacology text, but to supplement it for the key points of intersection between safe medication use and the aging process.

Absorption

For a drug to be effective it must be absorbed into the blood stream. The amount of time between the administration of the drug and its absorption depends on a number of factors, including the route of introduction (i.e., intravenous, oral, parenteral, transdermal, or rectal), bioavailability, and the amount of drug that passes into the body. The drug is delivered immediately to the blood stream with administration by intravenous route, and quickly with parenteral and transdermal routes and through mucous membranes such as the rectum and the oral mucosa. Orally administered drugs are absorbed the most slowly through the gastrointestinal tract.

Several normal age-related physiological changes have implications for differences in both the prescribing and the administration of medications for older adults (Table 8-1). The commonly seen increased gastric pH will retard the action of acid-dependent drugs. Delayed stomach emptying may diminish or negate the effectiveness of short-lived drugs that could become inactivated before reaching the small intestine. The absorption of some enteric-coated medications, such as enteric-coated aspirin, which are specifically meant to bypass stomach absorption, may be delayed so long that their action begins in the stomach and may produce gastric irritation or nausea. Absorption is also influenced by changes in gastrointestinal motility. If there is increased motility in the small intestine, drug effect is diminished because of shortened contact time and therefore decreased absorption and effectiveness. Conversely, slowed intestinal motility can increase the contact time and therefore the amount absorbed and the drug's effect. This increases the risk for adverse reactions or unpredictable effects.

Many medications commonly taken by older adults can also affect the absorption of other drugs. Antispasmodic drugs slow gastric and intestinal motility. In some instances the ingested drug's action may be useful, but

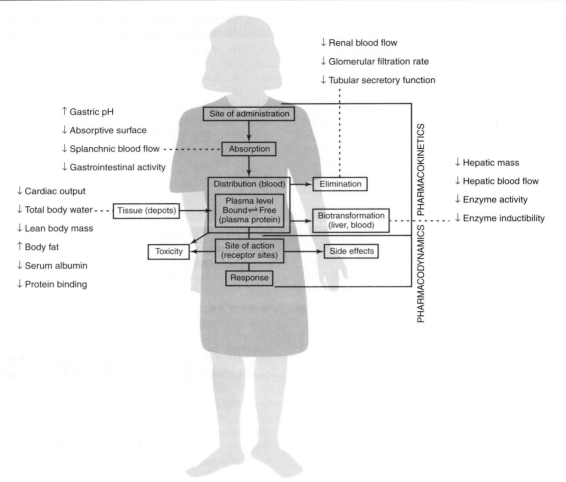

FIGURE 8-1 Physiological changes of aging and the pharmacokinetics and pharmacodynamics of drug use. (Data from Kane RL, Ouslander JG, Abrass IB: *Essentials of clinical geriatrics,* New York, 1984, McGraw-Hill; Lamy PP: Hazards of drug use in the elderly: commonsense measures to reduce them, *Postgrad Med* 76(1):50-53, 1984; Vestal RE, Dawson GW: Pharmacology and aging. In Finch CE, Schneider EL, editors: *Handbook of biology and aging,* New York, 1985, Van Nostrand Reinhold; Roberts J, Tumer N: Pharmacodynamic basis for altered drug action in the elderly, *Clin Geriatr Med* 4(1):127-149, 1988; Montamat SC, Cusack BJ, Vestal RE: Management of drug therapy in the elderly, *N Engl J Med* 321(5):303-309, 1989.)

when there are other medications involved, it is necessary to consider the problem of drug absorption alterations due to drug-drug interaction. Antacids or iron preparations affect the availability of some drugs for absorption by binding the drug with elements and forming chemical compounds. Drug-food interactions may either decrease or increase the amount absorbed. For example when a bisphosphonate such as Fosamax is taken with food of any kind, the absorption is reduced to only a few milligrams, and therefore the drug has no effect on the target organ, the bones; if thyroxin is taken at the same time

as any compounds such as calcium or magnesium, it is inactivated.

Distribution

When a drug is absorbed it must be transported to the receptor site on the target organ to have any effect. Distribution depends on the availability of plasma protein in the form of lipoproteins, globulins, and especially albumin. As drugs are absorbed, they bind with the protein and are distributed throughout the body. Normally, a predictable

TABLE **8-1**	Interaction of Aging and Drug Response, Select Medications	
Class	**Drug**	**Effect of Aging**
Analgesic	Morphine	↑ analgesia
Anticoagulant	Warfarin (Coumadin)	↑ blood time
Bronchodilator	Albuterol	↓ bronchodilation
Cardiovascular agents	ACE IIs	↑ BP reduction
	Enalapril	↑ BP reduction
	Diltiazem	↑ acute reduction in BP
	Verapamil	↑ acute reduction in BP
Diuretic	Furosemide (Lasix)	↓ maximum response
Other	Levodopa	↑ side effects

From Ruscin JM: Drug therapy in the elderly. In *The Merck manual for health professionals* – Epub. Last updated September 2009. Available at http://www.merckmanuals.com/professional/geriatrics/drug_therapy_ in_the_elderly/drug-related_problems_in_the_elderly.html#v1133742.

percentage of the absorbed drug is inactivated as it is bound to the protein. The remaining free drug is available in the blood stream and has therapeutic effect when an effective concentration is reached in the plasma. Many older adults have an insignificant reduction in the serum albumin level. In others, especially those with prolonged illness or malnutrition (such as residents in skilled nursing facilities), the serum albumin may become dramatically diminished. When this occurs, toxic levels of available free drug may accumulate unpredictably, especially of highly protein-bound medications with narrow therapeutic windows, such as phenytoin and warfarin (Ruscin, 2009).

Potential alterations of drug distribution in late life are related to changes in body composition, particularly decreased lean body mass, increased body fat, and decreased total body water (see Figure 8-1). Decreased body water leads to higher serum levels of water-soluble drugs, such as lithium, digoxin, ethanol, and aminoglycosides. Increased serum levels increase the risk for toxicity. Adipose tissue nearly doubles in older men and increases by one half in older women; therefore drugs that are highly lipid-soluble are stored in the fatty tissue, extending and possibly elevating the drug effect (Masoro & Austed, 2003). This affects drugs such as lorazepam, diazepam, chlorpromazine, phenobarbital, and haloperidol (Haldol).

Metabolism

Biotransformation or metabolism, is the process by which the body modifies the chemical structure of the drug.

Through this process the compound is converted to a metabolite that is later more easily excreted. A drug will continue to exert a therapeutic effect as long as it remains in either its original state or as an active metabolite. Active metabolites retain the ability to have a therapeutic effect, as well as the same or a greater chance of causing adverse effects. For example, the metabolites of acetaminophen (Tylenol) can cause liver damage with higher dosages (> 4 g/24 hr or more than four extra-strength products). The duration of drug action is determined by the metabolic rate and is measured in terms of half-life, or how long the drug remains active in the body.

A number of enzymes play an active part in drug metabolism. Among these are a group known as the cytochrome P450 (CYP450) monooxygenase system. The system is made up of about 50 isoforms, each of which has the potential to metabolize a drug by adding or subtracting part of the drug molecule. When this occurs the drug can be dramatically changed from its original state or even its intended effect. While age does not appear to affect the functioning of the CYP450 system, we now know that genetics have a great effect (Box 8-1).

BOX **8-1**   Focus on Genetics

As knowledge of genetics explodes, so does our ability to consider the possibility of what has come to be called "personalized medicine." Included in this is consideration of someday selecting medications and formulations consistent with the metabolic enzymes specific to the individual, which should optimize therapeutic effect while minimizing or eliminating any untoward effects. *Cytochrome P450* refers to a group of enzymes found primarily in the liver and responsible for the metabolism and excretion of the majority of drugs. Four phenotypic categories of persons relative to the speed of P450 metabolism have been identified. Someone who is a "poor" or "slow" metabolizer will excrete more slowly and therefore can achieve the same therapeutic effect with a low dose of a medication compared with the high dose needed by a "rapid" or even "ultrarapid" metabolizer. Among persons from the regions of northern Europe, 5% to 10% are poor metabolizers. This contrasts with persons from parts of Asia and Africa, among whom only 1% are poor metabolizers.

From Bartlett D: Drug therapy gets personal with genetic profiling. *Am Nurse Today* 6(5):23-28, 2011; Tiwari AK, Souza RP, Muller DJ: Pharmacogenetics of anxiolytic drugs. *J Neural Transm* 116:667, 2009.

The liver is the primary site of drug metabolism. With aging, the liver's activity, mass, volume, and blood flow are reduced and hepatic clearance may decrease by up to 30% to 40% (Ruscin, 2009). These changes result in a potential decrease in the liver's ability to metabolize drugs such as benzodiazepines (e.g., the tranquilizer lorazepam [Ativan]) (Table 8-2). These changes result in a significant increase in the half-life of these drugs. For example, the half-life of diazepam (Valium) in a younger adult is about 37 hours, but in an older adult extends to as long as 82 hours. If the dose and timing are not adjusted, the drug can accumulate, and the administration of a single dose can have significantly more effects (and longer) than in a younger person. Except in the rarest of circumstances Valium should not be used because of this (American Geriatrics Society [AGS], 2012).

TABLE 8-2	**Drugs to Watch: Examples of Commonly Used Medications Affected by Normal Changes with Aging**	
Class or category	**Affected by Decreased Hepatic Metabolism**	**Affected By Decreased Renal Excretion**
Analgesic/ antiinflamatory	Ibuprofen (Advil) Naproxen (Aleve) Morphine	
Antibiotics		Cipro Macrobid
Cardiovascular	Amlodipine (Norvasc) Diltiazem (Cardizem) Verapamil (Calan)	Captopril (Capoten) Digoxin (Lanoxin) Enalapril (Vasotec) Lisinopril (Zestril)
Diuretics		Furosemide (Lasix) HCTZ
Others	Levodopa	Glyburide Ranitidine (Axid)
Psychoactive drugs	Alprazolam (Xanax) Diazepam (Valium) Trazadone	Risperidone

From Ruscin JM: Drug therapy in the elderly. In *The Merck manual for health professionals* – Epub. Last updated September 2009. Available at http://www.merckmanuals.com/professional/geriatrics/drug_therapy_in_the_elderly/drug-related_problems_in_the_elderly.html#v1133742.

Excretion

Drugs and their metabolites are excreted in sweat, saliva, and other secretions but primarily through the kidneys. However, because kidney function declines significantly in aging (up to 50% decrease by the time one is 80 years of age), so does the ability to excrete or eliminate drugs in a timely manner (see Table 8-2). The considerably decreased glomerular filtration rate leads to prolongation of the half-life of drugs, or the amount of time required to eliminate the drug, again presenting opportunities for accumulation and increasing the potential for toxicity or other adverse events. Although renal function is highly individualized and cannot be estimated by the serum creatinine level, we approximate it by calculating the creatinine clearance (see equation). Reductions in dosages for drugs excreted by the kidneys (e.g., allopurinol, vancomycin) are needed when the creatinine clearance is reduced. Reductions in dosages may also be needed when the patient is very ill or dehydrated.

Estimated creatinine clearance (the Cockcroft-Gault equation):

$$\frac{(140 - age) \times wt\ (kg)\ (\times\ 0.85\ only\ if\ female)}{(serum\ creatinine\ \times\ 72)}$$

For alternative calculations, see http://nkdep.nih.gov/professionals/gfr_calculators.

Pharmacodynamics

Pharmacodynamics refers to the interaction between a drug and the body (see Figure 8-1). The older the person gets, the more likely there will be an altered or unreliable response of the body to the drug. Although it is not always possible to explain the change in response, several mechanisms are known. For example, the aging process causes a decreased response to beta-adrenergic receptor stimulators and blockers; decreased baroreceptor sensitivity; and increased sensitivity to a number of medications, especially anticholinergics, benzodiazepines, narcotic analgesics, warfarin (Coumadin), and the cardiac drugs diltiazem and verapamil (Briggs, 2005). If food-drug interactions occur, the problems are worsened. For example, drinking grapefruit juice at the same time as one takes a "statin" such as Lipitor or any number of antibiotics may cause an unreliable response. There is also a growing body of knowledge about the interaction of herbal preparations and currently prescribed medications (Table 8-3). For example, ginkgo biloba is commonly thought to enhance cognitive function.

TABLE 8-3	Selected Herb-Medication and Herb-Disease Interactions		
Herb	**Medication**	**Complication**	**Nursing Action**
Chamomile	Warfarin	May increase risk of bleeding	Advise to avoid teas and other products which contain the product
Garlic	Warfarin or any anticoagulant or antiplatelet drug NSAIDs	Risk of bleeding increases	Advise client not to take without provider approval
	Anticlotting drugs such as streptokinase and urokinase	May decrease effect	Advise against use
	Antihypertensives	May increase antihypertensive effect	Monitor BP
	Antihyperglycemic drugs	Serum glucose control may improve, lowering the amount of medication needed	Monitor blood glucose levels
Ginkgo	Aspirin Heparin and warfarin	Risk of bleeding increases	Teach client not to take without approval of provider
	Antihyperglycemic drugs	May alter blood glucose levels	Monitor blood glucose closely
	Antihypertensives Nifedipine	May cause increased effect	Monitor blood pressure
Ginseng	Antihyperglycemic drugs	May intensify effect	Monitor for hypoglycemia
	Anticoagulants and antiplatelet drugs	May increase bleeding	Advise use with caution
	Corticosteroids	May interfere with action	Advise against use
	Digoxin	May increase blood level	Advise against use
Green tea	Warfarin	May alter anticoagulant effects	Advise against use
Hawthorn	Digoxin	May cause a loss of potassium, leading to drug toxicity	Monitor blood levels
	Beta blockers and other drugs lowering blood pressure and improving blood flow	May be additive in effects	Monitor blood pressure meticulously; advise that this concern extends to erectile dysfunction drugs also
St. John's wort	HMG-CoA reductase inhibitors (e.g., Lipitor, simvistatin)	May decrease plasma concentrations of these drugs	Monitor levels of lipids
	Digoxin	Decreases the effects of the drug	Advise against use
	Alprazolam (Xanax)	May decrease effect of drug	Advise against use
	Efavirenz and other anti-HIVs	May decrease drug level	Advise against use
	Photosensitizing drugs (e.g., NSAIDs, some antibiotics)	Increased photosensitivity	Advise sun block use
	Tramadol	May increase risk of serotonin syndrome	Advise against use
	Olanzapine (Zyprexa)	May cause serotonin syndrome	Advise against use
	SSRIs (e.g., Xoloft)	Excessive sedation	Advise against use
	Albuterol	Decreases effect	Monitor drug effects
	Warfarin (Coumadin)	May decrease anticoagulant effect	Advise against use
	Amlodipine	Lowers efficacy of calcium channel	Advise against use

HIV, Human immunodeficiency virus; *HMG-CoA,* 3-hydroxy-3-methylglutaryl coenzyme A; *NSAIDs,* nonsteroidal antiinflammatory drugs; *SSRIs,* selective serotonin reuptake inhibitors.

From Basch E, Ulbricht C: *Natural standard herb & supplement handbook: the clinical bottom line,* St. Louis, 2005, Mosby; Jellin JM, editor: *Natural medicines comprehensive database* (2006). Available at www.naturaldatabase.com/; *NDH pocket guide to drug interactions,* Philadelphia, 2002, Lippincott, Williams & Wilkins; Yoon SL, Schaffer SD: Herbal, prescribed, and over-the-counter drug use in older women: prevalence of drug interactions, *Geriatr Nurs* 27(2):118-129, 2006; Merck Sharp & Dohme Corp: Some possible dietary supplement-drug interactions. In *The Merck manual for health care professionals* (2011). Available at http://www.merckmanuals.com/media/professional/pdf/Table_331-1.pdf.

However, it will increase the potential for bleeding when an anticoagulant such as Coumadin is used at the same time (Youngkin, 2012). In addition to the expected dry mouth, drugs with anticholinergic properties can cause confusion, constipation, blurred vision, orthostatic hypotension, urinary retention, or heat stroke, even at low doses (Ruscin, 2009). The use of benzodiazepines is associated with an increased risk for accidental injury, and they are on the "do-not-use" list for older adults (AGS, 2012).

Chronopharmacology

Another factor that affects both pharmacokinetics and pharmacodynamics are the normal biorhythms of the body. The relationship of biological rhythms to variations in the body's response to drugs is known as chronopharmacology. Although it has not yet been explored in aging, chronopharmacology is a developing science that may lead to more effective drug therapy (Ohdo, 2010). The best time to administer medications is now being considered in light of the biorhythms of various physiological processes. For example, if a cortisone tablet (e.g., from a Medrol dose pak) is taken in the morning it suppresses the adrenocortical system very little. If the same dose were given divided over the day, unwanted effects of the drug will occur from suppression of the hypothalamus-pituitary-adrenal axis.

As noted earlier, absorption depends on gastric acid pH, the level of motility of the gastrointestinal tract, and blood flow. All have been shown to have biorhythmical variations. Distribution of protein-bound drugs depends on albumin and glycoproteins produced by the liver. During the day, albumin levels are high, but they are low in the early morning. Drug metabolism is also biorhythmical due to changes in the liver over the course of the day. Renal elimination depends on kidney perfusion, glomerular filtration, and urine acidity and has shown rhythmic variation. The brain, the heart, and blood cells have also been found to have varied rhythmicity, resulting in a cyclical response for beta blockers, calcium channel blockers, angiotensin-converting enzyme (ACE) inhibitors, nitrates, and other, similar drugs. Table 8-4 shows some of the rhythmical influences on diseases and physiological processes.

As more is learned about chronotherapeutics, the potential for decreasing individual doses of medications and/or the frequency of administration is present. As we are able to do so we will be able to significantly decrease the potential for adverse drug events while maximizing therapeutic effects.

TABLE 8-4	Rhythmical Influences on Disease and Physiological Processes
Disease or Process	**Rhythmical Influence**
Allergic rhinitis	Symptoms worse in the morning
Arterial blood pressure	Circadian surge—morning hours
Asthma	Greatest respiratory distress overnight (during sleeping) Symptoms peak in early morning (4 to 5 AM)
Blood plasma	Plasma volume falls at night, thus hematocrit increases
Cancer	Tumor cells proliferate when normal cell miosis is low
Cardiac disease	Angina, myocardial infarction, thrombolytic stroke occur in the first 4 hours after waking (peak 9 AM) (through 10 PM) (Prinzmetal's angina—during sleep)
Catecholamines	Increase in early morning
Fibrinolytic activity	Increase in early morning
Platelet activation	May result from abnormality in circadian rhythm, which affects cortisol levels, body temperature, sleep-wake cycle
Gastric system	Gastric acid secretion peaks every morning (2 to 4 AM); circannual variability—incidence of gastric ulcers greater in winter
Osteoarthritis	Pain more severe in morning
Potassium excretion	Lowest in morning; highest in late afternoon
Rheumatoid arthritis	Pain more severe in late afternoon
Systemic insulin	Highest in afternoon

Medication-Related Problems and Older Adults

Polypharmacy

Although there is controversy about how many drugs are "too many," polypharmacy is the term used to indicate multiple drug use, and usually this implies the use of some drugs that are duplicated or unnecessary (Figure 8-2). Junius-Walker and colleagues (2007) define polypharmacy as taking more than five medications at the same time. In their study of German elders, the average number of prescribed

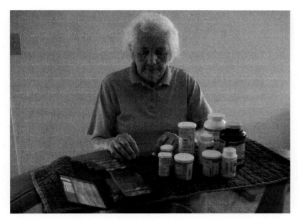

FIGURE 8-2 Polypharmacy. (Courtesy Shannon Perry, Phoenix, AZ.)

medications was 3.7 and the average number of over-the-counter (OTC) bioactive products was 1.4. They also found that almost 27% of those surveyed took over five medications; and, as the number increased, so did the likelihood of inclusion of inappropriate medications (ineffective, duplicative, or not indicated). Polypharmacy may occur "accidentally" if an existing drug regimen is not considered when new medications are prescribed or any number of the thousands of OTC preparations and supplements are added to the prescribed medications. The two major concerns with polypharmacy are the increased risk for drug interactions and the increased risk for adverse events. Adverse events include adverse drug interactions and reactions, adverse drug withdrawal, and therapeutic failures.

Drug Interactions

The more medications a person takes, the greater the possibility that one or more of them will interact with each other, with an herbal product, with a nutritional supplement, with food, or with alcohol. When two or more medications or foods are taken together or close together, the drugs may potentiate one another, or make one or both either more or less effective.

An interaction may result in altered pharmacokinetic activity, that is, alterations in the absorption, distribution, metabolism, or excretion of one or any of the medications. Absorption can be delayed by drugs exerting an anticholinergic effect. Tricyclic antidepressants act in this manner to decrease gastrointestinal motility and interfere with the absorption of other drugs. More than one drug may compete to simultaneously occupy the necessary binding receptors, preventing one or the other from reliably reaching the target organs and creating a varied bioavailability of one or both.

Interference with enzyme activity may alter metabolism and cause drug deficiencies or toxic and adverse responses from altered renal tubular function. Outside the body, interactions can occur any time that two medications or foods are mixed together before administration. For example, when delivering medications through a feeding tube, giving each one separately takes more time than is usually feasible. In haste the nurse may crush and deliver all of them simultaneously. The appropriate administration requires that the nurse know not only which medications are "crushable" but also which can be administered together. For example, Fosamax and the other bisphosphonates must be taken with a full glass of water 1 hour before any other medication, beverage, or food is ingested.

In pharmacodynamic interactions, one drug alters the patient's response to another drug without changing the pharmacokinetic properties. This can be especially dangerous for older adults when two or more drugs with the same effect are additive, that is, together they are more potent than each one taken separately. Unless attention is paid to what the overall drug list includes, when each drug is administered, and what other products are taken, a harmful situation of polypharmacy will occur. The nurse decreases the likelihood of this happening by monitoring the medications he or she administers and by encouraging the persons under their care to do the same. Although there is much that is unknown about the use of herbs and other bioactive substances, as studies are completed, the nurse will need to learn more and more about potential adverse reactions and interactions in order to safely manage medications.

Adverse Drug Reactions

An adverse drug reaction (ADR) or adverse drug event (ADE) is an unwanted pharmacological effect, ranging from a minor annoyance to death and including allergic reactions. These may be iatrogenic, drug-drug, drug-supplement, or drug-disease. It has been estimated that a person taking two different drugs has a 13% chance of having an ADR at some point, compared to 82% of those taking seven or more drugs (Constantiner, 2011). ADRs can sometimes be predicted from the pharmacological action of the drug (e.g., bone marrow depression from cancer chemotherapy; bleeding from Coumadin). Predictable ADRs can also occur when a patient is started on a drug at a dosage that is inappropriately high or one that necessitates laboratory monitoring and adjustment that is not done (e.g., lithium, Coumadin).

ADRs occur in all situations in which one takes or is administered medications. Older adults are four time more likely to be hospitalized for an ADR than younger persons (Ruscin, 2009). Page and Ruscin (2006) found that 31.9% of the elders studied experienced at least one ADR while hospitalized. In a review of several studies of ADRs in nursing homes, Handler and colleagues (2006) found the rate to range from 1.19 to 7.26 per 100 resident months. Atypical antipsychotics, warfarin, antidepressants, and sedative-hypnotics are most commonly associated with preventable ADRs in the nursing home setting, with hypoglycemic agents, nonsteroidal antiinflammatory agents (NSAIDs), and benzodiazepines in the community (Ruscin, 2009). All of these are frequently prescribed to older adults. Because of the large number of medications taken by most older adults in long-term care settings and their frequently altered nutritional and fluid status, the risk for adverse reactions is of special concern to nurses working in this setting. It is estimated that 27% of the ADRs in the community and 42% of those in the nursing home are preventable (AGS, 2012).

ADRs are not always predictable. An older patient who is well controlled on a stable dose of a drug may undergo a change in his or her physiology or environment and the body's response to the drug may be altered (e.g., levothyroxine [Synthroid]). Changes in diet can also have a profound impact on drug effect. For example, decreased fluid intake can cause lithium toxicity and increased intake of leafy green vegetables will counteract the anticoagulant effects of Coumadin and aspirin (Miller, 2008). Some drugs interfere with the body's ability to regulate temperature (e.g., antipsychotics, stimulants, anticholinergics) such that hot weather can lead more easily to heat stroke (Ruscin, 2009). Other drugs are photosensitizing, and an increase in sun exposure can lead more quickly to sunburn than expected (e.g., sulfa drugs, antidepressants, and many antipsycotics) (Semla et al., 2008). Older adults who have decreased fluid intake because of illness or because they cannot get to fluids, or who have inadequate intake during hot weather, may quickly become volume depleted and develop increased sensitivity to the orthostatic hypotensive effects of alpha blockers (e.g., phenothiazines, terazosin) or toxicity to antipsychotics (Jett, 2012).

One of the most troublesome ADRs for the older adult is drug-induced delirium and confusion. Polypharmacy with several psychoactive drugs exerting anticholinergic actions is perhaps the greatest precipitator of delirium as an adverse reaction. Too often delirium goes unrecognized as an ADR and instead is viewed as a worsening of preexisting dementia or even new-onset dementia (see Chapter 21). Any time there is a change in the person's cognitive abilities or mental status, the possibility of drug effect must be thoroughly evaluated. See Box 8-2 for a partial list of drugs with the potential to adversely affect cognitive functioning.

BOX 8-2　Common Medications with the Potential to Cause Cognitive Impairment

Alcohol
Analgesics
Anticholinergics
Antidepressants
Antihistamines
Antiparkinsonian agents
Antipsychotics
Benzodiazepines
Beta blockers
Digitalis, Lanoxin
Diuretics
Muscle relaxants
Sedatives, hypnotics

Another common adverse effect seen in older adults is lethargy, especially with the use of a number of the cardiovascular agents and antidepressants. Like confusion, lethargy can also be misinterpreted as a symptom of the worsening of cardiac, respiratory, or neurological conditions rather than as an ADR.

Among other troublesome effects are those related to sexual functioning. Although they are not detailed here, many medications interfere with or contribute to sexual dysfunction for adults of any age (see Chapter 24). The categories that are most responsible are cardiovascular drugs (some antihypertensives and ACE inhibitors) and some of the psychotropic drugs (e.g., antidepressants, phenothiazines).

Potentially Inappropriate Medication (PIM)

According to Ruscin (2009) a drug is inappropriate if "its potential for harm is greater than its potential for benefit." Kaur and colleagues (2009) define inappropriate prescribing as "when alternative therapy . . . is either more effective or associated with a lower risk to treat the same condition" (p. 1013). Due to multiple factors associated with aging, especially the increased number of drugs prescribed to older adults, the likelihood of receiving an inappropriate medication at some time is quite high. About 3% of all ER visits in persons at least 65 years of age are attributed to these, especially anticoagulants, antiplatelet drugs, hypoglygemic agents, and those with a narrow therapeutic index such as digoxin. Problems with digoxin, insulin, or warfarin (Coumadin) account for one third of ER visits. Taking PIMs have been found to lead to a number of problems, including gastrointestinal bleeding, falls, and delirium. While about 20% of community-living elders take at least one inappropriate medication, this number is higher for those in institutional care settings.

To address this problem, the first "Beers Criteria" was published in 1991 identifying the medications for which the risks needed careful consideration versus the benefits when prescribed to persons over 65 years of age. This was updated in 1997 and 2003 and most recently in March 2012 (Resnick & Fick, 2012). The new list identifies 53 medications or classes which are divided into three categories: potentially inappropriate medications and classes to avoid in older adults regardless of condition, those potentially inappropriate in certain disease states and syndromes, and those which should only be used with caution (AGS, 2012). Among the number of potentially inappropriate medications added to the 2003 list are Megace (megestrol), Micronase (glyburide), and sliding scale insulin. There are significant efforts underway at the national level to reduce the number of PIMs from being prescribed to older adults. For examples and information on accessing the entire list, see Table 8-5. The Beers list has been recommended as a "best practice" by the Hartford Institute for Geriatric Nursing (see www.consultgerirn.org).

Misuse of Drugs

The more drugs taken, the more likely misuse will occur. Forms of drug misuse include overuse, underuse, erratic use, and contraindicated use. Misuse can occur for any number of reasons, from inadequate skills of the nurse or the prescriber, to misunderstanding of instructions, or to inadequate funds to purchase prescribed medications. What if the elder is instructed but it is actually a caregiver who administers the medications? Although this is often referred to as noncompliance or nonadherence, "misuse" is a term that is more descriptive of what is happening. For older adults without medication insurance coverage, such as recent immigrants, the cost of necessary medication may be prohibitive.

Misuse by patients may be accidental, such as happens through misunderstanding or inability to read labels or understand instructions, or it may be deliberate, such as in an attempt to make a prescription last longer for financial reasons or because of beliefs that the dose is either too low or too high. For a striking example of misunderstandings and cultural differences between prescribers and patients related to medication use, the reader is referred to Anne Fadiman's (1998), *The Spirit Catches You and You Fall Down.*

TABLE 8-5	Examples of Drugs Considered Inappropriate for the Elderly
Drug	**Concern**
Alprazolam (Xanex)	Rapid addiction, prolonged sedation effects, potential for confusion and falling. Long-acting benzodiazepine
Amitriptyline (Elavil)	Strong anticholinergic and sedating properties, little effect on depression. With low does, sometimes effective for neurogenic pain
Chlorpropamide (Diabinese)	Long lasting, danger of hypoglycemia increased in elderly
Cimetidine (Tagamet)	Significant risk for ADR with many substances and medications
Cyclobenzaprine (Flexeril)	Anticholinergic side effects, sedation, weakness
Diazepam (Valium)	Long-acting benzodiazepines produce prolonged sedation, increasing fall risk and confusion risk (see alprazolam)
Diphenhydramine (Benedryl)	Excessive sedation, dry mouth, urinary retention, confusion
Dipyridamole (Persantine)	Orthostatic hypotension, no demonstrated effect on cognition
Disopyramide (Norpace)	May induce heart failure, strongly anticholinergic
Doxepin (Sinequan)	Strong anticholinergic and sedating properties
Meperidine (Demerol)	Metabolite accumulation in elderly, can cause tremors and seizures
Oxybutynin (Ditropan)	Strongly anticholinergic, confusion
Temazepam (Restoril)	Confusion, prolonged half-life

Adapted from multiple sources, all based on American Geriatric Society: American Geriatrics Society updated Beers Criteria for potentially inappropriate medication use in older adults, *J Am Geriatr Soc* 60(4):616-631, 2012. Available at http://www.americangeriatrics.org/health_care_professionals/clinical_practice/clinical_guidelines_recommendations/2012.

When a patient is labeled as noncompliant, the nurse and other health care personnel may become exasperated and angry at the individual for his or her failure to follow the established plan of care. In an attempt to help and do what they think is best for the patient, the nurse and other care providers tend to forget or ignore that one cannot and will not comply with a prescription or treatment plan under certain circumstances, such as when it is incompatible with the person's day-to-day life. For example, the individual cannot follow the instruction "take medication three times per day with meals" if he or she eats only two meals each day.

Memory failures associated with nonadherence to medication regimens are of two general types: forgetting the way to take medications correctly and "prospective" recall failure, which is failure to remember to take medication at the correct times (Miller, 2008). The more frequently a medication must be taken, the less anyone will comply. With more and more medications coming in once-daily dosing rather than three or four times each day, we can expect more people to take their medications as instructed.

Problems with health literacy also limit the ability to correctly take medications. Many older adults, especially those from minority groups or new immigrants, have low levels of literacy or no English literacy; written instructions should be at the third-grade level or below (see http://www.npsf.org/pchc/health-literacy.php; http://www.pfizerhealthliteracy.com/). Limitations in vision will interfere with the reading of instructions, especially of bottle labels. One can ask the pharmacist to use large type or symbols. The practice of nurses and doctors giving rapid-fire directions is not effective when addressing most persons, especially those with hearing impairments or the normal age-related need for slightly slower verbalizations; and the use of ambiguous terms such as "slowly increase" or "only in moderation" leads to further opportunities for misuse. The use of interpreters in giving health instructions to older adults must be modified from some standard practices (see Chapter 4).

Unfortunately, it is also common for the nurse to explain the treatment and give directions concerning medications when the patient is physically uncomfortable or is about to be discharged from a care facility; to explain in English even when the person has limited English proficiency; or to explain in a noisy or busy place. Background noise or an unfamiliar accent of the nurse, can significantly reduce understandability of speech for those with normal age-related hearing loss (see Chapter 16).

The individual must first comprehend and be committed to the treatment. The care provider must be able to communicate the information in a way that compensates for language differences and physical-sensory and cognitive changes so that the person understands. The person also must accept the need for the medication as it is prescribed to be willing to follow the treatment plan. The elder must be able to use what has been learned to obtain the prescribed medication, apply instructions, and adjust the regimen to his or her life patterns.

Implications for Gerontological Nursing and Healthy Aging

Assessment

The initial step in ensuring that elders use drugs safely and effectively is to conduct a comprehensive drug assessment. Although in some settings a clinical pharmacist collects the medication history, more often it is completed through the combined efforts of the licensed or registered nurse and the prescribing health care provider (a physician or a nurse practitioner).

In the outpatient, ambulatory care setting, it is best to use a "brown bag approach," or to ask the person to bring in all medications and other products they are currently taking. As each container is removed from the bag, the person is asked how he or she actually takes the medicine rather than depending on how the prescription is written, to begin to determine possible misunderstandings or misuse. An alternative method is a 24-hour medication recall, such as "Tell me everything you have taken in the last 24 hours." Two final approaches are associated with the review of systems or problems. These questions will be something like, "What do you take for your heart? circulation? breathing?" Or, if you know the person's major health problems, you may say, for example, "What do you take for headaches?" or "What do you use for indigestion?" Without the bag of medications or a list of some kind, patients often answer some of the above questions with descriptions (e.g., "a little blue pill" or "a bad-tasting one"), but it is a start.

In other settings obtaining accurate information is considerably more difficult. Transfers to the hospital are often in times of emergencies when information about medications is not available. In a cross-sectional study of medication following transfers to nursing homes discrepancies were found in almost 75% of patients (Marcum et al., 2010). Similar problems occur in the transfer between long-term care settings and back to home when the patient may have difficulty deciphering changes to previous drug regimens and may take the former medications instead of the new ones or both. When medical records become universally electronic a significant number of medication errors are expected to decrease and the ease and accuracy of the assessment will increase.

As the nurse learns the herbs, supplements, and OTC and prescribed medications that are taken, the assessment can continue. There is a great deal of information that is needed, but it is vital to the promotion of health. See Box 8-3 for examples of the information needed in a comprehensive medication history for all substances taken. Through this assessment the nurse can learn of discrepancies between the

---

BOX 8-3   Components of a Comprehensive Medication Assessment

Medications taken and prescribed, as described by patient, with names, doses, and frequency

Ability to self-administer medications

Diagnosis associated with each medication

Belief regarding effectiveness and necessity of medications

Over-the-counter and herbal preparations, with doses, frequency, and reason taken

Nutritional supplements, with doses, frequency, and reason taken

Medication-related problems, such as side effects, difficulty with adherence

Ability to pay for and obtain prescription medications

Source of prescriptions, including those borrowed from others

Persons involved in decision making regarding medications

Use of other drugs, such as tobacco or nicotine in gum, patch, or smoking

Use of social drugs, such as alcohol and caffeine, and nonprescription drugs

Recently discontinued drugs

History of allergies, interactions, and adverse drug reactions

Strategies used to remember when to take drugs as prescribed

Identification of malnutrition and hydration status

Recent drug blood levels as appropriate

Recent measurement of liver and calculation of renal functioning

---

BOX 8-4   Common Sources of Iatrogenic Drug Problems in Older Adults

Drug interactions

Inadequate monitoring

Inappropriate drug choice

Unnecessary treatment

Overtreatment or dosage

Undertreatment

BOX 8-5   Minimizing Iatrogenic Adverse Drug Reactions

Use electronic medical records whenever possible.

Stop and think whenever patient is prescribed a new medication:

Is it a potentially inappropriate medication or dosage?

What is the patient's renal function and will this affect the drug dose?

Is there a potential drug-drug interaction?

Is there a potential drug-disease interaction?

Is there a duplication of any other medications or supplements the patient is taking?

Consider potential effect of new medication on any change in the patient's condition.

Assure that appropriate monitoring diagnostic tests are ordered, completed, and reviewed as appropriate.

Monitor the patient's response. Is it potentially adverse? Is it not effective?

---

prescribed dosage and the actual dosage, potential drug-drug and food-drug interactions, and potential or actual ADRs. When potentially inappropriate products are identified, the prescriber can be consulted.

Monitoring and Evaluation

A significant part of the nurse's responsibilities is to monitor and evaluate the effectiveness of prescribed treatments and observe for signs of problems (ADRs, etc.)—either from a change in condition or what are known as iatrogenic complications (problems that are the result of something we have done or given to the person) (Box 8-4). This is particularly important in gerontological nursing due to the medical complexity of the patient and the polypharmacy that is often in place. Monitoring and evaluating involve making

astute observations and documenting those observations, noting changes in physical and functional status (e.g., vital signs, performance of activities of daily living, sleeping, eating, hydrating, eliminating) and mental status (e.g., attention and level of alertness, memory, orientation, behavior, mood, emotional display and affect, content and characteristics of interactions). Monitoring for iatrogenic effects also means ensuring that blood levels are measured as they are needed; such as scheduled thyroid-stimulating hormone (TSH) levels for all persons taking thyroid replacement, international normalized ratios (INRs) for all persons taking warfarin, or periodic hemoglobin A_{1c} levels for all persons with diabetes (Box 8-5). Care of a patient also means that the nurses promptly communicate their findings of potential problems to the patient's prescribing nurse practitioner or physician. The reader is referred to a geriatric pharmacology reference text for more detailed and thorough information. This information may also be available from specialized clinical pharmacists.

Patient Education

Usually the nurse is responsible for educating patients about medication use. Ideally, the nurse empowers the person to participate fully in goal setting and treatment planning (Box 8-6). Education relating to safe medication use can be accomplished on an individual basis or in small groups. In working with those with cognitive limitations this education must always include caregivers. Elders and their caregivers should be encouraged to exercise the right to question and know what they are taking, how it will affect them, and the alternatives available to them. Pamphlets and booklets written in lay terms and in appropriate language and reading level should be available. If there are none that are appropriate, the nurse can be creative and develop a booklet or information sheet that will meet the patient's needs. Information is best presented in a bulleted format rather than in paragraph form. Type should be large with contrasting colors.

Because of the complex needs of the older patient, education can be particularly challenging. The following tips may be helpful when the goal of the nurse is to promote healthy aging:

1. *Key persons:* Find out who, if anyone, manages the person's medications, helps the person, or assists with decision making; when applicable and with the elder's permission, make sure that the helper is present when any teaching is done.
2. *Environment:* Minimize distraction, and avoid competing with television or others demanding the patient's attention; make sure the person is comfortable and is not hungry, thirsty, tired, too warm or too cold, in pain, or in need of the toilet.
3. *Timing:* Provide the teaching during the best time of the day for the person, when he or she is most alert, engaged, and energetic. Keep the education sessions short and succinct.
4. *Communication:* Ensure that you will be understood. Make sure the elders have their glasses or hearing aids on if they are used. Use simple and direct language, and avoid medical or nursing jargon (e.g., "intake"). Remain respectful at all times, and do not allow negative stereotypes to cloud communication. Encourage questions. If the person is blind, voice or Braille instructions must be available (search "talking pill boxes").
5. *Reinforce teaching:* Provide memory aids to reinforce teaching. Have actual medications or containers handy to

---

BOX 8-6   Empowering the Patient for Safe Medication Practices: What Elders Should Know About Taking Their Medications

- What is the name of each drug?
- What is the purpose of each drug?
- What is the dose per administration?
- What is the number of doses every day?
- What is the best time to take the medication?
- How should the medication be taken?
- Can the medication be taken with other drugs?
- Which medications can and cannot be taken together?
- Are any special techniques, devices, or procedures necessary to administer the medication?
- For how long should the medication be taken?
- What are the common side effects?
- If side effects occur: What should the elder do? What changes in administration are necessary? When should the drug be stopped? When should the physician or pharmacist (or both) be called?
- What can be done at home to monitor for a therapeutic drug response?
- What should be done if a dose is missed?
- How many refills are allowed?
- How should the medication be stored?
- What are the nonprescription preparations that should not be used with the present drug therapy?
- Take all medications prescribed unless the physician states otherwise.
- Stop taking the medication and report if any new or unusual problems occur, such as shortness of breath, nausea, diarrhea, vomiting, sleepiness, dizziness, weakness, skin rash, or fever.
- Never take medication prescribed for another person.
- Do not take any medication more than 1 year old or past the expiration date on the container.
- Store medications in a safe place, preferably the kitchen, rather than the bathroom, where moisture from bathing, especially showers, may affect the medicine.
- Do not keep medicines, especially sedatives and hypnotics, on the bedside stand, because when you are sleepy, you may forget that you have already taken the medication earlier.
- Do not place different medicines in the same container.
- Take a sufficient supply of all medicines in their individual containers when traveling away from home.
- Find a way to keep track of medications taken.

visually illustrate directions. For persons who can read, use written charts and lists with large letters and simple language. For persons who cannot read, charts with pictures of the medications and symbols for times of the day or color coding can be used, such as a moon for evening use or a drawing of silverware for "with meals." If food is required with the medication or must be avoided, this should be indicated on the charts. Weekly calendars with pockets for medications indicating day, time, and date can be used; or a daily tear-off calendar to remind the elder to take daily medication can be used. Clear envelopes or sandwich bags containing the medication can be affixed to the dated square on a daily basis; each envelope or bag should state the name of the drug and dose and times it is to be taken that day. Commercial drug boxes are available for single or multiple doses by the day, week, or month, and some have alarms. Some pharmacies are equipped to fill prescriptions using such containers. After discharge from a hospital or nursing home, a follow-up phone call can help with assessing accurate medication usage or other problems with medications. A nurse's home visit to patients at high risk for problems, such as those with cognitive deficits or those with many medications for new conditions, reinforces medication information and provides assessment information.

6. *Evaluate teaching:* Have the patient repeat back instructions, including names of medications, purposes, side effects, times of administration, and method for remembering to take the medicines and to mark off their ingestion.

7. *Avoiding drug interactions:* Patients should be taught to obtain all their medications from the same pharmacy if possible. This will allow the pharmacist to monitor for drug duplications and interactions. When elders have no prescription drug coverage, they may need to shop around for the best prices, and this does increase the risk for problems. Additional information about recognizing and responding to early signs of ADR may save lives.

Medication Administration

Most elders who live in the community self-administer their own medications; others receive help from family, friends, or health care professionals. In nursing homes the administration of medications occupies nearly all of the "medication" nurses' time. In assisted living facilities, medication administration is an optional service and available only if permitted by local laws. Regardless of the setting or the persons involved, several skills are needed for safe administration.

Because of the high rate of arthritis and other debilitating conditions, it may be difficult or impossible for the person to remove a cap or break a tablet. If no children will have access to the medications, the patient can request alternative bottle caps that are easier to open. Either the person or the nurse can also ask the pharmacist to pre-break the pills or dispense a smaller dose. Pill cutters are commercially available but still call for fine motor dexterity to place the pill for cutting in the correct place.

Most medications are taken orally. Many tablets and capsules are difficult to swallow because of their size or because they stick to the tongue, especially if the mouth is dry as is a normal change with aging. Administration of a drug in liquid form is sometimes preferable and allows for flexible dosing; concentrations can be varied so that quantities of solution can be prepared and taken by the teaspoon, tablespoon, or ounce, simple and commonly used household measurements. Since household spoons vary greatly in actual volume, the nurse should ensure that the elder is using an accurate measure. Liquid self-administration will not likely be an option for the person with Parkinson's disease or any other type of tremor. Crushing tablets or emptying the powder from capsules into fluid or food should not be done unless specified by the pharmaceutical company or approved by a pharmacist, because it may interfere with the effectiveness of the drug (causing either underdose or toxicity) or create problems in administration, as well as injure the mouth or gastrointestinal tract. Some people have difficulty swallowing capsules. The person can be advised to place capsules on the front of the tongue and swallow a fluid; this should wash it to the back of the throat and down. Other persons do better with pills or capsules when taken with a semisolid food, such as applesauce, chocolate syrup, or peanut butter—as long as the substances do not interact.

Enteric-coated, extended-release, or sustained-release products are all used to allow absorption at different places in the gastrointestinal tract. These should never be crushed, broken, opened, or otherwise altered before administration. However, since the formulation of medications is rapidly changing, the reader is advised to contact a clinical pharmacist, consult a very current drug handbook or package insert (found in Physician's Desk References [PDRs]) for the changing list of "do-not-crush" products.

The transdermal patch, also called the transdermal delivery system (TDDS), is one of the newer of the approaches to medication administration, and more and more medications are being transformed to be administered by this route. The TDDS provides for a more constant rate of drug absorption and eliminates concern for gastrointestinal absorption variation, gastrointestinal tolerance, and drug interaction. TDDSs are not recommended for persons who are noticeably underweight because absorption is unpredictable owing to the reduced body fat.

When medications are being administered directly into the stomach or duodenum special precautions are needed via a feeding tube. Safe administration is a time-consuming task resulting in a high risk for medication errors. To administer enteral medications safely a detailed knowledge of their formulation is needed along with skills to prepare them appropriately. The outcomes of the errors include: occluded tube, reduced drug effect, drug toxicity, patient harm or patient death. The three most common errors are incompatible route, improper preparation, and improper administration (see Safety Alert).

SAFETY ALERT

Administration of Medications Through Enteral Feeding Tubes: The Three Most Common Errors

Incompatible route: Medications must be appropriate for the oral route for immediate action and crushable. All products intended for slow or extended release are not crushable as they are intended for only partial dissolution in the stomach; administration may lead to an excessive dose. Watch for extensions such as: CD, CR, ER, LA, SA, SE, TD, TR, XL, and XR as warnings for noncrushable drugs (this list is not inclusive). See the "do-not-crush" lists available from the pharmacy or online (http://www.ismp.org/Tools/DoNotCrush.pdf).

Improper preparation: Medications administered via an enteral feeding tube must be in a liquid or semiliquid form in order to pass through the tube and not adhere to the lining of the tube. Each medication should be dissolved individually in a product that will not change the product* and will not clog the tube. Watch for oral suspensions and tincture; drug remaining on tubing means reduced dose administered.

Improper administration: Be sure to know where the distal end of the tube is resting. A drug that requires partial absorption in the stomach cannot be used when it will be administered directly into the duodenum or jejunum. Do not combine with feeding unless directions are to "administer with food."

When more than one tablet is crushed or capsule opened and mixed together before administration, a new "product" has been prepared and may not have the same effect as the two products taken separately. Find "compatibility information" from pharmacists to determine which medications may be mixed in this way.

*See Medication Safety Alert at http://www.ismp.org/Newsletters/acutecare/articles/20100506.asp for more information.

Psychoactive Medications

Psychoactive or psychotropic medications are those that alter brain chemistry, emotions, and/or behavior. They include antipsychotics (neuroleptics), antidepressants, mood stabilizers, antianxiety agents (anxiolytics), and sedative-hypnotics. This section of the chapter provides an overview of some of the psychotropic medications used most often to treat symptoms that occur in disorders of behavior, cognition, arousal, and mood in the gerontological population. It is by no means exhaustive. A section is devoted to treating the movement disorders that may occur as a side effect from the use of antipsychotics.

In 1987 the Health Care Financing Administration mandated that residents of long-term care settings may only be prescribed psychotropic drugs for specific diseases or symptoms and that the use be monitored, reduced, or eliminated when possible. Prescribing physicians and nurse practitioners may exceed the recommended doses only if documentation reasonably explains the rationale for the benefit of the higher dose in restoring function or preventing dangerous behavior (Omnibus Budget Reconciliation Act [OBRA], 1987). Since that time the concern over the potential misuse of psychotropic medications or their effects continues to grow. For example, at one time an atypical antipsychotic such as resperidone was commonly prescribed for the patient with dementia who exhibited neuropsychiatric symptoms, especially agitation. Unless the agitation is specifically related to psychosis – this use is now not acceptable.

A patient should be prescribed a psychotropic medication only after thorough medical, psychological, and social assessments are done. Nursing assessment before medication intervention contributes knowledge and baseline information that can optimize the patient's medical and psychological improvement. At the same time assessments should be done quickly to enable the patient to receive the appropriate treatment as soon as possible. Pharmacological interventions should always be supplemented by nonpharmacological measures such as counseling, changes in the environment and other interventions which promote healthy aging. Issues to consider include the patient's medical status (and other medications that might interact with psychotropics), mental status, ability to carry out activities of daily living, and ability to participate in social activities and maintain satisfying relationships with others, as well as the potential for patient or caregiver compliance with any pharmacological or nonpharmacological recommendations.

The gerontological nurse, especially one working in a long-term care setting, is likely to care for older adults with psychiatric and cognitive problems, especially dementia, depression, anxiety, and psychosis. The rate of depression for older persons living in the community is significant, and even more so for those living in long-term care facilities (see Chapter 22). Anxiety is also common and when treated with benzodiazepines, increases the older person's risk for adverse effects and drug interactions. Unfortunately the use of psychotherapy is very limited, first because of the rarity of persons with a specialty training in gerontological psychiatry or counseling, and second because of the very low reimbursement rates established by Medicare and other insurance plans.

Finally a small group of elders, especially those with neurological conditions or any one of the dementias, may develop psychosis at some time in their illnesses. Psychosis is also seen in delirium from an infection or from an ADR and in the few elders with schizophrenia. Persons with psychoses are often treated with antipsychotics that call for special attention and skills from the gerontological nurse in cooperation with a psychiatrist or a psychiatric nurse practitioner specializing in geriatrics (see Chapter 22.)

Antidepressants

Antidepressants, as the name implies, are drugs used to treat depression. In the past, the major drugs used were monoamine oxidase inhibitors (MAOIs) and tricyclic antidepressants (TCAs), especially amitriptyline (Elavil) and doxepin (Sinequan). These drugs required high doses to be effective and had significant anticholinergic side effects such as dry mouth, constipation, sedation, and urinary retention. Since the development of the newer drugs, such as selective serotonin reuptake inhibitors (SSRIs) and SNRIs (serotonin-norepinephrine reuptake inhibitors), the MAOIs and TCAs are rarely seen for the treatment of depression in older adults. When the later drugs are seen they should be questioned.

The SSRIs (e.g., Zoloft, Prozac, Lexapro, Celexa, etc.) and SNRIs (e.g., Effexor) have been found to be highly effective, with minimal or manageable side effects, and are the drugs of choice for use in older adults. Most of these cause initial problems with nausea or a dry mouth. While effective, these must be used with caution especially related to serum sodium levels. The SSRIs should also be used with caution in persons with a history of falls due to the potential to produce ataxia or dizziness (AGS, 2012). One side effect of the SSRIs that does not resolve with time, if experienced, is sexual dysfunction. The SNRIs and other antidepressants are less likely to cause this problem and may be preferred by elders who are sexually active. Bupropion (under the brand name of Zyban) has also been found

to reduce nicotine cravings, and the combined effect may be very helpful to some; it cannot be used for persons with a history of seizures. When sleep is a problem, the patient may be prescribed the tetracyclic antidepressant mirtazapine (Remeron) which is often well tolerated in older adults. Most older adults are sensitive to these medications and may find significant relief from depression at low doses. Although it sometimes takes time to find the optimal dose, the nurse can help the elder monitor target symptoms and advocate for continued dose adjustments or changes until relief is obtained rather than the depression being simply reduced.

Antianxiety Agents

Drugs used to treat anxiety are referred to as anxiolytics or *antianxiety agents.* These agents include benzodiazepines, buspirone (BuSpar), and beta blockers. Antihistamines, especially diphenhydramine (Benadryl), are often used but **not recommended** owing to their significant and highly dangerous anticholinergic effects. The decision to treat anxiety pharmacologically is based on the degree to which the anxiety interferes with the person's ability to function and subjective feelings of discomfort.

Although they are usually contraindicated, the most frequently used agents are benzodiazepines. Despite the fact that benzodiazepines have been available for over 30 years, only minimal research has been done with older adults (Madhusoodanan & Bogunovic, 2004). What we do know is that older adults metabolize these drugs slowly and renal excretion is compromised, even in health, so they persist in the blood stream for long periods and can easily reach toxic levels more quickly than anticipated (see p. 109). Side effects include drowsiness, dizziness, ataxia, mild cognitive deficits, and memory impairment. Signs of toxicity include excessive sedation, unsteady gait, confusion, disorientation, cognitive impairment, memory impairment, agitation, and wandering. Because these symptoms resemble dementia, people can easily be misdiagnosed when they start taking benzodiazepines.

Benzodiazepines are highly addicting yet very popular because of their quick sedating effects for the highly anxious or agitated person. However, because of the problems noted earlier they should be avoided except in extreme cases. If necessary, lorazepam (Ativan) appears to be the least problematic, when prescribed in very low doses and for short periods. It has the shortest half-life of the benzodiazepines and no active metabolites.

Buspirone is a safer alternative. Although a side effect is dizziness, this is often dose-related and resolves with time. Buspirone is not addicting and may have an additive effect to some of the SSRIs, so lower doses can be used. No therapeutic effect may be felt by the patient or observed by the nurse for 5 to 7 days, and the drug may be mistakenly discontinued because of its apparent lack of effect. Buspirone is best used for chronic anxiety and is not indicated for acute needs (see Chapter 22.)

Antipsychotics (Neuroleptics)

The term "psychosis" covers a range of thinking and behavioral disorders that are based on responses of the ill person to a private reality—a reality that may be distressing and problematic for the patient and those around him or her. Characteristically, psychosis occurs in schizophrenia but can also occur in mania, depression, delirium, dementia, and paranoid states. When psychosis occurs in the person with dementia it is often seen in a cluster of neuropsychiatric symptoms, especially agitation, physical aggression, and wandering.

Antipsychotics, formerly known as *major tranquilizers and now often referred to as neuroleptics,* are drugs used to treat psychotic symptoms and used for their mood stabilizing effects. The second generation of these drugs is referred to as atypical (second generation) antipsychotics (e.g., resperidone, Seroquel, Zyprexa, etc.). Due to their danger, especially risk of cardiovascular events, stroke, and even death, they are used as drugs of last resort and can only be prescribed following a careful assessment and search for any potential underlying cause of the problem. Inappropriate use of antipsychotic medications is a significant problem in long-term care settings. In addition to the risk for ADR they may mask a reversible cause for the problem, such as a thyroid disturbance, infection, dehydration, fever, electrolyte imbalance, an ADR, or a sudden change in the environment (Bullock & Saharan, 2002).

However, when no other approaches have been successful they may be necessary and must be used very cautiously in true psychiatric disorders. Antipsychotics can provide a person with relief from what may be frightening and distressing symptoms. When used, drugs with the lowest side effects profile and at the lowest dose possible and for the shortest length of time should be prescribed. In most states the prescribing and use of antipsychotics in long-term care settings is carefully monitored.

There are different classes and potencies of antipsychotics. First generation antipsychotics (Thorazine, Prolixin, Mellaril, and Haldol) are less sedating than some of the second generation but cause more extrapyramidal reactions and are considered inappropriate medications (AGS, 2012). The older one is, the more susceptible one is to developing extrapyramidal reactions, particularly neuroleptic-induced parkinsonian symptoms. They can cause orthostatic hypotension, thereby increasing the risk for falls and the anticholinergic effects include dry mouth, constipation, urinary retention, hypotension, and confusion, all of which can significantly and negatively impact quality of life. A permanent side effect for this class of antipsychotics is tardive dyskinesia (see "Tardive Dyskinesia" later in this chapter).

Another potential concern with the use of neuroleptics is the rare but potentially life-threatening ADR *neuroleptic malignant syndrome* (NMS). The most typical symptoms are fever greater than 100.4° F, muscle rigidity, autonomic instability (e.g., labile BP, tachycardia), and altered mental status. Onset is rapid and unless treated appropriately and quickly death can ensue. The drugs most associated with NMS are the high-potency neuroleptics such as haloperidol, but others such as chlorpromazine (Compazine) and promethazine (Phenergan) have been implicated. While it occurs most often in the first 2 weeks of the start of treatment it must also be considered whenever a dose is increased. NMS is also seen if anti-Parkinson's medications are stopped abruptly. In most instances the person is hospitalized in an intensive care unit while being treated. The immediate response is to recognize that what is being seen may be an adverse reaction, stop the offending medication and promptly and safely cool the patient.

Appropriate preventive interventions include adequate hydration, activity in a cool area away from direct sunlight, and use of a fan or sponge bath if overheating should occur. The patient may or may not communicate his or her discomfort from the heat, so assessment for signs and symptoms is left to the nurse or other caregiver. Any circumstance resulting in dehydration greatly increases the risk of heatstroke with the morbidity and mortality increasing with age. Diuretics, coffee, alcohol, lithium, and uncontrolled diabetes decrease vascular volume, thereby decreasing the body's ability to handle antipsychotics. Concurrent use of medications with anticholinergic properties are especially contraindicated.

Movement Disorders

Although neuroleptic malignant syndrome is not commonly seen, the most significant potential side effects of antipsychotics (especially of first generation) are movement disorders, also referred to as *extrapyramidal syndrome (EPS)* reactions. These include acute dystonia, akathisia, parkinsonian symptoms, and tardive dyskinesia.

Acute Dystonia. An acute dystonic reaction is an abnormal involuntary movement consisting of a slow and continuous muscular contraction or spasm. Involuntary muscular contractions of the mouth, jaw, face, and neck are common. The jaw may lock (trismus), the tongue may roll back and block the throat, the neck may arch backward (opisthotonos), or the eyes may close. In an oculogyric crisis, the eyes are fixed in one position. Often this creates a feeling of needing to look up constantly without the ability to make the eyes come down. Dystonias can be painful and frightening. An acute dystonic reaction may occur hours or days following antipsychotic medication administration, or after dosage increases, and may last minutes to hours. It is considered a medical emergency.

Caregivers or others unfamiliar with these EPS reactions often become alarmed. Although frightening, acute dystonia is not usually dangerous and is quickly relieved by anticholinergic medication, such as benztropine (Cogentin), trihexyphenidyl (Artane), or diphenhydramine (Benadryl), providing relief within minutes if given intravenously, within 10 to 15 minutes if given intramuscularly, and within 30 minutes if given orally. These medications should be readily available to treat an EPS reaction for all persons taking antipsychotics. Although they are not recommended for use in persons over 65 years of age, anticholinergics and amantadine (Symmetrel), a dopamine agonist, are sometimes prescribed to prevent dystonic reactions, but because of slow onset of action, they are not used for acute treatment.

Akathisia. Akathisia refers to the compulsion to be in motion and may occur at any time during therapy. Patients describe feeling restless, being unable to be still, having an unrelenting desire to move, and feeling "like crawling out of my skin." Often this symptom is mistaken for worsening psychosis instead of the ADR that it is. Pacing, aimless walking, fidgeting, shifting weight from one leg to the other, and marked restlessness are characteristic behaviors for a person experiencing akathisia. Safety is the primary concern.

Parkinsonian Symptoms. The use of neuroleptics may cause a collection of symptoms that mimic Parkinson's disease. A bilateral tremor (as opposed to a unilateral tremor in true Parkinson's), bradykinesia, and rigidity may be seen, which may progress to the inability to move. The patient may have an inflexible facial expression and appear bored and apathetic and be mistakenly diagnosed as depressed. More common with the higher-potency antipsychotics (e.g., Haldol), parkinsonian symptoms may occur within weeks to months of the initiation of antipsychotic therapy.

Tardive Dyskinesia. When neuroleptics have been used continuously for at least 3 to 6 months, patients are at risk for the development of the irreversible movement disorder of *tardive dyskinesia (TD)*. Symptoms of TD usually appear first as wormlike movements of the tongue; other facial movements include grimacing, blinking, and frowning. Slow, maintained, involuntary twisting movements of limbs, trunk, neck, face, and eyes (involuntary eye closure) have been reported. There is no treatment that reverses the effect of TD; therefore it is essential that the nurse is attentive for early detection so that the health care provider can make prompt changes to the psychotropic regimen.

Response to treatment is the most important consideration when psychotropic medications are given. Subjective patient comments about feelings and symptoms and objective observations about the patient's behavior are important data for evaluating the effectiveness of a drug. Several tools are available to help the nurse monitor the patient taking antipsychotics. The Abnormal Involuntary Movement Scale (AIMS) was designed to quantify changes in movement. It has been shortened in the Abbreviated Dyskinesia Scale (Taksh, 2006). Other tools include the Barnes Rating Scale for Drug-Induced Akathisia (Barnes, 1989) and the Simpson-Angus Rating Scale for EPS (Simpson & Angus, 1970). All of these can be found on the Internet.

Mood Stabilizers

Mood stabilizers are the group of agents used for the treatment of bipolar disorders, which is seen as uncontrollable fluctuations in mood which affect the person's day-to-day life. Symptoms of a severe manic phase may include confusion, paranoia, labile affect, pressured speech and flight of ideas, morbid or depressive content of thought, increased psychomotor activity resembling agitated depression, and altered orientation and attention span. However, it is now recognized that instead many have periods of hypomania characterized by significantly increased energy and movement and somewhat diminished judgment. For the older adult in the long-term setting the symptoms of bipolar disorders are easily confused with others. For example, wandering is common for persons with moderate dementia, as is emotional lability.

The mood stabilizers include lamotrigine (Lamictal), lithium, and valproic acid (Depakote). Along with these, the anticonvulsants carbamazepine (Tegretol) and gabapentin (Neurontin) are used as well as several of the atypical antipsychotics (e.g., Abilify, Zyprexa, Seroquel) even when psychosis is not present. Each of these have very individualized drug-drug interaction profiles and several require blood level monitoring. The nurse who is caring for a patient with a bipolar disorder or who is taking a mood stabilizer should seek guidance from the person's psychiatrist regarding specific strategies to enhance the person's quality of life and which laboratory testing is required for monitoring. If the patient is taking lithium, this is especially important. Lithium interacts with other medications and certain foods and has a narrow therapeutic window. For example, a low-salt diet will elevate the lithium level, and a high-salt diet will decrease it. Likewise, thiazide diuretics and nonsteroidal antiinflammatory drugs (NSAIDs) will elevate the serum lithium level. Side effects include the following: confusion, disorientation, and memory loss; flattening of T waves on the electrocardiogram; polyuria and polydipsia; nausea, vomiting, and diarrhea; fine resting tremor; benign goiter; and ataxia.

Implications for Gerontological Nursing and Healthy Aging

All the medications presented in this chapter have indications, side effects, interactions, and individual patient reactions. The nurse's advocacy role includes education for the patient and the family or the caregiver. Further, the nurse must determine whether side effects are minimal and tolerable or serious. Asking the patient produces subjective data; and observing the patient's interactions, behavior, mood, emotional responses, and daily habits provides objective data. From this compilation of data, patient problems can be delineated, nursing diagnoses developed, outcome criteria planned, and interventions initiated.

Medications occupy a central place in the lives of many older persons; cost, acceptability, interactions, unacceptable side effects, and the need to schedule medications appropriately all combine to create many difficulties (Box 8-7). Although nurses, with the exception of advanced practice nurses, do not prescribe medications, we believe that their having a basic understanding of issues specific to the safe administration and consumption of medications by persons in late life will reduce the use of inappropriate medications and allow the nurse to observe more closely for adverse side effects and interactions. In the role of educator, the nurse might also decrease misuse through personally and culturally appropriate instructions.

The gerontological nurse is a key person in ensuring that the medication use is appropriate, effective, and as safe as possible. The knowledgeable nurse is alert for potential drug interactions and for signs or symptoms of ADRs. The nurse promotes the actions necessary to prevent drugs from becoming toxic and to treat toxicity promptly should it occur. Nurses in the long-term care setting are responsible for monitoring the overall health of the residents, including being alert for the need for laboratory tests and other measures to ensure correct dosage of several medications (e.g., Coumadin, vancomycin, thyroxin). The nurse must give prompt attention to changes in physiological function that are either the result of the medication regimen or are affected by the regimen, such as potassium level to minimize the likelihood of adverse and toxic reactions. The nurse is often the person to initiate assessment of medication use, evaluate outcomes, and provide the teaching needed for safe drug use and self-administration. In most settings the nurse is also in a position to influence the timing of prescribed doses so residents might more easily benefit from the findings from the developing knowledge of chronopharmacology (Barry et al., 2007). In all settings, a vital nursing function is to educate patients and to ensure that they understand the purpose of, the side effects of, and the time to call the provider regarding their medications.

KEY CONCEPTS

- As we age, the way our body responds to medications changes.
- Any medication has side effects. The therapeutic goal is to reduce the targeted symptoms without undesirable side effects.
- Drug-drug and drug-food incompatibilities are an increasing problem of which nurses must be aware.
- Polypharmacy is one of the most serious problems of elders today, and this is usually the first area to investigate when adverse physiological events occur.
- Drug misuse may be triggered by prescriber practices, individual self-medication, individual physiology, altered biodegradability, nutritional and fluid states, and inadequate assessment before prescribing.
- Nurses must consider the occurrence of a possible adverse medication effect immediately if a change in the person's condition is observed, including mental

---

BOX 8-7	The Right Medications for Older Adults

Efficacy is established
Compatible with other medications currently taking
Low likelihood of adverse events
Half-life no longer than 24 hours
No or minimally active metabolites
No adjustments needed for renal or hepatic functioning
Dosing once or twice a day
Strength and dosage available match that which is
    recommended for use in older adults
Patient is able to afford the medication

From Reuben DB, Herr KA, Pacala JT, et al.: *Geriatrics at your fingertips.* New York, 2008, American Geriatrics Society.

status changes in an individual who is normally alert and aware, or increasing confusion. Many drugs cause temporary cognitive impairment in older persons.

- Chronotherapy that uses biorhythms of the body for the most effective medication therapy has the potential to decrease dose, frequency, and cost of medication regimens and to improve adherence to drug therapy.
- The side effects of psychotropic medications vary significantly; thus these medications must be selected and prescribed for the older adult with care. This increases the nurse's responsibility in the administration and monitoring of these medications.
- The response of the elder to treatment with psychotropic medications should show reduced distress, clearer thinking, and more appropriate behavior.
- It is always expected that pharmacological approaches augment rather than replace nonpharmacological approaches.
- Older adults are particularly vulnerable to developing movement disorders (extrapyramidal symptoms, parkinsonism symptoms, akathisia, dystonias) with the use of antipsychotics.
- The Omnibus Budget Reconciliation Act (OBRA) restricts the use of psychotropic drugs in the long-term care setting unless they are truly needed for specific disorders and to maintain or improve function.
- Any time a behavior change is noted in a person, reversible causes must be sought and treated before medications are used.
- Dosages of medications must be carefully titrated for the individual, and the individual's responses must be accurately and consistently recorded.

ACTIVITIES AND DISCUSSION QUESTIONS

1. What are the age-related changes that occur in pharmacokinetics of the older adult?
2. What are the drug use patterns of older adults, and what can be done to correct or improve them?
3. Explain the role of the elder, the care provider, and the social network in reducing medication misuse.
4. List a variety of measures that the nurse can suggest to assist older adults with their medication use and adherence to a medication regimen.
5. What are the most troublesome side effects of antipsychotic medications?
6. Mrs. J. is calling out repeatedly for a nurse; other patients are complaining, and you simply cannot be available for long periods to quiet her. Considering the setting and the OBRA guidelines, what would you do to manage the situation?

REFERENCES

American Geriatric Society (AGS): American Geriatrics Society updated Beers Criteria for potentially inappropriate medication use in older adults, *J Am Geriatr Soc* 60(4): 616–631, 2012.

Barnes TR: A rating scale for drug-induced akathisia. *Brit J Psychtr* 154:672-676, 1989.

Barry PJ, O'Keefe N, O'Connor K, et al: Inappropriate prescribing in the elderly: a comparison of the Beers criteria and the improved prescribing in the elderly tool (IPET) in acutely ill elderly hospitalized patients, *J Clin Pharm Ther* 31(6):617–626, 2007.

Brandt L: Pharmcology and medication use. In Durso SC, Bowker LK, Price JD, et al, editors: *Oxford American handbook of geriatric medicine*, New York, 2010, Oxford University Press.

Briggs GC: Geriatric issues. In Younkgin E, Sawin KJ, Kissinger J, et al, editors: *Pharmacotherapeutics: a primary care guide*, Upper Saddle River, NJ, 2005, Prentice-Hall.

Bullock R, Saharan A: Atypical antipsychotics: experience and use in the elderly, *Int J Clin Pract* 56(7):515–525, 2002.

Constantiner M: *Mental health in older adults: medication issues.* From presentation at the 2011 Florida Medical Directors Association conference, best care practices for the geriatrics continuum.

Fadiman A: *The spirit catches you and you fall down*, New York, 1998, Farrar, Straus, and Giroux.

Gallagher PF, Barry PJ, Ryan C, et al: Inappropriate prescribing in an acutely ill population of elderly patients as determined by Beers' criteria, *Age Aging* 37(1):96–101, 2007.

Green JL, Hawley JN, Rask KJ: Is the number of prescribing physicians an independent risk factor for adverse drug events in an elderly outpatient populations? *Am J Geriatr Pharmacother* 5(1):31–39, 2007.

Handler SM, Wright RM, Ruby CM, et al: Epidemiology of medication-related adverse events in nursing homes, *Am J Geriatr Pharmacother* 4(3):264–272, 2006.

Jett K: Geropharmacology. In Touhy T, Jett K, editors: *Ebersole and Hess' toward healthy aging: human needs and nursing response*, St. Louis, 2012, Mosby.

Junius-Walker U, Theile G, Hummers-Pradier E: Prevalence and predictors of polypharmacy among older primary care patients in Germany, *Fam Pract* 24(1):14–19, 2007.

Kaur S, Mitchell G, Vitetta L, et al: Interventions that can reduce inappropriate prescribing in the elderly: a systematic review, *Drugs Aging* 26(12): 1013–1028, 2009.

Madhusoodanan S, Bogunovic OJ: Safety of benzodiazepine use in the geriatric population, *Expert Opin Drug Saf* 3(5): 485–493, 2004.

Marcum ZA, Handler SM, Boyce R, et al: Medication misadventures in the elderly: a year in review, *Am J Geriatr Pharmacother* 8(1):77–83, 2010.

Masoro EJ, Austed SN, editors: *Handbook of biology and aging*, ed 5, San Diego, 2003, Academic Press.

Miller CA: *Nursing for wellness in older adults*, ed 5, Philadelphia, 2008, Wolters Kluwer Health.

Ohdo S: Chronotherapeutic strategy: rhythm monitoring, manipulation and disruption, *Adv Drug Deliv Rev* 62(9-10): 859–875, 2010.

Omnibus Budget Reconciliation Act (OBRA) of 1987, House of Representatives, 100th Congress, 1st Session, Report 100-391, Washington, DC, 1987, U.S. Government Printing Office.

Page PL II, Ruscin JM: The risk of adverse drug events and hospital-related morbidity and mortality among older adults with potentially inappropriate medication use, *Am J Geriatr Pharmacother* 3(3):205–210, 2006.

Resnick B, Fick DM: 2012 Beers Criteria update: How should practicing nurses use the criteria? *Geriatric Nursing* 33(4): 253–255.

Ruscin JM: Drug therapy in the elderly (2009). Available at http://www.merckmanuals.com/professional/geriatrics/drug_therapy_in_the_elderly/drug-related_problems_in_the_elderly.html#v1133742.

Semla TP, editor: *Geriatric dosage handbook*, ed 17, Cleveland, 2012, Lexi-Comp, Inc.

Simpson GM, Angus JWS: A rating scale for extrapyramidal side effects. *Acta Psychiatr Scand* 212:11-19,1970.

Steinman MA, Landefeld CS, Rosenthal GE, et al: Polypharmacy and prescribing quality in older people, *J Am Geriatr Soc* 54(10):1516–1523, 2006.

Taksh U: A critical review of rating scales in the assessment of movement disorders in schizophrenia. *Curr Drug Targets* 7(9):1225–1229, 2006.

Youngkin E: The use of herbs and supplements in late life. In Touhy T, Jett K, editors: *Ebersole & Hess' toward healthy aging: human needs and nursing response,* St. Louis, 2012, Mosby.

CHAPTER 9

Nutrition and Hydration

Theris A. Touhy

evolve evolve.elsevier.com/Ebersole/gerontological

LEARNING OBJECTIVES

Upon completion of this chapter, the reader will be able to:

- Discuss nutritional requirements and factors affecting nutrition for older adults.
- Describe a nutritional screening and assessment.
- Identify interventions to promote adequate nutrition and hydration for older adults.
- Discuss assessment and interventions for older adults with dysphagia.
- List interventions that promote good oral hygiene for older adults.
- Develop a plan of care to assist an older person in developing and maintaining adequate nutrition and hydration.

GLOSSARY

Chemosenses The senses of taste and smell.

Dysphagia Sensation of impaired passage of food from the mouth to the esophagus and stomach; difficulty swallowing.

Gastroesophageal reflux disease (GERD) Backward flow of stomach contents into the esophagus.

Presbyesophagus Age-related change in the esophagus affecting motility.

Soul food Food possessing emotional significance and providing personal satisfaction; often has some cultural or traditional origins.

Xerostomia Dry mouth

THE LIVED EXPERIENCE

"If I do reach the point when I can no longer feed myself, I hope that the hands holding my fork belong to someone who has a feeling for who I am. I hope my helper will remember what she learns about me and that her awareness of me will grow from one encounter to another. Why should this make a difference? Yet, I am certain that my experience of needing to be fed will be altered if it occurs in the context of my being known . . . I will want to know about the lives of the people I rely on, especially the one who holds my fork for me. If she would talk to me, if we could laugh together, I might even forget the chagrin of my useless hands. We could have a conversation rather than a feeding."

From Lustbader W: Thoughts on the meaning of frailty, *Generations 13(4):*21-22, 1999.

Nutrition

Adequate nutrition is critical to preserving the health of older people. The quality and quantity of diet are important factors in preventing, delaying onset, and managing chronic illnesses associated with aging (American Dietetic Association [ADA], American Society for Nutrition [ASN], Society for Nutrition Education [SNE], 2010). About 87% of older adults have diabetes, hypertension, dyslipidemia, or a combination of these diseases that may have dietary implications. (ADA, ASN, SNE, 2010). This chapter discusses the dietary needs of older adults, age-related changes affecting nutrition, risk factors contributing to inadequate nutrition and hydration, obesity, and the effect of diseases and functional and cognitive impairments on nutrition. Dysphagia and oral care are included as additional concerns related to adequate nutrition in older adults. Readers are referred to a nutrition text for more comprehensive information on nutrition and aging and disease.

The *2010 Dietary Guidelines for Americans*, an evidence-based nutritional guideline published by the federal government, is designed to promote health, reduce the risk of chronic diseases, and reduce the prevalence of overweight and obesity through improved nutrition and physical activity (www.dietaryguidelines.gov). The guidelines focus on balancing calories with physical activity and encourage Americans to consume more healthy foods like vegetables, fruits, whole grains, fat-free and low-fat dairy products, and seafood, and to consume less sodium, saturated and *trans* fats, added sugars, and refined grains. In addition to the key recommendations, there are recommendations for specific population groups including older adults (U.S. Department of Agriculture [USDA], 2012). *Healthy People 2020* also provides goals for nutrition (see the Healthy People box).

 HEALTHY PEOPLE 2020
Nutrition and Weight Status

- Promote health and reduce chronic disease through the consumption of healthful diets and achievement and maintenance of body weight.
- Increase the proportion of primary care physicians who regularly measure the body mass index in their adult patients.
- Increase the proportion of physician office visits made by adult patients who are obese that include counseling or education related to weight reduction, nutrition, or physical activity.
- Increase the proportion of physician visits made by all child and adult patients that include counseling about nutrition or diet.
- Increase the proportion of adults who are at a healthy weight.
- Reduce household food insecurity and in so doing reduce hunger.

From U.S. Department of Health and Human Services, Office of Disease Prevention and Health Promotion: *Healthy people 2020* (2012). Available at http://www.healthypeople.gov/2020.

Age-Related Requirements
MyPlate for Older Adults

As part of the 2010 Guidelines, the new visual depiction of daily food intake, Choose MyPlate (ChooseMyPlate.gov), replaces the information formerly found on MyPyramid.gov. The USDA Human Nutrition Research Center on Aging at Tufts University has introduced the MyPlate for Older Adults that calls attention to the unique nutritional and physical activity needs associated with advancing years. The drawing features different forms of vegetables and fruits that are convenient, affordable, and readily available. Other unique components of the MyPlate for Older Adults include icons for regular physical activity and emphasis on adequate fluid intake, areas of particular concern for older adults (Figure 9-1).

Generally, older adults need fewer calories because they may not be as active and metabolic rates slow down. However, they still require the same or higher levels of nutrients for optimal health outcomes. The recommendations may need modification for the older adult with illness. The Dietary Approaches to Stop Hypertension (DASH) eating plan is another highly recommended eating plan to assist older adults with maintenance of optimal weight and management of hypertension. This plan consists of fruits, vegetables, whole grains, low-fat dairy products, poultry, and fish, and restriction of salt intake. Information on DASH can be found at http://www.nhlbi.nih.gov/health/health-topics/topics/dash/.

Other Dietary Recommendations

Fats
Similar to other age groups, older adults should limit intake of saturated fat and trans fatty acids. High fat diets cause obesity and increase the risk of heart disease and cancer. Recommendations are that 20% to 35% of total calories should be from fat, 45% to 65% from carbohydrates, and 10% to 35% from proteins. Monounsaturated fats, such as olive oil, are the best type of fat since they lower low-density lipoprotein (LDL) but leave the high-density lipoprotein (HDL) intact or even slightly raise it.

Protein
Presently, the Institute of Medicine's Recommended Dietary Allowance (RDA) for protein of 0.8 g/kg per day, based primarily on studies in younger men, may be inadequate for older adults. Results of a recent study (Beasley et al., 2010) suggest that higher protein consumption, as a fraction of total caloric intake, is associated with a decline

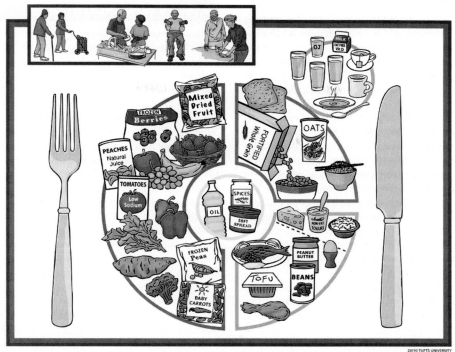

2011© TUFTS UNIVERSITY

FIGURE 9-1 MyPlate for older adults. Available at http://now.tufts.edu/news-releases/tufts-university-nutrition-scientists-unveil.

in risk of frailty in older adults. Protein intake of 1.5 g/kg per day, or 20% to 25% of total calorie intake, may be more appropriate for older adults at risk of becoming frail. Older people who are ill are the most likely segment of society to experience protein deficiency. Those with limitations affecting their ability to shop, cook, and consume food are at risk for protein deficiency and malnutrition.

Fiber

Fiber is an important dietary component that some older people do not consume in sufficient quantities. After age 50, women should receive around 21 g of dietary fiber daily, and men should receive around 30 g daily. However, even small amounts of fiber are beneficial (Academy of Nutrition and Dietetics, 2012). The benefits of fiber include the following: facilitates the absorption of water; helps control weight by delaying gastric emptying and providing a feeling of fullness; improves glucose tolerance by delaying movement of carbohydrate into the small intestine; prevents or reduces constipation by increasing the weight of the stool and shortening the transit time; helps prevent hemorrhoids and diverticulosis by decreasing pressure in the colon, shortening transit time, and increasing stool weight; reduces the risk of heart disease by binding with bile (which contains cholesterol) and causes its excretion; and protects against cancer.

It is better to get fiber from food rather than from fiber supplements such as Metamucil because supplements do not contain the essential nutrients found in high-fiber foods and their anticancer benefits are questionable. Ways to increase fiber intake include eating cooked dry beans, peas, and lentils; leaving skins on fruits and vegetables; eating whole fruit rather than drinking fruit juice; and eating whole-grain breads and cereals (National Institute on Aging, 2011). Those who have difficulty chewing could sprinkle oat bran on cereals or in soups, meat loaf, or casseroles. The quantity of bran depends on the individual, but generally, 1 to 2 tablespoons daily is sufficient. Individuals who have not used bran should begin with 1 teaspoon and progressively increase the quantity until the fiber intake is enough to accomplish its purpose. Fluid intake of 64 ounces daily is essential as well.

Vitamins and Minerals

Older people who consume five servings of fruits and vegetables daily will obtain adequate intake of vitamins A, C, and E, and potassium. But, Americans of all ages eat less than half of the recommended amounts of fruits and vegetables (Haber, 2010). After 50 years of age, the stomach produces less gastric acid, which makes vitamin B_{12} absorption less efficient. Vitamin B_{12} deficiency is a common and underrecognized condition that is estimated to occur in 12% to 14% of community-dwelling older adults and up to 25% of those residing in institutional settings (Ahmed & Haboubi, 2010).

Atrophic gastritis and pernicious anemia are the most common causes of vitamin B_{12} deficiency. Although intake of this vitamin is generally adequate, older adults should increase their intake of the crystalline form of vitamin B_{12} from fortified foods such as whole-grain breakfast cereals. Use of proton pump inhibitors for more than 1 year, as well as histamine H_2 receptor blockers, can lead to lower serum vitamin B_{12} levels by impairing absorption of the vitamin from food. Metformin, colchicine, and antibiotic and anticonvulsant agents may also increase the risk of vitamin B_{12} deficiency (Cadogan, 2010).

Calcium and vitamin D are essential for bone health and may prevent osteoporosis and decrease the risk of fracture. Chapter 18 discusses recommendations for calcium and vitamin D supplementation. Calcium is a difficult mineral to absorb, and some foods inhibit calcium absorption (e.g., spinach, green beans, peanuts, and summer squash) (Table 9-1). High levels of protein, sodium, or caffeine also cause more calcium to be excreted in the urine and should be avoided. For older adults with inadequate calcium intake from diet, supplemental calcium can be used.

TABLE **9-1**	**Calcium Content of Several Common Foods**	
Food Item	**Serving Size**	**Calcium (mg)**
Plain yogurt, fat-free	8 oz	452
American cheese	2 oz	312
Yogurt with fruit (low fat or fat-free)	8 oz	345
Milk	8 oz	300
Orange juice, calcium-fortified	8 oz	350
Dried figs	10 figs	269
Cheese pizza	1 slice	240
Ricotta cheese, part skim	1/2 cup	334
Ice cream, soft serve	4 oz	103
Spinach	4 oz	139
Cooked soybeans	1 cup	298

From National Institutes of Health: *Sources of calcium,* Washington, DC. Available at www.nichd.nih.gov/milk.

Obesity (Overnutrition)

Although most of the research on nutrition and older adults has centered on underweight and frailty, the increase in the prevalence of obesity in the general population, and in older adults, is getting increased attention. More than two thirds of all adults in the United States are overweight (BMI = 25 to 29.9) or obese (BMI $\geq$30), and the proportion of older adults who are obese has doubled in the past 30 years (Flicker et al., 2010). The obesity epidemic is occurring in parallel with the aging of the baby boomer generation. Adults over the age of 60 years are more likely to be obese than younger adults. Non-Hispanic black individuals have the highest rate (44.1%) followed by Mexican Americans (39.3%) and non-Hispanic whites (32.6%) (Ogden et al., 2012). Socioeconomic deprivation and lower levels of education have been linked to obesity.

Although there is strong evidence that obesity in younger people lessens life expectancy and has a negative effect on functionality and morbidity, it remains unclear whether overweight and obesity are predictors of mortality in older adults. In what has been termed the *obesity paradox,* for people who have survived to 70 years of age, mortality risk is lowest in those with a BMI classified as overweight (Felix, 2008, p. 36). Flicker and colleagues (2010) conclude that "BMI thresholds for overweight and obese are overly restrictive for older people. Overweight older people are not at greater mortality risk, and there is little evidence that dieting in this age group confers any benefit; these findings are consistent with the hypothesis that weight loss is harmful" (p. 239). For nursing home residents with severely decreased functional status, obesity may be regarded as a protective factor with regard to functionality and mortality (Kaiser et al., 2010).

At this time, maintaining weight in older persons seems to be a clinical recommendation, and any weight loss interventions in older persons must be "carefully considered on an individualized basis with special attention to the weight history and the medical conditions of each individual" (Bales & Buhr, 2008, p. 311). Maintaining a healthy weight throughout life can prevent many illnesses and functional limitations as a person grows older.

Malnutrition

Malnutrition is defined as "a state in which a deficiency, excess or imbalance of energy, protein and other nutrients causes adverse effects on body form, function, and clinical outcome" (Ahmed & Haboubi, 2010, p. 207). The rising incidence of malnutrition among older adults has been documented in acute care, long-term care, and the community. Between 16% and 30% of older adults are malnourished or at high risk, and about half of this population has protein levels consistent with malnutrition when they are admitted to hospitals (Duffy, 2010). Older adults in skilled nursing facilities and long-term nursing home residents also have a higher incidence of malnutrition. These figures are expected to rise dramatically in the next 30 years (Ahmed & Haboubi, 2010). Malnutrition among older people is clearly a serious challenge for health professionals in all settings.

Malnutrition has serious consequences, including infections, pressure ulcers, anemia, hypotension, impaired cognition, hip fractures, and increased mortality and morbidity. "Malnourished older adults take 40% longer to recover from illness, have two to three times as many complications, and have hospital stays that are 90% longer" (Haber, 2010, p. 211). Many factors contribute to the occurrence of malnutrition in older adults (Figure 9-2).

Protein-energy malnutrition (PEM) is the most common form of malnutrition in older adults. PEM is characterized by the presence of clinical signs (muscle wasting, low BMI) and biochemical indicators (albumin, cholesterol, or other protein changes) indicative of insufficient intake. Signs and symptoms of PEM are nonspecific, and it is important that other conditions such as malignancy, hyperthyroidism, peptic ulcer, and liver disease are ruled out. Comprehensive nutritional screening and assessment are essential in identifying older adults at risk for nutrition problems or who are malnourished.

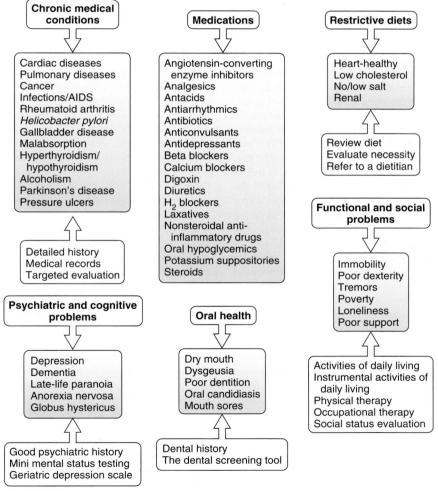

FIGURE 9-2 Risk factors for undernutrition illustrated by clinical approach. (From Omran M, Salem P: Diagnosing undernutrition, *Clin Geriatr Med 18:* 719-36, 2002)

Factors Affecting Fulfillment of Nutritional Needs

Fulfillment of the older person's nutritional needs is affected by numerous factors including changes associated with aging, lifelong eating habits, chronic disease, medication regimens, ethnicity and culture, socialization, socioeconomic deprivation, transportation, housing, and food knowledge.

Age-Associated Changes

Some age-related changes in the senses of taste and smell (chemosenses) and the digestive tract do occur as the individual ages and may affect nutrition. For most older people, these changes do not seriously interfere with eating, digestion, and the enjoyment of food. However, combined with other factors, they may contribute to inadequate nutrition and decreased eating pleasure (see Chapter 5).

Taste

The sense of taste has many components and primarily depends on receptor cells in the taste buds. Taste buds are scattered on the surface of the tongue, the cheek, the soft palate, the upper tip of the esophagus, and other parts of the mouth. Components in food stimulate taste buds during chewing and swallowing, and tongue movements enhance flavor sensation. Individuals have varied levels of taste sensitivity that seem predetermined by genetics and constitution, as well as age variations. Early studies suggested that a decline in the number of taste cells occurs with aging, but more recent studies suggest that "taste cells can regenerate but that the lag time of this turnover may account for the diminished taste response in older adults" (Miller, 2008, p. 363).

Age-related changes do not affect all taste sensations equally. With age, the inability to detect sweet taste seems to remain intact, whereas the ability to detect sour, salty, and bitter taste declines. Many denture wearers say they lose some of their satisfaction with food taste, possibly because dentures cover the palate and because texture is a very important element in food enjoyment. Difficulty in flavor appreciation comes from individual variables such as smoking, olfactory sensitivity, attitude toward food and eating, and the presence of moistening secretions. There are also aberrations in flavor sensation caused by certain medications and medical conditions. The addition of flavor enhancers (bouillon cubes) and concentrated flavors (jellies or sauces) can amplify both taste and smell. Fresh herbs and spices also give an extra boost to flavor and may increase enjoyment and interest in eating.

Smell

Age-related changes in the sense of smell and the consequent effect on nutrition is in need of further research. In the past, studies have shown a decline in the sense of smell as the individual ages. Research by Markovic and colleagues (2007) disputes this belief. Results of this study suggested that for perceived odors, olfactory pleasure increases at later stages in the life span, and the perceived intensity of odors remains stable. Decrease in the sense of smell may be related to many factors, including the following: nasal sinus disease, repeated injury to olfactory receptors through viral infections, age-related changes in central nervous system functioning, smoking, medications, and periodontal disease and other dentition problems. Changes in the sense of smell are also associated with Parkinson's disease and Alzheimer's disease (Cacchione, 2008).

Digestive System

Age-related changes in the oral cavity, the esophagus, the stomach, the liver, the pancreas, the gallbladder, and the small and large intestines may influence nutritional status in concert with other factors. However, these changes do not significantly affect function, and, in the absence of disease, the digestive system remains adequate throughout life. *Presbyesophagus, a decrease in the intensity of propulsive waves, may be an age-related change in the esophagus.* Some of these changes may be more attributable to pathological conditions rather than to age alone. The functional impact of presbyesophagus seems to be minimal, but combined with other conditions, may contribute to dysphagia.

Buccal Cavity

Age-related changes in the buccal cavity predispose older people to orodental problems that can significantly affect nutrition. Aging teeth become worn and darker in color and tend to develop longitudinal cracks. The dentin, or the layer beneath the enamel, becomes brittle and thickens so that pulp space decreases. People who are edentulous and are using complete dentures, continue to have oral health care needs. Ill-fitting dentures affect chewing and hence nutritional intake. People without teeth remain susceptible to oral cancer and other oral diseases. Oral care is discussed later in the chapter.

Another common oral problem among older adults is dry mouth (xerostomia). Approximately 25% to 40% of older adults experience xerostomia. More than 500 medications have the side effect of reducing salivary flow. A reduction in saliva and a dry mouth make eating, swallowing, and speaking difficult. It can also lead to significant problems of the teeth and their supporting structure (Jablonski, 2010). Artificial saliva preparations are available (avoid those containing sorbitol), and adequate fluid intake is also important when xerostomia occurs. Chewing on xylitol-flavored fluoride tablets, sugar-free candies, or sugar-free gum with xylitol 15 minutes after meals may stimulate saliva flow and promote oral hygiene (Miller, 2008). Medication review is also indicated to eliminate, if possible, medications contributing to xerostomia.

Regulation of Appetite

Appetite in persons of all ages is influenced by factors such as physical activity, functional limitations, smell, taste, mood, socialization, and comfort. With age, appetite and food consumption decline. Healthy older people are less hungry and are fuller before meals, consume smaller meals, eat more slowly, have fewer snacks between meals, and become satiated after meals more rapidly than younger people (Ahmed & Haboubi, 2010). There is some evidence that the endogenous opioid feeding and drinking drive may decline in aging and contribute to decreased appetite and risk for dehydration.

Lifelong Eating Habits

The nutritional state of a person reflects the individual's dietary history and present food practices. Lifelong eating habits are also developed out of tradition, ethnicity, and religion, all of which collectively can be called culture. Food habits established since childhood may influence the intake of older adults.

Eating habits do not always coincide with fulfillment of nutritional needs. Rigidity of food habits may increase with age as familiar food patterns are sought. Ethnicity determines if traditional foods are preserved, whereas religion affects the choice of foods possible. Members of a particular ethnic or religious group will have unique eating patterns, so individual assessment is important. Cultural preferences affect nutrition and culturally and religiously appropriate diets should be available in any institution or congregate dining program (see Chapter 4).

Lifelong habits of dieting or eating fad foods also echo through the later years. Older people may fall prey to advertisements that claim specific foods maintain youth and vitality or rid one of chronic conditions. Everyone can benefit from improved eating habits, and it's never too late to change dietary habits to improve health. Following the MyPlate for Older Adults (see Figure 9-1) is best for an ideal diet, with changes based on particular problems, such as hypercholesteremia. Older adults should be counseled to base their dietary decisions on valid research and consultation with their primary care provider. For the healthy older adult, essential nutrients should be obtained from food sources rather than relying on dietary supplements.

Socialization

The fundamentally social aspect of eating has to do with sharing and the feeling of belonging that it provides. All of us use food as a means of giving and receiving love, friendship, or belonging. Often, older adults may be isolated from the mainstream of life because of chronic illness, depression, and other functional limitations. When one eats alone, the outcome is often either overindulgence or disinterest in food. The presence of others during meals is a significant predictor of caloric intake (Locher et al., 2008).

Disinterest in food may also result from the effects of medication or disease processes. Misuse and abuse of alcohol are prevalent among older adults and are growing public health concerns. Excessive drinking interferes with nutrition. Drinking alcohol depletes the body of necessary nutrients and often replaces meals, thus making an individual susceptible to malnutrition (see Chapter 22).

The elderly nutrition program, authorized under Title III of the Older Americans Act (OAA), is the largest national food and nutrition program specifically for older adults. Programs and services include congregate nutrition programs, home-delivered nutrition services (Meals-on-Wheels), and nutrition screening and education. The program is not means-tested, and participants may make voluntary confidential contributions for meals. However, the OAA Nutrition Program reaches less than one third of older adults in need of its program and services, and those served receive only three meals a week. With the emphasis on community-based care rather than institutional care, expansion of nutrition services should be a priority. These programs enable older adults to avoid or delay costly institutionalization and allow them to stay in their homes and communities (ADA, 2010).

Chronic Diseases and Conditions

Many chronic diseases and their sequelae pose nutritional challenges for older adults. Functional impairments associated with chronic disease interfere with the person's abilities to shop, cook, and eat independently. For example, heart failure and chronic obstructive pulmonary disease (COPD) are associated with fatigue, increased energy expenditure, and decreased appetite. Dietary interventions for diabetes are essential but may also affect customary eating patterns and require lifestyle changes.

The side effects of medications prescribed for these conditions may further impair nutritional status. A number of prevalent disorders of the gastrointestinal (GI) tract are associated with nutritional concerns including gastroesophageal reflux disease (GERD), ulcers, constipation, diverticulosis, and colon cancer. Dysphagia, often a result of stroke or dementia, significantly affects nutrition. Diseases affecting function, such as arthritis and Parkinson's disease, may impair eating ability. Cancers and subsequent treatment impair appetite and ability to consume adequate nutrition.

Many medications affect appetite and nutrition. These include digoxin, theophylline, nonsteroidal anti-inflammatory drugs (NSAIDs), iron supplements, antidepressants, and psychotropics. There are clinically significant drug-nutrient interactions that result in nutrient loss, and evidence is accumulating that shows the use of nutritional supplements may counteract these possible drug-induced nutrient depletions. A thorough medication review is an essential component of nutritional assessment and individuals should receive education about the effects of prescription medications, as well as herbals and supplements, on nutritional status (see Chapter 8).

Socioeconomic Deprivation

There is a strong relationship between poor nutrition and socioeconomic deprivation. According to the federal government, fewer than 1 in 10 adults age 65 and older is living in poverty. However, poverty rates among older African Americans are nearly triple those of whites, and rates among Hispanics are more than double those of whites (Butrica, 2008). Older single women are also at high risk for poverty. Older adults with low incomes may need to choose among fulfilling needs such as food, heat, telephone bills, medications, and health care visits. Some older people eat only once per day in an attempt to make their income last through the month. Nurses need to be aware of resources in the community for socioeconomically disadvantaged older people and the local Area Agencies on Aging are good resources.

Transportation

Available and easily accessible transportation may be limited for older people. Many small, long-standing neighborhood food stores have been closed in the wake of the expansion of larger supermarkets, which are located in areas that serve a greater segment of the population. It may become difficult to walk to the market, to reach it by public transportation, or to carry a bag of groceries while using a cane or walker. Functional impairments also make the use of public transportation difficult for some older people.

Transportation by taxicab for an individual on a limited income is unrealistic, but sharing a taxicab with others who also need to shop may enable the older person to go where food prices are cheaper and to take advantage of sale items. Senior citizen organizations in many parts of the United States have been helpful in providing older adults with van service to shopping areas. In housing complexes, it may be possible to schedule group trips to the supermarket. Many urban communities have multiple sources of transportation available, but the older adult may be unaware of them. Resources in rural areas are more limited. It is important for nurses to be knowledgeable about resources in the community that are available to older people.

In addition, many older adults, particularly widowed men, may have never learned to shop and prepare food. Often, older adults have to rely on others to shop for them, and this may be a cause of concern depending on availability of support and the reluctance to be dependent on someone else, particularly family. For older adults who own a computer, shopping over the Internet and having groceries delivered offers advantages, although prices may be higher than in the stores.

Hospitalization and Long-Term Care Residence

Older adults in hospitals and long-term care settings are more likely to experience a number of the problems that contribute to inadequate nutrition. In addition to the risk factors mentioned earlier in the chapter, severely restricted diets, long periods of nothing-by-mouth (NPO) status, and insufficient time and staff for feeding assistance contribute to inadequate nutrition. Malnutrition is related to prolonged hospital stays, increased risk for poor health status, institutionalization, and mortality (DiMaria-Ghalili, 2012). Assessment of nutritional status to identify malnutrition and the risk factors for malnutrition is important and required by the Joint Commission. Sufficient time, care, and attention should be given to feeding dependent older people.

The incidence of eating disability in long-term care is high with estimates that 50% of all residents cannot eat independently (Burger et al., 2000). Inadequate staffing in long-term care facilities is associated with poor nutrition and hydration. In response to concerns about the lack of adequate assistance during mealtime in long-term care facilities, the Centers for Medicare and Medicaid Services (CMS) implemented a rule that allows feeding assistants with 8 hours of approved training to help residents with eating. Feeding assistants must be supervised by a registered nurse (RN) or licensed practical–vocational nurse (LPN-LVN). Family members may also be willing and able to assist at mealtimes and also provide a familiar social context for the patient. Nurses need to provide guidance and support on feeding techniques, supervise eating, and evaluate outcomes.

For many older adults residing in long-term care facilities, the benefits of less-restrictive diets outweigh the risks.

Restrictive diets (low salt, low cholesterol) often reduce food intake without significantly helping the clinical status of the individual (Pioneer Network and Rothschild Foundation, 2011). If caloric supplements are used, they should be administered at least 1 hour before meals or they interfere with meal intake. These products are widely used and can be costly. Often, they are not dispensed or consumed as ordered. Powdered breakfast drinks added to milk are an adequate substitute (Duffy, 2010).

Dispensing a small amount of calorically dense oral nutritional supplement (2 calories/mL) during the routine medication pass may have a greater effect on weight gain than a traditional supplement (1.06 calories/mL) with or between meals. Small volumes of nutrient-dense supplement may have less of an effect on appetite and will enhance food intake during meals and snacks. This delivery method allows nurses to observe and document consumption. Further studies and randomized clinical trials are needed to evaluate the effectiveness of nutritional supplementation (Doll-Shankaruk et al., 2008).

Attention to the environment in which meals are served is important. Feeding older people who have difficulty eating can become mechanical and devoid of feeling. The feeding process becomes rapid, and if it bogs down and becomes too slow, the meal may be ended abruptly, depending on the time the caregiver has allotted for feeding the person. Any pleasure derived through socialization and eating and any dignity that could be maintained is often absent (see "The Lived Experience" at the beginning of this chapter). Older adults accustomed to certain table manners may feel ashamed at their inability to behave in what they feel is an appropriate manner.

In addition to adequate staff, many innovative and evidence-based ideas can improve nutritional intake in institutions. Suggestions found in the literature include the following: restorative dining programs; homelike dining rooms; individualized menu choices, including ethnic foods; cafeteria style service; refreshment stations with easy access to juices, water, and healthy snacks; kitchens on the nursing units; availability of food around the clock; choice of mealtimes; liberal diets; finger foods; visually appealing pureed foods with texture and shape; music; touch; verbal cueing; hand-over-hand feeding; and sitting while assisting the person to eat. Other suggestions can be found in Box 9-1.

BOX 9-1   Suggestions to Improve Intake in Institutional Settings

- Serve meals with the person in a chair rather than in bed when possible.
- Provide analgesics and antiemetics on a schedule that provides comfort at mealtime.
- Determine food preferences; include culturally appropriate food.
- Make food available 24 hours/day—provide snacks between meals and at night.
- Avoid prolonged periods of NPO status and restore regular eating as soon as possible.
- Do not interrupt meals to administer medication if possible.
- Limit staff breaks to before and after mealtimes to ensure adequate staff are available to assist with meals.
- Walk around the dining area or the rooms at mealtime to determine if food is being eaten or if assistance is needed.
- Encourage family members to share the mealtimes for a heightened social situation.
- If caloric supplements are used, offer between meals or with the medication pass.
- Recommend an exercise program that may increase appetite.

- Ensure proper fit of dentures and denture use.
- Provide oral hygiene and allow the person to wash his or her hands.
- Have the person wear his or her glasses during meals.
- Sit while feeding the person who needs assistance, use touch, and carry on a social conversation.
- Provide soft music during the meal.
- Use small, round tables seating six to eight people. Consider using tablecloths and centerpieces.
- Seat people with like interests and abilities together and encourage socialization.
- Involve in restorative dining programs if in nursing home.
- Have OT evaluate for use of adaptive equipment.
- Make diets as liberal as possible depending on health status, especially for frail elders who are not consuming adequate amounts.
- Consider a referral to a speech-language pathologist for persons experiencing difficulties with eating and/or an occupational therapist for adaptive equipment.

Dementia

Older adults with dementia are particularly at risk for weight loss and inadequate nutrition. Weight loss often becomes a considerable concern in late-stage dementia. Significant weight loss affects 40% of individuals with dementia (Dunne et al., 2004). Some of the factors predisposing older people with dementia to nutritional inadequacy include lack of awareness of the need to eat, depression, loss of independence in self-feeding, agnosia, apraxia, vision impairments (deficient contrast sensitivity), and behavior disturbances. Modification of feeding techniques can assist in improving intake.

One of the best strategies for managing poor intake is establishing a routine so the older person does not have to remember time and places for eating. Caregivers should continue to serve foods and fluids that the person likes and has always eaten. Nutrient-dense foods are preferred. Attention to mealtime ambience is important, and the person should be able to take as much time as needed to eat the food. Food should be available 24 hours a day, and the person should be allowed to follow his or her accustomed eating schedule (e.g., late breakfast, early dinner). Other suggestions to enhance food intake for individuals with dementia are presented in Box 9-2. Amella and Lawrence (2007) provide a protocol: *Eating and Feeding Issues in Older Adults with Dementia* (see the Evidence-Based Practice box). Chapter 21 provides more discussion of dementia.

Implications for Gerontological Nursing and Healthy Aging

Nutritional Screening and Assessment

Older people are less likely than younger people to show signs of malnutrition and nutrient malabsorption. Evaluation of nutritional health can be difficult in the absence of severe malnutrition, but a comprehensive assessment can reveal deficits. A nutritional assessment that provides the most conclusive data about a person's actual nutritional state consists of the following steps: interview, physical examination, anthropometrical measurements, and biochemical analysis. The collective results provide the data needed to identify the immediate and the potential nutritional problems of the client so that plans for supervision, assistance, and education in the attainment of adequate nutrition for the older person can be implemented. Interprofessional team approaches are key to appropriate assessment and intervention and should involve medicine, nursing; dietary, physical, occupational, and speech therapy; and social work.

A Nutrition Screening Initiative checklist (Figure 9-3) can be used by older people or staff in any setting to identify risk factors for poor nutrition and determine the need for a more comprehensive assessment and nutritional interventions. The Mini Nutritional Assessment (MNA), developed by Nestlé of Geneva, Switzerland, is intended for use by professionals to screen for malnutrition (Figure 9-4).

BOX 9-2   Suggestions to Improve Intake for Individuals with Dementia

- Serve only one dish at a time.
- Provide only one utensil at a time.
- Consider using a "spork" (combination spoon-fork).
- Serve finger foods such as fried chicken, chicken strips, pizza in bite-size pieces, fish sticks, sandwiches.
- Serve soup in a mug.
- Remove any hot items or items that should not be eaten.
- Cut up foods before serving.
- Sit next to the person at their level.
- Demonstrate eating motions that the person can imitate.
- Use hand-over-hand feeding technique to guide self-feeding.
- Use verbal cueing and prompting (e.g., take a bite, chew, swallow).

- Use gentle tone of voice and avoid scolding or demeaning remarks.
- Provide verbal encouragement to participate in eating by talking about food taste and smell.
- Offer small amounts of fluid between bites.
- Help person focus on the meal at hand; turn off background noise, remove clutter from the table.
- Avoid patterned dishes or table coverings.
- Use red plates/glasses/cups (Dunne et al. (2004) found that food intake increased when food was served using high-contrast tableware).
- Use unbreakable dishes that won't slide around.
- Serve smaller, more frequent meals rather than expecting the person to complete a big meal.

From Dunne T, Neargarder S, Cipolloni P, et al: Visual contrast enhances food and liquid intake in advanced Alzheimer's disease, *Clinical Nutrition* 23(4):533-538, 2004; Spencer P: *How to solve eating problems common to people with Alzheimer's and other dementias.* Available at http://www.caring.com/articles/alzheimers-eating-problems.

Read the statements below. Circle the number in the Yes column for those that apply to you or someone you know. For each "yes" answer, score the number listed. Total your nutritional score.

	YES
I have an illness or condition that made me change the kind or amount of food I eat.	2
I eat fewer than two meals per day.	3
I eat few fruits, vegetables or milk products.	2
I have three or more drinks of beer, liquor, or wine almost every day.	2
I have tooth or mouth problems that make it hard for me to eat.	2
I don't always have enough money to buy the food I need.	4
I eat alone most of the time.	1
I take three or more different prescriptions or over-the-counter drugs each day.	1
Without wanting to, I have lost or gained 10 pounds in the past 6 months.	2
I am not always physically able to shop, cook, and/or feed myself.	2

Total Nutritional Score _____

0-2 indicates good nutrition
3-5 moderate risk
6+ high nutritional risk

FIGURE 9-3 Nutritional assessment and approaches. (Courtesy The Nutrition Screening Initiative, Washington, DC.)

The Minimum Data Set (MDS), used in long-term care facilities, includes assessment information that can be used to identify potential nutritional problems, risk factors, and the potential for improved function. Triggers for more thorough investigation of problems include weight loss, alterations in taste, medical therapies, prescription medications, hunger, parenteral or intravenous feedings, mechanically altered or therapeutic diets, percentage of food left uneaten, pressure ulcers, and edema. Other protocols and guidelines for nutritional assessment of older adults can be found in the Evidence-Based Practice box.

Interview

The interview provides background information and clues to the nutritional state and actual and potential problems of the older adult. Questions about the individual's state of health, social activities, normal patterns, and changes that

Evidence-Based Practice

Nutrition, Oral Care, Hydration

- Preventing aspiration in older adults with dysphagia:
  http://consultgerirn.org/uploads/File/trythis/try_this_20.pdf
- Assessing nutrition in older adults:
  http://consultgerirn.org/topics/nutrition_in_the_elderly/want_to_know_more
- Nursing Standard of Practice: Nutrition in Aging: DiMaria-Ghalili R: Nutrition. In Boltz M, Capezuti E, Fulmer T, et al: *Evidence-based geriatric nursing protocols for best practice,* New York, 2012, Springer.
- Eating and feeding issues in older adults with dementia. Part I and Part II—see eating and feeding issues:
  http://consultgerirn.org/resources/#issues_on_dementia
- Nursing Standard of Practice Protocol: Providing Oral Health Care to Older Adults:
  http://consultgerirn.org/topics/oral_healthcare_in_aging/want_to_know_more
- Nursing Standard of Practice Protocol: Oral Hydration Management:
  http://consultgerirn.org/topics/hydration_management/want_to_know_more
- Dehydration Risk Assessment Checklist:
  http://rgp.toronto.on.ca/torontobestpractice/Dehydrationriskappraisalchecklist.pdf
- O'Connor L: Oral health care. In Boltz M, Capezuti E, Fulmer T, Zwicker D: *Evidence-based geriatric nursing protocols for best practice,* New York, Springer, 2012.

Mini Nutritional Assessment
MNA®

**Nestlé
NutritionInstitute**

Last name:		First name:		
Sex:	Age:	Weight, kg:	Height, cm:	Date:

Complete the screen by filling in the boxes with the appropriate numbers. Total the numbers for the final screening score.

Screening

A Has food intake declined over the past 3 months due to loss of appetite, digestive problems, chewing or swallowing difficulties?
0 = severe decrease in food intake
1 = moderate decrease in food intake
2 = no decrease in food intake

B Weight loss during the last 3 months
0 = weight loss greater than 3 kg (6.6 lbs)
1 = does not know
2 = weight loss between 1 and 3 kg (2.2 and 6.6 lbs)
3 = no weight loss

C Mobility
0 = bed or chair bound
1 = able to get out of bed / chair but does not go out
2 = goes out

D Has suffered psychological stress or acute disease in the past 3 months?
0 = yes   2 = no

E Neuropsychological problems
0 = severe dementia or depression
1 = mild dementia
2 = no psychological problems

F1 Body Mass Index (BMI) (weight in kg) / (height in m2)
0 = BMI less than 19
1 = BMI 19 to less than 21
2 = BMI 21 to less than 23
3 = BMI 23 or greater

IF BMI IS NOT AVAILABLE, REPLACE QUESTION F1 WITH QUESTION F2.
DO NOT ANSWER QUESTION F2 IF QUESTION F1 IS ALREADY COMPLETED.

F2 Calf circumference (CC) in cm
0 = CC less than 31
3 = CC 31 or greater

Screening score (max. 14 points)

12-14 points: Normal nutritional status
8-11 points: At risk of malnutrition
0-7 points: Malnourished

References
1. Vellas B, Villars H, Abellan G, et al. Overview of the MNA® - Its History and Challenges. J Nutr Health Aging. 2006;10:456-465.
2. Rubenstein LZ, Harker JO, Salva A, Guigoz Y, Vellas B. Screening for Undernutrition in Geriatric Practice: Developing the Short-Form Mini Nutritional Assessment (MNA-SF). J. Geront. 2001;56A: M366-377.
3. Guigoz Y. The Mini-Nutritional Assessment (MNA®) Review of the Literature - What does it tell us? J Nutr Health Aging. 2006; 10:466-487.
4. Kaiser MJ, Bauer JM, Ramsch C, et al. Validation of the Mini Nutritional Assessment Short-Form (MNA®-SF): A practical tool for identification of nutritional status. J Nutr Health Aging. 2009; 13:782-788.
® Société des Produits Nestlé, S.A., Vevey, Switzerland, Trademark Owners © Nestlé, 1994, Revision 2009. N67200 12/99 10M
For more information: www.mna-elderly.com

FIGURE 9-4 Mini Nutritional Assessment. (Copyright Nestlé, 1994, Revision 2009, Glendale, Calif.)

have occurred should be asked. The nurse must explore the individual's needs, the manner in which food is obtained, and the client's ability to prepare food.

Information concerning the relationship of food to daily events will provide clues to the meaning and significance of food to that person. The older person who eats alone is considered a candidate for malnutrition. Information about occupation and daily activities will suggest the degree of energy expenditure and caloric intake most appropriate for the overall activity. One's economic status will have a direct bearing on nutrition. It is therefore important to explore the client's financial resources to establish the income available for food.

Medications being taken should be included in the nutrition history. Additional medical information should include the presence or absence of mouth pain or discomfort, visual difficulty, bowel and bladder function, and history of illness. Depression is a major cause of weight loss, so an evaluation for depression should be obtained (see Chapter 22).

Diet Histories

Frequently a 24-hour diet recall can provide an estimate of nutritional adequacy. When the older person cannot supply all of the information requested, it may be possible to obtain data from a family member or another source. There will be times, however, when information will not be as complete as one would like, or the older person, too proud to admit that he or she is not eating, will furnish erroneous information. Even so, the nurse will be able to obtain additional data from the other three areas of the nutritional assessment.

Keeping a dietary record for 3 days is another assessment tool. What one ate, when food was eaten, and the amounts eaten must be carefully recorded. Computer analysis of the dietary records provides information on energy and vitamin and mineral intake. Printouts can provide the older person and the health care provider with a visual graph of the intake. Accurate completion of 3-day dietary records in hospitals and nursing homes can be problematic, and intake may be either underestimated or overestimated. Standardized observational protocols should be developed to ensure accuracy of oral intake documentation as well as the adequacy and quality of feeding assistance during mealtimes. Nurses should ensure that direct caregivers are educated on the proper observation and documentation of intake and should closely monitor performance in this area.

Physical Examination

The physical examination furnishes clinically observable evidence of the existing state of nutrition. Data such as height and weight; vital signs; condition of the tongue, lips, and gums; skin turgor, texture, and color; and functional ability are assessed, and the overall general appearance is scrutinized for evidence of wasting. Height should always be measured and never estimated or given by self-report. If the person cannot stand, an alternative way of measuring standing height is knee-height using knee-height calipers. BMI should be calculated to determine if weight for height is within the normal range of 22 to 27. A BMI below 22 is a sign of undernutrition (DiMaria-Ghalili, 2012).

A detailed weight history should be obtained along with current weight. Weight loss is a key indicator of malnutrition, even in overweight older adults. History should include a history of weight loss, whether the weight loss was intentional or unintentional, and during what period it occurred. A history of anorexia is also important, and many older people, especially women, have limited their weight throughout life. Debate continues in the quest to determine the appropriate weight charts for an older adult. Although weight alone does not indicate the adequacy of diet, unplanned fluctuations in weight are significant and should be evaluated.

Procedures for weighing people in institutions should be established and followed consistently to obtain an accurate picture of weight changes. Weighing procedure should be supervised by licensed personnel, and changes should be reported immediately to the provider. One might meet correct weight values for height, but weight changes may be the result of fluid retention, edema, or ascites and merit investigation. An unintentional weight loss of more than 5% of body weight in 1 month, more than 7.5% in 3 months, or more than 10% in 6 months is considered a significant indicator of poor nutrition, as well as an MDS trigger indicating the need for further assessment.

Anthropometrical Measurements

Anthropometrical measurements include height, weight, midarm circumference, and triceps skinfold thickness. These are obtained by simple body measurement procedures, which take less than 5 minutes to perform. These measurements offer information about the status of the older person's muscle mass and body fat in relation to height and weight. Muscle mass measurements are obtained by measuring the arm circumference of the nondominant upper arm. The arm hangs freely at the side, and a measuring tape is placed around the midpoint of the upper arm, between the acromion of the scapula and the olecranon of the ulna. The centimeter circumference is recorded and compared with standard values.

Body fat and lean muscle mass are assessed by measuring specific skinfolds with Lange or Harpenden calipers.

Two areas are accessible for measurement. One area is the midpoint of the upper arm, the triceps area, which is also used to obtain arm circumference. The nondominant arm is again used. The nurse lifts the skin with the thumb and forefinger so that it parallels the humerus. The calipers are placed around the skinfold, 1 cm below where the fingers are grasping the skin. Two readings are averaged to the nearest half centimeter. If there is a neuropathological condition or hemiplegia following a stroke, the unaffected arm should be used for obtaining measurements.

Biochemical Examination

The final step in a nutritional assessment is the biochemical examination. A complete blood count, total lymphocyte count, thyroid level, comprehensive metabolic panel, and liver function tests help assess the presence of diseases known to affect weight loss or cause loss of appetite. Urinalysis to rule out infection, as well as a stool sample for fecal occult blood, should be included. Suggested biochemical parameters include serum albumin, cholesterol, hemoglobin, and serum transferrin. Although these parameters may also be abnormal in several conditions unassociated with malnutrition, they are useful as guides to interventions (Thomas, 2000). Serum proteins also decrease in an inflammatory reaction, infection, or liver disorder. In acute illness, hypoalbuminemia may occur but not be indicative of malnutrition; however, low serum protein levels need further investigation (Duffy, 2010). Serum albumin of more than 4 g/dL is desired; less than 3.5 g/dL is an indicator of poor nutritional state. Prealbumin level may be a better indicator of protein loss because it changes rapidly in the presence of malnutrition. Laboratory test results, although not definitive for malnutrition, provide important clues to nutritional status but should be evaluated in relation to the person's overall health status. Unintentional weight loss remains the most important indicator of a potential nutritional deficit (Ahmed & Haboubi, 2010).

Interventions

Interventions are formulated around the identified concerns. Nursing interventions are centered on techniques to increase food intake and to enhance and manage the environment to promote increased food intake (DiMaria-Ghalili, 2012). Collaboration with the interprofessional team is important in planning interventions. For the community-dwelling elder, nutrition education and problem solving with the elder and family members on how to best resolve the potential or actual nutritional deficit is important. Causes of poor nutrition are complex, and all of the factors emphasized in this chapter are important to assess when planning individualized interventions to ensure adequate nutrition for older people.

Pharmacological Therapy

Drugs that stimulate appetite (orexigenic drugs) can be considered to reverse resistant anorexia but only after all other interventions have been tried. They must be monitored closely for side effects and have had little evaluation in frail older people. Benefits are restricted to small weight gains without indication of decreased morbidity or mortality or improved quality of life or functional ability (Vitale et al., 2009).

Patient Education

Education should be provided to older adults on nutritional requirements for health, special diet modifications for chronic illness management, the effect of age-associated changes and medication on nutrition, and community resources to assist in maintaining adequate nutrition. Medicare covers nutrition therapy for select diseases, such as diabetes and kidney disease, which creates unprecedented opportunities for older Americans to access information.

Special Considerations in Nutrition for Older People: Hydration, Dysphagia, Oral Care

Several conditions warrant further discussion because they are frequently encountered in care of older adults and are related to adequate diet and nutritional status. These include dehydration, dysphagia, and oral health.

Hydration Management

Hydration management is the promotion of an adequate fluid balance, which prevents complications resulting from abnormal or undesirable fluid levels. Daily needs for water can usually be met by functionally independent older adults through intake of fluids with meals and social drinks. However, a significant number of older adults (up to 85% of those 85 years of age and over) drink less than 1 liter of fluid per day. Older adults, with the exception of those requiring fluid restrictions, should consume at least 1500 mL of fluid per day (Mentes, 2006).

Maintenance of fluid balance (fluid intake equals fluid output) is essential to health, regardless of a person's age

(Mentes, 2006). Age-related changes, medication use, functional impairments, and comorbid medical and emotional illnesses place some older adults at risk for changes in fluid balance, especially dehydration (Mentes, 2008). See the Evidence-Based Practice box for a hydration management guideline.

Dehydration

Dehydration is defined clinically as "a complex condition resulting in a reduction in total body water. In older people, dehydration most often develops as a result of disease, age-related changes, and/or the effects of medication and NOT primarily due to lack of access to water" (Thomas et al., 2008, p. 293). Dehydration is considered a geriatric syndrome that is frequently associated with common diseases (e.g., diabetes, respiratory illness, heart failure) and declining stages of the frail elderly (Crecelius, 2008). It is often an unappreciated comorbid condition that exacerbates an underlying condition such as a urinary tract infection, respiratory infection, or worsening depression (Thomas et al., 2008).

Dehydration is a problem prevalent among older adults in all settings. Dehydration is a significant risk factor for delirium, thromboembolic complications, infections, kidney stones, constipation, obstipation, falls, medication toxicity, renal failure, seizure, electrolyte imbalance, hyperthermia, and delayed wound healing. If not treated adequately, mortality from dehydration can be as high as 50% (Faes et al., 2007).

Thomas and colleagues (2008) comment that there are few diagnoses that generate as much concern about causes and consequences as does dehydration. Due to a lack of understanding of the pathogenesis and consequences of dehydration in older adults, the condition is often attributed to poor care by nursing home staff and/or physicians. However, the majority of older people develop dehydration as a result of increased fluid losses combined with decreased fluid intake, related to decreased thirst. The condition is rarely due to neglect (Thomas et al., 2008).

Risk Factors for Dehydration

Most healthy older adults maintain adequate hydration, but the presence of physical or emotional illness, surgery, trauma, or conditions of higher physiological demands increase the risk of dehydration. When the fluid balance of older adults is at risk, the limited capacity of homeostatic mechanisms becomes significant (Faes et al., 2007).

Age-related changes in the thirst mechanism, decrease in total body water (TBW), and decreased kidney function increase the risk for dehydration. The loss of muscle mass

with age increases the proportion of fat cells. This loss is greater in women because they have a higher percentage of body fat and less muscle mass than men. Because fat cells contain less water than muscle cells, older people have a decreased intracellular fluid volume.

Thirst sensation diminishes, resulting in the loss of an important defense against dehydration. In a mechanism that is not well understood, thirst in older adults is not "proportional to metabolic needs in response to dehydrating conditions" (Mentes, 2008, p. 371). Creatinine clearance also declines with age, and the kidneys are less able to concentrate urine. These changes are more pronounced in older people with illnesses affecting kidney function.

Other risk factors for dehydration include medications, particularly those that directly affect renal function and fluid balance (diuretics, laxatives, angiotensin-converting enzyme [ACE] inhibitors) and psychotropic medications that have anticholinergic effects (dry mouth, urinary retention, constipation). The use of four or more medications is also a risk factor (Faes et al., 2007).

Functional deficits, communication and comprehension problems, oral problems, dysphagia, delirium, depression, dementia, hospitalization, low body weight, diagnostic procedures necessitating fasting, inadequate assistance with fluid intake, diarrhea, fever, vomiting, infections, bleeding, draining wounds, artificial ventilation, fluid restrictions, high environmental temperature, and multiple comorbidities have all been noted as risk factors for dehydration in older people (Mentes, 2006; Faes et al., 2007). NPO requirements for diagnostic tests and surgical procedures should be as short as possible for older adults, and adequate fluids should be given once tests and procedures are completed. A 2-hour suspension of fluid intake is recommended for many procedures.

Implications for Gerontological Nursing and Healthy Aging

Assessment

Prevention of dehydration is essential, but assessment is complex in older people. Clinical signs may not appear until dehydration is advanced. Attention to risk factors for dehydration in older adults using a screen (Boxes 9-3 and 9-4) is very important. In addition, the MDS has triggers for dehydration/fluid maintenance. Education should be provided to older people and their caregivers on the need for fluids and the signs and symptoms of dehydration. Acute situations such as vomiting, diarrhea, or febrile episodes should be identified quickly and treated. Older adults over 85 years of

BOX 9-3	Simple Screen for Dehydration

Drugs, e.g., diuretics
End of life
High fever
Yellow urine turns dark
Dizziness (orthostasis)
Reduced oral intake
Axilla dry
Tachycardia
Incontinence (fear of)
Oral problems/sippers
Neurological impairment (confusion)
Sunken eyes

From Thomas D, Cote T, Lawhorne L, et al: Understanding clinical dehydration and its treatment, *Journal of the American Medical Directors Association 9(5)*:292-301, 2008.

age who have experienced volume deficits, weight loss, malnutrition, or infections, and those with dementia, delirium, and functional impairments are at high risk for dehydration.

Typical signs of dehydration may not always be present in older people, and most clinical signs and symptoms are not very sensitive or specific. "The large variability in the way different organs are affected by dehydration will cause symptoms to remain atypical in older adults" (Faes et al., 2007, p. 3). Skin turgor, assessed at the sternum and commonly included in the assessment of dehydration, is an unreliable marker in older adults because of the loss of subcutaneous tissue with aging. Dry mucous membranes in the mouth and nose, longitudinal furrows on the tongue, orthostasis, speech incoherence, extremity weakness, dry axilla, and sunken eye may indicate dehydration. However, the diagnosis of dehydration is biochemical (Thomas et al., 2008).

BOX 9-4	Ongoing Management of Oral Intake

1. Calculate a daily fluid goal.
   - All older adults should have an individualized fluid goal determined by a documented standard for daily fluid intake. At least 1500 mL of fluid/day should be provided.
2. Compare current intake to fluid goal to evaluate hydration status.
3. Provide fluids consistently throughout the day.
   - 75% to 80% of fluids delivered at meals and the remainder offered during nonmeal times such as medication times
   - Offer a variety of fluids and fluids that the person prefers
   - Standardize the amount of fluid that is offered with medication administration—for example, at least 6 oz
4. Plan for at-risk individuals.
   - Fluid rounds midmorning and midafternoon
   - Provide 2 8-oz glasses of fluid in the morning and evening
   - "Happy hour" or "tea time," when residents can gather for additional fluids and socialization
   - Modified fluid containers based on resident's abilities— for example, lighter cups and glasses, weighted cups and glasses, plastic water bottles with straws (attach to wheelchairs, deliver with meals)
   - Make fluids accessible at all times and be sure residents can access them—for example, filled water pitchers, fluid stations, or beverage carts in congregate areas
   - Allow adequate time and staff for eating or feeding. Meals can provide two thirds of daily fluids.
   - Encourage family members to participate in feeding and offering fluids
5. Perform fluid regulation and documentation.
   - Teach individuals, if they are able, to use a urine color chart to monitor hydration status
   - Document complete intake including hydration habits
   - Know volumes of fluid containers to accurately calculate fluid consumption
   - Frequency of documentation of fluid intake will vary among settings and is dependent on the individual's condition. In most settings, at least one accurate intake and output recording should be documented, including amount of fluid consumed, difficulties with consumption, and urine specific gravity and color. For individuals who are not continent, teach caregivers to observe incontinent pads or briefs for amount and frequency of urine, color changes, and odor and report variations from individual's normal pattern

Adapted from Mentes JC: Managing oral hydration. In Capezuti E, Zwicker D, Mezey M, et al, editors: *Evidence-based geriatric nursing protocols for best practice, ed 3,* New York, 2008, Springer; www.consultgerirn.org.

If dehydration is suspected, laboratory tests include blood urea nitrogen (BUN), sodium, creatinine, glucose, and bicarbonate. Osmolarity should be either directly measured or calculated. While most cases of dehydration have an elevated BUN, there are many other causes of an elevated BUN/creatinine ratio, so this test cannot be used alone to diagnose dehydration in older adults (Thomas et al., 2008). Mentes (2006) notes that "as is true with other standard tests, serum markers confirm a diagnosis of dehydration once it is too late to prevent it from occurring" (p. 5). Attention to risk factors is important to identify possible dehydration and to intervene early. Body weight changes should also be assessed as indicators of changes in hydration (Faes et al., 2007).

Urine color, which is measured using a urine color chart, has been suggested as helpful in assessing hydration status (not dehydration) in older individuals in nursing homes with adequate renal function (Mentes, 2008). The urine color chart has eight standardized colors, ranging from pale straw (number 1) to greenish brown (number 8) approximating urine specific gravities of 1.003 to 1.029 (Mentes, 2006, 2008). Urine color should be assessed and charted over several days. Pale straw–colored urine usually indicates normal hydration status, and as urine darkens, poor hydration may be indicated (after taking into account discoloration by food or medications). For older adults, a reading of 4 or less is preferred (Mentes, 2006). If a person's urine becomes darker than his or her usual color, fluid intake assessment is indicated, and fluids can be increased before dehydration occurs (Mentes, 2008).

Interventions

Interventions are derived from a comprehensive assessment and consist of risk identification and hydration management (Mentes, 2008) (see Boxes 9-3 and 9-4). Hydration management involves both acute and ongoing management of oral intake. Oral hydration is the first treatment approach for dehydration. Individuals with mild to moderate dehydration who can drink and do not have significant mental or physical compromise due to fluid loss may be able to replenish fluids orally (Thomas et al., 2008). Water is considered the best fluid to offer, but other clear fluids may also be useful depending on the person's preference.

Rehydration methods depend on the severity and the type of dehydration and may include intravenous or hypodermoclysis (HDC). A general rule is to replace 50% of the loss within the first 12 hours (or 1 L/day in afebrile elders) or sufficient quantity to relieve tachycardia and hypotension. Further fluid replacement can be administered more slowly over a longer period of time.

HDC is an infusion of isotonic fluids into the subcutaneous space. HDC is safe, easy to administer, and a useful alternative to intravenous administration for persons with mild to moderate dehydration, particularly those patients with altered mental status. HDC cannot be used in severe dehydration or for any situation requiring more than 3 L over 24 hours. Common sites of infusion are the lateral abdominal wall; the anterior or lateral aspects of the thighs; the infraclavicular region; and the back, usually the interscapular or subscapular regions with a fat fold of at least 1 inch thick (Mei & Auerhahn, 2009). Normal saline (0.9%), half-normal saline (0.45%), 5% glucose in water infusion (D_5W), or Ringer's solution can be used (Thomas et al., 2008). Hypodermoclysis can be administered in almost any setting, so hospital admissions may be avoided. Hypodermoclysis is "an evidence-based low-cost therapy in geriatrics" (Faes et al., 2007).

Dysphagia

Dysphagia, or difficulty swallowing, is a common problem in older adults. The prevalence of swallowing disorders is 16% to 22% in adults over 50 years of age, and up to 60% of nursing home residents have clinical evidence of dysphagia (Tanner, 2010). Dysphagia can be the result of behavioral, sensory, or motor problems and is common in individuals with neurologic disease and dementia. Dysphagia is a serious problem and has negative consequences, including weight loss, malnutrition, dehydration, aspiration pneumonia, and even death. Aspiration pneumonia is the leading cause of death and the second most common cause for hospitalization among nursing home residents (Sarin et al., 2008).

Implications for Gerontological Nursing and Healthy Aging
Assessment

It is important to obtain a careful history of the older adult's response to dysphagia and to observe the person during mealtime. Symptoms that alert the nurse to possible swallowing problems are presented in Box 9-5. Patients referred for a dysphagia evaluation ("swallowing study") must be assumed to be dysphagic and at risk for aspiration. NPO status should be maintained until the swallowing evaluation is completed. During this period, if necessary, nutrition and hydration needs can be met by intravenous, nasogastric, or gastric tubes (Tanner, 2010). A comprehensive evaluation by a speech-language pathologist, usually including a video fluoroscopic recording of a modified barium swallow, should be considered when dysphagia is suspected.

BOX 9-5   Risk Factors for Dysphagia

- Cerebrovascular accident
- Parkinson's disease
- Neuromuscular disorders (ALS, MS, myasthenia gravis)
- Dementia
- Head and neck cancer
- Traumatic brain injury
- Aspiration pneumonia
- Inadequate feeding technique
- Poor dentition

BOX 9-6   Interventions to Prevent Aspiration in Patients with Dysphagia: Hand Feeding

- Provide a 30-minute rest period before feeding; a rested person will likely have less difficulty swallowing.
- The person should sit at 90 degrees during all oral (PO) intake.
- Maintain 90-degree positioning for at least 1 hour after PO intake.
- Adjust rate of feeding and size of bites to the person's tolerance; avoid rushed or forced feeding.
- Alternate solid and liquid boluses.
- Follow speech therapist's recommendation for safe swallowing techniques and modified food consistency (may need thickened liquids, puree foods).
- If facial weakness is present, place food on the nonimpaired side of the mouth.
- Avoid sedatives and hypnotics that may impair cough reflex and swallowing ability.
- Keep suction equipment ready at all times.
- Supervise all meals.
- Monitor temperature.
- Observe color of phlegm.
- Visually check the mouth for pocketing of food in cheeks.
- Provide mouth care every 4 hours.

Adapted from Metheny N, Boltz M, Greenberg S: Preventing aspiration in older adults with dysphagia, *Am J Nurs 108(2)*:45-46, 2008.

Interventions

After the swallowing evaluation, a decision must be made about the person's potential for functional improvement of the swallowing disorder and their safety in swallowing liquid and solid food. The goal is safe oral intake to maintain optimal nutrition and caloric needs. Compensatory interventions include postural changes, such as chin tucks or head turns while swallowing, and modification of bolus volume, consistency, temperature, and rate of presentation (Easterling & Robbins, 2008). Neuromuscular electric stimulation has received clearance by the U.S. Food and Drug Administration for treatment of dysphagia. This therapy involves the administration of small electrical impulses to the swallowing muscles in the throat and is used in combination with traditional swallowing exercises.

Aspiration is the most profound and dangerous problem for older adults experiencing dysphagia. It is important to have a suction machine available at the bedside or in the dining room in the institutional setting. Suggested interventions helpful in preventing aspiration during hand feeding are presented in Box 9-6. The gerontological nurse must work closely with other members of the interprofessional team, such as dietitians and speech-language pathologists, in implementing suggested interventions to prevent aspiration. Research on the appropriate management of swallowing disorders in older people, particularly during acute illness and in long-term care facilities, is very limited, and additional study is essential. A comprehensive protocol for preventing aspiration in older adults with dysphagia and other resources, including a video presentation of assessment of dysphagia, can be found in the Evidence-Based Practice box.

Feeding Tubes

Comprehensive assessment of swallowing problems and other factors that influence intake must be conducted before initiating severely restricted diet modifications or considering the use of feeding tubes, particularly in older people with dementia or those at the end of life. The use of percutaneous endoscopic gastrostomy (PEG) feeding tubes has increased at an astonishing rate in older adults over recent years. No scientific study demonstrates improved survival, reduced incidence of pneumonia or other infections, improved function, or fewer pressure ulcers with the use of feeding tubes, particularly in older people with dementia or those at the end of life (Teno et al., 2010).

Few complications occur with insertion of a PEG tube, but numerous complications occur from having a PEG tube, including aspiration pneumonia, diarrhea, metabolic problems, and cellulitis. "Nearly 50% of patients die within 6 months following PEG insertion; the procedure is often overused and its value has been questioned" (Aparanji & Dharmarajan, 2010, p. 453). Box 9-7 presents myths and facts about PEG tube placement.

As discussed earlier in the chapter, food and eating are closely tied to socialization, comfort, pleasure, love, and the meeting of basic biological needs. Decisions about feeding tube placement are challenging and require thoughtful discussion with patients and caregivers, who should be free to make decisions without duress and with careful consideration of the patient's advance directives, if available. Aparanji and Dharmarajan (2010) suggest that decisions to place a feeding tube are often taken without completely exhausting means to maintain a normal oral intake and that discussions with the physician before insertion are often inadequate with room for improvement. Discussion about advance directives and feeding support should begin early in the course of the illness rather than waiting until a crisis develops. The best advice for individuals is to state preferences for the use of a feeding tube in a written advance directive.

Individuals have the right to use or not use a feeding tube but should be given information about the risks and benefits of enteral feeding, particularly in late-stage dementia. In difficult situations, an ethics committee may be consulted to help make decisions. It is important that everyone involved in the care of the patient be informed of the risks and benefits of tube feeding and the uncertainty of whether enteral feeding provides any benefit for the patient. The decision should never be understood as a question of tube feeding versus no feeding. No family member should be made to feel that they are starving their loved one to death if a decision is made not to institute enteral feeding. Efforts to provide nutrition should continue, and patients should be able to take any type of nutrition they desire any time they desire.

Excellent information for patients and families about enteral feeding can be found at http://www.chcr.brown.edu/dying/consumerfeedingtube.htm. The Northern California chapter of the Gerontological Nursing Advanced Practice Nurses Association has produced a brochure about nutrition and hydration for caregivers, families of persons with dementia, and the health care team (Hess, 2008). The New Dining Practice Standards, reflecting evidence-based research, provides comprehensive guidance for dysphagia interventions, including the use of feeding tubes (Pioneer Network and Rothschild Foundation, 2011).

Oral Care

Dental health of older adults is a basic need that is increasingly neglected with advanced age, debilitation, and limited mobility. Orodental health is integral to general health. *Healthy People 2020* addresses oral health (see the Healthy People box). Poor oral health is recognized

---

BOX 9-7   Myths and Facts about PEG Tubes

Myths
- PEGs prevent death from inadequate intake.
- PEGs reduce aspiration pneumonia.
- Not feeding people is a form of euthanasia and we can't let people starve to death.
- PEGs improve albumin levels and nutritional status.
- PEGs assist in healing pressure ulcers.
- PEGs provide enhanced comfort for people at the end of life.

Facts
- PEGs do not improve quality of life.
- PEGs do not reduce risk of aspiration, and they increase the rate of pneumonia development and the death rate.
- PEGs do not prolong survival in dementia.
- Nearly 50% of patients die within 6 months following PEG tube insertion.
- PEGs cause increased discomfort from both the tube presence and use of restraints.
- PEGs are associated with infections, gastrointestinal symptoms, and abscesses.
- PEG tube feeding deprives people of the taste of food and contact with caregivers during feeding.
- PEGs are popular because they are convenient and labor beneficial.

From Aparanji K, Dharmarajan T: Pause before a PEG: A feeding tube may not be necessary in every candidate, *J Am Med Dir Assoc* 11:453-456, 2010; Vitale C, Monteleoni C, Burke L, et al: Strategies for improving care for patients with advanced dementia and eating problems: optimizing care through physician and speech pathologist collaboration, *Ann Longterm Care* 17(5):32-39, 2009.

HEALTHY PEOPLE 2020
Dental Health Goals for Older Adults

- Prevent and control oral and craniofacial diseases, conditions, and injuries, and improve access to preventive services and dental care
- Reduce the proportion of adults with untreated dental decay
- Reduce the proportion of older adults 65 to 74 years of age with untreated coronal cavies
- Reduce the proportion of older adults 75 years of age and older with untreated root surface caries
- Reduce the proportion of adults who have ever had a permanent tooth extracted because of dental caries or periodontal disease
- Reduce the proportion of older adults 65 to 74 years of age who have lost all of their natural teeth
- Reduce the proportion of adults 45 to 74 years of age with moderate or severe periodontitis
- Increase the proportion of oral and pharyngeal cancers detected at the earliest stages

From U.S. Department of Health and Human Services, Office of Disease Prevention and Health Promotion: *Healthy people 2020* (2012). Available at http://www.healthypeople.gov/2020.

as a risk factor for dehydration and malnutrition, as well as a number of systemic diseases, including pneumonia, joint infections, cardiovascular disease, and poor glycemic control in type 1 and type 2 diabetes (Jablonski, 2010; O'Connor, 2012; Sarin et al., 2008).

The percentage of older people without natural teeth is more than 30%, primarily as a result of periodontitis, which occurs in about 95% of those older than 65 years (American Geriatrics Society [AGS], 2006). Prevalence of this disease is decreasing as knowledge increases and more people use fluorides, improve nutrition, engage in new oral hygiene practices, and take advantage of improved dental health care. However, older people may not have had the advantages of new preventive treatment, and those with functional and cognitive limitations may be unable to perform oral hygiene. Oral care is often lacking in institutions, and the "oral health status of nursing home residents has been described as deplorable" (Jablonski, 2010, p. 21). Access to dental care for older people may be limited as well as cost-prohibitive.

In the existing health care system, dental care is a low priority. Medicare does not provide any coverage for oral health care services, and few Americans 75 years of age or older have private dental insurance. Elders have fewer

dentist visits than any other age group. Older Americans with the poorest oral health are those who are economically disadvantaged, lack insurance, and are members of racial and ethnic minorities. Being disabled, homebound, or institutionalized increases the risk of poor oral health.

Implications for Gerontological Nursing and Healthy Aging

Assessment

Good oral hygiene and assessment of oral health are essentials of nursing care. In addition to identifying oral health problems, examination of the mouth can serve as an early warning system for some diseases and lead to early diagnosis and treatment. All persons, especially those over 50 years of age, with or without dentures, should have oral examinations on a regular basis. Federal regulations mandate an annual examination for residents of long-term care facilities. Although the oral examination is best performed by a dentist, nurses can provide basic screening examinations to persons using an instrument such as The Kayser-Jones Brief Oral Health Status Examination (BOHSE) (see the Evidence-Based Practice box).

Interventions

Prescribed oral hygiene for the individual with some or all teeth is to brush, floss, and use a fluoride dentifrice and mouthwash daily. There is evidence that cleaning the person's teeth with a toothbrush after meals lowers the risk of developing aspiration pneumonia (Metheny, 2007). Impaired manual dexterity may make it difficult for elders to adequately maintain their dental routine and remove plaque adequately. The hand grip of manual toothbrushes is too small to grasp and manipulate easily. Using a child's toothbrush or enlarging the handle of an adult-sized toothbrush by adding a foam grip or wrapping it with gauze to increase handle size has been effective in facilitating grasp. Caregivers may also bend a toothbrush handle back approximately 45 degrees to improve access in dependent older people or those who are resistant (Stein & Henry, 2009).

The ultrasonic toothbrush is an effective tool for elders or for those who must brush the teeth of elders. The base is large enough for easy grasp, and the ultrasonic movement of the bristles in concert with the usual brushing movement is very effective in plaque removal. Use of a commercial floss handle may provide the leverage and ease necessary for the person to continue flossing. Occupational therapists can be helpful in assessment of functional impairments and provision of adaptive equipment for oral care.

Foam swabs are available to provide oral hygiene but do not remove plaque as well as toothbrushes. Foam swabs may be used to clean the oral mucosa of an edentulous older adult. Lemon glycerin swabs should never be used for older people. In combination with decreased salivary flow and xerostomia, they dry the oral mucosa and erode the tooth enamel (O'Connor, 2012).

Infected teeth and poor oral hygiene are associated with pneumonia following aspiration of contaminated oral secretions. Research results indicate that tube feeding in older adults is associated with significant pathologic colonization of the mouth, greater than that observed in people who received oral feeding. Oral care should be provided every 4 hours for patients with gastrostomy tubes, and teeth should be brushed with a toothbrush after each feeding to decrease the risk of aspiration pneumonia (Metheny et al., 2008; O'Connor, 2012). The oral mucosa of unconscious or severely cognitively impaired patients should be hydrated using gauze soaked in physiological saline, and lips should be coated with petroleum jelly or lip balm (Gil-Montoya et al., 2006).

When the person is unable to carry out his or her dental/oral regimen, it is the responsibility of the caregiver to provide oral care (Box 9-8). Oral care is an often neglected part of daily nursing care and should receive the same priority as other kinds of care (Stein, 2009). Poor oral health and lack of attention to oral hygiene are major concerns in institutional settings and contribute significantly to poor nutrition and other negative outcomes such as aspiration pneumonia. Many reasons exist for this deficit, including inadequate knowledge of how to assess and provide care, difficulty providing oral care to dependent and cognitively impaired elders, inadequate training and staffing, and lack of appropriate supplies.

Older people with cognitive impairment may be resistive to mouth care, and this is one of the reasons caregivers may neglect oral care. Placing yourself at eye level and explaining all actions in step-by-step instructions with cues and gestures may decrease mouth care–resistive behavior. Even with individuals who need help, caregivers should encourage as much self-care as possible. Caregivers can have the person hold the toothbrush but place their hand over the person's hand (hand-over-hand technique) (Jablonski, 2010; Jablonski et al., 2009; Stein & Henry, 2009).

Many elders believe that there is no longer a need for oral care once they have dentures. Older adults with dentures should be taught the proper home care of their dentures and oral tissue to prevent odor, stain, plaque buildup, and oral infections. Care should include removal of debris under dentures to prevent pressure on and shrinkage of underlying support structures. Dentures and other dental appliances, such as bridges, should be rinsed after each meal and brushed thoroughly once a day, preferably at night (Box 9-9). Dentures should be worn constantly except at night (to allow relief of compression on the gums) and replaced in the mouth in the morning.

Dentures are very personal and expensive possessions. In communal living situations of nursing homes, hospitals,

---

BOX 9-8   Dental Care: Instructions for Caregivers

1. Explain all actions to the person; use gestures and demonstration as needed; cue and prompt to encourage as much self-care performance as possible.
2. If the patient is in bed, elevate his or her head by raising the bed or propping it with pillows, and have the patient turn his or her head to face you. Place a clean towel across the chest and under the chin, and place a basin under the chin.
3. If the patient is sitting in a stationary chair or wheelchair, stand behind the patient and stabilize his or her head by placing one hand under the chin and resting the head against your body. Place a towel across the chest and over the shoulders. (It may be helpful to secure it with a safety pin.) The basin can be kept handy in the patient's lap or on a table placed in front of or at the side of the patient. A wheelchair may be positioned in front of the sink.
4. If the patient's lips are dry or cracked, apply a light coating of petroleum jelly or use lip balm.
5. Brush and floss the patient's teeth as you have been instructed (use an electric toothbrush if possible, with sulcular brushing). It may be helpful to retract the patient's lips and cheek with a tongue blade or fingers in order to see the area that is being cleaned. Use a mouth prop as needed if the patient cannot hold his or her mouth open. If manual flossing is too difficult, use a floss holder or interproximal brush to clean the proximal surfaces between the teeth. Use a dentifrice-containing fluoride.
6. Provide the conscious patient with fluoride rinses or other rinses as indicated by the dentist or hygienist.

BOX 9-9   Instructions for Denture Cleaning

1. Rinse your denture or dentures after each meal to remove soft debris. Do not use toothpaste on dentures since it abrades denture surfaces.
2. Once each day, preferably before retiring, remove your denture and brush it thoroughly.
   a. Although an ordinary soft toothbrush is adequate, a specially designed denture brush may clean more effectively. (CAUTION: Acrylic denture material is softer than natural teeth and may be damaged by being brushed with very firm bristles.)
   b. Brush your denture over a sink lined with a facecloth and half-filled with water. This will prevent breakage if the denture is dropped.
   c. Hold the denture securely in one hand, but do not squeeze. Hold the brush in the other hand. It is not essential to use a denture paste, particularly if dentures are soaked before being brushed to

soften debris. Never use a commercial tooth powder, because it is abrasive and may damage the denture materials. Plain water, mild soap, or sodium bicarbonate may be used.

   d. When cleaning a removable partial denture, great care must be taken to remove plaque from the curved metal clasps that hook around the teeth. This can be done with a regular toothbrush or with a specially designed clasp brush.
3. After brushing, rinse your denture thoroughly; then place it in a denture-cleaning solution and allow it to soak overnight or for at least a few hours. (NOTE: Acrylic denture material must be kept wet at all times to prevent cracking or warping.) In the morning, remove your denture from the cleaning solution, rinse it thoroughly, and then insert it into your mouth. Use denture paste if necessary to secure dentures.

---

and other care centers, dentures have often been misplaced or mixed up with those of others. The utmost care should be taken when handling, cleaning, and storing dentures. Dentures should be marked, and many states require all newly made dentures to contain the client's identification. A commercial denture marking system called Identure, produced by the 3M Company, provides a simple, efficient, and permanent means of marking dentures.

Broken or damaged dentures and dentures that no longer fit because of weight loss are a common problem for older adults. Rebasing of dentures is a technique to improve the fit of dentures. Ill-fitting dentures or dentures that are not cleaned contribute to oral problems as well as to poor nutrition and reduced enjoyment of food. Both nursing students and nursing staff need to be knowledgeable about oral hygiene and techniques to care for teeth and dentures. Oral hygiene protocols and appropriate oral care equipment should be available in institutions. Patients and families also need education on the importance of good oral health in older adults and techniques for providing adequate oral care.

Implications for Gerontological Nursing and Healthy Aging

Maintenance of adequate nutritional health as a person ages is extremely complex. Knowledge of nutritional needs in later years and of the many factors contributing

to inadequate nutrition is essential for the gerontological nurse and should be a part of every assessment of an older person. Working with members of the interprofessional team in appropriate assessment and development of therapeutic interventions is a major role in community, hospital, and long-term care settings. Use of evidence-based practice protocols is important in determining nursing interventions to support and enhance nutrition and hydration status.

Prevention of undernutrition and malnutrition and the maintenance of dietary needs and food are also ethical responsibilities. No older person should be hungry or thirsty because he or she cannot shop, cook, buy and prepare food, or eat independently. Nor should any older person have to suffer because of a lack of assistance with these activities in whatever setting in which they may reside.

Application of Maslow's Hierarchy

Food is a basic human need for people of all ages. Attention must be paid to more than just adequate caloric intake to sustain life. Not only does adequate nutrition satisfy biological needs, but also the experience of eating provides opportunities for belonging. Being able to eat independently and enjoy meals or being provided with kind and competent assistance if unable to be independent promotes self-esteem and a feeling of worth.

KEY CONCEPTS

- Recommended dietary patterns for the older adult are similar to those of younger persons, with some reduction in the caloric intake based on decreased caloric requirements.
- Many factors affect adequate nutrition in late life, including lifelong eating habits, income, chronic illness, dentition, mood disorders, capacity for food preparation, and functional limitations.
- Protein-caloric malnutrition (PCM) is the most common form of malnutrition in older adults. Estimates indicate that 50% of nursing home patients, 50% of hospitalized patients, and 44% of home health patients over 65 years of age are malnourished.
- A comprehensive nutritional assessment is an essential component of the assessment of older adults.
- Making mealtime pleasant and attractive for the older adult who is unable to eat unassisted is a nursing challenge; mealtime must be made enjoyable, and adequate assistance must be provided.
- Dental health of older adults is a basic need that is increasingly neglected. Poor oral health is a risk factor for dehydration, malnutrition, and aspiration pneumonia.
- Age-related changes in the thirst mechanism, decrease in TBW, and decreased kidney function increase the risk for dehydration in older adults.
- Dysphagia is a serious problem and contributes to weight loss, malnutrition, dehydration, aspiration pneumonia, and death. Careful assessment of risk factors, observation for signs and symptoms, and collaboration with speech-language pathologists on interventions is essential.

ACTIVITIES AND DISCUSSION QUESTIONS

1. What are the factors affecting the nutrition of the older adult?
2. How can the nurse intervene to provide better nutrition for elders in the community, in acute care, and in long-term care settings?
3. What are the causes of malnutrition?
4. What is included in the nutritional assessment of an older person?
5. What are suggestions to encourage better oral care in hospitalized and institutionalized older adults?
6. How is dysphagia assessed, and what interventions may be helpful in preventing aspiration?
7. Develop a nursing care plan for an older adult at risk for malnutrition and dehydration using wellness and North American Nursing Diagnosis Association (NANDA) diagnoses.

REFERENCES

Academy of Nutrition and Dietetics: Fiber. Available at www.eatright.org/public/content.aspx?ID=6796#.ue-duoymy_M.

Ahmed T, Haboubi N: Assessment and management of nutrition in older people and its importance to health, *Clin Interv Aging* 5:207, 2010.

Amella E, Lawrence J: Eating and feeding issues in older adults with dementia (2007). Available at www.hartfordign.org.

American Dietetic Association [ADA], the American Society for Nutrition [ASN], and the Society for Nutrition Education [SNE]: Position of the American Dietetic Association, American Society for Nutrition and Society for Nutrition Education: Food and nutrition programs for community-residing older adults, *J Am Diet Assoc* 110:463, 2010.

American Geriatrics Society [AGS]: *Geriatrics at your fingertips*, New York, 2006, The Society.

Aparanji K, Dharmarajan T: Pause before a PEG: a feeding tube may not be necessary in every candidate, *J Am Med Dir Assoc* 11:453, 2010.

Bales C, Buhr G: Is obesity bad for older persons? A systematic review of the pros and cons of weight reduction in later life, *J Am Med Dir Assoc* 9(2):302–312, 2008.

Beasley J, LaCroix A, Neuhouser M, et al: Protein intake and incident frailty in the women's health initiative observational study, *J Am Geriatr Soc* 58:1063, 2010.

Burger S, Kayser-Jones J, Bell J: *Malnutrition and dehydration in nursing homes: key issues in prevention and treatment* (2000). Available at http://www.commonwealthfund.org/usr_doc/burger_mal_386.pdf.

Butrica B: Do assets change the racial profile of poverty among older adults? Urban Institute (2008). Available at http://www.urban.org/publications/411620.html.

Cacchione PZ: Sensory changes. In Capezuti E, Zwicker D, Mezey M, et al, editors: *Evidence-based geriatric nursing protocols for best practice*, New York, 2008, Springer.

Cadogan M: Clinical concepts: functional consequences of vitamin B12 deficiency, *J Gerontol Nurs* 36:18, 2010.

Crecelius C: Dehydration: myth and reality, *J Am Med Dir Assoc* 9:287, 2008.

DiMaria-Ghalili R: Nutrition. In Boltz M, Capezuti E, Fulmer T, et al: *Evidence-based geriatric nursing protocols for best practice*, New York, 2012, Springer.

Doll-Shankaruk M, Yau W, Oekle C: Implementation and effects of a medication pass nutritional supplement program in a long-term care facility, *J Gerontol Nurs* 34(5):45–50, 2008.

Duffy E: *Malnutrition in older adults*, Advance for NPs and PAs (2010). Available at http://nurse-practitioners-and-physician-assistants.advanceweb.com/article/malnutrition-in-older-adults.aspx.

Dunne T, Neargarder S, Cipolloni P, et al: Visual contrast enhances food and liquid intake in advanced Alzheimer's disease, *Clinical Nutrition* 23:533, 2004.

Easterling C, Robbins E: Dementia and dysphagia, *Geriatr Nurs* 29:275, 2008.

Faes MC, Spift MG, Olde, MG, et al: Dehydration in geriatrics, *Geriatric Aging* 10:590, 2007.

Felix H: Obesity, disability and nursing home admission, *Ann Longterm Care* 16:33, 2008.

Flicker L, McCaul K, Hankey G, et al: Body mass index and survival in men and women aged 70 to 75, *J Am Geriatr Soc* 58:234–241, 2010.

Gil-Montoya J, Ferreira A, Lopez I: Oral health protocol for the dependent institutionalized elderly, *Geriatr Nurs* 27(2):95–101, 2006.

Haber D: *Health promotion and aging*, ed 5, New York, 2010, Springer.

Ham R, Sloane P, Warshaw G, et al: *Primary care geriatrics: a case-based approach*, ed 4, St. Louis, 2007, Mosby.

Hess P: Artificial nutrition and hydration for the person with dementia: creation of a brochure, *Geriatr Nurs* 29(3):172–173, 2008.

Jablonski R: Examining oral health in nursing home residents and overcoming mouth-care resistive behaviors, *Ann Longterm Care* 18:21, 2010.

Jablonski R, Munro C, Grap M, et al: Mouth care in nursing homes: knowledge, beliefs, and practices of nursing assistants, *Geriatr Nurs* 30:99, 2009.

Kaiser R, Winning K, Uter W, et al: Functionality and mortality in obese nursing home residents: an example of "risk factor paradox?" *J Am Med Dir Assoc* 11:428, 2010.

Locher J, Ritchie C, Robinson C, et al: A multidimensional approach to understanding under-eating in homebound older adults: the importance of social factors, *Gerontologist* 48(2):223–234, 2008.

Lustbader W: Thoughts on the meaning of frailty, *Generations* 13(4):21–22, 1999.

Markovic K, Reulbach U, Vassiliadu A, et al: Good news for elderly persons: olfactory pleasure increases at later stages of the life span, *J Gerontol A Biol Sci Med Sci* 62(11):1287–1293, 2007.

Mei A, Auerhahn C: Hypodermoclysis: maintaining hydration in the frail older adult, *Ann Longterm Care* 17:28, 2009.

Mentes JC: Managing oral hydration. In Capezuti E, Zwicker D, Fulmer T, et al, editors: *Evidence-based geriatric nursing protocols for best practice*, New York, 2008, Springer.

Mentes JC: Oral hydration in older adults: greater awareness is needed in preventing, recognizing, and treating dehydration, *Am J Nurs* 106(6): 40–49, 2006.

Metheny M: Preventing aspiration in older adults with dysphagia (2007). Available at www.hartfordign.org/publications/trythis/issue_20.pdf.

Metheny M, Boltz M, Greenberg S: Preventing aspiration in older adults with dysphagia, *Am J Nurs* 108(2):45–46, 2008.

Miller C: *Nursing for wellness in older adults*, ed 5, Philadelphia, 2008, Wolters Kluwer–Lippincott Williams & Wilkins.

National Institute on Aging: *Healthy eating after 50* (2011). Available at www.nia.nih.gov/healthinformation/publications/healthyeating.htm.

Nutrition Screening Initiative, project of American Academy of Family Physicians, American Dietetic Association, and National Council on Aging. Grant from Ross-Abbott Laboratories, Inc, 1991.

O'Connor L: Oral health care. In Boltz M, Capezuti E, Fulmer T, et al: *Evidence-based geriatric nursing protocols for best practice*, New York, 2012, Springer.

Ogden CL, Carroll MD, Kit BK, et al: *Prevalence of obesity in the United States, 2009-2010*. NCHS Data Brief No. 82. Hyattsville, MD, 2012, National Center for Health Statistics.

Pioneer Network and Rothschild Foundation: *New dining practice standards* (2011). Available at http://www.pioneernetwork.net/Providers/DiningPracticeStandards/.

Sarin J, Balasubramanian R, Colcoran A: Reducing the risk of aspiration pneumonia among elderly patients in long-term care facilities through oral health interventions, *J Am Med Dir Assoc* 9(2):128–135, 2008.

Stein P, Henry R: Poor oral hygiene in long-term care, *Am J Nurs* 109:44, 2009.

Tanner D: Lessons from nursing home dysphagia malpractice litigation, *J Gerontol Nurs* 36:41, 2010.

Teno J, Mor V, DeSilva D, et al: Use of feeding tubes in nursing home residents with severe cognitive impairment, *JAMA* 287(24):3211–3212, 2002.

Teno J, Mitchell S, Gozalo P, et al: Hospital characteristics associated with feeding tube placement in nursing home residents with advanced cognitive impairment, *JAMA* 303:544, 2010.

Thomas D: Nutritional management in long-term care: development of a clinical guideline, *J Gerontol A Biol Sci Med Sci* 55(12):M725, 2000.

Thomas D, Cote T, Lawhorne L, et al: Understanding clinical dehydration and its treatment, *J Am Med Dir Assoc* 9:292, 2008.

U.S. Department of Agriculture [USDA]: *2010 Dietary guidelines for Americans* (2012). Available at http://www.cnpp.usda.gov/dietaryguidelines.htm.

Vitale C, Monteleoni C, Burke L, et al: Strategies for improving care for patients with advanced dementia and eating problems: optimizing care through physician and speech pathologist collaboration, *Ann Longterm Care* 17:32, 2009.

CHAPTER 10

Elimination

Theris A. Touhy

evolve evolve.elsevier.com/Ebersole/gerontological

LEARNING OBJECTIVES

Upon completion of this chapter, the reader will be able to:
- Define urinary and fecal incontinence.
- List factors contributing to urinary and fecal incontinence.
- Explain the types of urinary incontinence and their causes.
- Use evidence-based protocols in assessment and development of interventions for promotion of bowel and bladder health.

GLOSSARY

Detrusor A body part that pushes down, such as the bladder muscle
Incontinence The inability to control excretory function
Micturition Urination
Transient Temporary

THE LIVED EXPERIENCE

"UI (urinary incontinence) is like being a bad kid or a big baby."
"There's nothing that can be done. Well, I don't think there is anything else but a diaper."
"Sometimes I have to wet my bed before they get here, you know, and they are all busy and I have to wait for somebody, then I can't control it."
"I do something that is very wrong. I try not to drink too much but that's so wrong. So how can you drink a lot, you would be soaked all the time."

Comments from participants in a study of living with urinary incontinence in long-term care (MacDonald & Butler, 2007).

UI is a preventable and treatable condition and yet, "continence remains undervalued and UI remains underassessed. Even though UI is a basic nursing issue, nurses are not claiming it as one."

Comment from nurses in expert continence care (Mason et al., 2003, p. 3).

Elimination

The body must remove waste products of metabolism to sustain healthy function, but bladder and bowel activity are fraught with social implications. Bladder and bowel function in later life, although normally only slightly altered by the physiological changes of age, can contribute to problems severe enough to interfere with the ability to continue independent living and can seriously threaten the body's capacity to function and to survive. The effects of uncontrolled bladder and bowel action are a threat to the person's independence and well-being. Elimination is a private matter, not publicized socially. As children, correct behavior in dealing with our own body waste is taught early. Deviations from this are socially unacceptable and can lead to chastisement, ostracism, and social withdrawal. Nurses are in a key position to implement evidence-based assessment and interventions to enhance continence and improve function, independence, and quality of life for older people.

Bladder Function

Normal bladder function requires an intact brain and spinal cord, competent lower urinary tract function, the motivation to maintain continence, the functional ability to use a toilet, and an environment that facilitates the process. A full bladder increases pressure and signals the spinal cord and the brainstem center of the desire to micturate. Social training then dictates whether micturition should be attended to or should be postponed until there is an appropriate opportunity to seek out toilet facilities. However, when the bladder contents reach 500 mL or more, the pressure is such that it becomes more difficult to control the urge to void. As volume increases, emptying the bladder becomes an uncontrollable act.

Age-Related Changes

Bladder changes with aging include decreased capacity, increased irritability, contractions during filling, and incomplete emptying. In about 10% to 20% of well older adults, aging of the urinary tract is associated with an increased frequency of involuntary bladder contractions (Ham et al., 2007). These changes may lead to frequency, nocturia, urgency, and vulnerability to infection. The warning period between the desire to void and actual micturition is shortened. Postvoid residual urine volume increases to 75 to 100 mL in some cases. The first urge to void occurs at a lower bladder volume (150 to 300 mL) and total bladder capacity decreases to 300 to 600 mL (Ham et al., 2007). In combination with age-related changes, illness, cognitive impairments, difficulty in walking to the toilet or in handling a bedpan or urinal, and problems in manipulating clothing can affect an older person's ability to maintain continence. Drugs that increase urinary output and sedatives, tranquilizers, and hypnotics, which produce drowsiness, confusion, or limited mobility, promote incontinence by dulling the transmission of the desire to urinate.

Urinary Incontinence

Urinary incontinence (UI) is the involuntary loss of urine sufficient to be a problem (Dowling-Castronovo, 2008; Dowling-Castronovo & Bradway, 2012). UI is an important yet neglected geriatric syndrome. Because of the high prevalence and chronic but preventable nature of UI, it is most appropriately considered a public health problem (Lawthorne et al., 2008). UI is also a costly health problem with estimates that about 19.5 billion dollars are spent on UI care each year.

UI is a stigmatized, underreported, underdiagnosed, undertreated condition that is erroneously thought to be part of normal aging. About half of persons with UI have never discussed the concern with their primary care provider, and only one in eight who has experienced bladder control problems has been diagnosed. On average, women wait 6.5 years from the first time they experience symptoms until they obtain a diagnosis for their bladder control problems (Muller, 2005).

Individuals may not seek treatment for UI because they are embarrassed to talk about the problem or think that it is a normal part of aging. They may be unaware that successful treatments are available. Men may be unlikely to report UI to their primary care provider because they feel it is a woman's disease. Further research is necessary to explore the prevalence and experience of UI in men. A guideline for UI in men can be found in the Evidence-Based Practice box. Older people want more information about bladder control, and nurses must take the lead in implementing approaches to continence promotion and public health education about UI (Palmer & Newman, 2006).

Without an adequate knowledge base of continence care and use of evidence-based practice guidelines, nursing care will continue to consist of containment strategies, such as the use of pads and briefs, to manage UI (Dowling-Castronovo & Spiro, 2008). UI tends to be viewed as an inconvenience rather than a condition requiring assessment and treatment (MacDonald & Butler, 2007). Nurses in all practice settings with older adults should be prepared to assess data that relate to urine control and implement nursing interventions that promote continence (Dowling-Castronovo & Bradway, 2012). There is a growing role for nurses in continence care and advanced training and certification are available through specialty organizations such as the Society of Urologic Nurses and Associates (www.suna.org) and the Wound, Ostomy, and Continence Nurses Society (www.wocncb.org).

Prevalence of UI

UI affects millions of adults worldwide. Of those who experience UI, 75% to 80% are female; the prevalence of UI increases with age and functional dependency. Twenty-five percent of young women, 44% to 57% of middle-aged and postmenopausal women, and 75% of older women in nursing homes experience some involuntary urine loss

EVIDENCE-BASED PRACTICE

Continence Care

Bladder Continence/UTI

- Assessment and management of older adults with urinary incontinence: State of the Science papers:
  http://hartfordign.org/uploads/File/gnec_state_of_science_papers/gnec_incontinence.pdf
- Comprehensive toolkit for management of urinary incontinence in older adults in primary care:
  http://www.gericareonline.net/tools/eng/urinary/index.html
- Guideline for UI in men:
  www.guideline.gov/content.aspx?id514817
- Incontinence management useful to nurses in the long-term care setting:
  www.geronet.ucla.edu/centers/borun/modules/Incontinence_management/default.htm
- Nursing Standard of Practice Protocol: Urinary incontinence (UI) in older adults admitted to acute care (Dowling-Castronovo & Bradway, 2012)
- Urinary incontinence assessment in older adults: Part I: Transient urinary incontinence (Dowling-Castronovo & Spiro, 2013)
  http://consultgerirn.org/uploads/File/trythis/try_this_11_1.pdf
- Part II: Established urinary incontinence (Dowling-Castronovo & Spiro, 2008)
  http://consultgerirn.org/uploads/File/trythis/try_this_11_2.pdf
- Prevention of catheter-associated UTIs in acute care:
  http://www.guideline.gov/content.aspx?id513394&search5urinary1tract1 infections1acute1care1hospitals
- Nursing Standard of Practice: Prevention of Catheter-Associated Urinary Tract Infection Prevention: Wald H, et al: In Boltz M, Capezuti E, Fulmer T, et al: *Evidence-based geriatric nursing protocols for best practice,* New York, 2012, Springer.
- Video depicting a nurse assessing transient UI:
  http://consultgerirn.org/resources/media/?vid_id55003886#player_ container

Bowel Continence

- Prevention of urinary and fecal incontinence in adults (AHRQ):
  www.ahrq.gov/downloads/pub/evidence/pdf/fuiad/fuiad.pdf

(Agency for Healthcare Research and Quality, 2012). Some evidence suggests that European American women have higher rates of moderate and severe UI compared with African American and Asian women (Dowling-Castronovo & Bradway, 2012; Townsend et al., 2011).

Risk Factors for UI

Cognitive impairment, limitations in daily activities, and institutionalization are associated with higher risks of UI. Stroke, diabetes, obesity, poor general health, and comorbidities are also associated with UI (Shamliyan et al., 2007). Pregnancy, childbirth, menopause, and hysterectomy are other factors that contribute to UI. Older people with dementia are at high risk for UI. Hospital patients with dementia are more likely than other older people to develop new incontinence.

Dementia does not cause urinary incontinence but affects the ability of the person to find a bathroom and recognize the urge to void. Mobility problems and dependency in transfers are better predictors of continence status than dementia, suggesting that persons with dementia may have the potential to remain continent as long as they are mobile. Making toilets easily visible, providing assistance to the bathroom at regular intervals, and implementing prompted voiding protocols can assist in continence promotion for people with dementia. Box 10-1 presents risk factors for UI.

Consequences of UI

UI is identified as a marker of frailty in community-dwelling older adults. UI is associated with falls, skin irritations and infections, urinary tract infections (UTIs), pressure ulcers, and sleep disturbance. UI affects self-esteem and increases the risk for depression, anxiety, social isolation, and avoidance of sexual activity. Older adults with UI experience a loss of dignity, independence, and self-confidence, as well as feelings of shame and embarrassment (MacDonald & Butler, 2007; Dowling-Castronovo & Spiro, 2008). The psychosocial impact of UI affects the individual as well as the family caregivers.

BOX 10-1   Risk Factors for Urinary Incontinence

- Age
- Immobility, functional limitations
- Diminished cognitive capacity (dementia, delirium)
- Medications (those with anticholinergic properties, sedatives, diuretics)
- Smoking
- High caffeine intake
- Obesity
- Constipation, fecal impaction
- Pregnancy, vaginal delivery, episiotomy
- Low fluid intake
- Environmental barriers
- High-impact physical exercise
- Diabetes
- Stroke
- Parkinson's disease
- Hysterectomy
- Pelvic muscle weakness
- Childhood nocturnal enuresis
- Prostate surgery
- Estrogen deficiency
- Arthritis

Adapted from DeMaagd G: Urinary incontinence: treatment update with a focus on pharmacological management, *US Pharmacist* 32(6):34-44, 2007. Available at http://www.uspharmacist.com/content/d/featured_articles/c/10310/; Dowling-Castronovo A, Bradway C: Urinary incontinence. In Capezuti E, Zwicker D, Mezey M, et al, editors: *Evidence-based nursing protocols for best practice*, ed 3, New York, 2008, Springer.

Types of UI

Incontinence is classified as either *transient* (acute) or *established* (chronic). Transient incontinence has a sudden onset, is present for 6 months or less, and is usually caused by treatable factors such as UTIs, delirium, constipation and stool impaction, and increased urine production caused by metabolic conditions such as hyperglycemia and hypercalcemia. *Iatrogenic* (or treatment-induced) incontinence is a type of transient UI that results from the use of restraints, limited fluid intake, bed rest, or intravenous fluid administration. Use of medications such as diuretics, anticholinergic agents, antidepressants, sedatives, hypnotics, calcium channel blockers, and α-adrenergic agonists and blockers can also lead to transient UI (Dowling-Castronovo & Bradway, 2012).

Established UI may have either a sudden or gradual onset and is categorized into the following types: (1) urge; (2) stress; (3) urge, mixed, or stress UI with high postvoid residual (originally termed overflow UI); (4) functional UI; and (5) mixed UI.

Urge incontinence (overactive bladder) is defined as involuntary urine loss that occurs soon after feeling an urgent need to void. Overactive bladder is a syndrome that overlaps with urge UI. With overactive bladder syndrome, individuals have urinary frequency (more than eight voids in 24 hours), nocturia, urgency, with or without incontinence (Zarowitz & Ouslander, 2007). The bladder muscles are overactive and cause a sudden urge to void—the "Gotta Go Right Now" syndrome (Bucci, 2007). Defining characteristics of urge UI include loss of urine in moderate to large amounts before getting to the toilet and an inability to suppress the need to urinate. Postvoid residual urine reveals a low volume. Urge UI is the most common type of urinary incontinence in older adults.

Stress incontinence (outlet incompetence) is defined as an involuntary loss of less than 50 mL of urine associated with activities that increase intraabdominal pressure (e.g., coughing, sneezing, exercise, lifting, bending). Stress UI is more common in women because of short urethras and poor pelvic muscle tone. Stress UI occurs in men who have experienced prostatectomy and radiation. Postvoid residual urine is low.

Urge, mixed, or stress UI with high postvoid residual incontinence (formerly called overflow UI) occurs when the bladder does not empty normally and becomes overdistended with frequent and nearly constant urine loss (dribbling). Other symptoms include hesitancy in starting urination, slow urine stream, passage of infrequent or small volumes of urine, a feeling of incomplete bladder emptying, and large postvoid residuals. Persons with diabetes and men with enlarged prostates are at risk for this type of UI. Calcium channel blockers, anticholinergics, and adrenergics also contribute to symptoms.

Functional incontinence refers to a situation in which the lower urinary tract is intact but the individual is unable to reach the toilet because of environmental barriers, physical limitations, or severe cognitive impairment. Individuals may be dependent on others for assistance to the toilet but have no genitourinary problems other than incontinence. Older adults who are institutionalized have higher rates of functional incontinence (Dowling-Castronovo & Bradway, 2012). Functional UI may also occur in the presence of other types of UI.

Mixed incontinence is a combination of more than one urinary incontinence problem, usually stress and urge. Mixed UI is the most prevalent type of UI in women, and with increasing age older women with stress UI begin to experience urge UI (Shamliyan et al., 2007).

Implications for Gerontological Nursing and Healthy Aging

Assessment

Continence must be routinely addressed in the initial assessment of every older person, yet many older people do not bring up their concerns about incontinence, and many health professionals do not ask. Health care personnel must begin to change their thinking about incontinence and acknowledge that incontinence can be cured. If it cannot be cured, it can be treated to minimize its detrimental effects. Nurses are often the ones to identify urinary incontinence, but neither nurses nor physicians have been particularly aggressive in its management. "Nurses have long been the providers of personal hygiene information for those entrusted to their care. Therefore, it is essential that nurses play a leading role in assessing and managing UI . . ." (Dowling-Castronovo & Bradway, 2007, p. 7).

To begin the assessment, screening questions such as "Have you ever leaked urine? If yes, how much does it bother you?" are suggested (Dowling-Castronovo & Bradway, 2007). Assessment is multidimensional. It includes a health history, targeted physical examination (abdominal, rectal, genital), urinalysis, and determination of postvoid residual urine. For women, evaluation of the reproductive system and gynecological history and examination is recommended since gynecological factors may contribute to the urological problem. More extensive examinations are considered after the initial findings are assessed. Individuals who do not fit a simple pattern on UI should be referred promptly for urodynamic assessment (Ham et al., 2007).

A thorough health history should focus on the medical, neurological, gynecological, and genitourinary history. It should include functional assessment, cognitive assessment, psychosocial effects; strategies currently used to control UI; a medication review of both prescribed and over-the-counter drugs; a detailed exploration of the symptoms of the urinary incontinence; and associated symptoms and other factors. In care facilities, an environmental assessment including the accessibility of bathrooms, room lighting, and the use of aids such as raised toilet seats or commodes is also important. A link to a video of a nurse performing an assessment to evaluate transient incontinence can be found in the Evidence-Based Practice box.

In the nursing home, continence is assessed with the Minimum Data Set 3.0 (MDS) which provides a comprehensive overview of the assessment, treatment, and evaluation of bladder and bowel continence based on the new Centers for Medicare and Medicaid Services (CMS) guidelines (Johnson & Ouslander, 2006). All newly admitted nursing home residents should have a thorough assessment of continence status as well as ongoing evaluations during their length of stay (Figure 10-1). Both acute and long-term care facilities should perform comprehensive assessments of continence. Figure 10-2 presents a guide for the diagnostic assessment and management of UI in the nursing home setting.

One of the best ways to establish the presence of and describe incontinence problems is with a voiding diary. This is considered the "gold standard" for obtaining objective information about the person's voiding patterns and the UI episodes and their severity (Dowling-Castronovo & Bradway, 2007, p. 314) (Figure 10-3). The voiding diary can be used by both community-dwelling and institutionalized elders. The character of the urine (color, odor, sediment, or clear) and difficulty starting or stopping the urinary stream should be recorded. Activities of daily living (ADLs), such as ability to reach a toilet and use it and finger dexterity for clothing manipulation, should be documented.

Interventions

Behavioral

Urinary incontinence can be improved when appropriate care is provided. A number of behavioral interventions have a good basis in research and can be implemented by nurses without extensive and expensive evaluation. These treatments are viewed as healthy bladder behavior skills (HBBSs) (Dowling-Castronovo & Bradway, 2012). These interventions will do no harm and if there is no improvement, further evaluation can be sought. Before instituting HBBSs, the nurse should assess the motivation of the patient, informal caregiver, and/or nursing staff because behavior management is the premise of HBBSs. Behavioral techniques, such as scheduled voiding, prompted voiding, bladder training, biofeedback, and pelvic floor muscle exercises (PFMEs), are recommended as first-line treatment of UI.

Selection of a modality and interventions will depend on a comprehensive assessment, the type of incontinence and its underlying cause, and whether the outcome is to cure or to minimize the extent of the incontinence. Interventions for UI should be multidisciplinary, and everyone involved with the person's care should be involved in the treatment plan. If the person has mobility impairments, physical and occupational therapy and/or restorative nursing programs should be implemented as part of the treatment plan for UI. Box 10-2 lists the numerous modalities available in the treatment of incontinence. Nursing interventions focus primarily on the appropriate assessment

CHAMP TOOL

(Continence, History, Assessment, Medications, Mobility, Plan)

C Resident is continent? Yes ___ No ___

H Medical / Surgical History:

    a. Diagnosis often associated with continence? Yes ___ No ___

        ___ BPH (prostate) ___ Diabetes ___ MS

        ___ CHF ___ Fracture ___ Osteoporosis

        ___ Constipation ___ Heart Disease ___ Pain

        ___ Contractures ___ HTN ___ Parkinson's

        ___ CVA ___ Immobility ___ Spinal Cord Injury

        ___ Dementia ___ Kidney Stones ___ UTI (last 90 days)

        ___ Depression

    b. Recent Acute Medical Condition (last 30 days)? Yes ___ No ___

        If yes, date and type: _____

    c. Recent Surgery (last 30 days)? Yes ___ No ___

        If yes, date and type: _____

    d. Surgical History: Hysterectomy ___ Bladder Repair ___ Prostate (TURP) ___ Other ___

    e. Lab Data ___ Urodynamic Studies ___ Imaging Studies ___

        Date and type: _____

A Assessment of Urinary Incontinence:

    Trigger Event (surgery, accident, other)? Yes ___ No ___

    Leak urine when cough, sneeze, laugh, stand up, change position? Yes ___ No ___

    Urge to go (Need to be there NOW)? Yes ___ No ___

    Wet without feeling the need to go? Yes ___ No ___

    Number of night time voids? ___

    Leak only at night? Yes ___ No ___

    Difficult to start or stop stream? Yes ___ No ___

    Weak stream? Yes ___ No ___

    Dribbling? Yes ___ No ___

    Products used? _____

M1 Medications.

    a. Current Medication:

___ Anticholinergic	___ Diuretic	___ Narcotic
___ Antidepressant	___ Hypnotic	___ OTC Cold Remedies
___ Antihypertensive	___ Laxative	___ Sedative
___ Other:		

    b. Medications to treat Incontinence:

___ Antibiotic	___ Estrogen	___ Proscar
___ Detrol	___ Flomax	___ Sanctura
___ Ditropan	___ Imipramine	___ VESIcare
___ Enablex	___ Other:	

M2 Mobility Status: I Independent, A Assist, D Dependent

___ Ambulation	___ Dressing	___ Toileting
___ Transfer		

    Can access bedpan, BSC, urinal, toilet independently (Circle):___ Yes ___ No

P Plan of care:

    a. Resident is motivated to toilet: ___ Yes ___ No ___ Not oriented

    b. Resident is candidate for treatment program? Yes ___ No ___

    If no, reason: _____

    c. Care Plan interventions: (Circle Suggestions)

        ○ Incontinence, functional–Prompted voiding, behavioral modification (i.e., timed voiding), restorative toileting, physical and/or occupational therapy, environmental modifications

        ○ Incontinence, overflow–clean intermittent catheterization

        ○ Incontinence, stress–pelvic muscle exercises, behavior modification, medications

        ○ Incontinence, urge–pelvic muscle exercises, behavior modification, medication

        ○ Incontinence, mixed (stress and urge)–pelvic muscle exercises, behavior modification, medications

        ○ Incontinence, total–check and change

    d. Bladder treatment initiated (date):

    Nurse Signature: _____ Date: _____

FIGURE 10-1 CHAMMP tool. (From Bucci A: Be a continence champion: use the CHAMMP tool to individualize the plan of care, *Geriatr Nurs* 28(2):123, 2007.)

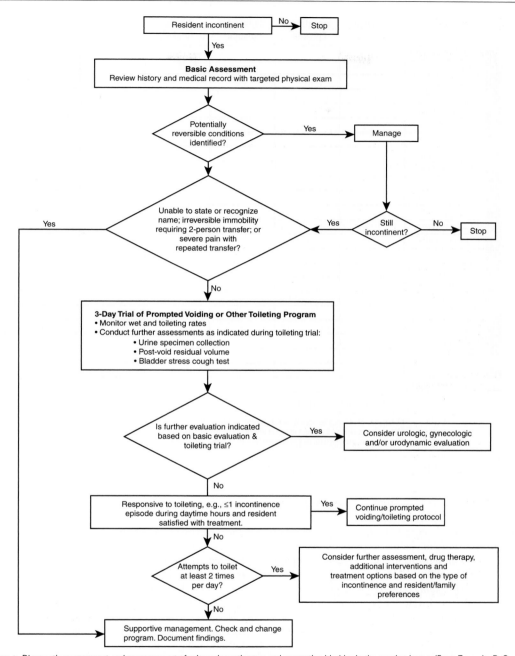

FIGURE 10-2 Diagnostic assessment and management of urinary incontinence and overactive bladder in the nursing home. (From Zarowitz B, Ouslander J: The application of evidence-based practice principles of care in older persons (Issue 6): Urinary Incontinence, *J Am Med Dir Assoc,* 8(1): 37, 2007.)

	Time Interval	Urinated in Toilet	Incontinent Episode[1]	Reason for Episode[1]	Liquid Intake[3]	Bowel Movement	Product Use[3]
A.M. HOURS	12:00–01:00 AM						
	01:00–02:00 AM						
	02:00–03:00 AM						
	03:00–04:00 AM						
	04:00–05:00 AM						
	05:00–06:00 AM						
	06:00–07:00 AM						
	07:00–08:00 AM						
	08:00–09:00 AM						
	09:00–10:00 AM						
	10:00–11:00 AM						
	11:00–12:00 PM						
P.M. HOURS	12:00–01:00 PM						
	01:00–02:00 PM						
	02:00–03:00 PM						
	03:00–04:00 PM						
	04:00–05:00 PM						
	05:00–06:00 PM						
	06:00–07:00 PM						
	07:00–08:00 PM						
	08:00–09:00 PM						
	09:00–10:00 PM						
	10:00–11:00 PM						
	11:00–12:00 AM						

[1] **Incontinent episodes:** (++) = SMALL: did not have to change pad/ clothing; (+++) = LARGE: needed to change pad/clothing
[2] **Examples of reasons for incontinent episodes:** leaked while sneezing; leaked while running to the bathroom
[3] **Examples of type and amount of liquid intake:** 12 oz can of cola, 2 cups regular coffee
[4] **Examples of product use:** pad, undergarment; track times you changed

FIGURE 10-3 Sample voiding or bladder diary. (Adapted from Fantl C, Newman DK, Colling J, et al: Urinary incontinence in adults: acute and chronic management. Clinical Practice Guideline No. 2. AHCPR Publication No. 96-0682. Rockville, MD, 1996, Agency for Health Care Policy and Research, U.S. Department of Health and Human Services.)

of continence and implementation and evaluation of supportive and therapeutic modalities to promote and restore continence and to prevent incontinence-related complications, such as skin breakdown.

Scheduled (timed) voiding is used to treat urge and functional UI in both cognitively intact and cognitively impaired older adults. The schedule or timing of voiding is based on the person's bladder diary patterns or common voiding patterns (voiding on arising, before and after meals, midmorning, midafternoon, and bedtime). In general, toileting is scheduled at 2- to 4-hour intervals. People can be taught to do this routinely or they can be assisted to the bathroom according to the scheduled intervals.

Prompted voiding (PV) combines scheduled voiding with monitoring, prompting, and verbal reinforcement.

The objective of PV is to increase self-initiated voiding and decrease the number of episodes of UI. The person is assisted to the toilet during waking hours if he or she requests it and receives positive feedback if he or she voids successfully. In a systematic review of randomized trials of interventions in nursing home residents with UI, Fink and colleagues (2008) concluded that prompted voiding is associated with modest short-term improvement in daytime UI in nursing home residents.

Newly admitted nursing home residents should receive a thorough assessment of continence, and those who are incontinent (and able to use the toilet) should receive a 3- to 5-day trial of prompted voiding. The trial can be helpful in demonstrating responsiveness to toileting and determining patterns of and symptoms associated with the

---

BOX 10-2 Therapeutic Modalities in the Treatment of Incontinence

Support Measures
- Appropriate attitude
- Accessible toilet substitutes (bedpan, urinal, commode)
- Avoidance of iatrogenic conditions (urinary tract infections, constipation/impaction, excessive sedation, inaccessible toilets, drugs adversely affecting the bladder or urethral function)
- Protective undergarments
- Absorbent bed pads
- Behavioral techniques: bladder training, scheduled (timed) voiding, prompted voiding, biofeedback, pelvic floor muscle exercises (PFMEs)
- Good skin care

Drugs
- Bladder relaxants
- Bladder outlet stimulants

Surgery
- Suspension of bladder neck
- Prostatectomy
- Prosthetic sphincter implants
- Urethral sling
- Bladder augmentation

Mechanical and Electrical Devices Catheters
- External (condom or "Texas" catheter)
- Intermittent
- Suprapubic
- Indewelling

---

incontinence. Residents who do not respond to prompted voiding but consistently attempt to toilet should receive further evaluation and may be appropriate candidates for drug therapy in addition to a PV program. Residents who are unresponsive to toileting programs or unable or unwilling to attempt toileting can be provided supportive management including absorbent pads and briefs, and attention to skin breakdown prevention (Zarowitz & Ouslander, 2007; Lawhorne et al., 2008) (see Figure 10-2).

Continence programs in nursing homes are both needed and required by CMS regulations (Johnson & Ouslander, 2006). Monitoring and documentation of continence status in relation to implemented continence care is a quality of care indicator for nursing homes (Shamliyan et al., 2007). Despite a growing body of evidence suggesting that toileting programs can be successful in long-term care, they are difficult to sustain. Barriers to implementation and continuation of toileting programs include inadequate staffing and lack of knowledge about UI and existing evidence-based protocols. A major advantage of PV programs is that they target residents who are likely to be successful and direct scarce staff resources to residents most likely to benefit.

Johnson and Ouslander (2006, p. 599) remind us that "cure of incontinence in nursing home residents is unusual and not a realistic goal for most." However, every resident who is incontinent deserves appropriate medical and nursing assessment and interventions that restore continence, if

possible, or provide supportive care and prevention of complications related to incontinence. Successful implementation of continence programs requires a systems-based approach with consideration of individual, group, organizational, and environmental level factors.

Bladder training aims to increase the time interval between the urge to void and voiding. This method is appropriate for people with urge UI who are cognitively intact and independent in toileting or after removal of an indwelling catheter. The person follows an established voiding schedule until UI episodes cease. When this is achieved, the interval between voidings is extended and techniques for overcoming the urge and postponing urination are taught (pelvic floor muscle exercises).

Pelvic floor muscle exercises (PFMEs), also called Kegel exercises, involve repeated voluntary pelvic floor muscle contraction. The targeted muscle is the pubococcygeal muscle, which forms the support for the pelvis and surrounds the vagina, the urethra, and the rectum. The goal of the repetitive contractions is to strengthen the muscle and decrease UI episodes. PFMEs are recommended for stress, urge, and mixed UI in older women. Combining PFME with bladder training is recommended to reduce UI, and PFME may also be important for young women and even girls to prevent future UI (Shamliyan et al., 2012).

Although there are some nursing home residents who may benefit from PFMEs and are capable of learning and practicing, the numbers may be insufficient to justify emphasis on this approach in this setting (Johnson & Ouslander, 2006). PFMEs have also been shown to be helpful for men who have undergone prostatectomy. Contractions should be repeated 30 to 100 times a day; the contraction is held for 10 seconds and followed by 10 seconds of relaxation.

Correct identification of the pelvic floor muscles and adherence to the exercise regimen are key to success. Improvement may not be noted until 2 to 4 weeks of exercises have been successfully completed. To help identify the correct muscle groups, it may be helpful to tell the person to try to tighten the anal sphincter (as if to control the passage of flatus or feces) and then tighten the urethral and/or vaginal muscles (as if to stop the flow of urine). Muscles of the stomach, thigh, and buttocks should not be contracted because this increases intraabdominal pressure. PFMEs may be taught during a vaginal or rectal examination when the clinician manually assists the person to identify the pelvic muscles by instructing the patient to squeeze around a gloved examination finger. Biofeedback may be helpful in identifying the correct muscle and visualizing the strength and time of the contraction.

Lifestyle Modifications

Several lifestyle factors are associated with either the development or exacerbation of UI. These include increased fluid intake, weight reduction, smoking cessation, bowel management, and physical activity. Recent research findings suggest that coffee and tea consumption has limited or no effect on incontinence but guidelines generally suggest limiting caffeine intake (Tettamanti et al., 2011). Box 10-3 presents other interventions helpful to noninstitutionalized elders to control or eliminate incontinence.

Urinary Catheters

Intermittent catheterization may be used in people with urinary retention related to a weak detrusor muscle (e.g., diabetic neuropathy), those with a blockage of the urethra (e.g., benign prostatic hypertrophy), or those with reflux incontinence related to a spinal cord injury. The goal is to maintain 300 mL or less of urine in the bladder. Most of the research on intermittent catheterization has been conducted with children or young adults with spinal cord injuries, but it may be useful for older adults who are able to self-catheterize. It provides an important alternative to indwelling catheterization.

Indwelling catheter use is not appropriate for long-term management (more than 30 days) except in certain clinical conditions. Continuous indwelling catheter use is

---

BOX 10-3 Helpful Interventions for Noninstitutionalized Elders to Control or Eliminate Incontinence

- Empty bladder completely before and after meals and at bedtime.
- Urinate whenever the urge arises; never ignore it.
- A schedule of urinating every 2 hours during the day and every 4 hours at night is often helpful in retraining the bladder. Use of an alarm clock may be necessary.
- Drink 1½ to 2 quarts of fluid a day before 8 pm. This helps the kidneys to function properly. Limit fluids after supper to ½ to 1 cup (except in very hot weather).
- Eliminate or reduce the use of coffee, tea, brown cola, and alcohol, because they have a diuretic effect.
- Take prescription diuretics in the morning upon rising.
- Limit the use of sleeping pills, sedatives, and alcohol because they decrease sensation to urinate and can increase incontinence, especially at night.
- If overweight, lose weight.
- Exercises to strengthen pelvic muscles that help support the bladder (PFMEs) are often helpful for women with stress, urge, and mixed UI. May also be helpful for men after prostatectomy
- Make sure the toilet is nearby with a clear path to it and good lighting, especially at night. Grab bars or a raised toilet seat may be needed.
- Dress protectively with cotton underwear and protective pants or incontinent pads if necessary.

---

indicated for urethral obstruction or urinary retention or in patients with the following conditions:

- When surgical or pharmacological interventions are inappropriate or unsuccessful
- If contraindications are present to intermittent catheterization to treat retention
- When changes of bedding, clothing, and absorbent products may be painful or disruptive for a patient with an irreversible medical condition, such as metastatic terminal disease, coma, or end-stage congestive heart failure
- For patients with severely impaired skin integrity
- For patients who live alone without a caregiver or with a caregiver who is unable to routinely change the person (Newman & Palmer, 2003; Johnson & Ouslander, 2006)

Regulatory standards in nursing homes follow these same guidelines, and the use of indwelling catheters must be justified on the basis of medical conditions and failure of other efforts to maintain continence. In hospitals, the use of indwelling catheters is often unjustified, and they are used inappropriately (convenience of staff) or left in place too long. Misuse of catheterization should be considered a medical error. About one in four indwelling catheters in hospitalized patients 70 years of age and older and one in three in patients 85 years of age and older turn out to be unnecessary (Inelmen et al., 2007). Cognitive impairment and the presence of pressure ulcers almost double the risk of receiving a catheter and severe functional decline is associated with a fourfold risk of catheter placement (Inelmen et al., 2007). Catheter care should consist of washing the meatal area with soap and water daily. A protocol to prevent catheter-associated urinary tract infections in acute care hospitals can be found in the Evidence-Based Practice box.

External catheters (condom catheters) are used in male patients who are incontinent and cannot be toileted. Long-term use of external catheters can lead to fungal skin infections, penile skin maceration, edema, fissures, contact burns from urea, phimosis, UTIs, and septicemia. The catheter should be removed and replaced daily and the penis cleaned, dried, and aired to prevent irritation, maceration, and the development of pressure ulcers and skin breakdown. If the catheter is not sized appropriately and applied and monitored correctly, strangulation of the penile shaft can occur.

SAFETY ALERT

Long-term catheter use increases the risk of recurrent urinary tract infections leading to urosepsis, urethral damage in men, urethritis, or fistula formation. Catheter-associated urinary tract infection is the most frequent health care–associated infection in the United States and Medicare no longer reimburses hospitals for this infection. One of the goals of *Healthy People 2020* is to prevent, reduce, and ultimately eliminate health care–associated infections. Indwelling catheters should be inserted only for appropriate conditions, must be removed as soon as possible, and alternatives should be investigated (e.g., condom catheters, intermittent catheterization, toileting programs).

Urinary Tract Infections

Urinary tract infections (UTIs) are the most common cause of bacterial sepsis in older adults and are 10 times more common in women than in men. The majority of UTIs in older adults are asymptomatic. Assessment and appropriate treatment of UTIs in older people, particularly nursing home residents, is complex. Cognitively impaired residents may not recall or report symptoms, older people frequently do not present with classic symptoms (fever, dysuria, flank pain), and other illnesses (e.g., pneumonia) may present with nonspecific symptoms similar to UTI. Changes in mental status, character of urine, decreased appetite, abdominal pain, chills, low back pain, urethral discharge in men, new onset of incontinence, or even respiratory distress may signal a possible UTI in older people (Juthani-Mehta et al., 2009).

Bacteremia plus pyuria alone are not sufficient to make a diagnosis of UTI in nursing home residents (Juthani-Mehta et al., 2009; Mouton et al., 2010). Both conditions will be present in approximately half of residents without a catheter and in almost all patients with a catheter (Genato & Buhr, 2012). Asymptomatic bacteria in the urine is considered benign in older people and should not be treated with antibiotics. Screening urine cultures should also not be performed in patients who are asymptomatic. Symptomatic UTIs necessitate antibiotic treatment, but it is important to pay attention to the range of symptoms older patients may present.

Absorbent Products

A variety of protective undergarments or adult briefs are available for the older adult who is incontinent. Disposable types come in several sizes, determined by hip and waist measurements, or as one size made to fit all. Many of these undergarments look like regular underwear and contribute more to dignity than the standard "diaper." Referring to protective undergarments as diapers is demeaning and infantilizing to older people and should be avoided. Some individuals may prefer to use absorbent products in addition to toileting interventions to maintain "social continence," and a wide variety of products are available.

Pharmacological

Pharmacological treatment may be indicated for urge UI and overactive bladder (OAB). OAB symptoms include urgency, frequency, and nocturia. Drugs for urge UI and OAB include anticholinergic (antimuscarinic) agents. Commonly prescribed medications include oxybutynin (Ditropan), tolterodine (Detrol), and darifenacin (Enablex), trospium (Sanctura), and solifenacin (Vesicare). Dosages should be started low in older adults and titrated slowly with careful attention to side effects and drug interactions. A trial of 4 to 8 weeks is adequate and recommended; there is no clear advantage in terms of efficacy between the various medications (DeMaagd, 2007; DuBeau, 2009). Undesirable side effects of anticholinergic medications such as dry mouth and eyes, constipation, confusion, or the precipitation of glaucoma are problematic in older people. These medications can be especially problematic for older adults with cognitive impairment (Barton et al., 2008). Medications are not considered first-line treatment but can be considered in combination with behavioral therapies in some cases.

Medications for the treatment of benign prostatic hypertrophy include α-adrenergic blockers and 5-α-reductase inhibitors. α-Adrenergic blockers are usually the therapy of choice in early, mild disease. Careful monitoring of side effects and drug interactions is necessary. The herbal saw palmetto, reported to have 5-α-reductase inhibitor activity, often used to treat lower urinary symptoms attributed to benign prostatic hypertrophy, has been found to have limited effectiveness (Barry et al., 2011).

Surgical

Surgical intervention may be appropriate for some conditions of incontinence. Augmentation cyctoplasty is the surgery most often performed for severe urge incontinence. In this surgery, a segment of the bowel is added to the bladder to increase bladder size and allow it to store more urine. Surgical suspension of the bladder neck (sling procedure) may be used in women who experience stress UI. Outflow obstruction incontinence secondary to prostatic hypertrophy is generally corrected by prostatectomy. Sphincter dysfunction resulting from nerve damage following surgical trauma or radical perineal procedures is 70% to 90% repairable through sphincter implantation.

Nonsurgical Devices

Stress UI can be treated with intravaginal support devices, pessaries, and urethral plugs. The pessary, used primarily to prevent uterine prolapse, is a device that is fitted into the vagina and exerts pressure to elevate the urethrovesical junction of the pelvic floor. The patient is taught to insert and remove the pessary, much like inserting and removing a diaphragm used for contraception. The pessary is removed weekly or monthly for cleaning with soap and water and then reinserted. Adverse effects include vaginal infection, low back pain, and vaginal mucosal erosion. Another concern is the danger of forgetting to remove the pessary.

Bowel Elimination

Bowel function of the older adult, although normally only slightly altered by the physiological changes of age, can be a source of concern and a potentially serious problem, especially for the older person who is functionally impaired.

Normal elimination should be an easy passage of feces, without undue straining or a feeling of incomplete evacuation or defecation.

Constipation is the most common gastrointestinal (GI) complaint made to the health care provider. The annual estimated expenditure for laxatives in the general population of the United States is $800 million annually. This figure is probably low because many people use over-the-counter medications before they seek prescription medications. The extensive use of laxatives among older adults in the United States can be considered a cultural habit. During earlier times, weekly doses of rhubarb, cascara, castor oil, and other types of laxatives were consumed and believed by many to promote health. The belief that cleaning out the colon and having a daily bowel movement is paramount to maintaining good health still persists in some groups.

Constipation is a symptom. It is a reflection of poor habits, postponed passage of stool, and many chronic illnesses—both physical and psychological—as well as a common side effect of medication. Diet and activity level play a significant role in constipation. Constipation and other changes in bowel habits can also signal more serious underlying problems, such as colonic dysmotility or colon cancer. Constipation in a hospitalized patient can lead to cognitive dysfunction and delirium with consequences of falls, prolonged hospitalization, and increased morbidity and mortality (Osei-Boamah et al., 2012). Thorough assessment is important, and these complaints should not be blamed on age alone. Numerous precipitating factors or conditions can cause or worsen constipation (Box 10-4).

Fecal Impaction

Fecal impaction is a major complication of constipation. It is especially common in incapacitated and institutionalized older people and is reported to occur in more than 40% of older adults admitted to the hospital (Roach & Christie, 2008). Symptoms of fecal impaction include malaise, urinary retention, elevated temperature, incontinence of bladder or bowel, alterations in cognitive status, fissures, hemorrhoids, and intestinal obstruction. Unrecognized, unattended, or neglected constipation eventually leads to fecal impaction. Paradoxical diarrhea, caused by leakage of fecal material around the impacted mass, may occur. Reports of diarrhea in older adults must be thoroughly assessed before the use of antidiarrheal medications, which further complicate the problem of fecal impaction. Digital rectal examination for impacted stool and abdominal x-rays will confirm the presence of impacted stool. Stool analysis for *Clostridium difficile* toxin should be ordered in patients who develop new-onset diarrhea. Continued

---

BOX 10-4   Precipitating Factors for Constipation

Physiological
Dehydration
Insufficient fiber intake
Poor dietary habits

Functional
Decreased physical activity
Inadequate toileting
Irregular defecation habits
Irritable bowel disease
Weakness

Mechanical
Abscess or ulcer
Fissures
Hemorrhoids
Megacolon
Pelvic floor dysfunction
Postsurgical obstruction
Prostate enlargement
Rectal prolapse
Rectocele
Spinal cord injury

Strictures
Tumors

Other
Lack of abdominal muscle tone
Obesity
Recent environmental changes
Poor dentition

Psychological
Avoidance of urge to defecate
Confusion
Depression
Emotional stress

Systemic
Diabetic neuropathy
Hypercalcemia
Hyperparathyroidism
Hypothyroidism
Hypokalemia
Porphyria
Uremia

Parkinson's disease
Cerebrovascular disease
Defective electrolyte transfer

Pharmacological
ACE inhibitors
Antacids: calcium carbonate,
    aluminum hydroxide
Antiarrhythmics
Anticholinergics
Anticonvulsants
Antidepressants
Anti-Parkinson's medications
Calcium channel blockers
Calcium supplements
Diuretics
Iron supplements
Laxative overuse
Nonsteroidal antiinflammatories
Opiates
Phenothiazines
Sedatives
Sympathomimetics

ACE, Angiotensin-converting enzyme.
Adapted from Allison OC, Porter ME, Briggs GC: Chronic constipation: assessment and management in the elderly, *J Am Acad Nurse Pract* 6(7):311, 1994;
Tabloski PA: *Gerontological nursing,* Upper Saddle River, NJ, 2006, Pearson/Prentice Hall.

---

obstruction by a fecal mass may eventually impair sensation, leading to the need for larger stool volume to stimulate the urge to defecate, which contributes to megacolon.

Removal of a fecal impaction is at times worse than the misery of the condition. Management of fecal impaction requires the digital removal of the hard, compacted stool from the rectum with use of lubrication containing lidocaine jelly. In general, this is preceded by an oil-retention enema to soften the feces in preparation for manual removal. Use of suppositories is not effective, because their action is blocked by the amount and size of the stool in the rectum. Suppositories do not facilitate the removal of stool in the sigmoid, which may continue to ooze when the rectum is emptied.

Several sessions or days may be necessary to totally cleanse the sigmoid colon and rectum of impacted feces. When this is achieved, attention should be directed to planning a regimen that includes adequate fluid intake, increased dietary fiber, administration of stool softeners if needed, and many of the suggestions presented for prevention of constipation.

For patients who are hospitalized or residing in long-term care settings, accurate bowel records are essential; unfortunately, they are often overlooked or inaccurately completed. Education about the importance of bowel function, and the accurate reporting of size, consistency, and frequency of bowel movements, should be provided to all direct care providers. This is especially important for frail or cognitively impaired elders to prevent fecal impaction, a serious and often dangerous condition for older people.

Implications for Gerontological Nursing and Healthy Aging

Assessment

The precipitants and causes of constipation must be included in the evaluation of the patient. A review of these factors will also determine whether the patient is at risk for altered bowel function. Older people at high risk for constipation and subsequent fecal impaction are those who have hypotonic colon function, who are immobilized and debilitated, or who have central nervous system lesions. It is important to note that alterations in cognitive status, incontinence, increased temperature, poor appetite, or unexplained falls may be the only clinical symptoms of constipation in the cognitively impaired or frail older person.

Recognizing constipation can be a challenge because there may be a significant disconnect between patient definitions of constipation and those of clinicians. Constipation has different meanings to different people. Assessment begins with clarification of what the patient means by constipation. It is important to obtain a bowel history including usual patterns, frequency of bowel movements, size, consistency, and any changes. The Rome III criteria for defining chronic functional constipation in adults can be used to guide the evaluation and treatment of constipation (Box 10-5). The Bristol Stool Form Scale can also be used to provide a visual depiction of stool appearance (Lewis & Heaton, 1997).

A physical examination is needed to rule out systemic causes of constipation such as neurological, endocrine, or metabolic disorders. Symptoms that may suggest the presence of an underlying GI disorder are abdominal pain, nausea, cramping, vomiting, weight loss, melena, rectal bleeding, rectal pain, and fever. A review of food and fluid intake may be necessary to determine the amount of fiber and fluid ingested. Questions should be asked about the level of physical activity and the use of medications, including over-the-counter products, herbs, and supplements. A psychosocial history with attention to depression, anxiety, and stress management is also indicated.

The abdomen is examined for masses, distention, tenderness, and high-pitched or absent bowel sounds. A rectal examination is important to reveal painful anal disorders, such as hemorrhoids or fissures, that will impede the evacuation of stool and to evaluate sphincter tone, rectal prolapse, stool presence in the vault, strictures, masses, anal reflex, and enlarged prostate. Biochemical tests should include a complete blood count, fasting glucose, chemistry panel, and thyroid studies. Other diagnostic studies such as flexible sigmoidoscopy, colonoscopy, computed tomography (CT) scan of the abdomen, or abdominal x-ray study may also be indicated.

Interventions

The first intervention is to examine the medications the person is taking and eliminate those that are constipation-producing, preferably changing to medications that do not carry that side effect. Medications are the leading cause of constipation, and almost any drug can cause it. Drugs that affect the central nervous system, nerve conduction, and smooth muscle function are associated with the highest frequency of constipation. Anticholinergics, pain opiates, and many psychoactive medications can be especially problematic.

Nonpharmacological interventions for constipation that have been implemented and evaluated can be grouped into four areas: (1) fluid- and fiber-related, (2) exercise, (3) environmental manipulation, and (4) a combination of these. Adequate hydration is the cornerstone of constipation therapy, with fluids coming mainly from water. A low-fiber diet and insufficient fluid intake contribute to constipation, and the importance of dietary fiber to adequate nutrition and bowel function is discussed in Chapter 9.

Exercise

Exercise is important as an intervention to stimulate colon motility and bowel evacuation. Daily walking for 20 to 30 minutes is helpful, especially after a meal. Pelvic tilt exercises and range of motion (passive or active) exercises are beneficial for those who are less mobile or who are

---

BOX 10-5   Rome III Criteria for Defining Chronic Functional Constipation in Adults

Chronic constipation is defined by symptoms that have persisted for the last 3 months with an onset at least 6 months before diagnosis. All three of the following criteria must be met:

- At least two of the following:
    - Hard or lumpy stool in ≥25% of defecations
    - Straining during ≥25% of defecations
    - Sensation of incomplete evacuation in ≥25% of defecations
    - Sensation of anorectal obstruction or blockage for ≥25% of defecations
    - Manual maneuvers (e.g., digital evacuation or pelvic floor support to facilitate ≥25% of defecations)
    - Fewer than three defecations per week
- Loose stools rarely present without the use of laxatives. However, it is important to check for impaction if loose stools are present.
- Insufficient criteria for irritable bowel syndrome (IBS)

Adapted from Cash B: Chronic constipation—defining the problem and clinical impact, *Medscape Gerontol* 7(1), 2005. Available at www.medscape.com/viewarticle/501467_print; Longstreth GF, Thompson WG, Chey WD, et al: Functional bowel disorders, *Gastroenterology* 130(5):1480-1491, 2006.

bedridden. Exercise and physical activity is discussed in Chapters 11 and 13.

Positioning

The squatting or sitting position, if the patient is able to assume it, facilitates bowel function. A similar position may be obtained by leaning forward and applying firm pressure to the lower abdomen or by placing the feet on a stool. Massaging the abdomen may help stimulate the bowel.

Regularity

Establishing a routine for toileting promotes or normalizes bowel function (bowel retraining). The gastrocolic reflex occurs after breakfast or supper and may be enhanced by a warm drink. Given privacy and ample time (a minimum of 10 minutes), many will have a daily bowel movement. However, any urge to defecate should be followed by a trip to the bathroom. Older people dependent on others to meet toileting needs should be assisted to maintain normal routines and provided opportunities for routine toilet use. Box 10-6 presents a bowel-training program.

Laxatives

When changes in diet and lifestyle are not effective, the use of laxatives is considered. Older persons receiving opiates need to have a constipation prevention program in place, because these drugs delay gastric emptying and decrease peristalsis. Correction of constipation associated with opiate use calls for a senna or osmotic laxative to overcome the strong opioid effect. Stool softeners and bulking agents alone are inadequate.

Laxatives commonly used in chronic constipation include the following:
- Bulking agents (e.g., psyllium, methylcellulose)
- Stool softeners (surfactants) (e.g., docusate sodium)
- Osmotic laxatives (e.g., lactulose, sorbitol)
- Stimulant laxatives (e.g., senna, bisacodyl)
- Saline laxatives (e.g., magnesium hydroxide [Milk of Magnesia])

Bulk laxatives are often the first prescribed because of their safety. Bulk laxatives absorb water from the intestinal lumen and increase stool mass. Adequate fluid intake is essential, and use of these laxatives is contraindicated in the presence of obstruction or compromised peristaltic

---

BOX 10-6   Bowel Training Program

1. Obtain bowel history, and establish a schedule for the bowel training program that is normal and comfortable for the patient and conforms to his or her lifestyle.
2. Ensure adequate fiber and fluid intake (normalize stool consistency).
   a. Fiber.
      (1) Add high-fiber foods to diet (dried fruit, dried beans, vegetables, and wheat products).
      (2) Suggest adding 1 to 3 tbsp bran or Metamucil to diet one or two times each day. (Titrate dosage based on response.)
   b. Fluid.
      (1) Two to three L daily (unless contraindicated).
      (2) Four oz of prune, fig, or pear juice (or a warm fluid) may be given daily as a stimulus (e.g., 30-60 min before the established time for defecation).
3. Encourage exercise program.
   a. Pelvic tilt, modified sit-ups for abdominal strength.
   b. Walking for general muscle tone and cardiovascular system.
   c. More vigorous program if appropriate.
4. Establish a regular time for the bowel movement.
   a. Established time depends on patient's schedule.
   b. Best times are 20 to 40 min after regularly scheduled meals, when gastrocolic reflex is active.
   c. Attempts at evacuation should be made daily within 15 min of the established time and whenever the patient senses rectal distention.
   d. Instruct patient in normal posture for defecation. (The patient normally sits on the toilet or bedside commode; for the patient who is unable to get out of bed, the left side-lying position is best.)
   e. Instruct the patient to contract the abdominal muscles and "bear down."
   f. Have the patient lean forward to increase the intraabdominal pressure by use of compression against the thighs.
   g. Stimulate anorectal reflex and rectal emptying if necessary.
5. (a) Insert a rectal suppository or mini-enema into the rectum 15 to 30 min before the scheduled bowel movement, placing the suppository against the bowel wall, or (b) insert a gloved, lubricated finger into the anal canal and gently dilate the anal sphincter.

activity. It may take 1 to 3 days before a bulk-forming laxative starts to work. Bulk-forming agents can decrease absorption of other medications, particularly aspirin, warfarin, and carbamazepine, and may also affect blood glucose levels (Osei-Boamah et al., 2012). A saline or osmotic laxative can be added if the bulk laxative is not effective. Use of saline laxatives should be avoided in patients with poor renal function or congestive heart failure because they may cause electrolyte imbalances.

Stimulant laxatives should be used when other laxatives are ineffective. The emollient laxative, mineral oil, should be avoided because of the risk of lipoid aspiration pneumonia. Stool softeners (surfactants) are frequently used as laxatives. They are poorly absorbed and have a detergent-like effect of reducing the water–oil interface in the stool. Studies of surfactants, such as docusate, have reported minimal effectiveness, particularly in older adults with limited mobility. Because stool softeners do not increase bowel activity, their use may result in certain individuals having a bowel filled with soft stool (Osei-Boamah et al., 2012). Use should be limited to patients in whom excessive straining or painful defecation occurs, or for individuals at high risk for developing constipation, in combination with other types of laxatives and bowel programs.

Combinations of natural fiber, fruit juices, and natural laxative mixtures are often recommended in clinical practice, and some studies have found an increase in bowel frequency and a decrease in laxative use when these mixtures are used. The Beverley-Travis natural laxative recipe and an additional recipe for an alternative natural laxative mixture are presented in Box 10-7.

Enemas

Enemas of any type should be reserved for situations in which other methods produce no response or when it is known that there is an impaction. Enemas should not be used on a regular basis. Soapsuds enemas should not be used because they can produce mucosal damage to the rectum.

 SAFETY ALERT

Sodium phosphate enemas (Fleets) should not be used because they may lead to severe metabolic disorders associated with high mortality and morbidity (Ori et al., 2012). Oil retention enemas are used for refractory constipation and in the treatment of fecal impaction.

BOX 10-7   Natural Laxative Recipes

1. Beverley-Travis Natural Laxative Mixture
Ingredients
1 cup raisins
1 cup pitted prunes
1 cup figs
1 cup dates
1 cup currants
1 cup prune concentrate

Directions
Combine contents together in grinder or blender to a thickened consistency. Store in refrigerator between uses.

Dosage
Administer 2 tablespoons (tbs) twice a day (once in the morning and once in the evening). May increase or decrease according to the frequency of bowel movements.

Nutritional Composition
Each 2-tbs dose contains the following:
61 calories
137 mg potassium
8 mg sodium
11.9 g sugar
0.5 g protein
1.4 g fiber

2. Power Pudding
Ingredients
1 cup wheat bran
1 cup applesauce
1 cup prune juice

Directions
Mix and store in refrigerator. Start with administration of 1 tbs/day. Increase **slowly** until desired effect is achieved and no disagreeable symptoms occur.

From Hale E, Smith E, St. James J, et al: Pilot study of the feasibility and effectiveness of a natural laxative mixture, *Geriatr Nurs* 28(2):104-111, 2007.

A program to prevent as well as treat constipation that incorporates a high-fiber diet, liberal fluid intake, daily exercise, and environmental modifications that promote a regular pattern of bowel elimination must be developed for each client. Interventions in any setting are based on a thorough assessment. Assessment and management of bowel function are an important nursing responsibility.

Fecal Incontinence

Fecal incontinence (FI) is defined as "continuous or recurrent uncontrolled passage of fecal material for at least one month in a mature person" (Stevens & Palmer, 2007). Estimates are that more than 6.5 million Americans have fecal incontinence. Accurate estimates are difficult to obtain because many people are reluctant to discuss this disorder and many primary care providers do not ask about it. Prevalence varies with the study population: 2% to 17% in community-dwelling older people, 50% to 65% in older adults in nursing homes, and 33% in hospitalized older adults. Fecal incontinence is a significant risk factor for nursing home placement. Higher prevalence rates are found among patients with diabetes, irritable bowel syndrome, stroke (new onset, 30%; 15% at three years post-stroke), multiple sclerosis, and spinal cord injury (Roach & Christie, 2008; Grover et al., 2010).

Often FI is associated with urinary incontinence and as many as 50% to 70% of patients with UI also carry the diagnosis of FI. FI can be transient (episodes of diarrhea, acute illness, fecal impaction) or persistent. Fecal incontinence, like urinary incontinence, has devastating social ramifications for the individuals and families who experience it. UI and FI share similar contributing factors, including damage to the pelvic floor as a result of surgery or trauma, neurological disorders, functional impairment, immobility, and dementia.

Implications for Gerontological Nursing and Healhty Aging

Assessment

Assessment should include a complete client history as in urinary incontinence (described earlier in this chapter) and investigation into stool consistency and frequency, use of laxatives or enemas, surgical and obstetrical history, medications, effect of FI on quality of life, focused physical examination with attention to the gastrointestinal system, and a bowel record. A digital rectal examination should be performed to identify any presence of a mass, impaction, or occult blood.

Interventions

Nursing interventions are aimed at managing and/or restoring bowel continence. Therapies similar to those used to treat urinary incontinence such as environmental manipulation (access to toilet), diet alterations, habit-training schedules, improving transfer and ambulation ability, sphincter-training exercises, biofeedback, medications, and/or surgery to correct underlying defects are effective.

Keeping accurate bowel records and identifying triggers that influence incontinence are important. For example, eating a meal stimulates defecation 30 minutes after completion of the meal, or defecation occurs after the morning cup of coffee. If the fecal incontinence occurs only once or twice each day, it can be controlled by being prepared. Placing the individual on the toilet, commode, or bedpan at a given time after the trigger event facilitates defecation in the appropriate place at the appropriate time (see Box 10-6). The judicious use of nonirritant laxatives can help to maintain bowel function and prevent constipation.

The effectiveness of interventions in fecal incontinence will be self-evident but will take time. As in the treatment of urinary incontinence, goals must be realistic. It cannot be stated too often or too strongly that the nurse must always provide immaculate skin care to persons with incontinence, because self-esteem and skin integrity depend on it.

Application of Maslow's Hierarchy

Meeting elimination needs is basic to the maintenance of biological and physiological integrity, but its importance reaches far higher on the hierarchy. Often nurses are key to ensuring that these basic needs are met. Inadequate attention to this basic need can cause excess disability and insecurity, affect safety, cause social isolation and curtailment of meaningful activities and relationships, and interfere with the ability of the older person to achieve a meaningful and fulfilling life.

KEY CONCEPTS

- Urinary incontinence is not a part of normal aging. UI is a symptom of an underlying problem and calls for thorough assessment.
- Urinary incontinence can be minimized or cured, and there are many therapeutic modalities available for treatment of UI that nurses can implement.
- Health promotion teaching, identification of risk factors, comprehensive assessments of UI, education of informal and formal caregivers, and use of evidence-based interventions are basic continence competencies for nurses.
- A number of interventions for urinary incontinence are applicable to the management of bowel incontinence.

ACTIVITIES AND DISCUSSION QUESTIONS

1. Discuss risk factors for UI in older adults.
2. Conduct a UI history with a partner or with an older adult.

3. What measures can be taken to cure or decrease urinary incontinence in the community and long-term care settings?

4. Devise a nursing care plan for an older adult with urinary incontinence or fecal incontinence.

REFERENCES

Agency for Healthcare Research and Quality: Experts seek better diagnosis and treatment for women's urinary incontinence and chronic pelvic pain, *AHRQ Research Activities* 383, 2012.

Barry MJ, Meleth S, Lee JY, et al: Effect of increasing doses of saw palmetto extract on lower urinary tract symptoms: a randomized trial, *JAMA* 28 (305):1344–1351, 2011.

Barton C, Sklenicka J, Sayegh P, et al: Contraindicated medication use among patients in a memory disorders clinic, *Am J Geriatr Pharmacother* 6(3):147–152, 2008.

Bucci A: Be a continence champion: use the CHAMMP tool to individualize the plan of care, *Geriatr Nurs* 28(2):120–124, 2007.

DeMaagd G: *Urinary incontinence: treatment update with a focus on pharmacological management* (2007). Available at http://www.uspharmacist.com/content/d/feature/c/10310/.

Dowling-Castronovo A, Bradway C: Urinary incontinence. In Boltz M, Capezuti E, Fulmer T, et al, editors: *Evidence-based geriatric nursing protocols for best practice,* New York, 2012, Springer.

Dowling-Castronovo A, Spiro E: *Urinary incontinence assessment in older adults: Part I—Transient urinary incontinence* (2013). Available at http://consultgerirn.org/uploads/File/trythis/issue11-1.pdf.

Dowling-Castronovo A, Spiro E: *Urinary incontinence assessment in older adults: Part II—Established urinary incontinence* (2008). Available at http://consultgerirn.org/uploads/File/trythis/issue11-2.pdf.

DuBeau CE: Therapeutic/pharmacologic approaches to urinary incontinence in older adults, *Clinical Pharmacology* 85:98, 2009.

Fink HA, Taylor BC, Tacklind JW, et al: Treatment interventions in nursing home residents with urinary incontinence: a systematic review of randomized trials, *Mayo Clin Proc* 83(12):1332–1343, 2008.

Genato L, Buhr W: Urinary tract infections in older adult residing in long-term care facilities, *Ann Longterm Care* 20(4):33–38, 2012.

Grover M, Busby-Whitehead J, Palmer MH, et al: Survey of geriatricians on the effect of fecal incontinence on nursing home referral, *J Am Geriatr Soc* 58:1058, 2010.

Ham R, Sloane P, Warshaw G, et al: *Primary care geriatrics: a case-based approach*, ed 4, St. Louis, 2007, Mosby.

Inelmen E, Giuseppe S, Giuliano E: When are indwelling catheters appropriate in elderly patients? *Geriatrics* 62(10):18–22, 2007.

Johnson T, Ouslander J: The newly revised F-Tag 315 and surveyor guidance for urinary incontinence in long-term care, *J Am Med Dir Assoc* 7(9):594–600, 2006.

Juthani-Mehta M, Quagliarello V, Perrelli E, et al: Clinical features to identify urinary tract infection in nursing home residents: a cohort study, *J Am Geriatr Soc* 57: 963, 2009.

Lawhorne L, Ouslander J, Parmelee P, et al: Urinary incontinence: a neglected geriatric syndrome in nursing facilities, *J Am Med Dir Assoc* 9(1):9–35, 2008.

Lewis SJ, Heaton KW: Stool Form Scale as a useful guide to intestinal transit time, *Scand J Gastroenterol* 32:920, 1997.

MacDonald C, Butler L: Silent no more: elderly women's stories of living with urinary incontinence in long-term care, *J Gerontol Nurs* 33(1):14–20, 2007.

Mason DJ, Newman DK, Palmer MH: Changing UI practice, *Am J Nurs* 3(Suppl):2–3, 2003.

Mouton C, Adenuga B, Vijayan J: Urinary tract infections in long-term care, *Ann Longterm Care* 18:35, 2010.

Muller N: What Americans understand and how they are affected by bladder control problems: highlights of recent nationwide consumer research, *Urol Nurs* 25(2):109–115, 2005.

Newman DK, Palmer MH, editors: The state of the science on urinary incontinence, *Am J Nurs* 3(Suppl):1–58, 2003.

Ori Y, Rozen-Zvi B, Chagnac A, et al: Fatalities and severe metabolic disorders associated with use of sodium phosphate enemas, *Arch Intern Med* 172(3):263–265, 2012.

Osei-Boamah E, Chui J, Diaz C, et al: Constipation in the hospitalized older patient. *Clinical Geriatrics* 20(10):20–26, 2012.

Palmer MH, Newman D: Bladder control educational needs of older adults, *J Gerontol Nurs* 32(10):28–32, 2006.

Roach M, Christie J: Fecal incontinence in the elderly, *Geriatrics* 63(2):13–22, 2008.

Robinson JP, Shea JA: Development and testing of a measure of health-related quality of life for men with urinary incontinence, *J Am Geriatr Soc* 50(5):935–945, 2002.

Shamliyan T, Wyman J, Bliss DZ, et al: *Prevention of fecal and urinary incontinence in adults*, Rockville, MD, 2007, Agency for Healthcare Research and Quality.

Shamliyan T, Wyman J, Kane RL: *Nonsurgical treatments for urinary incontinence in adult women: diagnosis and comparative effectiveness* (2012). Available at www.effectivehealthcare.ahrq.gov/reports/final.cfm.

Stevens T, Palmer R: Fecal incontinence in LTC patients, *LTC Clin Interface* 8(4):35–39, 2007.

Tettamanti G, Altman D, Pedersen NL, et al: Effects of coffee and tea consumption on urinary incontinence in female twins, *BJOG An International Journal of Obstetrics and Gynaecology* 2011.

Townsend M, Curhan G, Resnik N, et al: Rates of remission improvement, and progression of urinary incontinence in Asian Black, and white women, *Am J Nurs* 111(4):26–33, 2011.

Zarowitz B, Ouslander J: The applications of evidence-based principles of care in older persons (issue 6): urinary incontinence, *J Am Med Dir Assoc* 8:35, 2007.

CHAPTER 11

Rest, Sleep, and Activity

Theris A. Touhy

evolve   evolve.elsevier.com/Ebersole/gerontological

LEARNING OBJECTIVES

Upon completion of this chapter, the reader will be able to:
- Identify age-related changes that affect rest, sleep, and activity.
- Discuss the importance of sleep and activity to the health and well-being of older adults.
- Describe the beneficial effects of exercise and appropriate exercise regimens for older adults.
- Use evidence-based protocols in assessment and development of interventions for rest, sleep, and promotion of activity.

GLOSSARY

Circadian rhythm Regular recurrence of certain phenomena in cycles of approximately 24 hours.
Insomnia Disturbed sleep pattern in presence of adequate opportunity and circumstances for sleep.
Non–rapid eye movement (NREM) sleep First four stages of sleep.
Obstructive sleep apnea Repetitive cessation (>10 seconds) of respiration during sleep.
Rapid eye movement (REM) sleep Wakeful and active form of sleep during which dreaming occurs or tension is discharged.

THE LIVED EXPERIENCE

You know, I never get a decent night's sleep. I wake up at least 4 times every night, and I just know I won't get back to sleep. I really don't want to keep taking pills for sleep, but when I lie there awake, I just think of all the difficult times and situations I can't manage. After a while, I'm really in a stew about everything.

Richard, a 67-year-old recent retiree

This is really beginning to tire me out. Richard keeps waking me at night because he can't sleep. I try to tell him to get up and read or something. I really need my sleep if I'm going to get to work on time. I wonder if Richard needs to see a doctor. Maybe he is depressed about being retired and alone while I'm at work. I'll talk to him about it.

Clara, Richard's wife

Rest, sleep, and activity depend on one another. Inadequacy of rest and sleep affects any activity, whether it is considered strenuous exertion or falls under the heading of the activities of daily living. Activity, in turn, is necessary to maintain physical and physiological integrity (e.g., cardiopulmonary endurance and function; musculoskeletal strength, agility, and structure) and it helps a person obtain adequate sleep. Rest, sleep, and activity contribute greatly to overall physical and mental well-being.

Rest and Sleep

The human organism needs rest and sleep to conserve energy, prevent fatigue, provide organ respite, and relieve tension. Sleep is an extension of rest, and both are physiological and mental necessities for survival. Sleep is a basic need. Rest occurs with sleep in sustained unbroken periods. Sleep occupies a third of our lives and is a vital function and basic need. Sleep deprivation and fragmentation of sleep in older adults may adversely affect cognitive, emotional, and physical functioning as well as quality of life (Martin et al., 2010; Teodorescu & Husain, 2010). Because of the public health burden of chronic sleep loss and sleep disorders, and the low awareness of poor sleep health, *Healthy People 2020* includes sleep health as a special topic area. Goals for adults are presented in the Healthy People box.

 HEALTHY PEOPLE 2020

Sleep Health
Goals:
- Increase public knowledge of how adequate sleep and treatment of sleep disorders improve health, productivity, wellness, quality of life, and safety on roads and in the workplace.
- Increase the proportion of persons with symptoms of obstructive sleep apnea who seek medical evaluation.
- Increase the proportion of adults who get sufficient sleep.

From U.S. Department of Health and Human Services, Office of Disease Prevention and Health Promotion: *Healthy people 2020* (2012). Available at http://www.healthypeople.gov/2020.

Biorhythm and Sleep

Our lives proceed in a series of rhythms that influence and regulate physiological function, chemical concentrations, performance, behavioral responses, moods, and the ability to adapt. Biorhythms vary between individuals and age-related changes in biorhythms (circadian rhythms) are relevant to health and the process of aging. With aging, there is a reduction in the amplitude of all circadian endogenous responses (e.g., body temperature, pulse, blood pressure, hormonal levels). The most important biorhythm is the circadian sleep-wake rhythm. As people age, the natural circadian rhythm may become less responsive to external stimuli, such as changes in light during the course of the day.

Sleep and Aging

The predictable pattern of normal sleep is called sleep architecture. The body progresses through the five stages of the normal sleep pattern consisting of rapid eye

movement (REM) sleep and non–rapid eye movement (NREM) sleep. Sleep structure is shown in Box 11-1. Most of the changes in sleep architecture in healthy adults begin between the ages of 40 and 60 years. The age-related changes include less time spent in stages 3 and 4 sleep and more time spent awake or in stage 1 sleep. Declines in stage 3 and 4 sleep begin between 20 and 30 years of age and are nearly complete by the age of 50 to 60 years. The amount of deep sleep in stages 3 and 4 contributes to how rested and refreshed a person feels the next day. Time spent in REM sleep also declines with age, and transitions between stages 1 and 2 are more common. The changes that occur in sleep with aging are summarized in Box 11-2.

BOX 11-1   Sleep Structure

Four Stages of Non–Rapid Eye Movement (NREM) Sleep
Stage 1
  Lightest level
  Easy to awaken
  Comprises 5% of sleep in young

Stage 2
  Decreases with age
  Low-voltage activity on electroencephalogram (EEG)
  May cease in old age

Stage 3
  Decreases with age
  High-voltage activity on EEG
  May cease in old age

Stage 4
  Decreases with age
  High-voltage activity on EEG
  Comprises 15% of sleep in elders

Rapid Eye Movement (REM) Sleep
  Alternates with NREM sleep throughout the night
  Rapid eye movements are the key feature
  Breathing increases in rate and depth
  Muscle tone relaxed
  85% of dreaming occurs in REM sleep

Adapted from Beers MH, Berkow R: *The Merck manual of geriatrics,* ed 3, Whitehouse Station, NJ, 2000, Merck Research Laboratories.

- More time spent in bed awake before falling asleep
- Total sleep time and sleep efficiency are reduced
- Awakenings are frequent, increasing after age 50 (>30 minutes of wakefulness after sleep onset in >50% of older subjects)
- Daytime napping
- Changes in circadian rhythm (early to bed, early to rise)
- Sleep is subjectively and objectively lighter (more stage 1, little stage 4, more disruptions)
- Rapid eye movement (REM) sleep is short, less intense, and more evenly distributed.

Adapted from Subramanian S, Surani S: Sleep disorders in the elderly, *Geriatrics* 62(12):10-32, 2007.

Older adults with good general health, positive moods, and engagement in more active lifestyles and meaningful activities report better sleep and fewer sleep complaints. Results of a recent large study of 155,877 participants exploring the prevalence of sleep-related complaints across age groups found that on average, older adults reported sleeping better than younger adults. Sleep complaints are usually linked to other health problems and sleep disorders. Poor sleep is not an inevitable consequence of aging but rather an indicator of health status and calls for investigation (Grandner et al., 2012).

Sleep Disorders

Insomnia

Insomnia is defined as "a complaint of disturbed sleep in the presence of an adequate opportunity and circumstance for sleep" (Bloom et al., 2009, p. 6). The diagnosis of insomnia requires that the person has difficulty falling asleep for at least 1 month and that impairment in daytime functioning results from difficulty sleeping. Insomnia is classified as either primary or comorbid. Primary insomnia implies that no other cause of sleep disturbance has been identified. Comorbid insomnia is more common and is associated with psychiatric and medical disorders, medications, and primary sleep disorders, such as obstructive sleep apnea or restless legs syndrome. Comorbid insomnia does not suggest that these conditions cause insomnia but that insomnia and the other conditions co-occur and each may require attention and treatment (Bloom et al., 2009). Insomnia has a higher prevalence in older adults and

there are many influencing factors, both physiological and behavioral (Box 11-3).

Prescription and nonprescription medications also create sleep disturbances. Drugs and alcohol use are thought to account for 10% to 15% of cases of insomnia (Ham et al., 2007). Problematic drugs include serotonin reuptake inhibitors (SSRIs), antihypertensives (clonidine, beta blockers, reserpine, methyldopa), anticholinergics, sympathomimetic amines, diuretics, opiates, cough and cold medications, thyroid preparations, phenytoin, cortisone, and levodopa. The times of day that medications are given can also contribute to sleep problems—for example, a diuretic given before bedtime or sedating medication given in the morning (Rose & Lorenz, 2010).

Sleep Apnea

Sleep apnea is a condition in which people stop breathing while asleep. Apneas (complete cessation of respiration)

- Age-related changes in sleep architecture
- Comorbidities (cardiovascular disease, diabetes, pulmonary disease, musculoskeletal disorders), CNS disorders (Parkinson's disease, seizure disorder, dementia), GI disorders (hiatal hernia, GERD, PUD), urinary disorders (incontinence, BPH)
- Depression, anxiety, delirium, psychosis
- Pain
- Polypharmacy
- Life stressors
- Limited exposure to sunlight
- Environmental noises, institutional routines
- Poor sleep hygiene
- Lack of exercise
- Excessive napping
- Caregiving for a dependent elder
- Sleep apnea
- Restless legs syndrome
- Periodic leg movement
- Rapid eye movement behavior disorder
- Alcohol
- Smoking

BPH, Benign prostatic hyperplasia; *CNS*, central nervous system; *GI*, gastrointestinal; *GERD*, gastroesophageal reflux disease; *PUD*, peptic ulcer disease. Adapted from Subramanian S, Surani S: Sleep disorders in the elderly, *Geriatrics* 62(12):10-32, 2007.

and hypopneas (partial decrease in respiration) result in hypoxemia and changes in autonomic nervous system activity. The result is increases in systemic and pulmonary arterial pressure and changes in cerebral blood flow. The episodes are generally terminated by an arousal (brief awakening), which results in fragmented sleep and excessive daytime sleepiness. Other symptoms of sleep apnea include loud periodic snoring, gasping and choking on awakenings, unusual nighttime activity such as sitting upright or falling out of bed, morning headache, poor memory and intellectual functioning, and irritability and personality change. If the person has a sleeping partner, it is often the person who reports the nighttime symptoms.

The two types of sleep apnea are obstructive sleep apnea (OSA) and central sleep apnea (CSA). OSA, caused by obstruction of the upper airway, is the most common; CSA is due to central nervous system or cardiac dysfunction. Sleep apnea affects an estimated 20% of older men and women in the United States (Rajki, 2012).

In long-term care facilities, the prevalence of OSA has been estimated to be as high as 70% to 80% (Rose & Lorenz, 2010). The age-related decline in the activity of the upper airway muscles, which results in compromised pharyngeal patency, predisposes older adults to OSA. Older adults with sleep apnea demonstrate significant cognitive decline compared with younger people with the same disease severity. The diagnosis of sleep apnea is often delayed in older adults and symptoms are blamed on age (Subramanian & Surani, 2007). Risk factors for sleep apnea are listed in Box 11-4.

Assessment. Assessment includes information from the sleeping partner, and a sleep study is usually considered. A sleep study or polysomnogram (PSG) is a multiple-component test that electronically transmits and records specific physical activities during sleep. The data obtained is analyzed by a qualified physician to determine whether the person has a sleep disorder. Recognition of OSA in older adults may be more difficult because many are widowed and may not have a sleeping partner to report symptoms. If there is a sleeping partner, he or she may move to another room to sleep because of the disturbance to his or her own rest.

Interventions. Therapy will depend on the severity and type of sleep apnea, as well as the presence of comorbid illnesses. Specific treatment of sleep apnea may involve weight loss, avoidance of alcohol and sedatives, cessation of smoking, and avoidance of supine sleep positions. There should be risk counseling about impaired judgment from sleeplessness and the possibility of accidents when driving. Continuous positive airway pressure (CPAP) is the most effective treatment and the treatment of choice for older adults. The CPAP device delivers pressurized air through tubing to a nasal mask or nasal pillows, which are fitted around the head. The pressurized air acts as an airway splint and gently opens the patient's throat and breathing passages, allowing them to breathe normally, but only through their nose. CPAP has been shown to be well tolerated and effective for OSA in older adults with dementia (Rose & Lorenz, 2010). Another therapy for mild cases of OSA is the use of a dental appliance that moves the jaw forward, preventing the throat from closing (Rajki, 2012).

Restless Legs Syndrome

Restless legs syndrome (RLS) is a sensorimotor neurological disorder characterized by unpleasant leg sensations that disrupt sleep. RLS is categorized as primary or secondary. Primary (idiopathic) develops at a younger age with no predisposing factors and probably has a genetic basis. Secondary RLS can result from a variety of medical conditions that have iron deficiency in common, the most common being iron deficiency anemia, end-stage renal disease, and pregnancy. Impairment in dopamine transport in the substantia nigra due to reduced intracellular iron seems to play a critical role in the disease.

Individuals with RLS have an uncontrollable need to move the legs, often accompanied by discomfort in the legs. Other symptoms include paresthesias; creeping sensations; crawling sensations; tingling, cramping, and burning sensations; pain; or even indescribable sensations. RLS has a circadian rhythm, with the intensity of the symptoms

---

BOX 11-4   Risk Factors for Sleep Apnea

- Increasing age
- Increased neck circumference
- Male sex
- Anatomical abnormalities of the upper airway
- Upper airway resistance and/or obstruction
- Family history
- Excess weight
- Use of alcohol, sedatives, or tranquilizers
- Smoking
- Hypertension

Data from Phillips B: Sleep apnea, periodic leg movement, restless legs syndrome and cardiovascular complications. In Sleep disorders in the geriatric population: implications for health, *Clin Geriatrics* (Suppl Dec): 2005, American Geriatrics Society.

becoming worse at night and improving toward the morning. It may be temporarily relieved by movement.

The estimated prevalence of RLS among people over 65 years of age is 10% to 20%, and it affects women more than men (Bloom et al., 2009). Other sleep disorders, periodic limb movements of sleep (PLMS), and periodic limb movement disorder (PLMD), are often associated with RLS. These movement disorders of sleep are sometimes called nocturnal myoclonus or periodic leg movements and involve repeated rhythmical extensions of the big toe and dorsiflexion of the ankle. Disrupted sleep is the reason people with these disorders seek help.

Antidepressants and neuroleptic medications can aggravate RLS symptoms. Increased body mass index, caffeine use, tobacco, and sedentary lifestyle are also contributing factors. Diagnosis of RLS includes ruling out and/or treating as indicated any medical condition. Oral iron supplements should be prescribed for patients with serum iron levels lower than 45 µg/L (Winkelman et al., 2007). Dopamine receptor agonists (pramipexole, ropinirole) are the drugs of choice for RLS. Gabapentin may also be effective for individuals with comorbid RLS and peripheral neuropathy (Winkelman et al., 2007; Bloom et al., 2009). Nonpharmacological therapy includes stretching the lower extremities, mild to moderate physical activity, hot baths, and relaxation techniques, and avoidance of alcohol.

Rapid Eye Movement Sleep Behavior Disorder

Rapid eye movement sleep behavior disorder (RBSD) is a sleep disorder common in older adults. The mean age at emergence is 60 years, and RBSD is more common in males. Characteristics of RBSD are loss of normal voluntary muscle atonia during REM sleep associated with complex behavior while dreaming (Subramanian & Surani, 2007). Patients report elaborate enactment of their dreams, often with violent content, during sleep. This may include violent behaviors, such as punching and kicking, with the potential for injury of both the patient and the bed partner.

RBSD may be primary or secondary to neurodegenerative diseases such as Parkinson's disease, diffuse Lewy body disease, Alzheimer's disease, and progressive supranuclear palsy. It may also be idiopathic (Bloom et al., 2009). RBSD may be an early sign of Parkinson's disease. Within 5 to 8 years of being diagnosed with RBSD, 60% to 80% of individuals develop Parkinson's disease (Brooks & Peever, 2008). Caffeine and some medications (SSRIs, tricyclic antidepressants) may also contribute to RBSD. Interventions include neurological examination, removal of aggravating medications, and counseling related to safety measures in the sleep environment. Clonazepam and/or melatonin may be effective in treating RBSD.

Circadian Rhythm Sleep Disorders

In circadian rhythm sleep disorders (CRSDs) relatively normal sleep occurs at abnormal times. Two clinical presentations are seen: advanced sleep phase disorder (ASPD) and irregular sleep–wake disorder (ISWD). In ASPD, the individual begins and ends sleep at unusually early times (e.g., going to bed as early as 6 or 7 PM and waking up between 2 and 5 AM). Not all individuals with an advanced sleep phase have ASPD. If they are not bothered by their sleep phases and have no functional impairment, we may just consider them "morning" people. In irregular sleep–wake disorder, sleep is dispersed across the 24-hour day in bouts of irregular length. Factors contributing to these disorders are age-related changes in sleep and circadian rhythm regulation combined with decreased levels of light exposure and activity.

A combination of good sleep hygiene practices and methods to delay the timing of sleep and wake times are recommended as treatment for ASPD. Bright light therapy (2500 to 10,000 lux) for 1 to 2 hours at about 7 to 8 PM can help normalize or delay circadian rhythm patterns (Bloom et al., 2009).

In ISWD, the individual may obtain enough sleep over the 24-hour period, but time asleep is broken into at least three different periods of variable length. Erratic napping occurs during the day, and nighttime sleep is severely fragmented and shortened. Chronic insomnia and/or daytime sleepiness are present. ISWD is most commonly encountered in individuals with dementia, particularly those who are institutionalized. Sleep disturbances of individuals with dementia are often among the reasons for nursing home placement. Treatment consists of increasing the duration and intensity of light exposure during the daytime and avoiding exposure to bright light in the evening. Structured activity during the day and a quiet sleeping environment may also improve ISWD (Bloom et al., 2009).

Implications for Gerontological Nursing and Healthy Aging

Assessment

Sleep habits should be reviewed with older adults in all settings. Many people do not seek treatment for insomnia and may blame poor sleep on the aging process. Nurses are in an excellent position to assess sleep and suggest interventions to improve the quality of the older person's sleep. Night shift nursing staff in institutions have the opportunity to assess sleep patterns and implement appropriate interventions to enhance sleep (Kerr & Wilkinson, 2010). Assessment for sleep disorders and contributing factors to poor sleep (pain, chronic illness, medications, alcohol use, depression, anxiety) are important.

Subjective and objective measures included in sleep assessment that are available to nurses include visual analog scales, subjective rating scales (e.g., 0 to 10 or 0 to 100), questionnaires that determine whether one's sleep is disturbed, interviews, and daily sleep charts/diaries (Box 11-5). Resources are shown in the Evidence-Based Practice box.

🔍 EVIDENCE-BASED PRACTICE

Sleep

- Excessive sleepiness (Epworth Sleepiness Scale): http://consultgerirn.org/topics/sleep/want_to_know_more
- Nursing Standard of Practice: Excessive Sleepiness: Chasens E, Umlauf M: Excessive Sleepiness. In Boltz M, Capezuti E, Fulmer T, et al, editors: *Evidence-based geriatric nursing protocols for best practice.* New York, 2012, Springer.
- Practice parameters for the clinical evaluation and treatment of circadian rhythm sleep disorders: http://www.guideline.gov/content.aspx?id= 12112&search=sleep
- Clinical guideline for the evaluation, management and long-term care of obstructive sleep apnea in adults: http://www.guideline.gov/content.aspx?id=15298&search= sleepAHRQ

The nurse should learn how well the person sleeps at home, how many times the person is awakened at night, what time the person retires, and what rituals occur at bedtime. Rituals include bedtime snacks, watching television, listening

---

BOX 11-5 Sleep Diary

Instructions: Record the following for 2 to 4 weeks. To be completed by the person or caregiver if the person is unable.
1. The number of times a call for assistance to the bathroom or for pain medication or subjective symptoms of inability to sleep (e.g., anxiety) occur
2. Whether the person appears to be asleep or awake when checked during the night
3. If sleep medication was given and if repeated
4. The time the person awakens in the morning (approximation)
5. Where the person falls asleep in the evening
6. Daytime naps

---

to music, or reading—activities whose execution is crucial to the individual's ability to fall asleep. Other assessment data should include the amount and type of daily exercise; favorite position when in bed; room environment, including temperature, ventilation, and illumination; activities engaged in several hours before bedtime; medications taken for sleep as well as information about all medications taken. Additional assessment data include information about the individual's involvement in hobbies, life satisfaction, perception of health status, and assessment for depression. The patient's bed partner, caregivers, and/or family members can also provide valuable information about the person's sleep habits and lifestyle.

Interventions

Nonpharmacological Treatment

Interventions begin after a thorough sleep history has been recorded and, if possible, a sleep log obtained. Management is directed at identifiable causes. Pharmacological treatment should be considered an adjuvant treatment to nonpharmacological interventions. Attention to sleep hygiene principles is important to promote good sleep habits (Box 11-6). Cognitive behavioral therapy using stimulus control, sleep restriction therapy, relaxation therapy, and exercise is effective and produces sustained positive effects. These administered behavior treatments have been reported to be an effective and practical treatment for chronic insomnia in older adults (Buysse et al., 2011). T'ai Chi Chih can be considered a useful nonpharmacological approach for sleep complaints (Irwin et al., 2008).

In hospital and institutional settings, promotion of a good sleep environment is important. A sleep improvement protocol, including do-not-disturb periods; provision of usual bedtime routines; and use of soft music, relaxation techniques, massage, and aromatherapy might improve sleep in hospital and nursing home settings. A multidisciplinary approach to identify sources of noise and light, such as equipment and staff interactions, could result in modification without compromising safety and quality of patient care. "Because a full sleep cycle of 90 minutes can have a positive influence on sleep effectiveness," efforts to allow sufficient time for a full sleep cycle are important (Missildine, 2008; Missildine et al., 2010). Suggested interventions to reduce daytime sleepiness and enhance nighttime sleep among residents of long-term care facilities are presented in Box 11-7.

Pharmacological Treatment

Medications may be recommended for short-term sleep problems. They should be used in combination with

---

BOX 11-6	**Steps to Good Sleep Hygiene**

1. Make sure the bedroom is restful and comfortable.
2. Use the bedroom only for sleep and intimate relations; do not watch television from bed or work in bed.
3. Have a regular bedtime and wake-up time even on weekends.
4. Avoid naps. If you must nap, sleep no longer than 30 minutes in early afternoon (before 3 PM).
5. Get regular exercise, but avoid exercising within 4 hours of bedtime.
6. Get regular exposure to natural light.
7. Limit caffeine (tea, cola, coffee, chocolate), nicotine, and diuretics, especially late in the day.
8. Avoid alcohol for at least 2 hours before bedtime, and don't use alcohol to promote sleep.
9. Avoid large meals before bedtime. Avoid being too hungry or too full at bedtime.
10. Give attention to the bed environment (comfortable bed, pillows between the knees, quiet, darkness, comfortable temperature).
11. Practice a relaxing bedtime routine (relaxation techniques, guided imagery).
12. Avoid spending too much time in bed.
13. Do not watch the clock, which increases anxiety and pressure to sleep; if anxious, take a warm bath.
14. Avoid working on the computer before bedtime.
15. If you cannot fall asleep, get up and go to another room. Stay up as long as needed to feel sleepy. Return to bed when sleepy. If unable to sleep again after 10 minutes, repeat and get up as long as needed.

BOX 11-7	**Suggestions to Promote Sleep in Nursing Homes**

- Limit intake of caffeine and other fluids in excess before bedtime.
- Provide a light snack or warm beverage before bedtime.
- Maintain a quiet environment: soft lights, quiet music, and limited noise and staff intrusions when possible.
- Reduce nursing interruptions for medication administration by modifying dose schedule if possible.
- Discontinue invasive treatments when possible (Foley catheters, percutaneous gastrostomy tubes [PEG] tubes, intravenous lines).
- Encourage and assist to the bathroom before bed and as needed.
- Give pain medication before bedtime for patients with pain.
- Provide regular exercise or walking programs.
- Allow resident to stay out of bed and out of the room for as long as possible before bed if tolerated.
- Institute same time for resident to arise and get out of bed every morning.
- Maintain comfortable temperature in room; provide blankets as needed.
- Provide meaningful activities during the daytime.

behavioral interventions and must be chosen carefully, started at the lowest possible dosage, and monitored closely to avoid untoward effects in older adults. Patients should be educated on the proper use of medications and their side effects. Sedatives and hypnotics, including benzodiazepines and barbiturates, should be avoided. Over-the-counter (OTC) drugs such as diphenhydramine (Benadryl) or Tylenol PM (which contains diphenhydramine), often thought to be relatively harmless, should be avoided because of antihistaminic and anticholinergic side effects.

Benzodiazepine receptor agonists, such as zolpidem, eszopiclone, and zaleplon, have shorter half-lives and more favorable safety profiles for older adults. However, they also have undesirable effects and a narrow safety margin and should be used short-term only. Because of the rapid action of these drugs, they should be taken immediately before bedtime. Recent research results report that hospitalized patients who took zolpidem had a fall rate more than 4 times higher than those who did not take the drug. Fall precautions should be in place for individuals who take sleeping medications (Kolla et al., 2012). Ramelteon, a melatonin receptor agonist that promotes sleep via action on the circadian system, can be used for individuals who have difficulty falling asleep.

Activity

Regular physical activity throughout life is likely to enhance health and functional status as people age while also decreasing the number of chronic illnesses and functional limitations often assumed to be a part of growing older. The frail health and loss of function we associate with aging is in large part due to physical inactivity. Few factors contribute as much to health in aging as being physically active. The old adage "use it or lose it" certainly applies to our muscles and physical fitness.

Despite a large body of evidence about the benefits of physical activity to maintain and improve function, only about one third of men and 25% of women 65 to 74 years of age engage in leisure-time activity. With advancing age participation is even lower, with 16% of men and 11% of women 75 years of age and older engaged in leisure-time strengthening activities (lifting weights, calisthenics) (Centers for Disease Control and Prevention [CDC], 2011). Older African-American women are the least physically active race-sex subgroup in the United States (Duru et al., 2011). Physical activity is a topic area for *Healthy People 2020* and goals for adults are presented in the Healthy People box.

 HEALTHY PEOPLE 2020

Physical Activity
- Reduce the proportion of adults who engage in no leisure-time physical activity
- Increase the proportion of adults who engage in aerobic physical activity or at least moderate intensity for at least 150 minutes/week, or 75 minutes/week of vigorous intensity, or an equivalent combination.

From U.S. Department of Health and Human Services, Office of Disease Prevention and Health Promotion: *Healthy people 2020* (2012). Available at http://www.healthypeople.gov/2020.

Older people are also less likely to receive exercise counseling from their primary care providers than younger individuals. The levels of physical activity among older adults have not improved over the past decade in the United States. Many older people mistakenly believe that they are too old to begin a fitness program. Physical activity is important for all older people, not just active healthy elders. Even a small amount of time (at least 30 minutes of moderate activity several days a week) can improve health.

Physical activity is also associated with better cognitive functioning in old age. For women, physical activity at any time during the life course, especially as teenagers, is associated with a lower likelihood of cognitive impairment in later life (Middleton et al., 2010). Erickson and colleagues (2010) reported that people 65 years of age and over who walked at least 6 miles a week had greater gray matter volume and halved their risk of developing memory problems. Once weekly progressive strength training

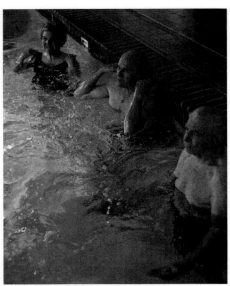

Aquatic exercise. Aquatic exercise programs are beneficial for elders with mobility problems. They improve circulation, muscle strength, and endurance, and they provide socialization and relaxation. (Copyright © Getty Images.)

exercise programs have also been shown to improve cognitive abilities in women 65 to 75 years of age (Davis et al., 2010).

Studies have found that increasing physical activity improves health outcomes in persons with chronic illnesses (regardless of severity) and in those with functional impairment (Sherrington et al., 2008; Yeom et al., 2009). The benefit of exercise (improvement in walking speed, strength, functional ability) of frail nursing home residents with diagnoses ranging from arthritis to lung disease and dementia has also been shown (Heyn et al., 2008). Physical activity can also improve emotional health and quality of life. Regardless of age or situation, the older person can find some activity suitable for his or her condition. It is important to keep older people moving any way possible for as long as possible.

Implications for Gerontological Nursing and Healthy Aging

Assessment

Assessment of functional abilities and screening should be included as part of the health assessment of all older adults. The purpose of screening is to (1) identify medical problems while allowing the individual to achieve the maximal benefit from physical activity; (2) identify functional limitations that will be addressed in the exercise program; and (3) minimize injury or other serious adverse effect.

The Exercise and Screening for You (EASY) tool (www.easyforyou.info) is a screening tool that can be used to determine a safe exercise program for older adults on the basis of underlying physical problems. The programs recommended on this website have all been reviewed and endorsed by national organizations such as the National Institute on Aging (Bethesda, MD) and can be printed and given to the person (Resnick, 2009). There are many resources available on the Internet that provide excellent information on physical activity in a usable format.

Frail older adults will need more comprehensive assessment and close monitoring to ensure benefit without compromising safety. Exercise goals for the frail older adult are different from those for younger adults. Exercise in younger adults helps prevent disease and increases life expectancy. For frail older people, exercise is important to minimize the effects of aging, reverse the effects of disuse, and maximize psychological health. Absolute contraindications to exercise testing and training include recent electrocardiogram changes or myocardial infarction; unstable angina; and uncontrolled arrhythmias, third-degree heart block, and acute heart failure. Poorly controlled diabetes, severe hypertension, respiratory disease, acute musculoskeletal pain, and arthritis are other conditions that warrant careful assessment before exercise programs are begun. Exercise programs may need to be adapted depending on the condition of the individual (e.g., pool exercise programs rather than resistance activities, such as lifting weights or using stretchy bands, if the elder has arthritis).

Interventions

Guidelines for Physical Activity

Recommendations for all adults are participation in 30 minutes of moderate-intensity physical activity for five or more days of the week. People do not have to be active for 30 minutes at a time but can accumulate 30 minutes over 24 hours. As little as 10 minutes of exercise has health benefits and three 10-minute bouts of activity have the same fitness effects as one 30-minute bout. Health care practitioners should counsel all patients on how to incorporate exercise into their daily routines (CDC, 2011).

Guidelines for physical activity for adults 65 years of age or older who are generally fit and have no limiting health conditions are as follows:

- Two hours and 30 minutes (150 minutes) of moderate-intensity aerobic activity (e.g., brisk walking, swimming,

bicycling) every week AND muscle-strengthening activities on two or more days that work all major muscle groups (legs, hips, abdomen, chest, shoulders, and arms) (CDC, 2011). See www.cdc.gov/physicalactivity/everyone/guidelines/olderadults.html for video presentations of exercise as well as an explanation of guidelines and tips for physical activity.
- Stretching (flexibility) and balance exercises (particularly for older people at risk of falls) are also recommended. Yoga and T'ai Chi exercises have been shown to be of benefit to older people in terms of improving flexibility and balance as well as pain reduction and improved psychological well-being (Rogers et al., 2010). T'ai Chi can be adapted for level of function and mobility status. Home-based balance-training exercise programs are also available.

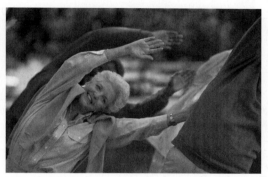

Stretching. © 2010 Photos.com, a division of Getty Images. All rights reserved.)

One does not have to invest in expensive equipment or gym memberships or follow a structured exercise regimen to benefit from increased activity. The older person may be able to integrate activity into daily life rather than doing a specific exercise. Examples include walking to the store instead of driving, golfing, raking leaves, gardening, washing windows or floors, washing and waxing the car, and swimming. The Wii game system offers other possibilities for exercise at all levels and is increasingly being used in nursing homes and assisted living facilities to encourage physical activity and enjoyable entertainment.

Special Considerations

Nonambulatory older people can also engage in physical activity and may benefit most from an exercise program in terms of function and quality of life. "Muscle weakness and atrophy are probably the most functionally relevant and reversible aspects to exercise in nonambulatory older adults" (Resnick et al., 2006, p. 174). Suggested exercises might include upper extremity cycling, marching in place, stretching, range of motion, use of resistive bands, and chair yoga. At the Louis and Anne Green Memory and Wellness Center at Florida Atlantic University (Boca Raton, FL), 90-year-old Vera Paley leads groups of cognitively impaired elders as well as caregivers in chair yoga sessions. See the resources on the Evolve website for this book for more information about Vera's yoga program.

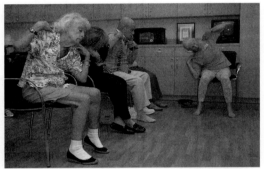

Yoga. Vera Paley leads yoga class. (Courtesy of Louis and Anne Green Memory & Wellness Center, Boca Raton, FL.)

Exercise Prescription

Prescribing an exercise plan that includes the specific exercises the individual should do as well as the reasonable short- and long-term goals and safety tips is suggested. As suggested by the CDC, the program should include endurance, strength, balance, and flexibility (Table 11-1). Examples of strength-training exercises that can be done at home are presented in Figure 11-1. Varied activities that involve interaction with peers and fit the person's lifestyle and culture will encourage participation. The individual should be informed of resources in the community, and communities should be encouraged to provide accessible and affordable options for physical activity.

Motivational interventions are important when encouraging older adults to begin and sustain a physical activity program. Collaborate with individuals on the goals they hope to achieve. Most older people are interested in how physical activity will improve the quality of their life and enhance their functional ability. The immediate benefits that can be expected should be emphasized—for example,

improving walking ability or decreasing risk of falls. Specific types of exercises that are to be done daily as well as daily and long-term goals can be written down. Individuals can also keep a journal or diary of their exercises and goals.

Implications for Gerontological Nursing and Healthy Aging

This chapter has looked separately at the need for rest and sleep and the need for activity. In summary, it is apparent that each area influences the function of the other. The quality and the overall perception of life can be augmented when the nurse monitors these specific functions and provides support or assistance according to identified problems. Gerontological nurses must be knowledgeable about age-related changes in sleep and activity and the effect of lifestyle on these changes. Many older people may have misconceptions about sleep and exercise, and the nurse can assess beliefs and understanding and provide education to enhance optimal wellness.

Assessment of sleep, the chosen level of activity, and the design of interventions must be grounded in evidence-based knowledge and applied to meet the needs of each unique individual. Common practices such as the use of hypnotics for sleep without a thorough assessment or being confined to a wheelchair because there is no one to help maintain walking skills lead to disabling and preventable problems for older people. Adequate sleep and activity are essential to physical, emotional, and cognitive functioning. Poor sleep and decline in functional capacity affect the ability to perform activities of daily living, compromise independence, and lead to disability and illness. Improvement of function is possible for even the most frail elder and gerontological nurses must incorporate the health promotion activities discussed in this chapter into any plan of care for an older adult.

Application of Maslow's Hierarchy

Sleep and activity needs must be met not only to maintain biological integrity, but also to meet higher-level needs such as safety and security, belonging and attachment, self-esteem and self-efficacy, and self-actualization and transcendence. The older adult would not survive if these needs were not met independently or with the assistance of others. Ineffective sleep, rest, and activity patterns contribute to depression, loneliness, and loss of independence and self-esteem, as well as physical and cognitive illnesses.

TABLE 11-1	Guidelines for Teaching Older Adults About Exercise				
Exercise	**Description**	**Benefits**	**Intensity**	**Frequency**	**Examples**
Moderate-intensity aerobic activity	Continuous movement involving large muscle groups that is sustained for a minimum of 10 minutes	Improves cardiovascular functioning, strengthens heart muscle, decreases blood glucose and triglycerides, increases HDL, improves mood	On a 10-point scale, where sitting is 0 and working as hard as you can is 10, moderate-intensity aerobic activity is a 5 or 6. You will be able to talk but not sing the words to your favorite song	30 minutes on 5 days/week. Perform for at least 10 minutes at a time	Biking, swimming, dancing, brisk walking, lifestyle activities that incorporate large muscle groups (pushing a lawn mower, climbing stairs)
Muscle strengthening activities that involve moving or lifting some type of resistance and work all major muscle groups (legs, hip, back, abdomen, chest, shoulders, arms)	Activities that involve moving or lifting some type of resistance and work all major muscle groups (legs, hip, back, abdomen, chest, shoulders, arms)	Increase muscle strength, prevent sarcopenia, reduce fall risk, improve balance, modify risk factors for cardiovascular disease and type 2 diabetes	To gain health benefits, muscle strengthening activities need to be done to the point where it's hard for you to do another repetition without help. A repetition is one complete movement of an activity like lifting a weight. Try to do 8-12 repetitions per activity that count as 1 set. Try to do at least 1 set	2 days a week but not consecutive days to allow muscles to recover between sessions	Lifting weights, working with resistance bands, exercises that use your body weight for resistance (push-ups, sit-ups), heavy gardening (digging, shoveling), yoga
Stretching (flexibility)	A therapeutic maneuver designed to elongate shortened soft tissue structures and increase flexibility	Facilitates ROM around joints, prevents injury	Stretch muscle groups but not past the point of resistance or pain	At least 2 days a week	Yoga, ROM exercises
Balance exercises	Movements that improve the ability to maintain control of the body over the base of support to avoid falling	Improve lower body strength, improve balance, help prevent falls	Safety precaution essential (holding onto a chair, working with another person)	Can be incorporated into regularly scheduled strength exercises. More formal balance programs may be appropriate for those at high risk for falls	T'ai Chi Exercises such as standing on one leg, walking heel toe (see http://www.nia.nih.gov/HealthInformation/Publications/ExerciseGuide/04d_balance.htm for pictorial description)

HDL, High-density lipoprotein; *ROM,* range of motion.

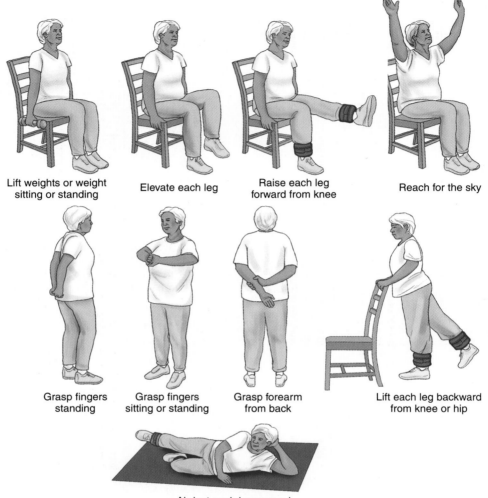

Lift weights or weight sitting or standing

Elevate each leg

Raise each leg forward from knee

Reach for the sky

Grasp fingers standing

Grasp fingers sitting or standing

Grasp forearm from back

Lift each leg backward from knee or hip

Abduct each leg upward

FIGURE 11-1 Examples of strength-training exercises. (Modified from Centers for Disease Control and Prevention. *Growing stronger: strength training for older adults: Exercises: stage 1*. Available at www.cdc.gov/nccdphp/dnpa/physical/growing_stronger/exercises/index.htm).

Maintaining adequate sleep and activity allows the older person to continue to find fulfillment in activities, and in life itself, despite limitations that may be associated with aging and illness.

KEY CONCEPTS

- Many chronic conditions often interfere with the quality and quantity of sleep. Rest and sleep are restorative, recuperative, and necessary for the preservation of life.

Sleep is a barometer of health and can be considered one of the vital signs.

- Complaints of sleep difficulties should be thoroughly investigated and not attributed to age. Nonpharmacological interventions should always be considered in any plan of care to improve sleep.
- Activity is an indication of an individual's health and wellness; inability to exercise, do physical work, or perform activities of daily living is one of the first indicators of decline.

- Lack of physical activity increases the risk for many medical conditions experienced by elders. Exercise can be done by elders who are ambulatory, chair-bound, or bedridden and should include endurance exercises, strength training, balance exercises, and flexibility exercises.
- The benefits of exercise are that it maintains functional ability, enhances self-confidence and self-sufficiency, decreases depression, improves one's general lifestyle, maintains mental functional capacity, and decreases the risk of medical problems.
- Exercise counseling and an exercise prescription should be included in assessment of all older adults.

ACTIVITIES AND DISCUSSION QUESTIONS

1. What age-related changes affect rest, sleep, and activity in older adults?
2. How would you assess an elder for adequacy or inadequacy of rest, sleep, and activity?
3. Develop an exercise prescription for an older adult residing in the community.
3. Discuss the nursing interventions to promote rest, sleep, and activity.
4. Develop a nursing care plan for an older adult who is complaining of difficulty sleeping using wellness and North American Nursing Diagnosis Association (NANDA) diagnoses.

REFERENCES

Bloom H, Ahmed I, Alessi C, et al: Evidence-based recommendations for the assessment and management of sleep disorders in older persons, *J Am Geriatr Soc* 57:761, 2009.

Brooks P, Peever J: Glycinergic and GABA$_A$–mediated inhibition of somatic motor neurons does not mediate rapid eye movement sleep motor atonia, *J Neurosci* 28(14):3535–3545, 2008.

Buysse D, Germain A, Moul D, et al: Efficacy of brief behavioral treatment for chronic insomnia in older adults, *Arch Intern Med* 535:E1–E8, 2010.

Centers for Disease Control and Prevention: *How much physical activity do older adults need?* (2011). Available at http://www.cdc.gov/physicalactivity/everyone/guidelines/olderadults.html.

Davis J, Marra C, Beattie L, et al: Sustained cognitive and economic benefits of resistance training among community-dwelling senior women: a 1-year follow-up study of the brain power study, *Arch Intern Med* 170(22):2036–2038, 2010.

Duru O, Sarkisian C, Leng M, et al: Sisters in motion: a randomized controlled trial of a faith-based physical activity intervention, *J Am Geriatr Soc* 58:1863–1869, 2010.

Erickson KI, Raji CA, Lopez OL, et al: Physical activity predicts gray matter volume in late adulthood, *Neurology* 75:1415–1422, 2010.

Grandner M, Martin J, Patel N, et al: *Age and sleep disturbances among American men and women: data from the U.S. behavioral risk factor surveillance system* (2012). Available at http://www.journalsleep.org/.

Ham R, Sloane P, Warshaw G, et al: *Primary care geriatrics: a case-based approach*, ed 4, St. Louis, 2007, Mosby/Elsevier.

Heyn PC, Johnson KE, Kramer AF: Endurance and strength training outcomes on cognitively impaired and cognitively intact older adults: a meta-analysis, *J Nutr Health Aging* 12:401, 2008.

Irwin MR, Olmstead R, Motivala SJ: Improving sleep quality in older adults with moderate sleep complaints: a randomized controlled trial of Tai Chi Chih, *Sleep* 31:1001, 2008.

Kerr D, Wilkinson H: *Providing good care at night for older people*, London, 2010, Jessica Kingsley Publishers.

Kolla B, Lovely J, Mansukhani M, et al: Zolpidem is independently associated with increased risk of inpatient falls, *J Hosp Med*, 19 Nov 2012. [Epub.] Available at http://www.medpagetoday.com/HospitalBasedMedicine/General HospitalPractice/36033.

Martin J, Fiorentino L, Jouldjian S, et al: Sleep quality in residents of assisted living facilities: effect on quality of life, functional status, and depression, *J Am Geriatr Soc* 58:829, 2010.

Middleton L, Barnes D, Lui L, et al: Physical activity over the life course and its association with cognitive performance and impairment in old age, *J Am Geriatr Soc* 58(7):1322–1326, 2010.

Missildine K: Sleep and the sleep environment of older adults in acute care settings, *J Gerontol Nurs* 34(6):15–21, 2008.

Missildine K, Bergstrom N, Meininger J, et al: Sleep in hospitalized elders: a pilot study, *Geriatr Nurs* 31:263, 2010.

Rajki M: Sleep problems in older adults (2012). Available at http://occupational-therapy.advanceweb.com/Features/Articles/Sleep-Problems-in-Older-Adults.aspx.

Resnick B: Promoting exercise for older adults, *J Am Acad Nurse Pract* 21:77, 2009.

Resnick B, Ory M, Rogers M, et al: Screening and prescribing exercise for older adults, *Geriatr Aging* 9(3):174–182, 2006.

Rogers C, Keller C, Larkey L: Perceived benefits of meditative movement in older adults, *Geriatr Nurs* 31:37, 2010.

Rose K, Lorenz R: Sleep disturbances in dementia: what they are and what to do, *J Gerontol Nurs* 36:9, 2010.

Sherrington C, Whitney J, Lord S, et al: Effective exercise for the prevention of falls: a systematic review and meta-analysis, *J Am Geriatr Soc* 56:2234, 2008.

Subramanian S, Surani S: Sleep disorders in the elderly, *Geriatrics* 62(12):10–32, 2007.

Teodorescu M, Husain N: Nonpharmacological approaches to insomnia in older adults, *Ann Longterm Care* 18:36, 2010.

Winkelman J, Allen R, Tenzer P, et al: Restless legs syndrome: nonpharmacologic and pharmacologic treatments, *Geriatrics* 62(10):13–16, 2007.

Yeom H, Keller C, Fleury J: Interventions for promoting mobility in community-dwelling older adults, *J Am Acad Nurse Pract* 21:95, 2009.

CHAPTER 12

Promoting Healthy Skin and Feet

Theris A. Touhy

evolve evolve.elsevier.com/Ebersole/gerontological

LEARNING OBJECTIVES

Upon completion of this chapter, the reader will be able to:
- Identify age-related changes of the integument and feet.
- Identify skin and foot problems commonly found in late life.
- Identify preventive, maintenance, and restorative measures for skin and foot health.
- Identify risk factors for pressure ulcers and design interventions for prevention and evidence-based treatment.

GLOSSARY

Debride To remove dead or infected tissue, usually of a wound.
Emollient An agent that softens and smoothes the skin.
Eschar Black, dry, dead tissue.
Hyperemia Redness in a part of the body caused by increased blood flow, such as in area of an infection.
Maceration Tissue that is overhydrated and subject to breakdown.
Slough Dead tissue that has become wet, appearing as yellow to white and fibrous.
Tissue tolerance The amount of pressure a tissue (skin) can endure before it breaks down, as in a pressure ulcer.
Xerosis Very dry skin.

THE LIVED EXPERIENCE

I can't thank you enough for helping me with my feet. I have been to the podiatrist, but no one has made them, and me, feel so good. I feel like I can walk forever now—you are an angel.

Tom, age 86

Gerontological nurses have an instrumental role in promoting the health of the skin and the feet of the persons who seek their care. These areas of function may often be overlooked when the focus is on management of disease or acute problems. However, preservation of the integrity of the skin and the functioning of the feet is essential to well-being. In order to promote healthy aging, the nurse needs information about common problems encountered by the older adult and skill in developing effective interventions for both acute and chronic conditions.

Skin

The skin is the largest organ of the body. Exposure to heat, cold, water, trauma, friction, and pressure notwithstanding, the skin's function is to maintain a homeostatic environment. Healthy skin is durable, pliable, and strong enough to protect the body by absorbing, reflecting, cushioning, and restricting various substances and forces that might enter and alter its function; yet it is sensitive enough to relay subtle messages to the brain. When the integument malfunctions or is overwhelmed, discomfort, disfigurement, or death may ensue. However, the nurse can both promptly recognize and help to prevent many of the sources of danger to a person's skin in the promotion of the best possible health.

Many skin problems are seen with aging, both in health and when compromised by illness or mobility limitations. The skin problems seen in older adults are influenced by the environment and age-related changes. The most common skin problems of aging are xerosis (dry skin), pruritus, seborrheic keratosis, herpes zoster, and cancer. Those who are immobilized or medically fragile are at risk for fungal infections and pressure ulcers, both major threats to wellness.

Common Skin Problems

Xerosis

Xerosis is extremely dry, cracked, and itchy skin. Xerosis is the most common skin problem experienced by older people. Xerosis occurs primarily in the extremities, especially the legs, but can affect the face and the trunk as well. The thinner epidermis of older skin makes it less efficient, allowing more moisture to escape. Inadequate fluid intake worsens xerosis as the body will pull moisture from the skin in an attempt to combat systemic dehydration.

Exposure to environmental elements such as artificial heat, decreased humidity, use of harsh soaps, and frequent hot baths or hot tubs contributes to skin dryness. Nutritional deficiencies and smoking lead to dehydration of the outer layer of the epidermis. Dry skin may be just dry skin, but it may also be a symptom of more serious systemic disease (e.g., diabetes mellitus, hypothyroidism, renal disease) or dehydration.

To prevent excessive loss of moisture and natural oil during bathing, only tepid water temperatures and super-fatted soaps or skin cleansers without hexachlorophene or alcohol should be used. Products such as Cetaphil, Basis, Dove, Tone, and Caress soaps or Jergens, Neutrogena, and Oil of Olay bath washes are effective in helping to prevent the loss of the protective lipid film from the skin surface. Most lubricants such as creams, lotions, and emollients work by trapping moisture and are most effective when applied to towel-patted, damp skin immediately after a bath. Bath oils and other hydrophobic preparations may also be used to hold in moisture. Light mineral oil is as effective and more economical than commercial brands of lotions and oils. However, oils poured directly into a tub or shower increase the risk for falls. It is safer and more effective to apply the oil directly to the moist skin. Water-laden emulsions without perfumes or alcohol are best.

Pruritus

One of the consequences of xerosis is *pruritus,* that is, itchy skin. It is a symptom, not a diagnosis or disease, and is a threat to skin integrity because of the attempts to relieve it by scratching. It is aggravated by perfumed detergents, fabric softeners, heat, sudden temperature changes, pressure, sweating, restrictive clothing, fatigue, exercise, and anxiety. If rehydration of the stratum corneum is not sufficient to control itching, cool compresses, or oatmeal or Epsom salt baths may be helpful. Failure to control the itching increases the risk for eczema, excoriations, cracks in the skin, inflammation, and infection. Pruritus also may accompany systemic disorders such as chronic renal failure, biliary or hepatic disease, and iron deficiency anemia. The nurse should be alert to signs of infection.

Scabies

Scabies is a skin condition that causes intense itching, particularly at night. Scabies is caused by a tiny burrowing mite called *Sarcoptes scabiei.* Scabies is contagious and can spread quickly through close physical contact in a family, child care group, school class, or other close communal living facilities such as nursing homes. To diagnose scabies, a close skin examination is conducted to look for signs of mites, including their characteristic burrows. A scraping may be taken from an area of skin for microscopic examination to determine the presence of mites or their eggs.

Scabies treatment involves eliminating the infestation with prescribed lotions and creams (Elimite, Lindane). Treatment is usually provided to family members, caregivers, and other close contacts even if they show no signs of scabies infestation. Medication kills the mites but itching may not stop for several weeks. The oral medication ivermectin (Stromectol) may be prescribed for individuals with altered immune systems, for those with crusted scabies, or for those who do not respond to prescription lotions and creams. All clothes and linen used at least three times before treatment should be washed in hot, soapy water and dried with high heat.

Purpura

Thinning of the dermis leads to increased fragility of the dermal capillaries and to blood vessels rupturing easily with minimal trauma. Extravasation of the blood into the surrounding tissue, commonly seen on the dorsal forearm and hands, is called *purpura.* These are not related to a bleeding disorder, and individuals who are prone to purpura should be advised to protect the skin against trauma and friction. Health care personnel must be advised to be gentle when handling the skin of older patients because even minor trauma can cause purpura. Long-sleeved shirts reduce shear and friction, and protect the skin against trauma. If a skin tear occurs, use nonadherent dressings secured with tubular retention bandages.

Keratoses

There are two types of keratosis: seborrheic and actinic. *Actinic keratosis* is a precancerous lesion and is discussed later in the chapter. *Seborrheic keratosis* is a benign growth that appears mainly on the trunk, the face, the neck, and the scalp as single or multiple lesions. One or more lesions are present on nearly all adults older than 65 years of age and are more common in men. An individual may have dozens of these benign lesions. Seborrheic keratosis is a waxy, raised, verrucous lesion, flesh-colored or pigmented in various sizes. The lesions have a "stuck on" appearance, as if they could be scraped off. Seborrheic keratoses may be removed by a dermatologist for cosmetic reasons. A variant seen in darkly pigmented persons occurs mostly on the face and appears as numerous small, dark, possibly taglike lesions (see www.dermatlas.com).

Herpes Zoster

Herpes zoster (HZ), or shingles, is a viral infection frequently seen in older adults. HZ is caused by reactivation of latent varicella-zoster virus (VZV) within the sensory neurons of the dorsal root ganglion decades after initial VZV infection is established. HZ occurs most commonly in adults over 50 years of age, those who have medical conditions that compromise the immune system, or people who receive immunosuppressive drugs. HZ always occurs along a nerve pathway, or *dermatome*. The more dermatomes involved, the more serious the infection, especially if it involves the head. When the eye is affected it is always a medical emergency. Most HZ occurs in the thoracic region but it can also occur in the trigeminal area and cervical, lumbar, and sacral areas. HZ vesicles never cross the midline.

The onset may be preceded by itching, tingling, or pain in the affected dermatome several days before the outbreak of the rash. It is important to differentiate HZ from herpes simplex. Herpes simplex does not occur in a dermatome pattern and is recurrent. During the healing process, clusters of papulovesicles develop along a nerve pathway. The lesions themselves eventually rupture, crust over, and resolve. Scarring may result, especially if scratching or poor hygiene leads to a secondary bacterial infection. HZ is infectious until it becomes crusty. HZ may be very painful and pruritic.

Prompt treatment with the oral antiviral agents acyclovir, valacyclovir, and famciclovir decreases the severity and duration of acute pain from zoster. Zoster vaccine (Zostavax) is recommended for all persons 60 years of age and over who have no contraindications, including persons who report a previous episode of zoster or who have chronic medical conditions. Before administration of the vaccine, patients do not need to be asked about their history of varicella or have serologic testing to determine varicella immunity.

A common complication of HZ is postherpetic neuralgia (PHN), a chronic, often debilitating pain condition that can last months or even years. The risk of PHN in patients with HV is 10% to 18%. Another complication of HZ is eye involvement, which occurs in 10% to 25% of zoster episodes and can result in prolonged or permanent pain, facial scarring, and loss of vision. The pain of PHN is difficult to control and can significantly affect one's quality of life. The American Academy of Neurology (2012) treatment guidelines for PHN include the use of tricyclic antidepressants, anticonvulsants, steroids, lidocaine skin patches, and opioids, as well as nonpharmacological treatments such as stress reduction techniques and behavioral cognitive therapy. Assessment and management of pain are discussed in Chapter 15.

Photo Damage of the Skin

Although exposure to sunlight is necessary for the production of vitamin D, the sun is also the most common cause of skin damage and skin cancer. "Photo-damage, not the aging process, has been estimated to account for 90% of age-associated cosmetic problems" (Ham et al., 2007, p. 616). The damage (photo or solar damage) comes from prolonged exposure to ultraviolet (UV) light from the environment or in tanning booths. Although the amount of sun-induced damage varies with skin type and genetics, much of the associated damage is preventable. Ideally, preventive measures begin in childhood, but clinical evidence has shown that some improvement can be achieved at any time by limiting sun exposure and using sunscreens regularly.

Skin Cancers

Cancer of the skin (including melanoma and nonmelanoma skin cancer) is the most common of all cancers. The exact number of basal and squamous cell cancers is not known for certain because they are not reported to cancer registries, but it is estimated that there are more than two million basal and squamous cell skin cancers found each year. Most of these are basal cell cancers. Squamous cell cancer is less common. Most of these are curable but melanoma, which accounts for less than 5% of skin cancer cases, has the greatest potential to cause death.

Actinic Keratosis

Actinic keratosis is a precancerous lesion that may become a squamous cell carcinoma. It is directly related to years of overexposure to UV light. Risk factors are older age and fair complexion. It is found on faces, lips, hands, and forearms, areas of chronic sun exposure in everyday life. Actinic keratosis is characterized by rough, scaly, sandpaper-like patches, pink to reddish-brown on an erythematous base. Lesions may be single or multiple; they may be painless or mildly tender. The person with actinic keratoses should be monitored by a dermatologist every 6 to 12 months for any change in appearance of the lesions. Early recognition, treatment, and removal of these lesions is easy and important. Removal is aimed at preventing the possible conversion to a malignant lesion.

Basal Cell Carcinoma

Basal cell carcinoma is the most common malignant skin cancer. It occurs mainly in older age groups but is occurring more and more in younger persons. It is slow-growing, and metastasis is rare. A basal cell lesion can be triggered by extensive sun exposure, especially burns, chronic irritation, and chronic ulceration of the skin. It is more prevalent in light-skinned persons. It usually begins as a pearly papule with prominent telangiectasias (blood vessels) or as a scarlike area with no history of trauma. Basal cell carcinoma is also known to ulcerate. It may be indistinguishable from squamous cell carcinoma and is diagnosed by biopsy. Early detection and treatment are necessary to minimize disfigurement.

Squamous Cell Carcinoma

Squamous cell carcinoma is the second most common skin cancer. However, it is aggressive and has a high incidence of metastasis if not identified and treated promptly. Squamous cell cancer is more prevalent in fair-skinned, older men who live in sunny climates and is usually found on the head, the neck, or the hands. Individuals in their mid-60s who have been or are chronically exposed to the sun are prime candidates for this type of cancer. The lesion begins as a firm, irregular, fleshy, pink-colored nodule that becomes reddened and scaly, much like actinic keratosis, but it may increase rapidly in size. It may also be hard and wartlike with a gray top and horny texture, or it may be ulcerated and indurated with raised, defined borders. Because it can appear so differently, it is often overlooked or thought to be insignificant. The best advice to give older patients, especially those who live in sunny climates, is that they should be regularly screened by a dermatologist.

Melanoma

Melanoma, a neoplasm of the melanocytes, accounts for less than 5% of skin cancer cases, but it causes most skin cancer deaths. The number of new cases of melanoma in the United States has been increasing for at least 30 years. In recent years, the increases have been most pronounced in young white women and in older white men. It is one of the most common cancers in people under 30 years of age. Melanoma is more than 10 times more common in white Americans than in African Americans and slightly more common in men than in women (American Cancer Society, 2012).

Persons with a history of frequent blistering sunburns, use of tanning beds, skin cancer, or exposure to carcinogenic materials, or with sun sensitivity or a depressed immune system, are at particular risk. Increasing age along with a history of sun exposure increases one's risk even further. White individuals with fair skin, freckles, and red or blond hair have a higher risk for melanoma. The legs and backs of women, and the backs of men, are the most common sites of melanoma. Melanoma has a high mortality rate because of its ability to metastasize quickly (American Cancer Society, 2012).

Melanoma has a classical multicolor, raised appearance with an asymmetrical, irregular border. It may appear to be of any size, but the surface diameter is not necessarily reflective of the size beneath the surface, similar in concept to an iceberg. It is treatable if caught early, before it has a chance to invade surrounding tissue. If the nurse finds any questionable lesions, the individual should be referred to a dermatologist immediately. The "ABCD" approach to assessing such potential lesions is used (Box 12-1).

Cancer

The nurse has an active role in the prevention and early recognition of skin cancers. This role may include working with community awareness and education programs,

---

BOX 12-1   **ABCD Rules of Melanoma**

*A*symmetry: One half does not match the other half.
*B*order irregularity: The edges are ragged, notched, or blurred.
*C*olor: The pigment is not uniform in color, having shades of tan, brown, or black, or a mottled appearance with red, white, or blue areas.
*D*iameter: The diameter is greater than the size of a pencil eraser or increasing in size.

screening clinics, and direct care. In promoting skin health, the nurse is vigilant in observing skin for the changes that require further evaluation.

Age-related skin changes, such as thinning and diminished melanocytes, significantly increase the risk for solar damage and subsequent skin cancer. By far, the most important preventive nursing intervention is to provide education regarding the risks of photo and smoke damage. Preventive strategies include the use of sunscreens and protective clothing and limiting sun exposure.

Secondary prevention is in the form of early diagnosis. After a thorough clinical screening, the elder and his or her intimate partner can be taught to perform regular "checks" of each other's skin, watching for signs of change and the need to contact a primary care provider or dermatologist promptly. For the person with keratosis and multiple freckles (nevi), photographing the body parts may be a useful reference. The adage "when it doubt, get it checked" is an important one and regular screenings should be a part of the health care of all older adults.

Other Skin Conditions

Combined with the skin changes discussed previously, older people who are more frail or physically ill and in hospitals or nursing homes are at more risk for the development of pressure ulcers as well as fungal skin infections.

Candidiasis (Candida albicans)

The fungus *Candida albicans* (referred to as "yeast") is present on the skin of healthy persons of any age. However, under certain circumstances and in the right environment, a fungal infection can develop. Persons who are obese, malnourished, receiving antibiotic or steroid therapy, or have diabetes are at increased risk. *Candida* grows especially well in areas that are moist, warm, and dark, such as in skinfolds, in the axilla and the groin, and under pendulous breasts. It can also be found in the corners of the mouth associated with the chronic moisture of angular cheilitis. In the vagina it is also called a "yeast infection." If this is found in an older woman, it may mean that her diabetes either has not yet been diagnosed or is in poor control.

Inside the mouth a *Candida* infection is referred to as "thrush" and is associated with poor hygiene and immunocompromise, such as those with long-term steroid use, who are receiving chemotherapy, or who test positive for or are infected with human immunodeficiency virus (HIV) or have acquired immunodeficiency syndrome (AIDS). In the mouth, candidiasis appears as irregular, white, flat to slightly raised patches on an erythematous base that cannot be scraped off. The infection can extend down into the throat and cause swallowing to be painful. In severely immunocompromised persons the infection can extend down the entire gastrointestinal tract.

On the skin, *Candida* is usually maculopapular, glazed, and dark pink in persons with less pigmentation and grayish in persons with more pigmentation. If it is advanced, the central area may be completely red and/or dark, and weeping with characteristic bright red and/or dark satellite lesions (distinct lesions a short distance from the center). At this point the skin may be edematous, itching, and burning.

The best approach to managing fungal infections is to prevent them, and the key to prevention is limiting the conditions that encourage fungal growth. Prevention is prioritized for persons who are obese, bedridden, incontinent, or diaphoretic. Attention is given to the adequate drying of bodily target areas after bathing, the prompt management of incontinent episodes, the use of loose-fitting cotton clothing and underwear, the changing of clothing when damp, and the avoidance of incontinence products that are tight or have plastic that touches the skin.

One of the best ways to dry hard-to-reach, vulnerable areas is with a hair dryer set on low. A folded, dry washcloth or cotton sanitary pad can be placed under the breasts or between skinfolds to promote exposure to air and light. Cornstarch should never be used because it promotes the growth of *Candida* organisms. Optimizing nutrition and glycemic control is also important.

The goal of treatment is to eradicate the infection. This includes not only the use of prescribed antifungal medication, but also the active involvement of the nurse to reduce or eliminate the conditions that created the problem. The affected area of the skin must be cleansed carefully and dried thoroughly before antifungal preparations are applied. A mild soap or cleansing agent, such as Cetaphil, should be used. Antifungal preparations come as powders, creams, and lotions. Because the latter two trap moisture, the powder is recommended. They are usually needed for 7 to 14 days or until the infection is completely cleared.

Antifungal medications include miconazole (Micatin), clotrimazole (Lotrimin), nystatin (Mycostatin), and econazole (Spectazole). Treatment of oral *Candida* infection includes mouth swishing and swallowing with an antifungal suspension and/or sucking on antifungal troches. Angular cheilitis is treated by application of a topical antifungal ointment to the corners of the mouth. If the *Candida* cannot be eliminated in the usual course of therapy, it may be necessary to use ketoconazole or fluconazole systemically for a prescribed period.

Pressure Ulcers

Definition

The European Pressure Ulcer Advisory Panel (EPUAP) and the National Pressure Ulcer Advisory Panel (NPUAP) constitute an international collaboration convened to develop evidence-based recommendations to be used throughout the world to prevent and treat pressure-related wounds. According to this group, a pressure ulcer is "an injury to the skin and/or underlying tissue resulting from pressure or in combination with shear, usually over a bony prominence" (EPUAP & NPUAP, 2009). As tissue is compressed, blood is diverted and blood vessels are forcibly constricted by the persistent pressure on the skin and underlying structures; thus cellular respiration is impaired and cells die from ischemia and anoxia. Intervention at any point in this development can stop the advancement of the pressure ulcer.

Just how much pressure can be endured by tissue (tissue tolerance) is highly variable from body location to location and person to person. Tissue tolerance is inversely affected by moisture, amount of pressure, friction, shearing, and age and is directly related to malnutrition, anemia, and low arterial pressure.

Prevalence

Older people account for 70% of all pressure ulcers (Jamshed & Schneider, 2010). Several studies have reported a higher prevalence and incidence of pressure ulcers among African Americans in nursing homes than other race groups, and these differences remain after adjustment for clinical risk factors and sociodemographic and facility characteristics (Cai et al., 2010; Howard & Taylor, 2009; Li et al., 2011).

Pressure ulcers occur in all settings across the continuum, with the highest incidence reported in hospitalized vulnerable older people undergoing orthopedic procedures (9% to 19%) and individuals with quadriplegia (33% to 60%). Baumgarten and colleagues (2009) reported that approximately one third of hip fracture patients develop at least one new pressure ulcer, at stage 2 or higher, within 32 days of hospital admission. The NPUAP reported that the prevalence of pressure ulcers in acute care settings ranged from 10% to 18%, with 2.3% to 28% in long-term care and 0% to 29% in home care. There is wide variability among institutions. Differences in sample characteristics and study methodologies affect these statistics, but it is clear that pressure ulcers are a significant problem in all settings (Jamshed & Schneider, 2010; Plawecki et al., 2010). *Healthy People 2020* (U.S. Department of Health and Human Services, 2012) includes a goal of reducing the rate of pressure ulcer–related hospitalizations among older adults.

Cost and Regulatory Requirements

Prevention of pressure ulcers is seen as a "key quality indicator of nursing care and pressure ulcers are widely supported as a nursing sensitive outcome" (Jull & Griffiths, 2010, p. 531). Pressure ulcers are recognized as a geriatric syndrome and efforts at prevention have always been considered an essential nursing intervention, particularly in long-term care (Armstrong et al., 2008). "Though nursing homes have been grappling with increasingly tight regulatory standards regarding wound care for two decades, there have been no similar regulatory incentives for hospitals" (Levine, 2008).

In 2008, the Centers for Medicare & Medicaid (CMS) included hospital-acquired pressure ulcers as one of the eight preventable adverse events. Hospitals will no longer receive additional reimbursement to care for a patient who has acquired pressure ulcers under the hospital's care. Estimated annual costs for pressure ulcer treatment are from $9 to $11.6 billion per year in the United States. Medicare estimated in 2007 that each pressure ulcer added $43,180 in costs to a hospital stay (Agency for Healthcare Research and Quality [AHRQ], 2012).

Characteristics

Pressure ulcers can develop anywhere on the body but are seen most frequently on the posterior aspects, especially the sacrum, the heels, and the greater trochanters. Secondary areas of breakdown include the lateral condyles of the knees and the ankles. The pinna of the ears is another area subject to breakdown, as are the elbows and the scapulae. Heels are particularly prone to the development of pressure ulcers because they are small surfaces that receive a high degree of pressure. Older adults with diabetes are prone to the development of foot ulcers and are at higher risk of earlier death compared to those without diabetes (Brownrigg et al., 2012). Attention to foot care is essential when caring for an older adult with diabetes. More information on diabetes can be found in Chapter 17, and a discussion of foot care is included later in this chapter.

Classification

The EPUAP and NPUAP recommend a four-category classification of pressure ulcers. The NPUAP also describes two additional categories for the United States that do not fall into one of the established or classifiable categories: suspected deep tissue injury and unstageable or unclassified wound (Figure 12-1). Suspected deep tissue injury is defined by a localized area of intact skin or blood-filled blister, maroon or purple in color, caused by damage of the underlying soft tissue from shear and/or pressure (Plawecki et al., 2010).

Stage I

Erythema not resolving within thirty (30) minutes of pressure relief. Epidermis remains intact. REVERSIBLE WITH INTERVENTION.

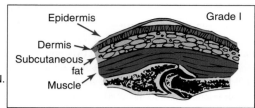

Stage II

Partial-thickness loss of skin layers involving epidermis and possibly penetrating into but not through dermis. May present as blistering with erythema and/or induration; wound base moist and pink; painful; free of necrotic tissue.

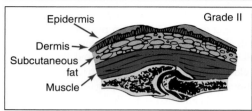

Stage III

Full-thickness tissue loss extending through dermis to involve subcutaneous tissue. Presents as shallow crater unless covered by eschar. May include necrotic tissue, undermining, sinus tract formation, exudate, and/or infection. Wound base is usually not painful.

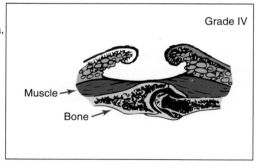

Stage IV

Deep tissue destruction extending through subcutaneous tissue to fascia, possibly involving muscle layers, joint, and/or bone. Presents as a deep crater. May include necrotic tissue, undermining, sinus tract formation, exudate, and/or infection. Wound base is usually not painful.

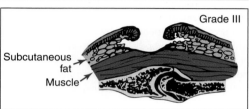

Unstageable

A wound that is covered by eschar or slough, preventing the visualization of the wound bed.

FIGURE 12-1 Pressure ulcer development.

Unstageable wounds are characterized by full-thickness tissue loss in which the base of the ulcer is covered by slough (yellow, tan, gray, green, or brown) and/or eschar (tan, brown, or black) in the wound bed. Until enough slough and/or eschar is removed to expose the base of the wound, the true depth and stage cannot be determined, but it will be either a category III or IV. However, NPUAP recommends that treatment with off loading and dressings appropriate for category III or IV wounds be utilized until stage can be determined following debridement (NPUAP, 2012).

The ulcer is always classified by the highest stage "achieved," and reverse staging is never used. This means that the wound is documented as the stage representing the maximal damage and depth that has occurred. As the wound heals, it fills with granulation tissue composed of endothelial cells, fibroblasts, collagen, and an extracellular matrix. Muscle, subcutaneous fat, and dermis are not replaced. A stage IV pressure sore that is healing does not revert to stage III and then stage II. It remains defined as a healing stage IV pressure ulcer.

Risk Factors

Many factors increase the risk of pressure ulcers in older adults including changes in the skin, comorbid illnesses, nutritional status, cognitive deficits, and reduced mobility. "The primary risk factors for pressure ulcer development are immobility and limited activity with positioning that exerts unrelieved pressure on tissue confined between nonpliable surfaces" (Ham et al., 2007, p. 374). Individuals confined to bed or chair, who are unable to shift weight or reposition themselves at regular intervals, are at greatest risk. Tissue tolerance, in addition to unrelieved pressure, contributes to the risk of a pressure ulcer. Tissue tolerance is related to the ability of the tissue to distribute and compensate for pressure exerted over bony prominences. Factors that affect tissue tolerance include moisture, friction, shear force, nutritional status, age, sensory perception, and arterial pressure (de Souza et al., 2010).

Prevention

Although often repeated, prevention is the key to pressure ulcer treatment. Systematic prevention programs have been shown to decrease hospital-acquired pressure ulcers by 34% to 50% (Armstrong et al., 2008). However, "despite a number of national prevention initiatives and existing evidence-based protocols, pressure ulcer frequency has not declined in recent years and pressure ulcers continue to have a negative impact on patient outcomes and health care costs in a variety of care settings" (Baumgarten et al., 2009, p. 253). Several studies have reported that compliance with evidence-based protocol recommendations is a concern (Spillsbury et al., 2007; Baumgarten et al., 2009).

Early identification of risk status is critical so that timely interventions can be designed to address specific risk factors. The Braden Scale for Predicting Pressure Sore Risk is widely used and clinically validated. This scale assesses the risk of pressure ulcers on the basis of a numerical scoring system of six risk factors: sensory perception, moisture, activity, mobility, nutrition, and friction/shear. For a video on the use of the Braden Scale and other resources see the Evidence-Based Practice box.

Because the Braden Scale does not include all of the risk factors for pressure ulcers, it is recommended that it be used as an adjunct rather than in place of clinical judgment. A thorough patient history to assess other risk factors such as age, medications, comorbidities (diabetes, peripheral vascular disease [PVD]), history of pressure ulcers, and other factors is important to fully address the risk of pressure ulcer development so that appropriate preventive interventions can be developed (Armstrong et al., 2008; Jull & Griffiths, 2010).

🔍 EVIDENCE-BASED PRACTICE

Pressure Ulcers

- Nursing Standard of Practice Protocol: Pressure ulcer prevention and skin tear prevention:
  http://consultgerirn.org/topics/pressure_ulcers_and_skin_tears/want_to_know_more
- Nursing Standard of Practice: Pressure ulcer prevention: Ayello E, Sibbald R: Preventing pressure ulcers and skin tears. In Boltz M, Capezuti E, Fulmer T, et al, editors: *Evidence-based geriatric nursing protocols for best practice,* New York, 2012, Springer.
- Video demonstrating use of the Braden Scale:
  http://consultgerirn.org/resources/media/?vid_id=4200956#player_container
- National Pressure Ulcer Advisory Panel:
  http://www.npuap.org/
- American Medical Directors Association Clinical Practice Guideline: Pressure ulcers:
  http://www.amda.com/tools/cpg/pressureulcer.cfm
- Pressure Ulcer Prevention and Treatment Protocol:
  http://www.guideline.gov/content.aspx?id=36059

A consensus paper from the International Expert Wound Care Advisory Panel (Armstrong et al., 2008) provides recommendations for prevention of pressure ulcers that include patient education, clinician training for all members of the health care team, strategies in developing communication and terminology materials, implementation of toolkits and protocols (prevention bundles), documentation checklists, outcome evaluation, quality improvement efforts, evidence-based treatment protocols, and appropriate products. It is important to note that not all pressure ulcers may be avoidable. Gravely ill patients facing multiple organ failure, reduced tissue perfusion, and no mobility (e.g., at the end of life) are especially at high risk. Armstrong and colleagues (2008) note: "the skin, like any other organ in the body, can fail."

Consequences

Pressure ulcers are costly to treat and prolong recovery and extend rehabilitation. Complications include the need for grafting or amputation, sepsis, or even death, and may lead to legal action by the individual or his or her representative against the caregiver. The personal impact of a pressure ulcer on health and quality of life is also significant and not well understood or researched. Findings from a study exploring patients' perceptions of the impact of a pressure ulcer and its treatment on health and quality of life suggest that pressure ulcers cause suffering, pain, discomfort, and distress that is not always recognized or adequately treated by nursing staff. Pressure ulcers had a profound impact on the patients' lives, physically, socially, emotionally, and mentally (Spillsbury et al., 2007).

Implications for Gerontological Nursing and Healthy Aging

The treatment and prevention of pressure ulcers is complex. A team approach that involves primary care providers, nursing staff, physical therapists, nutritionists, and other clinicians is the most effective (Armstrong et al., 2008). Nursing staff, as direct caregivers, are key team members who perform skin assessment, identify risk factors, and implement numerous preventive interventions. The nurse alerts the health care provider of the need for prescribed treatments, recommends treatments, and administers and evaluates the changing status of the wound(s) and adequacy of treatments.

Assessment

Assessments are performed on admission and whenever there is a change in the status of the patient. Assessment begins with a history, detailed head-to-toe skin examination, nutritional evaluation, and analysis of laboratory findings. Laboratory values that have been correlated with risk for the development and the poor healing of pressure ulcers include those that reflect anemia and poor nutritional status. Visual and tactile inspection of the entire skin surface with special attention to bony prominences is essential. Inspection is best accomplished in nonglare daylight or, if that is not possible, with focused lighting. Special attention should be directed to affected areas when an individual uses orthotic devices such as corsets, braces, prostheses, postural supports, splints, slings, or casts.

The nurse looks for any interruption of skin integrity or other changes, including redness or hyperemia. If pressure is present, it should be relieved and the area reassessed in 1 hour. In darker-pigmented persons, redness and blanching may not be observed. The wound may appear like a bruise. Observe for induration, darkening, change in color from surrounding skin, or a shadowed appearance of the skin. The affected skin area, when compared with adjacent tissues, may be firm, warmer, cooler, or painful (Plawecki et al., 2010).

It is necessary to look for induration, darkening, or a shadowed appearance of the skin and to feel for warmth or a boggy texture to the affected tissue compared with the surrounding tissue. Pressure areas and surrounding tissue should be palpated for changes in temperature and tissue resilience. Blisters or pimples with or without hyperemia and scabs over weight-bearing areas in the absence of trauma should be considered suspect.

Ulcers are assessed with each dressing change for worsening, with a detailed assessment repeated on a weekly, biweekly, and as-needed basis (Box 12-2). The purpose is to specifically and carefully evaluate the effectiveness of treatment. If there are no signs of healing from week to week or worsening of the wound is seen, then either the treatment is insufficient or the wound has become infected; in both cases, treatment must be changed.

Lastly, careful and detailed documentation of the condition of the skin is required. The PUSH tool (Pressure Ulcer Scale for Healing) provides a detailed form that covers all aspects of assessment, but contains only three items and takes only a short time to complete (Gardner et al., 2005). Most institutions have special forms or screens on their computer software for recording skin assessments. The Agency for Healthcare Research and Quality (AHRQ) provides the On-Time Pressure Ulcer Healing Project (http://www.ahrq.gov/research/pressureulcerhealing/) as well as a toolkit for preventing pressure ulcers in hospitals (http://www.ahrq.gov/research/ltc/pressureulcertoolkit/putool1.htm). For patients admitted with pressure ulcers, photographic documentation is highly recommended both at the onset of the problem and at intervals during its treatment (Ahn & Salicido, 2008). The reader is referred to the NPUAP website (www.npuap.org) for more information.

Interventions

The goal of nurses is to help maintain skin integrity against the various environmental, mechanical, and chemical assaults that are potential causes of breakdown. In promoting healthy aging of all persons, nurses focus on prevention,

---

BOX 12-2 Key Aspects of Assessment of a Pressure Ulcer

1. Location and exact size (width, depth, length)
2. Condition of the surrounding tissue
3. Condition of the wound edges: for example, smooth and white or irregular and pink
4. Wound bed: warmth, moisture, color, odor, amount, and color of exudate

taking action to eliminate friction and irritation to the skin, such as from shearing; to reduce moisture so that tissues do not macerate; and to displace body weight from prominent areas to facilitate circulation to the skin. The nurse should be familiar with the types of supportive surfaces and types of dressings so that the most effective products are used. The nurse should assess the frequency of position change, adding pillows so that skin surfaces do not touch, and establish a turning schedule if needed.

Nutritional intake should be monitored, as well as the serum albumin, hematocrit, and hemoglobin levels. Caloric, protein, vitamin, and/or mineral supplementation can be considered if there is evidence of deficiencies of these nutrients. Routine use of higher than the recommended daily allowance of vitamin C and zinc for the prevention and/or treatment of pressure ulcers is not supported by evidence (Jamshed & Schneider, 2010).

Although a full discussion of the treatment options and indications for their use in the nursing care and treatment of pressure ulcers is beyond the scope of this text, key points in the promotion of healing can be found in Box 12-3. The type of dressing selected is based on the condition of the ulcer; the presence of granulation, necrotic tissue, and slough; the amount of drainage; microbial status; and the quality of the surrounding skin. "Too frequently, aggressive and expensive interventions are implemented without attention to basic care practices such as provision of adequate nutrition, good hygiene, and proper positioning" (Ham et al., 2007, p. 375).

Provision of education to patients, families, and professional staff must also be included in any skin care program. Consultation with a wound care specialist is advisable for wounds that are extensive or nonhealing. Specialized nurses such as enterostomal therapists or nurse practitioners may work with wound centers or surgeons to provide consultation in nursing homes, offices, or clinics.

BOX 12-3   Promoting Wound Healing

- Keep wound warm at all times.
- Keep clean and moist at all times.
- Protect from further injury.
- Promptly absorb exudate and fill dead space with a biofriendly material.
- Do not subject tissue to caustic products (e.g., Betadine).

Healthy Feet

Feet influence one's physical, psychological, and social well-being. Feet carry one's body weight, hold the body erect, coordinate and maintain balance in walking, and must be rigid yet loose and adaptable enough to conform to changing walking surfaces. Little attention is given to one's feet until they interfere with walking and moving and ultimately the ability to remain independent. Foot problems in older people often are unrecognized and untreated, leading to considerable dysfunction (Anderson et al., 2010). Yet, promoting healthy feet and good care of the feet can alleviate disability and pain, and decrease the risk for falling.

Common Foot Problems

The human foot is a complex structure with many bones, joints, tendons, muscles, and ligaments. Some foot irregularities and problems are genetically inherited; however, many problems occur because of ill-fitting shoes, wear and tear, and misuse of feet.

Older feet, subjected to a lifetime of stress, may not be able to continue to adapt, and inflammatory changes in bone and soft tissue can occur. Many older adults are limited by foot problems; approximately 90% of adults 65 years of age and older have some form of altered foot integrity such as nail fungus, dry skin, and corns and calluses (Anderson et al., 2010). Foot health and function may reflect systemic disease or give early clues to physical illness. Sudden or gradual changes in the condition of the nails or the skin of the feet or the appearance of recurring infections may be precursors of more serious health problems. Rheumatological disorders such as the various forms of arthritis usually affect other joints but can also affect the feet. Both diabetes and PVD commonly cause problems in the lower extremities that can quickly become life-threatening.

Major abnormalities occur gradually. Without proper care and treatment, these conditions become disabling and threatening to the person's mobility and independence. Care of the foot takes a team approach, including the person, the nurse, the podiatrist, and the person's primary health care provider. Nurses have the opportunity to promote healthy aging by applying their knowledge of the common problems of the feet and their skills in foot care.

Corns, Calluses, and Bunions
Corns and calluses are both growths of compacted skin that occur as a result of prolonged pressure, usually from ill-fitting, tight shoes. Corns are cone-shaped and develop on

the top of the toe joints from the rubbing of the shoe on the joint. Soft corns form between opposing surfaces of the toes from prolonged squeezing. Both can interfere with the ability to walk and wear shoes comfortably. When formed, continued pressure on the corn will cause pain. Unless the friction and pressure are relieved, they will continue to enlarge and cause increasing pain.

Many elders self-treat corns and calluses by following what they or their parents have done for years. Over-the-counter preparations may remove the corn temporarily but may also burn the surrounding healthy tissue. Chemical burns and ulcerations from these products can result in the loss of toes or a leg for the person with diabetes, with neurological impairment, or with poor circulation in the lower extremity. Some people use razor blades and scissors to remove the affected tissue; this is dangerous and is never recommended.

For persons with PVD and diabetes, foot care should be performed only by a nurse with expertise in foot care, a doctor, or a podiatrist. Padding and protecting the affected area is the best practice. Oval corn pads, moleskin, or lamb's wool, with a hole cut in the center for the corn, can be used for more proper treatment. This can be placed around the corn, protecting it from pressure without restricting circulation to healthy tissue. Newer pads of a gel type are also useful to protect against friction and pressure. For persons prone to calluses, daily lubrication of the feet is important.

Bunions are bony deformities that also develop from long-standing squeezing together of the first (great) and second toes. Bony prominences develop over the medial aspect of the joint of the great toe and, at times, at the lateral aspect of the fifth metatarsal head (the joint of the little toe). There may be a hereditary factor in their development. Walking can be markedly compromised with any of these. Bunions may be treated with corticosteroid injections or antiinflammatory pain medications. A custom-made shoe should be considered. Shoes that provide forefront space (e.g., running shoes) work well. Surgery is an option as well.

Hammer Toes

A *hammer toe* is permanently flexed with a clawlike appearance; the condition is a result of muscle imbalance and pressure from the big toe slanting toward the second toe. The toe then contracts, leaving a bulge on top of the joint. It is aggravated, again, by poor-fitting shoes and is often seen in conjunction with bunions. This condition limits the ability to walk and restricts balance and comfort. As with bunions, treatment includes professional orthotics or specially designed protective devices; properly fitting, nonconstricting shoes; and/or surgical intervention.

Fungal Infections

Fungal infections are common on the aging foot, and the incidence increases with age. A fungal infection may affect the skin of the foot as well as the nails. Nail fungus, or *onychomycosis,* the most common nail disorder, is characterized by degeneration of the nail plate with color changes to yellow or brown and opaque, brittleness, and thickening of the nail. A fine powdery collection of fungus forms under the center of the nail, separating the layers and pushing it up, causing the sides of the nail to dig into the skin like an ingrown toenail. Culturing is the only definitive way to diagnose onychomycosis. Hands should be washed each time feet with a fungal infection are handled.

When nails are involved, cure is difficult to impossible because of the limited circulation to the nails. Several oral medications are available, but all are expensive and of limited effectiveness, are taken for long periods of time (3 to 12 months), and are potentially toxic to the liver and heart. A promising treatment is photodynamic therapy (PDT). In PDT, near infrared, dual wave length optical energy is pulsed on the skin using special equipment. While further study is necessary to support the use of PDT for superficial fungal infections of the skin and nails, the technology is well established for other dermatological conditions with good outcomes (Anderson et al., 2010).

Fungal infection of the foot *(tinea pedis)* is due to many of the same causes as *Candida* infections elsewhere on the body. *Tinea pedis* is treated similarly to any other fungal infections. Feet, especially the areas between the toes, should be kept dry and clean and regularly exposed to sun and air. Topical application of antifungal powders, in addition to the hygiene measures already noted, is the usual treatment. If exacerbated by diabetes, glycemic control is an additional goal.

Implications for Gerontological Nursing and Healthy Aging

Assessment

The gerontological nurse is an advocate for promoting the best foot health possible. Foot care is a prime factor in the maintenance of mobility and independence. Nursing care of the person with foot problems should be directed toward optimal comfort and function, removing possible mechanical irritants, and decreasing the likelihood of infection. The nurse has the important function of assessing the feet for clues of functional ability and their owner's well-being—not just bathing and applying lotion to the feet (Box 12-4). Nurses can identify potential and actual problems and make referral to or seek assistance as needed from the primary care provider or podiatrist for any changes in the feet.

BOX 12-4 Essential Aspects of Foot Assessment

Observation of Mobility
- Gait
- Use of assistive devices
- Footwear type and pattern of wear

Past Medical History
- Neuropathies
- Musculoskeletal limitations
- PVD
- Vision problems
- History of falls
- Pain affecting movement

Bilateral Assessment
- Color
- Circulation and warmth
- Pulses
- Structural deformities
- Skin lesions
- LE edema
- Evidence of scratching
- Rash or excessive dryness
- Condition and color of toenails

PVD, Peripheral vascular disease; *LE,* lower-extremity.

Assessment also includes observation of gait, postural deformities, physical limitations, position of the foot with the heel strike, and the type of shoe worn and its condition, including sole wear. Inspect feet for irritation, abrasions, and other lesions; check for hazards to the maintenance of adequate circulation to the lower extremities and the existing circulatory status; and observe the individual's general mobility. Routine assessment of the feet is especially important for persons with diabetes, heart disease, PVD, and thyroid or renal conditions as well as any neurological impairment, such as reduced or absent sensation resulting from a stroke.

Interventions

Care of the Toenails

Care of the feet and nails of persons in the long-term care setting falls to the nurse. Poor close vision, difficulty bending, obesity, or increased nail thickness make self-care difficult. Normal nails that become too long will begin to interfere with stockings, hose, or shoes. Ideally, toenails should be trimmed after the bath or shower when they are softened, but if this is not possible, soaking the feet for 20 to 30 minutes before care is sufficient. They should be clipped straight across and even with the top of the toe, with the edges filed slightly to remove the sharpness but not to the point of rounding (Figure 12-2). Diabetic foot care should be done only by a podiatrist or registered nurse (RN) with some experience, with special care to prevent accidental damage or trauma to the skin. Diabetic nail care can never be delegated to the licensed practical nurse (LPN) or certified nurse assistant (CNA). Persons with diabetes or peripheral neuropathy should never have pedicures from commercial establishments.

An ingrown toenail is a fragment of nail that pierces the skin at the edge of the nail. Often this problem is a consequence of the hypertrophy of the nail with onychomycosis, of improper cutting of the nail, or of pressure exerted on the toes by tight hosiery or shoes. Ingrown toenails should be referred to the podiatrist because of the risk of infection. Temporary relief can be provided by inserting a small piece of cotton under the affected nail corner.

Nursing interventions include assisting the older person to understand the necessity of appropriate footwear and how to obtain it. Shoes should be functional, that is, they should cover, protect, and stabilize the foot and provide maximal toe space. They must also be the right size. One foot is usually larger than the other, and feet lengthen slightly with age and are largest in the afternoons. Shoes should be fitted to the largest foot, and afternoon purchases are advised,

Slip-on shoes are helpful for those who are unable to bend or lace shoes, but care must be taken that the

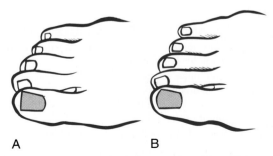

FIGURE 12-2 Cutting toenails. **A,** Correct angle and shape. **B,** Incorrect angle and shape.

person will not accidentally "slip out" of the shoe, which can lead to a fall. Velcro closures are useful for those who have limited finger dexterity. Older people should be advised that walking with shoes of low heel height and high surface contact area may reduce the risk of falls. Rubber-soled shoes such as sneakers, often recommended for older people, may increase the risk of stumbling while walking, particularly if the person is not accustomed to this type of shoe. This type of shoe may provide too much "sway" and may not promote good balance (American Geriatrics Society, 2010). Orthotic and orthopedic shoes may be indicated for certain foot problems and can greatly enhance mobility and comfort. At the time of this writing, Medicare will cover the cost of one pair of orthotic shoes per year for persons with diabetes when purchased from an approved vendor.

KEY CONCEPTS

- The skin is the largest and most visible organ of the body; it has multiple roles in maintaining one's health.
- Maintaining adequate oral hydration and skin lubrication will reduce the incidence of xerosis and other skin problems.
- The best way to minimize the risk of skin cancer is to avoid prolonged sun exposure.
- Mobility is fundamental to independence; therefore care of the feet and toenails is an important area for the gerontological nurse.
- A pressure ulcer is documented by stage, which reflects the greatest degree of tissue damage; and as it heals, reverse staging is not appropriate.
- A pressure ulcer that is covered in dead tissue (eschar or slough) cannot be staged until it has been debrided.
- Darkly pigmented persons will not display the "typical" erythema of a stage I pressure ulcer or early PVD; therefore, closer vigilance is necessary.

ACTIVITIES AND DISCUSSION QUESTIONS

1. Describe the common skin and foot problems an older adult is more likely to experience.
2. What is the nurse's responsibility in health promotion related to maintaining skin integrity?
3. What evidence-based protocols can the nurse utilize for prevention of pressure ulcers?
4. Develop a nursing care plan for an older adult at risk for pressure ulcers using wellness and North American Nursing Diagnosis Association (NANDA) diagnoses.

REFERENCES

Agency for Healthcare Research and Quality [AHRQ]: *Preventing pressure ulcers in hospitals: a toolkit for improving quality of care* (2012). Available at http://www.ahrq.gov/research/ltc/pressureulcertoolkit/putool1.htm.

Ahn C, Salicido RS: Advances in wound photography and assessment methods, *Adv Skin Wound Care* 21(2):94–95, 2008.

American Academy of Neurology: *Shingles* (2012). Available at http://www.aan.com/apps/disorders/index.cfm?event=database:disorder.view&disorder_id=1061.

American Cancer Society [ACS]: *What are key statistics about melanoma?* (2012). Available at http://www.cancer.org/Cancer/SkinCancer-Melanoma/DetailedGuide/melanoma-skin-cancer-key-statistics.

American Geriatrics Society: *2010 AGS/BGS clinical practice guideline: prevention of falls in older persons* (2010). Available at http://www.americangeriatrics.org/health_care_professionals/clinical_practice/clinical_guidelines_recommendations/2010/.

Anderson J, White K, Kelechi T: Managing common foot problems in older adults, *J Gerontol Nurs* 36(10):9–14, 2010.

Armstrong D, Ayello E, Capitulo K, et al: Opportunities to improve pressure ulcer prevention and treatment: implementation of the CMS inpatient hospital care present on admission (POA) indicators/hospital acquired conditions (HCA) policy, *Wounds* 20:A14, 2008. Available at http://www.medscape.com/viewarticle/581767.

Baumgarten M, Margolis D, Orwig D, et al: Use of pressure-redistributing support surfaces among elderly hip fracture patients across the continuum of care: adherence to pressure ulcer prevention guidelines, *The Gerontologist* 50:253, 2009.

Brownrigg J, Davey J, Holt P, et al: The association of ulceration of the foot with cardiovascular and all-cause mortality in patients with diabetes: a meta-analysis, *Diabetologia*, 4 Aug 2012. [Epub.]

Cai S, Mukamel DB, Temkin-Greener H: Pressure prevalence among black and white nursing homes residents in New York state: evidence of racial disparity? *Med Care* 48(3):233–239, 2010.

de Souza DM, Santos V, Iri H, et al: Predictive validity of the Braden Scale for pressure ulcer risk in elderly residents of long-term care facilities, *Geriatr Nurs* 31:95, 2010.

European Pressure Ulcer Advisory Panel and National Pressure Ulcer Advisory Panel [EPUAP & NPUAP]: *Pressure ulcer treatment: quick reference guide* (2009). Available at http://nationalpres750.corecommerce.com/cart.html.

Gardner SE, Frantz RA, Bergquist S, et al: A prospective study of the Pressure Ulcer Scale for Healing (PUSH). *J Gerontol A Biol Sci Med Sci* 60:93–97, 2005.

Ham R, Sloane P, Warshaw G, et al: *Primary care geriatrics: a case-based approach*, ed 4, St. Louis, 2007, Mosby.

Howard D, Taylor Y: Racial and gender differences in pressure ulcer development among nursing home residents in the southeastern United States, *J Women Aging* 21:266, 2009.

Jamshed N, Schneider E: Is the use of supplemental vitamin C and zinc for the prevention and treatment of pressure ulcers evidence-based? *Ann Longterm Care* 18:28, 2010.

Jull A, Griffiths P: Is pressure sore prevention a sensitive indicator of the quality of nursing care? a cautionary note, *International J Nurs Stud* 47:531, 2010.

Levine J: What hospitals can learn about pressure ulcers from long-term care clinicians, *Caring for the Ages* 9(11): 6, 2008.

Li Y, Yin J, Cai X, et al: Association of race and sites of care with pressure ulcers in high-risk nursing home residents, *JAMA* 306(2):179–186, 2011.

National Pressure Ulcer Advisory Panel [NPUAP]: *Unstageable pressure ulcers: NPUAP commentary for CMS* (2012). Available at www.npuap.org.

Plawecki L, Amrhein D, Zortman T: Under pressure: nursing liability and skin breakdown in older patients, *J Gerontol Nurs* 36:23, 2010.

Spillsbury K, Nelson A, Cullum N, et al: Pressure ulcers and their treatment and effects on quality of life: hospital inpatient perspectives, *J Adv Nurs* 57:494, 2007.

U.S. Department of Health and Human Services, Office of Disease Prevention and Health Promotion: *Healthy People 2020* (2012). Available at http://www.healthypeople.gov/2020.

CHAPTER 13

Promoting Safety

Theris A. Touhy

evolve   evolve.elsevier.com/Ebersole/gerontological

LEARNING OBJECTIVES

Upon completion of this chapter, the reader will be able to:

- Discuss the importance of prevention of injuries and accidents and promotion of a culture of safety in all settings for older adults.
- Identify older adults who are at risk for falls and list several measures to reduce fall risk.
- Discuss the use of assistive technologies to promote self-care, safety, and independence.
- Understand the effects of restraints and discuss appropriate alternatives for safety promotion.
- Identify factors in the environment that contribute to the safety and security of the older person.
- Develop a nursing care plan appropriate for an elder at risk of falling.

GLOSSARY

Orthostatic (postural) hypotension A drop in blood pressure occurring when a person assumes an upright position after being in a lying-down position.

Proprioception Sensations from within the body regarding spatial position and muscular activity.

THE LIVED EXPERIENCE

After that fall last year when I slipped on the urine in the bathroom, I feel so insecure. I find myself taking small, shuffling steps to avoid falling again, but it makes me feel awkward and clumsy. When I was younger, I never worried about falling, but now I'm so afraid I will break a bone or something.

Betty, age 75

Promotion of Safety

Promotion of safety and fall prevention are public health issues and are addressed in many national initiatives including those from the Centers for Disease Control and Prevention (CDC), National Council on Aging (NCOA), Joint Commission, National Center for Patient Safety, and Quality and Safety Education for Nurses (QSEN). For older adults, promotion of a safe environment and prevention of falls, accidents, and injuries in all settings is essential to optimal function and quality of life. This chapter focuses on falls and fall risk reduction, measures to promote safety without the use of restraints, aids and interventions that are useful when mobility is impaired, and assistive technologies to enhance self-care, safety, and independence. Issues related to transportation and driving as essential aspects of environmental mobility are also included. Activity and exercise are discussed in Chapter 11 and bone and joint problems affecting mobility are discussed in Chapter 18.

Falls and Fall Risk Reduction

Falls are one of the most important geriatric syndromes and the leading cause of morbidity and mortality for people older than 65 years of age. Thirty to forty percent of people 65 years of age or older fall at least once each year (U.S. Preventive Services Task Force [USPSTF], 2012). Nursing home residents, who are more frail, fall frequently (Quigley et al., 2010). Falls among nursing home residents are estimated at 2.6 per year (Gray-Micelli, 2010).

Falls are a significant public health problem. Falls rank as the seventh leading cause of unintentional injury fatality among older adults and the most common cause of nonfatal injuries and hospital admissions for trauma (Gray-Micelli & Quigley, 2012; CDC, 2010a). Falls and their subsequent injuries result in physical and psychosocial consequences. Twenty percent to 30% of people who fall suffer moderate to severe injuries (bruises, hip fractures, traumatic brain injury [TBI]). Estimates are that up to two thirds of falls may be preventable (Lach, 2010). *Healthy People 2020* (U.S. Department of Health and Human Services, 2012) includes several goals related to falls (see the Healthy People box). Box 13-1 presents statistics of falls and fall-related concerns.

Falls are considered a nursing-sensitive quality indicator. Patient falls have been reported to account for at least

---

HEALTHY PEOPLE 2020

Falls, Fall Prevention, Injury

- Reduce the rate of emergency department visits due to falls among older adults
- Reduce fatal and nonfatal injuries
- Reduce hospitalizations for nonfatal injuries
- Reduce emergency department visits for nonfatal injuries
- Reduce fatal and nonfatal traumatic brain injuries

From U.S. Department of Health and Human Services, Office of Disease Prevention and Health Promotion: *Healthy people 2020* (2012). Available at http://www.healthypeople.gov/2020.

SAFETY ALERT

The Quality and Safety Education for Nurses (QSEN) project has developed quality and safety measures for nursing and proposed targets for the knowledge, skills, and attitudes to be developed in nursing prelicensure and graduate programs. Education on falls and fall risk reduction is an important consideration in the QSEN safety competency, which addresses the need to minimize risk of harm to patients and providers through both system effectiveness and individual performance (http://www.qsen.org/competencies.php).

BOX 13-1   Statistics on Falls and Fall-Related Concerns

- One third of people older than 65 years of age fall at least one time each year, and about half of those fall repeatedly.
- Every 15 seconds, an older adult is treated in the emergency room for a fall; every 29 minutes, an older adult dies following a fall.
- Of those who fall, 20% to 30% suffer moderate to serious injuries, such as hip fractures or head traumas.
- Falls account for 40% of nursing home admissions annually.
- Older adults 75 years of age and older have the highest rates of traumatic brain injury (TBI)-related hospitalization and death. TBIs account for 46% of fatal falls among older adults.
- Men are more likely to die from a fall.
- Rates of fall-related fractures among older adults are more than twice as high for women as for men. White women have significantly higher rates of fall-related hip fractures than black women.
- More than 95% of hip fractures among older adults are caused by falls.
- Between 18% and 33% of older patients with hip fractures die within 1 year of the fracture.
- Up to 25% of adults who lived independently before the hip fracture have to stay in a nursing home for at least 1 year after the injury.
- The financial toll for older adult falls is expected to increase as the population ages and may reach $54.9 billion by 2020.

From Centers for Disease Control and Prevention: *Falls among older adults: an overview* (2012). Available at http://www.cdc.gov/home-andrecreationalsafety/falls/adultfalls.html/; Lach H: The costs and outcomes of falls: what's a nursing administrator to do? *Nurs Admin Q* 34:147, 2010; National Council on Aging: *Falls prevention fact sheet*. Available at www.ncoa.org.

40% of all hospital adverse occurrences (Ireland et al., 2010). All falls in the nursing home setting are considered sentinel events and must be reported to the Centers for Medicare & Medicaid Services (CMS). The Joint Commission (JC) has established national patient safety goals (NPSG) for fall reduction in all JC-approved institutions across the health care continuum (Capezuti et al., 2008). In the hospital, falls with resultant fractures, dislocations, and crushing injuries are considered one of the 10 hospital-acquired conditions (HACs) that are not covered under

Medicare (www.cms.gov/HospitalAcqCond/06_Hospital-Acquired_Conditions.asp).

Falls are a symptom of a problem and are rarely benign in older people. The etiology of falls is multifactorial; falls may indicate neurological, sensory, cardiac, cognitive, medication, or musculoskeletal problems or impending illness. Episodes of acute illness or exacerbations of chronic illness are times of high fall risk. The presence of dementia increases risk for falls twofold, and individuals with dementia are also at increased risk of major injuries (fracture) related to falls (Oliver et al., 2007).

Consequences of Falls

Hip Fractures

More than 95% of hip fractures among older adults are caused by falls. Hip fracture is the second leading cause of hospitalization for older people, occurring predominantly in older adults with underlying osteoporosis (Andersen et al., 2010). Hip fractures are associated with considerable morbidity and mortality. Only 50% to 60% of patients with hip fractures will recover their prefracture ambulation abilities in the first year postfracture. Older adults who fracture a hip have a five to eight times increased risk of mortality during the first 3 months after hip fracture. This excess mortality persists for 10 years after the fracture and is higher in men. Existing research also suggests that mortality and morbidity limitations are higher in nonwhite people as compared with white people. Most research on hip fractures has been conducted with older women, and further studies of both men and racially and culturally diverse older adults are necessary (Andersen et al., 2010; CDC, 2010a; Haentjens et al., 2010).

Traumatic Brain Injury

Older adults (75 years of age and older) have the highest rates of TBI-related hospitalization and death. TBI has been called the "silent epidemic" and older adults with TBI are an even more silent population within this epidemic. Falls are the leading cause of TBI for older adults. Advancing age negatively affects the outcome after TBI, even with relatively minor head injuries (Timmons & Menaker, 2010). A new CDC initiative, *Help Seniors Live Better Longer: Prevent Brain Injury,* provides educational resource materials on TBI for older adults, caregivers, and health care professionals in both Spanish and English (http://www.cdc.gov/traumaticbraininjury/seniors.html.)

Factors that place the older adult at greater risk for TBI include the presence of comorbid conditions, use of aspirin and anticoagulants, and changes in the brain with age. Brain changes with age, although clinically insignificant, do increase the risk of TBIs and especially subdural hematomas, which are much more common in older adults. There is a decreased adherence of the dura mater to the skull, increased fragility of bridging cerebral veins, and increases in the subarachnoid space and atrophy of the brain, which creates more space within the cranial vault for blood to accumulate before symptoms appear (Timmons & Menaker, 2010). Falls are the leading cause of TBI, but older people may experience TBI with seemingly more minor incidents (e.g., sharp turns or jarring movement of the head). Some patients may not even remember the incident.

In cases of moderate to severe TBI, there will be cognitive and physical sequelae obvious at the time of injury or shortly afterward that will require emergency treatment. However, older adults who experience a minor incident with seemingly lesser trauma to the head often present with more insidious and delayed symptom onset. Because of changes in the aging brain, there is an increased risk for slowly expanding subdural hematomas. TBIs are often missed or misdiagnosed among older adults (CDC, 2010b).

Health professionals should have a high suspicion of TBI in an older adult who falls and strikes the head or experiences even a more minor event, such as sudden twisting of the head. For older adults who are receiving warfarin and experience minor head injury with a negative CT scan, a protocol of 24-hour observation followed by a second CT scan is recommended (Menditto et al., 2012). Manifestations of TBI are often misinterpreted as signs of dementia, which can lead to inaccurate prognoses and limit implementation of appropriate treatment (Flanagan et al., 2006). Table 13-1 presents signs and symptoms of TBI.

Fallophobia

Even if a fall does not result in injury, falls contribute to a loss of confidence that leads to reduced physical activity, increased dependency, and social withdrawal (Rubenstein et al., 2003; Hill et al., 2010). Fear of falling (fallophobia) may restrict an individual's life space (area in which an individual carries on activities). Fear of falling is an important predictor of general functional decline and a risk factor for future falls. Resnick (2002) suggests that nursing staff may also contribute to fear of falling in their patients by telling them not to get up by themselves or by using restrictive devices to keep them from independently moving about. More appropriate nursing responses include assessing fall risk and designing individual interventions and safety plans that will enhance mobility and independence, as well as reduce fall risk.

TABLE 13-1	Signs and Symptoms of Traumatic Brain Injury (TBI) in Older Adults	

Symptoms of Mild TBI	Symptoms of Moderate to Severe TBI
Low-grade headache that won't go away	Severe headache that gets worse or does not go away
Having more trouble than usual remembering things, paying attention or concentrating, organizing daily tasks, or making decisions and solving problems	Repeated vomiting or nausea
	Seizures
	Inability to wake from sleep
Slowness in thinking, speaking, acting, or reading	Dilation of one or both pupils
Getting lost or easily confused	Slurred speech
Feeling tired all of the time, lack of energy or motivation	Weakness or numbness in the arms or legs
Change in sleep pattern (sleeping much longer than usual, having trouble sleeping)	Loss of coordination
	Increased confusion, restlessness, or agitation
Loss of balance, feeling light-headed or dizzy	
Increased sensitivity to sounds, lights, distractions	
Blurred vision or eyes that tire easily	
Loss of sense of taste or smell	
Ringing in the ears	
Change in sexual drive	
Mood changes (feeling sad, anxious, listless or becoming easily irritated or angry for little or no reason)	

NOTE: Older adults taking blood thinners should be seen immediately by a health care provider if they have a bump or blow to the head, even if they do not have any of the symptoms listed above.

From Centers for Disease Control and Prevention: *Preventing traumatic brain injury in older adults* (2010). Available at www.cdc.gov/BrainInjuryInSeniors.

Factors Contributing to Falls

Individual risk factors can be categorized as either intrinsic or extrinsic. Intrinsic risk factors are unique to each patient and are associated with factors such as reduced vision and hearing, unsteady gait, cognitive impairment, acute and chronic illnesses, and effect of medications. Extrinsic risk factors are external to the patient and related to the physical environment and include lack of support equipment by bathtubs and toilets, height of beds, condition of floors, poor lighting, inappropriate footwear, improper use of or inadequate assistive devices (Tzeng & Yin, 2008).

Falls in the young-old and the more healthy old occur more frequently because of external reasons; however, with increasing age and comorbid conditions, internal and locomotor reasons become increasingly prevalent as factors contributing to falls. The risk of falling increases with the number of risk factors. Most falls occur from a combination of intrinsic and extrinsic factors that come together at a certain point in time (Table 13-2).

In institutional settings, factors such as limited staffing, lack of toileting programs, and restraints and side rails also interact to increase fall risk. Inadequate staff communication and training, incomplete patient assessments and reassessments, environmental issues, incomplete care planning or delayed care provision, and an inadequate organizational culture of safety have been reported as factors contributing to falls in hospitals (Tzeng & Yin, 2008).

Gait Disturbances

Gait disturbances are frequently seen in older people, especially those 85 years of age and older. Marked gait disorders are not normally a consequence of aging alone but are more likely indicative of an underlying pathological condition. Arthritis of the knee may result in ligamentous weakness and instability, causing the legs to give way or collapse. Diabetes, dementia, Parkinson's disease, stroke, alcoholism, and vitamin B deficiencies may cause neurological damage and resultant gait problems.

Foot Deformities

Foot deformities and ill-fitting footwear also contribute to gait problems. Care of the feet is an important aspect of mobility, comfort, and a stable gait, and is often neglected (see Chapter 12). Some older persons are unable to walk comfortably, or at all, because of neglect of corns, bunions, and overgrown nails. Other causes of problems may be traced to loss of fat cushioning and resilience with aging, diabetes, ill-fitting shoes, poor arch support, excessively repetitive weight-bearing activities, obesity, or uneven distribution of weight on the feet. As many as 35% of persons living at home may have significant foot disability that goes untended.

Postural and Postprandial Hypotension

Declines in depth perception, proprioception, vibratory sense, and normotensive response to postural changes are important factors that contribute to falls, although the majority of falls occur in individuals with multiple medical problems. Appropriate assessment of postural changes in pulse and blood pressure is important. Clinically significant postural hypotension (orthostasis) is detected in up to

TABLE 13-2	Fall Risk Factors for Elders	
Conditions		**Situations**
Sedative and alcohol use, psychoactive medications, opioids, diuretics, anticholinergics, antidepressants, cardiovascular agents, anticoagulants, bowel preparations		Urinary incontinence, urgency, nocturia
Four or more medications		Environmental hazards
Unrelieved pain		Recent relocation, unfamiliarity with new environment
Previous falls and fractures		Inadequate response to transfer and toileting needs
Female, 80 years of age or older		Assistive devices used for walking
Acute and recent illness		Inadequate or missing safety rails, particularly in bathroom
Cognitive impairment (delirium, dementia)		Poorly designed or unstable furniture
Diabetes		High chairs and beds
Chronic pain		Uneven floor surfaces
Dehydration		Glossy, highly waxed floors
Weakness of lower extremities		Wet, greasy, icy surfaces
Abnormalities of gait and balance		Inadequate visual support (glare, low wattage bulbs, lack of nightlights)
Unsteadiness, dizziness, syncope		General clutter
Foot problems		Inappropriate footwear/clothing
Depression, anxiety		Pets that inadvertently trip an individual
Decreased vision or hearing		Electrical cords
Fear of falling		Loose or uneven stair treads
Orthostatic hypotension		Throw rugs
Postprandial drop in blood pressure		Reaching for a high shelf
Decreased weight		Inability to reach personal items, lack of access to call bell or inability to use it
Sleep disorders		Side rails, restraints
Skeletal and neuromuscular changes that predispose to weakness and postural imbalance		Lack of staff training in fall risk–reduction techniques
Functional limitations in self-care activities		
Inability to rise from a chair without using the arms		
Slow walking speed		
Wheelchair-bound		

30% of older people (Tinetti, 2003). Postural hypotension is considered a decrease of 20 mm Hg (or more) in systolic pressure or a decrease of 10 mm Hg (or more) in diastolic pressure.

Assessment of postural hypotension in everyday nursing practice is often overlooked or assessed inaccurately. Postural hypotension is more common in the morning, and therefore assessment should occur then. All older persons should be cautioned against sudden rising from sitting or supine positions, particularly after eating.

Postprandial hypotension (PPH) occurs after ingestion of a carbohydrate meal and may be related to the release of a vasodilatory peptide. PPH is more common in people with diabetes and Parkinson's disease but has been found in approximately 25% of persons who fall. Lifestyle modifications such as increased water intake before eating or substituting six smaller meals daily for three larger meals may be effective, but further research is needed (Luciano et al., 2010).

Cognitive Impairment

Older adults with cognitive impairment, such as dementia and delirium, are at increased risk for falls. Fall risk assessments may need to include more specific cognitive risk factors, and cognitive assessment measures may need to be more frequently scheduled for at-risk individuals. One study (Harrison et al., 2010) reported that use of the Confusion Assessment Method (CAM) to screen for delirium (see Chapter 21), and the symptom of inattention, has the potential to improve early detection of fall risk in cognitively impaired hospitalized individuals.

Vision and Hearing

Formal vision and hearing assessments are important interventions to identify remediable problems. Although a significant relationship exists between visual problems and falls and fractures, little research has been conducted on interventions for visual problems as part of fall–risk reduction programs. Hearing ability is also directly related to fall risk. For someone with only a mild hearing loss, there is a threefold increased chance of having falls (Lin & Ferrucci, 2012).

Implications for Gerontological Nursing and Healthy Aging

Screening and Assessment

The American Geriatrics Society/British Geriatrics Society *Clinical Practice Guideline: Prevention of Falls in Older Persons* (2010) recommends that all older individuals should be asked whether they have fallen in the past year and whether they experience difficulties with walking or balance. In addition, ask about falls that did not result in an injury and the circumstances of a near fall, mishap, or misstep because this may provide important information for prevention of future falls (Zecevic et al., 2006). Older people may be reluctant to share information about falls for fear of losing independence, so the nurse must use judgment and empathy in eliciting information about falls, assuring the person that there are many modifiable factors to increase safety and help maintain independence.

If the person reports a fall, they should be asked about the frequency and circumstances of the fall(s) and should be evaluated for gait and balance (Figure 13-1). Multifactorial fall risk assessments may be performed depending on the individual circumstances but are not automatically recommended to prevent falls in community-dwelling older adults because the likelihood of benefit is small. They may be appropriate for older people who are frail, ill, or have had prior falls (USPSTF, 2012).

Patients who fall present a complex diagnostic challenge and require multifactorial assessment. In the acute and long-term care settings, an interprofessional team (physician, nurse, health care provider, risk manager, physical and occupational therapist, and other designated staff) should be involved in planning care on the basis of findings from an individualized assessment. Attention to modifying risk factors through appropriate medical management is essential, and this may include medication reduction, treatment of cardiac irregularities, cataract surgery, and management of pain.

Assessment is an ongoing process that includes "multiple and continual types of assessment, reassessment, and evaluation following a fall or intervention to reduce the risk of a fall. Assessment includes: (1) assessment of the older adult at risk; (2) nursing assessment of the patient following a fall; (3) assessment of the environment and other situational circumstances upon admission and during institutional stays; (4) assessment of the older adult's knowledge of falls and their prevention, including willingness to change behavior, if necessary, to prevent falls" (Gray-Micelli, 2008, p. 164).

Fall Risk Assessment Instruments

Fall risk is formally assessed through administration of fall risk tools. Instruments that have been evaluated for reliability and validity should be used rather than creating new instruments (Gray-Micelli, 2008; Gray-Micelli & Quigley, 2012). The National Center for Patient Safety recommends the Morse Falls Scale, but not for use in long-term care. The Hendrich II Fall Risk Model (Hendrich et al., 2003) (see Figure 13-1), recommended by the Hartford Foundation for Geriatric Nursing (New York, NY), is an example of an instrument that has been validated with skilled nursing and rehabilitation populations. In the skilled nursing facility, the Minimum Data Set (MDS 3.0) includes information about history of falls and hip fractures as well as an assessment of balance during transitions and walking (moving from seated to standing, walking, turning around, moving on and off toilet, and transfers between bed and chair or wheelchair) (see Chapter 7).

Fall risk assessments provide first-level assessment data as the basis for comprehensive assessment but comprehensive postfall assessments (PFAs) must be used to identify multifactorial, complex fall and injury risk factors in those who have fallen (Gray-Micelli & Quigley, 2012). All assessment data on an individual's risk for falls must be tailored with individual assessment so that appropriate fall risk–reduction interventions can be developed and modifiable risk factors identified and managed.

The following concerns have been identified related to fall risk assessment instruments:

- In institutions, nurses often complete these assessments every shift in a routine manner and risk factors identified may not be addressed. In addition, risk factors may not be known due to lack of assessment and knowledge of patient's history.
- The scores used to identify patients at high risk may not be based on research.
- So many patients are considered at high risk that nurses may become desensitized to fall risks and have difficulty prioritizing interventions.
- Nurses' clinical judgment is not considered and may be as effective at identifying high-risk patients as use of fall-risk screening tools (Harrison et al., 2010; Lach, 2010).

Hendrich II Fall Risk Model™

Confusion Disorientation Impulsivity		4	
Symptomatic Depression		2	
Altered Elimination		1	
Dizziness Vertigo		1	
Male Gender		1	
Any Administered Antiepileptics		2	
Any Administered Benzodiazepines		1	
Get Up & Go Test			
Able to rise in a single movement – No loss of balance with steps		0	
Pushes up, successful in one attempt		1	
Multiple attempts, but successful		3	
Unable to rise without assistance during test (OR if a medical order states the same and/or complete bedrest is ordered) * If unable to assess, document this on the patient chart with the date and time		4	
A Score of 5 or Greater = High Risk		**Total Score**	

FIGURE 13-1 The Hendrich II Fall Risk Model, a fall risk assessment tool recommended by the Hartford Institute for Geriatric Nursing. (© 2012 AHI of Indiana, Inc. All Rights Reserved. U.S. Patent Nos. 7,282,031 and 7,682,308. Federal laws prohibit the replication, distribution, or clinical use expressed or implied without written permission from AHI of Indiana, Incorporated.

Lach (2010) reported that "the problems with fall risk assessment tools caused one author to wonder whether these tools should be 'put to bed'" (p. 152). Additional research is needed to develop valid, reliable instruments to differentiate levels of fall risk in various settings.

Postfall Assessment

Determination of why a fall occurred (postfall assessment [PFA]) is vital and provides information on underlying fall etiologies so that appropriate plans of care can be instituted. Incomplete analysis of the reasons for a fall can result in repeated incidents. "When important details are overlooked,

missing information leads to an inappropriate plan of care" (Gray-Micelli, 2008, p. 33). The purpose of the PFA is to identify the clinical status of the person, verify and treat injuries, identify underlying causes of the fall when possible, and assist in implementing appropriate individualized risk-reduction interventions.

PFAs include a fall-focused history; fall circumstances; medical problems; medication review; mobility assessment; vision and hearing assessment; neurological examination (including cognitive assessment); and cardiovascular assessment (orthostatic B/P, cardiac rhythm irregularities) (Gray-Micelli & Quigley, 2012). If the older adult cannot tell you about the circumstances of the fall, information should be obtained from staff or witnesses. Because complications of falls may not occur immediately, all patients should be observed for 48 hours after a fall and vital signs and neurological status monitored for 7 days or more, as clinically indicated. Standard "incident report" forms do not provide adequate postfall assessment information. The Department of Veterans Affairs National Center for Patient Safety (http://www.patientsafety.gov/SafetyTopics/fallstoolkit/index.html) provides comprehensive information about fall assessment, fall risk reduction, and policies and procedures. Box 13-2 presents information for a PFA that can be used in health care institutions.

Interventions

Randomized controlled trials support the effectiveness of multicomponent fall prevention strategies in reducing fall risks (Tinetti et al., 2008; Cameron et al., 2010). However, Frick and colleagues (2010) suggest that multifactorial approaches aimed at all older people, or high-risk elders, are not necessarily more cost-effective or better than focused intervention approaches and that further research is needed. The U.S. Preventive Services Task Force recommends exercise or physical therapy and vitamin D supplementation to prevent falls in community-dwelling older adults (USPSTF, 2012).

Choosing the most appropriate interventions to reduce the risk of falls depends on appropriate assessment at various intervals depending on the person's changing condition and tailoring to individual cognitive function and language (American Geriatrics Society and British Geriatrics Society, 2010). A one-size-fits-all approach is not effective and further research is needed to determine the type, frequency, and timing of interventions best suited for specific populations (community-living, hospital and institutionalized, and racially and culturally diverse older adults).

BOX 13-2   Postfall Assessment Suggestions

History

Description of the fall from the resident or witness
Resident's opinion of the cause of the fall
Circumstances of the fall (trip or slip)
Person's activity at the time of the fall
Presence of comorbid conditions, such as a previous stroke, Parkinson's disease, osteoporosis, seizure disorder, sensory deficit, joint abnormalities, depression, cardiac disease
Medication review
Associated symptoms, such as chest pain, palpitations, lightheadedness, vertigo, fainting, weakness, confusion, incontinence, or dyspnea
Time of day and location of the fall
Presence of acute illness

Physical Examination

Vital signs: postural blood pressure changes, fever, or hypothermia
Head and neck: visual impairment, hearing impairment, nystagmus, bruit
Heart: arrhythmia or valvular dysfunction
Neurological signs: altered mental status, focal deficits, peripheral neuropathy, muscle weakness, rigidity or tremor, impaired balance
Musculoskeletal signs: arthritic changes, range of motion (ROM), podiatric deformities or problems, swelling, redness or bruises, abrasions, pain on movement, shortening and external rotation of lower extremities

Functional Assessment

Observe and inquire about the following:
Functional gait and balance: observe resident rising from chair, walking, turning, and sitting down
Balance test, mobility, use of assistive devices or personal assistance, extent of ambulation, restraint use, prosthetic equipment
Activities of daily living: bathing, dressing, transferring, toileting

Environmental Assessment

Staffing patterns, unsafe practice in transferring, delay in response to call light
Faulty equipment
Use of bed, chair alarm
Call light within reach
Wheelchair, bed locked
Adequate supervision
Clutter, walking paths not clear
Dim lighting
Glare
Uneven flooring
Wet, slippery floors
Poor-fitting seating devices
Inappropriate footwear
Inappropriate eye wear

Ireland and colleagues (2010) also suggest that each institution needs to design strategies to meet organizational needs and to match patient population needs and clinical realities of the staff. Use of the Acute Care of the Elderly (ACE) units; Nurses Improving Care for Healthsystem Elders (NICHE) program; and the Geriatric Resource Nurse (GRN) model, which utilize a system-level quality improvement approach, including educational programs for staff, realized a decrease in fall rate by 5.8% (Gray-Micelli & Quigley, 2012) (see Chapter 3).

Box 13-3 presents an innovative fall risk–reduction program, designed by a nurse in an acute care facility that has been adopted around the country and included in fall risk–reduction guidelines. Other innovative programs in nursing homes include the Visiting Angels and neighborhood watch teams. In the Visiting Angels program, alert residents visit and converse with cognitively impaired residents in the late afternoon and evening when fall risk starts to rise. Neighborhood watch teams involve the evening and night staff in morning reviews of any fall or incident that happened during the night (Kilgore, 2010). The components most commonly included in efficacious interventions are shown in Box 13-4. There are many excellent sources of information for both consumers and health care professionals on interventions to reduce fall risk (see the Evidence-Based Practice box).

 EVIDENCE-BASED PRACTICE

Fall Risk Reduction and Restraint Alternatives

- American Geriatrics Society/British Geriatrics Society Clinical Practice Guideline for Prevention of Falls in Older Persons:
  http://www.americangeriatrics.org/health_care_professionals/clinical_practice/clinical_guidelines_recommendations/2010/
- Dementia Series: Tools and strategies in the assessment of older adults with dementia (includes avoiding restraints in older adults with dementia in print and video):
  http://consultgerirn.org/resources/#issues_on_dementia
- National Center for Patient Safety:
  http://www.patientsafety.gov/SafetyTopics/fallstoolkit/index.html
- National Guideline Clearing House: Fall Management Guideline:
  http://www.guideline.gov/summary/summary.aspx?doc_id513484
- The Nursing Standard of Practice: Fall Prevention:
  www.consultgerirn.org/topics/falls/want_to_know_more
- Side rail utilization assessment:
  http://www.fallsinltc.ca/physicalrestraints/siderails.htm
- Use of physical restraints with elderly patients:
  http://consultgerirn.org/topics/physical_restraints/want_to_know_more/

BOX 13-3   The Ruby Slipper Fall Intervention Program

Nurse Ginny Goldner of St. Joseph's Hospital in Tucson, Arizona, started the "Ruby Slipper" program to identify patients at risk for falling and to help prevent falls in older patients. Patients at risk for falls wear red socks with non-slip treads so that anyone from a housekeeper to a head nurse who sees them walking around or trying to get out of bed will know to stay with them until they are safely back in bed. Education on fall risk reduction, identification of patients at high risk, and Ruby Slipper rounds on high-risk patients to see if they need anything, such as to go to the bathroom, are included in the program as well. The program has reduced patient falls by nearly 75%. Ginny was awarded the March of Dimes Arizona Innovation and Creativity Nurse of the Year Award for the program. The Ruby Slipper program has been adopted by many hospitals across the country and is included in the evidence-based guideline for fall prevention from the Institute for Clinical Systems Improvement: Health Care Protocol Prevention of Falls (Acute Care) (http://www.icsi.org/falls__acute_care___prevention_of__protocol_/falls__acute_care___prevention_of__protocol__24255.html).

Data from Arizona Hospital and Healthcare Association, www.azhha.org. For information, contact Ginny Goldner RN, MS at (520) 873-3722 or email vgoldner@carondelet.org.

BOX 13-4	Selected Components of Fall Risk–Reduction Interventions

- Withdrawal or minimization of psychoactive medications
- Withdrawal or minimization of other medications
- Management of postural hypotension
- Continence programs such as prompted voiding
- Management of foot problems and footwear
- Exercise, particularly balance, strength, and gait training
- Staff and patient education

From American Geriatrics Society: *Prevention of falls in older persons.* Available at http://www.americangeriatrics.org/health_care_professionals/clinical_practice/clinical_guidelines_recommendations/2010; Nursing Standard of Practice Protocol: Fall Prevention. Available at www.consultgerirn.org/topics/falls/want_to_know_more.

Medication Review

Medications implicated in increasing fall risk include those causing potentially dangerous side effects including drowsiness, mental confusion, problems with balance or loss of urinary control, and sudden drops in blood pressure with standing. These include psychotropics (benzodiazepines, sedatives/hypnotics, antidepressants, neuroleptics, antiarrhythmics, digoxin, and diuretics (Gray-Micelli & Quigley, 2012). All medications, including over-the-counter (OTC) and herbals, should be reviewed and limited to those that are absolutely essential. Risk of falls increases with the use of four or more medications, particularly neuroleptics and benzodiazepines.

In a study of the cost-effectiveness of fall prevention programs that reduce hip fracture in older adults, Frick and colleagues (2010) reported that management of psychotropics was the most effective and least expensive falls management option of those considered. Home modifications, group T'ai Chi, and assessment and treatment of osteoporosis (see Chapter 18) were also reported to be effective and cost-efficient interventions.

The use of low-potency opioids for chronic pain, particularly codeine combinations, is increasing among older adults (see Chapter 15). Higher doses of these medications result in twice the risk of injury from falls ((Buckeridge et al, 2010). Further research is needed but if these medications are being used, patient teaching should be provided related to fall risk, appropriate dosing and use of other medications, such as benzodiazepines, as well as alcohol use.

Environmental Modifications

Environmental modifications alone have not been shown to reduce falls, but when included as part of a multifactorial program, they may be of benefit in risk reduction. However, a home environmental assessment including mitigation of hazards and interventions to promote the safe performance of daily activities is recommended (Table 13-3). Another valuable resource for older adults is the Check for Safety

TABLE 13-3	Assessment and Interventions of the Home Environment for Older Persons
Problem	**Intervention**
Bathroom	
Getting on and off toilet	Raised seat; side bars; grab bars
Getting in and out of tub	Bath bench; transfer bench; hand-held shower nozzle; rubber mat; hydraulic lift bath seat
Slippery or wet floors	Nonskid rugs or mats
Hot water burns	Check water temperature before bath; set hot water thermostat to 120° F or less Use bath thermometer
Doorway too narrow	Remove door and use curtain; leave wheelchair at door and use walker
Bedroom	
Rolling beds	Remove wheels; block against wall
Bed too low	Leg extensions; blocks; second mattress; adjustable-height hospital bed

Continued

TABLE 13-3	Assessment and Interventions of the Home Environment for Older Persons—cont'd
Problem	**Intervention**
Lighting	Bedside light; night-light; flashlight attached to walker or cane
Sliding rugs	Remove; tack down; rubber back; two-sided tape
Slippery floor	Nonskid wax; no wax; rubber-sole footwear; indoor-outdoor carpet
Thick rug edge/doorsill	Metal strip at edge; remove doorsill; tape down edge
Nighttime calls	Bedside phone; cordless phone; intercom; buzzer; lifeline
Kitchen	
Open flames and burners	Substitute microwave; electric toaster oven
Access items	Place commonly used items in easy-to-reach areas; adjustable-height counters, cupboards, and drawers
Hard-to-open refrigerator	Foot lever
Difficulty seeing	Adequate lighting; utensils with brightly colored handles
Living Room	
Soft, low chair	Board under cushion; pillow or folded blanket to raise seat; blocks or platform under legs; good armrests to push up on; back and seat cushions
Swivel and rocking chairs	Block motion
Obstructing furniture	Relocate or remove to clear paths
Extension cords	Run along walls; eliminate unnecessary cords; place under sturdy furniture; use power strips with breakers
Telephone	
Difficult to reach	Cordless phone; inform friends to let phone ring 10 times; clear path; answering machine and call back
Difficult to hear ring	Headset; speaker phone
Difficult to dial numbers	Preset numbers; large button and numbers; voice-activated dialing
Steps	
Cannot handle	Stair glide; lift; elevator; ramp (permanent, portable, or removable)
No handrails	Install at least on one side
Loose rugs	Remove or nail down to wooden steps
Difficult to see	Adequate lighting; mark edge of steps with bright-colored tape
Unable to use walker on stairs	Keep second walker or wheelchair at top or bottom of stairs
Home Management	
Laundry	Easy to access; sit on stool to access clothes in dryer; good lighting; fold laundry sitting at table; carry laundry in bag on stairs; use cart; use laundry service
Mail	Easy-to-access mailbox; mail basket on door
Housekeeping	Assess safety and manageability; no-bend dust pan; lightweight all-surface sweeper; provide with resources for assistance if needed
Controlling thermostat	Mount in accessible location; large-print numbers; remote-controlled thermostat
Safety	
Difficulty locking doors	Remote-controlled door lock; door wedge; hook and chain locks
Difficulty opening door and knowing who is there	Automatic door openers; level doorknob handles; intercom at door
Opening and closing windows	Lever and crank handles
Cannot hear alarms	Blinking lights; vibrating surfaces
Lighting	Illumination 1-2 feet from object being viewed; change bulbs when dim; adequate lighting in stairways and hallways; night-lights

TABLE **13-3**	Assessment and Interventions of the Home Environment for Older Persons—cont'd
Problem	**Intervention**
Leisure	
Cannot hear television	Personal listening device with amplifier; closed captioning
Complicated remote	Simple remote with large buttons; universal remote control; voice control–activated remote control; clapper
Cannot read small print	Magnifying glass; large-print books
Book too heavy	Read at table; sit with book resting on lap pillow
Glare when reading	Place light source to right or left; avoid glossy paper for reading material; black ink instead of blue ink or pencil
Computer keys too small	Replace keyboard with one with larger keys

Modified from Rehabilitation Engineering Research Center on Aging (RERC-Aging), Center for Assistive Technology, University at Buffalo.

available at http://www.cdc.gov/ncipc/pub-res/toolkit/Falls_ToolKit/DesktopPDF/English/booklet_Eng_desktop.pdf.

In institutional settings, the patient care environment should be assessed routinely for extrinsic factors that may contribute to falls and corrective action taken. Patients should be able to access the bathroom or be provided with a bedside commode, routine assistance to toilet, and programs such as prompted voiding (see Chapter 10). The majority of falls in acute care occur in patient rooms (79.5%) followed by bathrooms (11%) and hallways (9.5%) (Tzeng & Yin, 2008).

The following is a list of important areas to check for safety:

- Outdoor grounds and indoor floor surfaces for spills, wet areas, and unevenness
- Proper illumination and functioning of lights, including night lights
- Tabletops, furniture, and beds are sturdy and in good repair
- Grab rails and nonskid appliqués or mats are in place in the bathroom
- Appropriate shoe wear is available and used
- Adaptive aids work properly and are in good repair
- Bed rails do not collapse when used for transitioning or support
- Patient gowns/clothing do not cause tripping; proper footwear is provided
- IV poles are sturdy if used during ambulation and tubing does not cause tripping

Assistive Devices

Research on multifactorial interventions including the use of assistive devices has demonstrated benefits in fall risk reduction. It is important to provide instruction and supervision on the correct use of assistive devices. Assist the person in obtaining a written prescription for the assistive device because Medicare may cover up to 80% of the cost of the device; other insurance coverage varies.

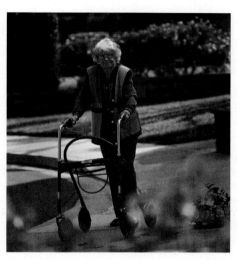

Maintaining ambulation and safety with appropriate assistive devices. (Courtesy Corbis Images.)

When an assistive device is obtained, the individual will need assistance in learning to use it correctly. Following are some general principles for walker and cane use:

- Place your cane firmly on the ground before you take a step, and do not place it too far ahead of you. Put all of your weight on your unaffected leg, and then move the cane and your affected leg at a comfortable distance forward. With your weight supported on both the cane and your affected leg, step through with your unaffected leg.
- Always wear low-heeled, nonskid shoes. It is best to have the person wear the kind of shoes they are accustomed to wearing and consideration should be given to properly fitted orthotic shoes as appropriate.
- When using a cane on stairs, step up with the unaffected leg and down with the affected leg. Use the cane as support when lifting the affected leg. Bring the cane

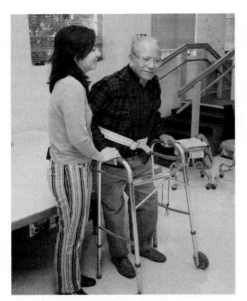

A physical therapist helping a client to ambulate. (From Ignatavicius DD, Workman ML: *Medical-surgical nursing: patient-centered collaborative care,* ed 6, St. Louis, 2010, Saunders.)

up to the step just reached before climbing another step. When descending, place the cane on the next step down, move the affected leg down, and then move the unaffected leg down.

- When using a walker, stand upright and lift or roll the walker with both hands a step's length ahead of you. Lean slightly forward, and hold the arms of the walker for support. Step toward it with the weaker leg, and then bring the stronger leg forward. Do not climb stairs with a walker.
- Every assistive device must be adjusted to individual height; the top of the cane should align with the crease of the wrist.
- Choose a size and shape of cane handle that fits comfortably in the palm; like a tight shoe, it will be a constant irritant if it is not properly fitted.
- Cane tips are most secure when they are flat at the bottom and have a series of rings. Replace tips frequently because they wear out, and a worn tip is insecure.

Wheelchairs are a necessary adjunct at some level of immobility and for some individuals, but are overused in nursing homes, with up to 80% of residents spending time sitting in a wheelchair every day. Often, the individual is not assessed for therapeutic treatment and restorative ambulation programs to improve mobility and function.

Improperly maintained or ill-fitting wheelchairs can cause pressure ulcers, skin tears, bruises and abrasions, nerve impingement, and account for 16% of nursing home falls (Gavin-Dreschnack et al., 2010). It is important that a professional evaluate the wheelchair for proper fit and provide training on proper use as well as evaluate the resident for more appropriate mobility and seating devices and ambulation programs. There are many new assistive devices that could replace wheelchairs, such as small walkers with wheels and seats and automatic brakes.

All nursing homes need to implement programs that promote ambulation and improve function. Brief walks and repeated chair stands four times a day improved walking and endurance in frail, deconditioned, cognitively impaired nursing home residents. Tappen and colleagues (2000) reported that a combination of assisted walking with conversation reduced decline in functional ability and improved mood in nursing home residents with Alzheimer's. If the person is unable to ambulate without assistance, they should be seated in comfortable chairs with frequent repositioning and wheelchairs should be used for transport only.

Emerging Technologies to Enhance Safety of Older Adults

Advancements in all types of technology hold promise for improving quality of life, decreasing the need for personal care, and enhancing independence and the ability to live safely at home and age-in-place (Daniel et al., 2009). Assistive technology is any device or system that allows a person to perform a task independently or that makes the task easier and safer to perform. Assistive technology is decreasing the number of older people who depend on others for personal care in activities of daily living (ADLs) and presents cost-effective alternatives to human services and institutionalization (Daniel et al., 2009). Delaying the need to send people from their homes to assisted living or nursing facilities by even one month can save $1.12 billion annually (Bezaitis, 2009).

Gerotechnology is the term used to describe assistive technologies for older people and is expected to significantly influence how we live in the future. Health care technologies, telemedicine, mobility and ADL aids, and environmental control systems (smart houses/intelligent homes) are some examples of assistive technology.

Telemedicine offers exciting possibilities for managing medical problems in the home or other setting, reducing health care costs, and promoting self-management of illness. The number of telemedicine programs is increasing, and these programs offer exciting possibilities for nurses, particularly advanced practice nurses. Smart medical homes (http://www.urmc.rochester.edu/future-health/validation/smart-home.cfm) are being studied as a way to aid in the prevention and early detection of disease through the use of sensors and monitors. These devices keep data on vital signs and other measures such as gait, behavior, and sleep and provide an interactive medical-advising system. Devices to monitor gait and detect balance problems, such as the iShoe and the "smart carpet" (a sensor system embedded in carpet that detects gait abnormalities that may predispose to falls, and detects falls and summons assistance), are being developed (Aud et al., 2010; Rantz et al., 2008). See http://www.agingtech.org/imagine_video.aspx for a video depicting home technology for older adults.

On the horizon are technology developments such as household robots that can help lift things, check a person's vital signs, and assist with baths and meals. A child-size therapist robot on wheels with a humanlike torso is being developed for use in homes and long-term care facilities to assist with the high level of attention individuals with dementia require for safety and function. Wheelchair technology that enables the user to go down stairs, move to an upright position, be reminded to change positions to alleviate pressure, or use mechanical arms to change a light bulb or get things out of the refrigerator are other developing technologies.

As the baby boomers and future generations age, comfort with technology will be increased, and people will seek options for better, safer, and more independent ways not yet imagined. At this time, many of the assistive technologies can be cost-prohibitive for older people, but with more development they may be more accessible and affordable for more people. Research is needed on assistive technologies and their acceptance among older people. It is important for nurses to be aware of available technology to improve safety.

Restraints and Side Rails

Definition and History

A physical restraint is defined as any manual method, physical or mechanical device, material, or equipment that immobilizes or reduces the ability of a patient to move his or her arms, legs, body, or head freely. A chemical restraint is when a drug or medication is used as a restriction to manage the patient's behavior or restrict the patient's freedom of movement and is not a standard treatment or dosage for the patient's condition. Historically, restraints and side rails have been used for the "protection" of the patient and for the security of the patient and staff. Originally, restraints were used to control the behavior of individuals with mental illness considered to be dangerous to themselves or others (Evans & Strumpf, 1989).

The problem of restraint use was first brought to the forefront of nursing attention by a request from Doris Schwartz, one of the gerontological nursing pioneers, for information from practicing nurses regarding their observations and concerns about restraint usage. Research over the last 20 years by nurses such as Lois Evans, Neville Strumpf, and Elizabeth Capezuti has shown that the practice of physical restraint is ineffective and hazardous. Through research, increased knowledge about restraint alternatives, advocacy groups' efforts, and changed standards and regulations concerning restraints, there has been a significant reduction in restraint use, particularly in long-term care settings. According to the Agency for Healthcare Research and Quality (2011) *2010 National Healthcare Quality and Disparities Report*, the number of residents in nursing homes who were physically restrained dropped by more than half from 1999 to 2007 in long-term care (http://www.ahrq.gov/research/sep10/0910RA33.htm).

Consequences of Restraints

Physical restraints, intended to prevent injury, do not protect patients from falling, wandering, or removing tubes and other medical devices. Physical restraints may actually exacerbate many of the problems for which they are used and can cause emotional and physical problems as well as serious injury and death. "The most common mechanism of restraint-related death is by asphyxiation—that is, the person is suspended by a restraint from a bed or chair and the ability to inhale is inhibited by gravitational chest compression" (Wagner et al., 2008, p. 168). Physical restraints are associated with higher mortality rates, injurious falls, health care–acquired infections, incontinence, contractures, pressure ulcers, agitation, and depression. Although prevention of falls is most frequently cited as the primary reason for using restraints, restraints do not prevent serious injury and may even increase the risk of injury and death. Injuries occur as a result of the patient attempting to remove the restraint or attempting to get out of bed while restrained.

Side Rails

Side rails are no longer viewed as simply attachments to a patient's bed but are considered restraints with all the accompanying concerns just discussed. Side rails are defined as restraints or restrictive devices when used to impede a person's ability to voluntarily get out of bed and the person cannot lower them by themselves. Restrictive side rail use is defined as two full-length or four half-length raised side rails. If the patient uses a half- or quarter-length upper side rail to assist in getting in and out of bed, it is not considered a restraint (Talerico & Capezuti, 2001).

There is no evidence to date that side rail use decreases the risk or rate of fall occurrence. There are numerous reports and studies documenting the negative effects of side rail use, including entrapment deaths and injuries that occur when the person slips through the side rail bars or between split side rails, the side rail and the mattress, or between the head or footboard, side rail, and the mattress (Talerico and Capezuti, 2001; Wagner et al., 2008).

The Centers for Medicare & Medicaid Services (CMS) require nursing homes to conduct individualized assessments of residents, provide alternatives, or clearly document the need for restrictive side rails. A side rail utilization assessment can be found at http://www.fallsinltc.ca/physical-restraints/siderails.htm.

Restraint-Free Care

Restraint-free care is now the standard of practice and an indicator of quality care in all health care settings, although transition to that standard is still in progress, particularly in acute care settings. The Hartford Geriatric Nursing Institute provides an evidence-based protocol on physical restraints (see the Evidence-Based Practice box) and a guideline for restraint use in acute care has been developed by Park and Hsiao-Chen Tang (2007) (Figure 13-2).

Flaherty (2004) remarked that a "restraint-free environment should be held as the standard of care and anything less is substandard. The fact that it is done in some European hospitals (de Vries et al., 2004) and in some U.S. hospitals, even among delirious patients, and in skilled nursing facilities should be evidence enough that it can be done everywhere" (p. 919). Implementing best practice nursing in fall risk reduction and restraint-free care is a complex clinical decision-making process and calls for recognition, assessment, and intervention for physical and psychosocial concerns contributing to patient safety, knowledge of restraint alternatives, interdisciplinary teamwork, and institutional commitment.

Antonelli (2008) described a comprehensive restraint management program in acute care that was successful in improving care practices and reducing restraint use. Included in the program were the development of a restraint prevention cart to increase the accessibility of alternatives to restraints, rounds and consultation led by a geriatric nurse practitioner, the use of college and high school students as activity assistants, and staff education.

Removing restraints without careful attention to underlying fall risk factors and effective alternative strategies can jeopardize safety. The use of advanced practice nurse consultation in implementing alternatives to restraints has been most effective (Bourbonniere & Evans, 2002; Capezuti, 2004). Wagner and colleagues (2008) suggest the following important areas of focus derived from research on advanced practice nurse consultations: (1) compensating for memory loss (e.g., improving behavior); (1) anticipating needs, providing visual and physical cues; (3) improving impaired mobility; (4) reducing injury potential; (5) evaluating nocturia/incontinence; and (6) reducing sleep disturbances. The key to successful implementation of restraint-free fall prevention interventions is conducting careful individualized assessments. What works for one individual may not necessarily be effective for another (pp. 134, 138).

Staff education is also important and one study reported increased knowledge, attitude change, and reduction of the use of physical restraints without any change in the incidence of falls or use of psychoactive medications after a six-month education program (Pellfolk et al., 2010). Many of the suggestions on safety and fall risk reduction in this chapter can be used to promote a safe and restraint-free environment. Fall risk reduction and alternative strategies to restraints are presented in Boxes 13-5 and 13-6. A list of resources can be found in the Evidence-Based Practice box.

Implications for Gerontological Nursing and Healthy Aging

Gerontological nurses need to be knowledgeable about fall risk factors and fall risk–reduction interventions in all settings. Health promotion interventions to maintain fitness and mobility; appropriate assessment of fall risk; teaching older adults, their caregivers, and staff about fall risk factors; fall risk–reduction interventions; and restraint–free care are important nursing responses. For community-dwelling older adults, nurses need to have knowledge of home, community, and environmental safety factors, as well as assistive devices and technology, environmental modifications, and resources to aid in maintaining independence and functional abilities. Accidents and injuries among older adults in all settings are significant in terms of morbidity and mortality, and using evidence-based practice can ensure improvement of many modifiable and preventable injuries, as well as mobility limitations and functional decline.

Environmental Safety

A safe environment is one in which one is capable, with reasonable caution, of carrying out activities of daily living (ADLs) and instrumental activities of daily living (IADLs), as well as the activities that enrich one's life, without fear of attack, accident, or imposed interference. Vulnerability to environmental risks increases as people become less physically or cognitively able to recognize or cope with real or potential hazards. The following section discusses the influences of changing health and disability on the safety and security of older adults. Included is vulnerability to temperature extremes, natural disasters, and driving safety.

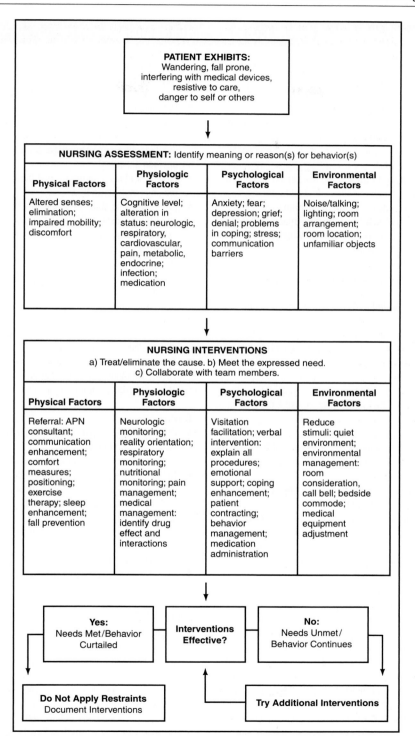

FIGURE 13-2 Decision algorithm: behavior management and restraint-free care. (From Park M, Hsiao-Chen Tang J: Evidence-based guidelines: changing the practice of physical restraint use in acute care, *J Gerontol Nurs* 33[2]:9-16, 2007.)

BOX 13-5 **Suggestions for Fall Risk Reduction and Restraint Alternatives**

- Work with the interdisciplinary team; nurses cannot manage these complicated challenges alone.
- Fall-risk screening, gait, balance and mobility assessment; multifactorial assessment as indicated.
- Assess ambulation ability; refer to physical therapy for walking and/or strengthening.
- Check for postural hypotension (orthostasis) and post-prandial hypotension.
- Use a behavior log to track when the person is trying to get up and/or when he or she seems agitated.
- Assess mental status (delirium/dementia).
- Assess vision and hearing; if the person wears glasses, hearing aid, or dentures, see that they are worn.
- Assess continence status.
- Assess for pain and ensure that pain is well managed.
- Involve family and all staff in fall risk–reduction education and activities.
- Inform all staff of fall risk, and put fall risk and fall risk–reduction interventions on care plan.
- Use identification bracelet or door sign to indicate patients at risk for falling; use red socks with treads to identify patient at risk.

Patient Room
- Lower the bed to the lowest level, or use a bed that is especially designed to be low to the floor.
- Use concave mattress.
- Use bed boundary markers to mark edges of bed such as mattress bumpers, rolled blanket, or "swimming noo-dles" under sheets.
- If the person is (or has been married), line spouse's side of the bed with pillows or bolsters.
- Place soft floor mat or a mattress by the bed to cushion any falls.
- Use water mattress to reduce movement to edge of bed.
- Have person at risk sleep on mattress on the floor.
- Remove wheels from bed.
- Clear the floor of debris, excessive furniture; make sure it is not wet or slippery.
- Place nonskid strips on floor next to bed; ensure that floors are nonskid.
- Use night lights in room and bathroom.
- Place call bell within reach, and make sure the patient can use it—attach call bell to garment or obtain adapted call device.
- Provide visual reminders to encourage the patient to use call bell.
- Have purse (empty or without harmful items or important papers or money) in bed with the person, if a woman.

- Ensure all personal items are within reach.
- Have ambulation devices within reach, and make sure pa-tient knows how to use them properly.
- Use bed, chair, or wrist alarms (the best alarm tells you only that there is an emergency; still need frequent checks, supervised areas). Apply patient-worn sensor (lightweight alarm worn above the knee that is position-sensitive).
- Provide trapeze or patient-assist handles (transfer bars) to enhance mobility in bed.
- If the person is able, he or she should walk at every opportunity possible. If the patient walked in or could walk before hospitalization, make every effort to keep the patient walking during hospitalization.
- Do frequent bed checks, especially in evening and at night.
- Be especially alert at change-of-shift times.
- Understand that very few people spend all day in bed; activity is necessary.
- Provide diversional activities (catalogues, puzzles, therapeutic activity kit) (http://consultgerirn.org/uploads/File/trythis/try_this_d4.pdf).
- Know sleeping patterns—if the person is usually up during the night, get him or her up in a chair and keep at nursing station or involve in activities.

Bathroom
- Establish toileting plan, and take the person to the bathroom frequently.
- Have the person use bedside commode.
- Make sure the person knows the location of the bathroom—leave door open so he or she can see the toi-let, or put a picture of a toilet on the door; clear path to bathroom.
- Provide grab bars in bathroom and shower, shower chair with suction bottom.
- Provide elevated toilet seat.
- Have the person wear clothing that is easy to pull down for toileting.

On the Unit
- Assess for environmental hazards.
- Keep person in supervised area or room within view of the nursing station.
- Have the person sit in a reclining chair, chair with a deep seat, bean bag chair, rocker—keep close to nurses' sta-tion in the chair.
- Consider OT evaluation for seating devices.
- Provide a supervised area and meaningful activities.

BOX 13-5	Suggestions for Fall Risk Reduction and Restraint Alternatives—cont'd

- If the person is wandering or trying to exit, create a grid with masking tape on floor in front of doorway, use black half-rug, and camouflage exit doors with wallpaper, window treatments, etc.
- Provide hip protectors, helmets, and arm pads for high-risk individuals.

- Investigate the Hospital Elder Life Program (HELP) and consider implementing (http://elderlife.med.yale.edu/public/public-main.php).
- Provide a restraint-management cart with alternative restraint products arranged in order of least restrictive measures as described by Antonelli (2008).

BOX 13-6	Tips for Dealing with Tubes, Lines, and Other Medical Devices

- Assessment: First question: "Is the device really necessary?" Remove as soon as possible.
- Preoperative teaching and showing the tubes and explaining may be effective in decreasing anxiety about devices.
- Use guided exploration and a mirror to help patient understand what is in place and why.
- Provide comfort care to the site—oral and nasal care, anchoring of tubing, topical anesthetic on site.
- Foley catheters should be used only if patient needs intensive output monitoring or has an obstruction.
- Weigh risks and benefits of restraint versus therapy. Are alternatives available? For example, replace intravenous (IV) tubing with heparin lock, deliver medications intramuscularly (IM), consider intermittent IV administration or hypodermoclysis.
- Use camouflage: clothing or elastic sleeves, temporary air splint (occupational therapy [OT] can be helpful), skin sleeves to prevent IV tube dislodgement.
- Use mitts instead of wrist restraints; roll belts instead of vest restraints.
- Use diversional activity aprons (zipping-unzipping, threading exercises, dials and knobs), busy box, or

therapeutic activity kit (http://consultgerirn.org/uploads/File/trythis/try_this_d4.pdf).
- Hide lines by placing in unobtrusive place; place tubing behind patient out of his or her view; have patient wear long sleeves or double surgical gowns with cuffs to prevent access.
- Hang IV bags behind the patient's field of vision.
- Nasogastric (NG) tubes—replace with percutaneous endoscopic gastrostomy (PEG) tube if necessary but obtain comprehensive speech therapy (ST) swallowing evaluation. If NG tube is used, use as small a lumen as possible to minimize irritation; consider taping with occlusive dressings.
- Cover PEG tube or abdominal incisions and other tubes with abdominal binder, sweat pants.
- For men with Foley catheters—shave area just above pubis, and tape catheter to pubis. NEVER secure catheter to leg (causes discomfort and can cause a fistula). Run tubing around back and down leg to a leg bag. Patient should wear underpants and pajama pants.
- Take restraints off while working with patient.
- Use modified soft collar for tracheotomy protection.

Vulnerability to Environmental Temperatures

Given the nation's growing problems with supply and costs of energy, many older adults are exposed to temperature extremes in their own dwellings. Environmental temperature extremes impose a serious risk to older persons with declining physical health. Preventive measures require attentiveness to impending climate changes, as well as protective alternatives. Early intervention in extreme temperature exposure is crucial because excessively high or low body temperatures further impair thermoregulatory function and can be lethal.

Thermoregulation

Neurosensory changes in thermoregulation delay or diminish the older person's awareness of temperature changes and may impair behavioral and thermoregulatory response to dangerously high or low environmental temperatures (see Chapter 5). These changes vary widely among individuals and are related more to general health than to age.

Additionally, many of the drugs taken by older people affect thermoregulation by affecting the ability to vasoconstrict or vasodilate, both of which are thermoregulatory mechanisms. Other drugs inhibit neuromuscular activity (a significant source of kinetic heat production), suppress metabolic heat generation, or dull awareness (tranquilizers, pain medications). Alcohol is notorious for inhibiting thermoregulatory function by affecting vasomotor responses in either hot or cold weather.

Economic, behavioral, and environmental factors may combine to create a dangerous thermal environment in which older persons are subjected to temperature extremes from which they cannot escape or that they cannot change. Caregivers and family members should be aware that persons are vulnerable to temperature extremes if they are unable to shiver, sweat, control blood supply to the skin, take in sufficient liquids, move about, add or remove clothing, adjust bedcovers, or adjust the room temperature. A temperature that may be comfortable for a young and active person may be too cold or too warm for a frail elder.

Economic conditions often play a role in determining whether an older person living in the community can afford air conditioning or adequate heating. More older people die from excessive heat than from hurricanes, lightning, tornadoes, floods, and earthquakes combined (CDC, 2006). Local governments and communities must coordinate response strategies to protect the older person. Strategies may include providing fans and opportunities to spend part of the day in air-conditioned buildings, and identification of high-risk older people.

Temperature Monitoring in Older Adults. Diminished thermoregulatory responses and abnormalities in both the production and response to endogenous pyrogens may contribute to differences in fever responses between older and younger patients in response to an infection. Up to one third of older people with acute infections may present without a robust febrile response, leading to delays in diagnosis and appropriate treatment, as well as increased morbidity and mortality (Outzen, 2009). Careful attention to temperature monitoring in older adults is very important, and often this technical task is not given adequate attention by professional nurses.

Hyperthermia

When body temperature increases above normal ranges because of environmental or metabolic heat loads, a clinical condition called heat illness, or *hyperthermia*, develops. Diuretics and low intake of fluids exacerbate fluid loss and can precipitate the onset of hyperthermia in hot weather. Hyperthermia is a temperature-related illness and is classified as a medical emergency. Annually, there are numerous deaths among elders from temperature extremes, and these could be almost entirely prevented with education and caution. Although most of these problems occur in the home among individuals who do not have air conditioning during temperature extremes, older adults with multiple physical problems residing in institutions may be especially vulnerable to temperature changes. Elders with cardiovascular disease, diabetes, or peripheral vascular disease and those taking certain medications (anticholinergics, antihistamines, diuretics, beta blockers, antidepressants, antiparkinsonian drugs) are at risk. Interventions to prevent hyperthermia when ambient temperature exceeds 90° F (32° C) are presented in Box 13-7.

Hypothermia

Nearly 50% of all deaths from hypothermia occur in older adults (Ham et al., 2007). Hypothermia is produced by exposure to cold environmental temperatures and is defined as a core temperature of less than 35° C (95° F). Hypothermia is a medical emergency requiring comprehensive assessment of neurological activity, oxygenation, renal function, and fluid and electrolyte balance.

During cold weather, two situations tend to produce hypothermia: (1) exposure involving a healthy individual in severely cold environmental conditions for a prolonged period; or (2) exposure involving a person with impaired thermoregulatory ability in room temperature without

---

⚡ SAFETY ALERT

A temperature of 98.6° F may indicate fever in frail older people. Because of thermoregulatory changes, up to one third of older people with acute infections may present without a febrile response. Additionally, baseline temperatures in frail older people may be lower than the expected 98.6° F. If the baseline temperature is 97° F, a temperature of 98° F is a one-degree elevation and may be significant. Temperatures reaching or exceeding 100.94° F are very serious in older people and are more likely to be associated with serious bacterial or viral infections. Careful attention to temperature monitoring in older adults is very important and can prevent morbidity and mortality. Accurate measurement and reporting of body temperature requires professional nursing supervision.

BOX 13-7   Interventions to Prevent Hyperthermia

- Drink 2 to 3 L of cool fluid daily.
- Minimize exertion, especially during the heat of the day.
- Stay in air-conditioned places, or use fans when possible.
- Wear hats and loose clothing of natural fibers when outside; remove most clothing when indoors.
- Take tepid baths or showers.
- Apply cold wet compresses, or immerse the hands and feet in cool water.
- Evaluate medications for risk of hyperthermia.
- Avoid alcohol.

protection. The more severe the impairment or prolonged the exposure, the less able are thermoregulatory responses to defend against heat loss. Older adults are particularly predisposed to hypothermia because the opportunity for heat loss frequently coexists with the decline in heat generation and conservation responses. Such coexistence occurs frequently among persons who are homeless or cognitively impaired; persons who are injured in falls or from trauma; and persons with cardiovascular, adrenal, or thyroid dysfunction, and diabetes. Other risk factors include excessive alcohol use, exhaustion, poor nutrition, inadequate housing, as well as the use of sedatives, anxiolytics, phenothiazines, and tricyclic antidepressants.

Unfortunately, a dulling of awareness accompanies hypothermia, and persons experiencing the condition rarely recognize the problem or seek assistance. For the very old and frail, environmental temperatures below 65° F (18° C) may cause a serious drop in core body temperature to 95° F (35° C). Factors that increase the risk of hypothermia are numerous, as shown in Box 13-8. Box 13-9 lists factors that may induce low basal body temperatures in elders.

When exposed to cold temperatures, healthy persons conserve heat by vasoconstriction of superficial vessels, shunting circulation away from the skin where most heat is lost. Heat is generated by shivering and increased muscle activity, and a rise in oxygen consumption occurs to meet aerobic muscle requirements. Circulatory, cardiac, respiratory,

or musculoskeletal impairments affect either the response to or function of thermoregulatory mechanisms. Older persons with some degree of thermoregulatory impairment, when exposed to cold temperatures, are at high risk for hypothermia if they undergo surgery, are injured in a fall or accident, or are lost or left unattended in a cool place.

All body systems are affected by hypothermia, although the most deadly consequences involve cardiac arrhythmias and suppression of respiratory function. Correctly conducted rewarming is the key to good management, and the guiding principle is to warm the core before the periphery and raise the core temperature 0.5° C to 2° C per hour. Heating blankets and specially designed heating vests are used in addition to warm humidified air by mask, warm intravenous boluses, and other measures depending on the severity of the hypothermia (Ham et al., 2007).

Detecting hypothermia among community-dwelling older adults is sometimes difficult, because unlike in the clinical setting, no one is measuring body temperature. For persons exposed to low temperatures in the home or the environment, confusion and disorientation may be the first overt signs. As judgment becomes clouded, a person may remove clothing or fail to seek shelter, and hypothermia can progress to profound levels. For this reason, regular contact with home-dwelling elders during cold weather is crucial. For those with preexisting alterations in thermoregulatory ability, this surveillance should include even mildly cool

---

BOX 13-8   Factors That Increase the Risk of Hypothermia in Older Adults

Thermoregulatory Impairment

Failure to vasoconstrict promptly or strongly on exposure to cold
Failure to sense cold
Failure to respond behaviorally to protect oneself against cold
Diminished or absent shivering to generate heat
Failure of metabolic rate to rise in response to cold

Conditions That Decrease Heat Production

Hypothyroidism, hypopituitarism, hypoglycemia, anemia, malnutrition, starvation
Immobility or decreased activity (e.g., stroke, paralysis, parkinsonism, dementia, arthritis, fractured hip, coma)
Diabetic ketoacidosis

Conditions That Increase Heat Loss

Open wounds, generalized inflammatory skin conditions, burns

Conditions That Impair Central or Peripheral Control of Thermoregulation

Stroke, brain tumor, Wernicke's encephalopathy, subarachnoid hemorrhage
Uremia, neuropathy (e.g., diabetes, alcoholism)
Acute illnesses (e.g., pneumonia, sepsis, myocardial infarction, congestive heart failure, pulmonary embolism, pancreatitis)

Drugs That Interfere with Thermoregulation

Tranquilizers (e.g., phenothiazines)
Sedative-hypnotics (e.g., barbiturates, benzodiazepines)
Antidepressants (e.g., tricyclics)
Vasoactive drugs (e.g., vasodilators)
Alcohol (causes superficial vasodilation; may interfere with carbohydrate metabolism and judgment)
Others: methyldopa, lithium, morphine

BOX 13-9   Factors Associated with Low Body Temperature in the Elderly

Aging
Increases risk of thermoregulatory dysfunction.
Increases risk of acute and chronic conditions that
predispose to hypothermia.

Low Environmental Temperature
Risk of hypothermia increased below 65° F.

Thinness and Malnutrition
Very thin people have less thermal insulation, higher surface
area/volume ratios.
Prolonged malnutrition can decrease the metabolic rate by
20% to 30%.

Poverty
Increases risk of thinness and malnutrition, inadequate
clothing, low environmental temperature secondary to
poor housing conditions and inadequate heat.

Living Alone
Associated with poverty, delayed detection of hypothermia,
delayed rescue if person falls.

Nocturia/Night Rising
Associated with falls; if rescue delayed and person lies
immobilized for a long time, hypothermia may develop as
heat is conducted away from the body to the cold floor.

Orthostatic Hypotension
An indicator of autonomic nervous system impairment;
dizziness and postural instability are associated with
falls.

---

weather. Because heating costs are high in the United States, the Department of Health and Human Services provides funds to help low-income families pay their heating bills. Specific interventions to prevent hypothermia are shown in Box 13-10.

Implications for Gerontological Nursing and Healthy Aging

Recognition of clinical signs and severity of hypothermia and hyperthermia are important nursing responsibilities. Nurses are responsible for keeping frail elders in environments with appropriate temperatures for comfort and prevention of problems. It is important to closely monitor body temperature in older people and pay particular attention to lower or higher than normal readings compared with the person's baseline. The potential risk of hypothermia and its associated cardiorespiratory and metabolic exertion makes prevention important and early recognition vital. Nurses must advocate for resources in the community to insure appropriate temperatures in the homes of older people and surveillance when temperature changes occur.

Vulnerability to Natural Disasters

Natural disasters such as hurricanes, tornadoes, floods, and earthquakes claim the lives of many people worldwide each year. In addition, human-made or human-generated disasters include chemical, biological, radiological, and nuclear terrorism and food and water contamination. The events of September 11, 2001, have prompted much thought and planning related to human-generated disasters. Older people are at great risk during and after disasters, and the older population had the highest casualty rate during disaster events when compared to all other age groups (Burnett et al., 2008).

Older adults at most risk include, but are not limited to, those who depend on others for daily functioning; those with limited mobility; and those who are socially isolated, cognitively impaired, or institutionalized (Brown, 2008). Older people may be less likely to seek formal or informal help during disasters and may not get as much assistance as younger individuals. Nursing home residents compose a particularly vulnerable group due to their frailty and nursing homes need to be prepared for disasters. Rhoads and Clayman (2008) provide a guide to preparing long-term care facilities for disasters.

Implications for Gerontological Nursing and Healthy Aging

Gerontological nurses must be knowledgeable about disaster preparedness and assist in the development of plans to address the unique needs of older adults, as well as educate

---

BOX 13-10   Nursing Interventions to Prevent Cold Discomfort and the Development of Accidental Hypothermia in Frail Elders

Desired Outcomes
- Hands and limbs warm
- Body relaxed, not curled
- Body temperature >97° F
- No shivering
- No complaints of cold

Interventions
- *Maintain a comfortably warm ambient temperature* no lower than 65° F. Many frail elders will require much higher temperatures.
- *Provide generous quantities of clothing and bedcovers.* Layer clothing and bedcovers for best insulation. Be careful not to judge your patient's needs by how you feel working in a warm environment.
- *Limit time patients sit by cold windows or air conditioners* to short periods in which they are adequately dressed and covered.
- *Provide a head covering* whenever possible—in bed, out of bed, and particularly out-of-doors.

- *Cover patients well during bathing.* The standard—a light bath blanket over a naked body—is not enough protection for frail elders.
- *Cover naked patients with heavy blankets for transfer to and from showers;* dry quickly and thoroughly before leaving shower room; cover head with a dry towel or hood while wet. Shower rooms and bathrooms should have warming lights.
- *Dry wet hair quickly* with warm air from an electric dryer. Never allow the hair of frail elders to air-dry.
- *Use absorbent pads* for incontinent patients rather than allow urine to wet large areas of clothing, sheets, and bedcovers. Avoid skin problems by changing pads frequently, washing the skin well, and applying a protective cream.
- *Provide as much exercise as possible* to generate heat from muscle activity.
- *Provide hot, high-protein meals and bedtime snacks* to add heat and sustain heat production throughout the day and as far into the night as possible.

---

fellow professionals, older adult clients, and community agencies about disaster preparedness. Comprehensive planning is necessary to respond to the needs of the aging population in emergency situations around the world. The U.S. Department of Health and Human Services provides resources for emergency and disaster preparedness for special populations, including older adults (http://sis.nlm. nih.gov/outreach/specialpopulationsanddisasters.html).

Transportation Safety

Available transportation is a critical link in the ability of older adults to remain independent and functional. The lack of accessible transportation may contribute to other problems, such as social withdrawal, poor nutrition, or neglect of health care. Even when municipal transportation service is available, elders may not use it. Urban buses and subways can be physically hazardous and often dangerous. A "crisis in mobility" exists for many older people because of the lack of an automobile, an inability to drive, limited access to public transportation, health factors, geographical location, and economic considerations.

County, state, or federally subsidized transportation is being provided in certain areas to assist older people in

reaching social services, nutrition sites, health services, emergency care, recreational centers, day care programs, physical and vocational rehabilitation, continuing education, grocery, and library services. Although transportation can often be found for special needs, it is virtually impossible to locate transportation for pleasure or recreation. Senior centers offer a wide range of activities for older people, as well as transportation services. Nurses can refer older people to local social service and aging organizations, such as Area Agencies on Aging, for information on transportation resources and financial assistance for services.

Driving

Driving is one of the instrumental activities of daily living (IADLs) for most elders because it is essential to obtaining necessary resources. Driving is a highly complex activity that requires a variety of visual, motor, and cognitive skills (Mathias & Lucas, 2009). Assessments of functional capacities often neglect this important activity. We should evaluate whether an individual can drive, feels safe driving, and has a driver's license. Giving up mobility and independence afforded by driving one's own car has many psychological ramifications and inconveniences. Giving up driving is a major loss for an older person both in terms of independence and pleasure, as well as feelings of competence and self-worth. Driving cessation has been associated with decreased social integration, decreased out-of-home activities, increased depressive and anxiety symptoms, decreased quality of life, and increased risk of nursing home placement (Carr & Ott, 2010; Siren & Hakamies-Blomqvist, 2009).

For many older people, alternate transportation is not available, and consequently, they may continue driving beyond the time when it is safe. Almost 90% of people 65 years of age and older continue to drive, and these numbers are expected to grow as "baby boomers" age and more people live into their 80s and 90s. Older men seem to place more value on the ability to drive, as well as owning a car, than older women. Therefore, one can expect more stress involved with the decision not to drive for older men. Specialized driving cessation support groups aimed at the transition from driver to non-driver may also be beneficial in decreasing the negative outcomes associated with this decision (Dobbs et al., 2009).

Driving Safety

Older drivers typically drive fewer miles than younger drivers and tend to drive less at night, during adverse weather conditions, or in congested areas. Generally, they choose familiar routes, and fewer older drivers speed or drive after drinking alcohol than drivers of other ages. However, when compared with younger age-groups, older people have more accidents per mile driven, and older drivers and passengers are three times more likely to die than younger people following an auto crash. The leading cause of injury-related deaths among drivers 65 to 74 years of age is a motor vehicle accident; for those older than 75 years of age, motor vehicle accidents are the second leading cause of death, after falls (Hooyman & Kiyak, 2011). Age-related changes in driving skills, including vision changes, cognitive impairment, and various medical illnesses and functional impairments, are factors related to driving safety for older adults.

Driving and Dementia

Driving has been identified as one of the top 10 tough ethical issues associated with dementia (Dobbs et al., 2009). Dementia, even in the early stages, can impair cognitive and functional skills required for safe driving. Evidence from some studies of motor vehicle crashes suggests that drivers with dementia have at least a two-fold risk of crashes compared to those without cognitive impairment (Carr & Ott, 2010; Gray-Vickrey, 2010a).

As many as 30% of older individuals with dementia continue to drive (Carr & Ott, 2010; Gray-Vickrey, 2010b). Many individuals early in the course of dementia are still able to pass a driving performance test, so a diagnosis of dementia should not be the sole justification for revocation of a driver's license (Carr & Ott, 2010). However, discussions should begin about the inevitability of driving cessation. Additionally, driving evaluations should be conducted every six months or as needed as the disease progresses.

The legal regulations regarding driver's license renewal in older drivers and the responsibility of medical practitioners to identify unsafe drivers vary from state to state and country to country (Mathias & Lucas, 2009). Driver's license renewal procedures may include accelerated renewal cycles, renewal in person rather than electronically or by mail, and vision and road tests. Additional information can be found at www.iihs.org/laws/state_laws/older_drivers.html. The issues of driving in the older adult population are the subject of a great deal of public discussion. Many older drivers and their families struggle with issues related to continued safety in driving and when and how to tell older people they are no longer safe to drive.

Driving Cessation

Planning for driving cessation should occur for all older adults before their mobility situations become urgent (Carr & Ott, 2010). Health care providers should encourage open discussion of issues related to driving with the older person and his or her family and should identify impairments that affect safe driving, correct them when possible, and offer alternatives for transportation. It is generally agreed that voluntarily giving up a driver's license, rather than having it revoked, is associated with more positive outcomes (Oxley & Charlton, 2009). Jett and colleagues (2005) provide useful strategies for driving counseling for people with dementia from a qualitative study involving guided interviews with participants (Box 13-11).

Implications for Gerontological Nursing and Healthy Aging

Suggestions for easing the transition from driving to not driving are to encourage the individual to modify driving habits such as not driving on unfamiliar roads, during rush hour, at dusk or at night, in inclement weather, or in heavy traffic. Other strategies to decrease the need to drive include home-delivered groceries, prescriptions, and meals; personal services provided in the home; asking a caregiver to obtain needed supplies or act as a copilot; and exploring

---

BOX 13-11   Action Strategies Used to Bring About Driving Cessation

Imposed Type

Report person to division of motor vehicles for possible license suspension.

Use of deception or threats such as false keys, disabling the car, saying car was stolen.

Attempts to order control, such as provider writing a prescription, commands from children to stop driving.

Involved Type

All family members and individuals discuss the situation and come to a mutual agreement of the problem.

Dialogue is ongoing from the earliest signs of cognitive impairment about the eventuality of the need to stop driving.

Arrangements are made for alternative transportation plans that are available when needed and acceptable to the individual

From Jett K, Tappen R, Roselli M: Imposed versus involved: different strategies to effect driving cessation in cognitively impaired older adults, *Geriatr Nurs* 26(2):111-116, 2005.

BOX 13-12   Adaptations for Safer Driving

- Wider rear-view mirrors
- Pedal extensions
- Less complicated, larger, and legible instrument panels
- Electronic detectors in front and back that signal when the car is too close to other cars
- Better protection on doors
- Booster cushions for shorter-stature drivers
- "Smart" driving assistants (under development) that automatically plans a safe driving route based on the person's driving habits
- GPS devices

Modified from Hooyman N, Kiyak H: *Social gerontology,* Boston, 2011, Allyn & Bacon.

---

community resources for transportation (Gray-Vickrey, 2010b). Additional suggestions include asking the provider to "prescribe" driving cessation, use medical conditions other than dementia (impaired vision, slowed reaction time) as the reason to stop driving, and request the family lawyer to discuss financial and legal implications of crash or injury (Carr & Ott, 2010). Disabling the car in some way (such as replacing keys with ones that will not start the vehicle, disabling the ignition, and removing the car) is another suggestion, but often the older person can circumvent these strategies by hiring a mechanic to repair the car or buying a new vehicle.

Vehicle adaptations (Box 13-12), sensory aids, elder driving training, and driving assessment programs are helpful in promoting safe driving (Gillian & Schwartzberg, 2005; Perkinson et al., 2005). There is no gold standard for determining driving competency, but driving evaluations are offered by driver rehabilitation specialists through local hospitals and rehabilitation centers and private or university-based driving assessment programs. State Departments of Motor Vehicles (DMVs) also conduct performance-based road tests.

The American Medical Association, in partnership with the National Highway Traffic Safety Administration,

provides the *Physician's Guide to Assessing and Counseling Older Drivers,* with step-by-step plans for assessing older driver safety (www.ama-assn.org/ama/pub/category/10791.html). The National Institutes of Health has an online resource for older drivers and families, which includes information on how aging may affect driving, safety issues, and ways older drivers can cope when driving skills change (http://nihseniorhealth.gov/olderdrivers/howagingaffectsdriving/01.html).

Many states have implemented the Silver Alert system. Similar to Amber Alerts for missing children, the Silver Alert is designed to create a widespread lookout for older adults who have wandered from their surroundings. Silver Alert features a public notification system to broadcast information about missing persons, especially older adults with Alzheimer's disease or other mental disabilities, in order to aid in their return. Silver Alert uses a wide array of media outlets, such as commercial radio stations, television stations, and cable TV, to broadcast information about missing persons. Silver Alert also uses message signs on roadways to alert motorists to be on the lookout for missing elders and provides the car's make, model, and license information.

Application of Maslow's Hierarchy

Feeling safe and secure in one's environment is essential to the attainment of all levels of needs as conceived by Maslow. Safety and security needs include personal security, financial security, health and well-being, and safety against accident/illness and their adverse impacts. As individual's age, threats to safety and security can be frequent due to health challenges and environmental threats. The nurse's role is to insure safe environments in all settings and provide interventions that decrease risks so that the individual can function at his or her highest level.

KEY CONCEPTS

- A thorough nursing assessment must include assessment of fall risk, balance, and gait; intrinsic, extrinsic, and iatrogenic factors; and postfall assessments.
- Implementation of individualized fall risk–reduction interventions is one of the most important proactive considerations to preserve health and function for older adults.
- Physical restraints are not appropriate for "safety" and increase injuries related to falls. Restraint-free care, fall risk–reduction interventions, and a safe environment are essential to best practice care for elders.
- Thermoregulatory changes, chronic illness, and medications may predispose the older adult to hypothermia and hyperthermia. Careful attention must be paid to temperature monitoring and provision of adequate heat and cooling in weather extremes.
- Transportation for older adults is critical to their physical, psychological, and social health.

ACTIVITIES AND DISCUSSION QUESTIONS

1. Put your shoes on the wrong feet, and then ask another student to analyze your gait.
2. Borrow a pair of bifocals from someone, and then attempt to go up and down stairs.
3. Evaluate the safety of your living quarters or the living quarters of your parents/grandparents, using Table 13-3 as a guide.
4. Discuss falls you have had and their consequences. Consider how it might have been different if you were 80 years old.
5. Obtain a wheelchair, and sit in it for 20 minutes with a restraining belt around your waist. Discuss your feelings with a partner. Reverse the process with your partner.
6. Discuss the various reasons why you might need to ensure safety for a hospitalized elder, and identify several alternatives that might be appropriate. Are these alternatives available in the acute care setting where you study?

REFERENCES

Agency for Healthcare Research and Quality: *2010 National healthcare quality and disparities report* (2011). Available at http://www.ahrq.gov/qual/qrdr10.htm.

American Geriatrics Society [AGS], British Geriatrics Society: *Clinical practice guideline: prevention of falls in older persons* (2010). Available at http://www.americangeriatrics.org/health_care_professionals/clinical_practice/clinical_guidelines_recommendations/2010/.

Andersen D, Osei-Boamah E, Gambert S: Impact of trauma-related hip fractures on the older adult, *Clin Geriatr* 18:18, 2010.

Antonelli M: Restraint management: moving from process to outcome, *J Nurs Care Qual* 23:227, 2008.

Aud M, et al: Smart carpet: developing a sensor system to detect falls and summon assistance, *J Gerontol Nurs* 36:8–12, 2010.

Bezaitis A: Robot technologies: exciting new frontier, *Aging Well* 2:10, 2009.

Bourbonniere M, Evans LK: Advanced practice nursing in the care of frail older adults, *J Am Geriatr Soc* 50:2062, 2002.

Brown L: Issues in mental health care for older adults after disasters, *Generations* 31(4):21–26, 2008.

Buckeridge D, Huang A, Hanley J, et al: Risk of injury associated with opioid use in older adults, *J Am Geriatr Soc* 58(9):1664–1670, 2010.

Burnett J, Dyer C, Pickins S: Rapid needs assessments for older adults in disasters, *Generations* 31(4):10–15, 2008.

Cameron I, Murray G, Gillespie L, et al: Interventions for preventing falls in older people in nursing facilities and hospitals, *Cochrane Database Syst Rev* 1:CD005465, 2010.

Capezuti E: Building the science of falls-prevention research, *J Am Geriatr Soc* 52(3):461–462, 2004.

Capezuti E, Zwicker D, Mezey M, et al: *Evidence-based geriatric nursing protocols for best practice*, ed 3, New York, 2008, Springer.

Carr D, Ott B: The older adult driver with cognitive impairment: "it's a very frustrating life," *JAMA* 303:1632–1641, 2010.

Centers for Disease Control and Prevention [CDC]: Heat-related deaths—United States, 1999-2003, *MMWR Morb Mortal Wkly Rep* 55:796-798, 2006.

Centers for Disease Control and Prevention [CDC]: *Hip fractures among older adults* (2010a). Available at http://www.cdc.gov/HomeandRecreationalSafety/Falls/adulthipfx.html.

Centers for Disease Control and Prevention [CDC]: *Preventing traumatic brain injury in older adults* (2010b). Available at http://cdc.gov/BrainInjuryinSeniors.

Daniel K, et al: Emerging technologies to enhance the safety of older people in their homes, *Geriatric Nursing* 30:384–389, 2009.

deVries OJ, Ligthart GJ, Nikolaus T, on behalf of the participants of the European Academy of Medicine of Ageing—Course III: Differences in period prevalence of the use of physical restraints in elderly inpatients of European hospitals and nursing homes [Letter], *J Gerontol Med Sci* 59(9)9:922–923, 2004.

Dobbs B, Harper L, Woods A.: Transitioning from driving to driving cessation: the role of specialized driving cessation support groups for individuals with dementia, *Top Geriatr Rehabil* 25:73-86, 2009.

Evans LK, Strumpf NE: Tying down the elderly: a review of the literature on physical restraint, *J Am Geriatr Soc* 37(1):65–74, 1989.

Flaherty J: Zero tolerance for physical restraints: difficult but not impossible, *J Gerontol A Biol Sci Med Sci* 59A(9):M919–920, 2004.

Flanagan S, Hibbard M, Riordan B, et al: Traumatic brain injury in the elderly: diagnostic and treatment challenges, *Clin Geriatr Med* 22:449, 2006.

Frick K, Kung J, Parrish J, et al: Evaluating the cost-effectiveness of fall prevention programs that reduce fall-related hip fractures in older adults, *J Am Geriatr Soc* 58:136, 2010.

Gavin-Dreschnack D, Volicer L, Morris C: Prevention of overuse of wheelchairs in nursing homes, *Ann Longterm Care* 18:34, 2010.

Gillian C, Schwartzberg J: Addressing the at-risk older driver, *Clin Geriatr Med* 13:27–34, 2005.

Gray-Micelli D: Falls in the environment. 1. Faulty footwear or footing? an interdisciplinary case-based perspective, *Ann Longterm Care* 18:32, 2010.

Gray-Micelli D: Preventing falls in acute care. In Capezuti E, Zwicker D, Mezey M, et al, editors: *Evidence-based geriatric nursing protocols for best practice*, New York, 2008, Springer.

Gray-Micelli D, Quigley P: Fall prevention: assessment, diagnoses, and intervention strategies. In Boltz M, Capezuti E, Fulmer T, et al, editors: *Evidence-based geriatric nursing protocols for best practice*, New York, 2012, Springer.

Gray-Vickrey P: Enhancing driver safety in dementia, *Alzheimer's Care Today* 11:147–148, 2010a.

Gray-Vickrey P: Research updates: driving and dementia, *Alzheimer's Care Today* 11:149–150, 2010b.

Haentjens P, Magaziner J, Colon-Emeric C, et al: Meta-analysis: excess mortality after hip fracture among older men and women, *Ann Intern Med* 152:380, 2010.

Ham R, et al: *Primary care geriatrics: a case-based approach*, ed 5, St. Louis, 2007, Elsevier.

Harrison B, Ferrari M, Campbell C, et al: Evaluating the relationship between inattention and impulsivity-related falls in hospitalized older adults, *Geriatr Nurs* 31:8, 2010.

Hendrich AL, Bender PS, Nyhuis A: Validation of the Hendrich II fall risk model: a large concurrent case/control study of hospitalized patients, *Applied Nursing Research* 16:9, 2003.

Hill K, Womer M, Russell M, et al: Fear of falling in older fallers presenting at emergency departments, *J Adv Nurs* 66:1769, 2010.

Hooyman N, Kiyak H: *Social gerontology: a multidisciplinary perspective*, Boston, 2011, Allyn & Bacon.

Ireland S, Lazar T, Mavrak C, et al: Designing a falls prevention strategy that works, *J Nurs Care Qual* 25:198, 2010.

Jett K, Tappen R, Roselli M: Imposed versus involved: different strategies to effect driving cessation in cognitively impaired older adults, *Geriatr Nurs* 26(2):111–116, 2005.

Kilgore C: Fall-prevention efforts must be multifaceted, *Caring for the Ages* 11:26, 2010.

Lach H: The costs and outcomes of falls: what's a nursing administrator to do? *Nurs Adm Q* 34:147, 2010.

Lin F, Ferrucci L: Hearing loss and falls among older adults in the United States, *Arch Intern Med* 172(4):369–371, 2012.

Luciano G, Brennan M, Rothberg M: Postprandial hypotension, *Am J Med* 123(3):281.e1–6, 2010.

Mathias J, Lucas L: Cognitive predictors of unsafe driving in older drivers: a meta-analysis, *Inter Psychogeriatrics* 21:637–653, 2009.

Mendito V, Lucci M, Polonara S, et al: Management of minor head injury in patients receiving oral anticoagulant therapy: a prospective study of a 24-hour observation protocol, *Ann Emerg Med* 59(6):451–455, 2012.

Oliver D, Connelly J, Victor C, et al: Strategies to prevent falls and fractures in hospitals and care homes and effect of cognitive impairment: systematic review and meta-analyses, *BMJ* 334:82, 2007. Available at https://www.ncbi.nlm.nih.gov/pmc/articles/PMC1767306/.

Outzen M: Management of fever in older adults, *J Gerontol Nurs* 35:17–23, 2009.

Oxley J, Charlton J: Attitudes to and mobility impacts of driving cessation, *Top Geriatr Rehabil* 25:43–54, 2009.

Park M, Hsiao-Chen Tang J: Evidence-based guidelines: changing the practice of physical restraint use in acute care, *J Gerontol Nurs* 33(2):9–16, 2007.

Pellfolk T, Gustafson Y, Bucht G, et al: Effects of a restraint minimization program on staff knowledge, attitudes, and practice: a cluster randomized trial, *J Am Geriatr Soc* 58:62, 2010.

Perkinson M, Berg-Weger M, Carr D, et al: Driving and dementia of the Alzheimer type: beliefs and cessation strategies, *Gerontologist* 45(5):676–685, 2005.

Quigley P, Bulat T, Kurtzman E, et al: Fall prevention and injury protection for nursing home residents, *J Am Med Dir Assoc* 11:284, 2010.

Rantz M, Aud M, Alexander G: et al: Falls, technology, and stunt actors, *J Nurs Care Qual* 23:195–201, 2008.

Resnick B: In Henkel G: Beyond the MDS: team approach to falls assessment, prevention and management, *Caring for the Ages* 3(4):15–20, 2002.

Rhoads J, Clayman A: Learning from Katrina: preparing long-term care facilities for disasters, *Geriatric Nursing* 29:253–258, 2008.

Rubenstein T, Alexander N, Hausdoff J: Evaluating fall risk in older adults: steps and missteps, *Clin Geriatr* 11(1):52–61, 2003.

Siren A, Hakamies-Blomqvist L: Mobility and well-being in old age, *Top Geriatr Rehabil* 25:3–11, 2009.

Talerico K, Capezuti E: Myths and facts about side rails, *Am J Nurs* 101:43, 2001.

Tappen R, Roach K, Applegate E, et al: Effect of a combined walking and conversation intervention on functional mobility of nursing home residents with Alzheimer's disease, *Alzheimer Dis Assoc Disord* 14:196–201, 2000.

Timmons T, Menaker J: Traumatic brain injury in the elderly, *Clinical Geriatrics* 18:20, 2010.

Tinetti ME: Preventing falls in elderly persons, *N Engl J Med* 348(1):42–49, 2003.

Tinetti ME, Baker DI, King M, et al: Effect of dissemination of evidence in reducing injuries from falls, *N Engl J Med* 359(3):252–261, 2008.

Tzeng H, Yin C: The extrinsic risk factors for inpatient falls in hospital patient rooms, *J Nurs Care Qual* 23:233, 2008.

U.S. Department of Health and Human Services, Office of Disease Prevention and Health Promotion: *Healthy People 2020.* (2012). Available at http://www.healthypeople.gov/2020.

U.S. Preventive Services Task Force: *Prevention of falls in community-dwelling older adults* (2012). Available at http://www.uspreventiveservicestaskforce.org/uspstf/uspsfalls.htm.

Wagner LM, Capezuti E, Brush BL, et al: Contractures in frail nursing home residents, *Geriatr Nurs* 29:259, 2008.

Zecevic A, Salmoni A, Speechley N, et al: Defining a fall and reasons for falling: comparisons among the views of seniors, health care providers, and the research literature, *Gerontologist* 46(3):367–376, 2006.

CHAPTER 14

Living with Chronic Illness

Theris A. Touhy

℮volve evolve.elsevier.com/Ebersole/gerontological

LEARNING OBJECTIVES

Upon completion of this chapter, the reader will be able to:

- Define chronic illness and explain the differences between chronic illness and acute illness.
- Discuss the factors that influence the experience of chronic illness.
- Identify competencies to improve care for chronic conditions.
- Discuss models to enhance self-care management of chronic illness.
- Discuss nursing interventions to maximize wellness in the presence of chronic illness.

GLOSSARY

Exacerbation A worsening. In medicine, exacerbation may refer to an increase in the severity of a disease or its signs and symptoms.

Exorbitant Exceeding that which is usual or proper.

Trajectory The path followed by a body or an event moved along by the action of certain forces.

THE LIVED EXPERIENCE

"Because you understand my disease, you don't understand me. To understand that I am ill does not mean that you understand how I experience my illness. I am unique. I think and feel and behave in a combination that is unique to me. You do not understand me because you have a label for my disease or a plan for my treatment. It is not my disease or treatment that you need to understand. It is me. This could happen to you…You are just a diagnosis away from being a patient."

Jevne, 1993, p. 121

Chronic Illness

Scope of the Problem

The rising prevalence and associated costs of chronic illness is a global health concern. Chronic illness accounts for over half the global health burden. By 2020, estimates are that chronic illness will account for nearly 80% of worldwide disease. Seven out of 10 deaths among Americans each year are from chronic diseases, with heart disease, cancer, and stroke accounting for more than 50% of all deaths each year. Vulnerable and socially disadvantaged people get sicker and die sooner as a result of chronic illness than people of higher social positions. A host of social determinants, especially education, income, gender, and ethnicity influence levels of chronic illness (World Health Organization [WHO], 2012).

Three out of four U.S. health care dollars are spent to care for individuals with chronic illnesses and they account for 80% of the Medicare program's annual expenditures (Boult & Wieland, 2010). By the year 2020, 25% of the American population will be living with multiple chronic conditions, and costs for managing these conditions will reach $1.07 trillion. Chronic illnesses also exact significant personal costs and burden due to diminished quality of life for both the individual and his or her family and significant others. Access to care, quality outcomes, and patient satisfaction remain issues of concern despite spending. The current health care system excels at responding to immediate medical needs such as accidents, severe injury, and sudden bouts of illness. American health care is less expert at providing ongoing care to people with chronic conditions and improving their day-to-day lives.

Older adults are at high risk for developing chronic illnesses and related disabilities. These chronic conditions include diabetes, arthritis, congestive heart failure, and dementia. Preventing the onset of chronic illness and, after it is diagnosed, reducing the infirmity and disability that can result, remains central to the goal of improving function, well-being, and quality of life for older adults. This chapter discusses chronic illness and the implications for gerontological nursing and healthy aging. Information on specific chronic illnesses and associated symptoms can be found in Chapters 15 to 22.

Chronic and Acute Illnesses

Chronic illnesses are "conditions that last a year or more and require ongoing medical attention and/or limit activities of daily living (Hwang et al., 2001, p. 268). From a nursing perspective, "chronic illness is the irreversible presence, accumulation, or latency of disease states or impairments that involve the total human environment for supportive care and self-care, maintenance of function and prevention of further disability" (Curtin & Lubkin, 2006, pp. 6-7). Chronic disorders and acute illness cannot really be separated, because so many conditions are intricately intertwined; acute disorders have chronic sequelae, and many of the commonly identified chronic disorders tend to flare up intermittently into acute problems and then to go into remission.

A chronic illness continues indefinitely, is managed rather than cured, and necessitates that the individual "learn to live with it" (Lundman & Jansson, 2007, p. 109). By definition, it is always present although not always visible. If not triggered by an acute event, the onset may be insidious and identified only during a health screening. Symptoms of the effects of the illness, including disabilities, may not appear for years. For example, the person with hypertension develops enough heart damage to cause an acute episode of heart failure.

The person with a chronic illness may have episodic exacerbations or remain in remission with no symptoms for a long time. People with chronic illnesses often continue to work and perform their usual activities early in their diseases. Later, and with increasing age, the effects of the limitations increase. Many elders have several chronic disorders simultaneously (comorbidities) and have great difficulty managing the complexity of the overlapping and often contradictory demands.

Symptoms of chronic illness interfere with many normal activities and routines, make medical regimens necessary, disrupt patterns of living, and frequently make it necessary for the individual to make significant lifestyle changes. Physical suffering, loss, worry, grief, depression, functional impairment, and increased dependence on family or friends for support are among the negative consequences of chronic illnesses. One of the greatest fears of older people is being dependent on others as a result of chronic illness (Zauszniewski et al., 2007).

Chronic Illness and Aging

Many factors influence the rapid rise in the number of individuals with chronic illnesses including the aging of the population, advances in medical sciences in extending the life span and in treating illness, a rise in conditions such as asthma and diabetes, and obesity in younger people. Additional factors include the changing trajectory of illnesses such as HIV/AIDS, cancer, and dementia which are becoming chronic illnesses to live with for extended periods of time, and less than adequate prevention and health promotion efforts across the life span, particularly for diverse populations.

Chronic illnesses are common among older adults. About 88% of older adults have at least one chronic illness, and 50% have at least two (Zauszniewski et al., 2007). By the time a person has lived 50 years, he or she is likely to have at least one chronic condition. It may be slight arthritis at the site of an old football injury, hypertension, diabetes mellitus, obesity, or any one of a number of illnesses. The most common chronic condition for all ages is sinusitis, whereas for persons older than 65 years of age, the most common chronic conditions are arthritis and hypertension (Figure 14-1). For the older adult, the presence or absence of a chronic illness is not as important as its effect on one's functioning. The effect may be as little as an inconvenience or as great as an impairment of one's ability to perform activities of daily living (ADLs), or instrumental activities of daily living (IADLs) (Figure 14-2).

The term *compressed morbidity* proposes that premature death will be minimized, and disease and functional decline will be compressed into a period of three to five years before death. There is some evidence that this is already occurring because major diseases such as arthritis, arteriosclerosis, and respiratory problems now appear 10 to 25 years later than for past cohorts (Fries, 2002; Hooyman & Kiyak, 2011). The current generation of older people is generally healthier than

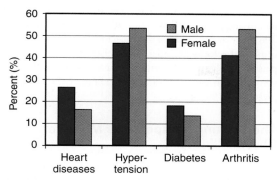

FIGURE **14-1** Chronic health conditions among the population 65 years of age and over, by sex, 2007–2008. (Redrawn from Federal Interagency Forum on Aging-Related Statistics: *Older Americans 2010: key indicators of well-being,* Washington DC, 2010, U.S. Government Printing Office.)

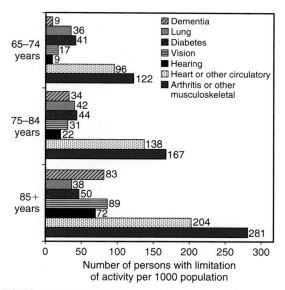

FIGURE **14-2** Activity limitation caused by chronic conditions among older adults, 2006-2007. (From National Center for Health Statistics: *Health, United States, 2009: with special feature on medical technology,* Hyattsville, MD, 2010.)

earlier cohorts, and rates of disability are declining or stabilizing (Manton et al., 2008). Future cohorts of older people may be healthier and more functional well into their eighties and nineties, but the obesity epidemic has the potential to reduce these gains. However, rates of disability and chronic illness continue to be higher among racially and ethnically diverse older adults and need continued attention (see Chapter 4). Key strategies for improving the health of older people are presented in Box 14-1.

BOX **14-1**   **Key Strategies for Improving the Health of Older People**

- Healthy lifestyle behaviors at all ages
- Injury prevention
- Delivery of culturally appropriate clinical preventive services
- Immunizations and preventive screenings
- Increased funding for prevention and health promotion at all ages
- Address cognitive impairment
- Address issues related to mental health
- Attention to quality end-of-life care and palliative care programs
- Implementation and evaluation of chronic illness management programs
- Include public health, aging, prevention and chronic illness management in education of health care professionals

Prevention

Research has shown that chronic illness and poor health are not inevitable consequences of aging. Many chronic illnesses are preventable through lifestyle choices or early detection and management of risk factors. Risk factors for chronic illness begin early in life and continue through adulthood so a life span approach is essential. Health promotion activities and attention to healthy lifestyle habits throughout life can postpone and reduce morbidity for older people.

Four modifiable health risk behaviors: lack of physical activity, poor nutrition, tobacco use, and excessive alcohol consumption are responsible for much of the illness, suffering, and early death related to chronic diseases (Centers for Disease Control and Prevention [CDC], 2012). Exciting research in the field of epigenetics is leading to new understanding of the effect of environmental factors and lifestyle habits such as diet, stress, smoking, and prenatal nutrition on life expectancy for individuals and their children (see http://ww.epigenome.org/). *Healthy People 2020* (U.S. Department of Health and Human Services, 2012) recognizes this and includes attention to the effect of early life factors, together with late life factors, on health outcomes.

Wellness in Chronic Illness

High-level wellness is an integrated method of functioning that maximizes the individual's unique potential (Dunn, 1972). Physical manifestations of chronic illness are often multiple and serious but need not kill the spirit or define the person. The wellness approach suggests that every person has an optimal level of functioning to achieve a good and satisfactory existence (well-being). Even in chronic illness and dying, an optimum level of wellness and well-being is attainable for each individual.

Theoretical Frameworks for Chronic Illness

Several theoretical frameworks have been used to understand the effect of chronic illness and organize the nurse's response to calls from persons with chronic illness: the Chronic Illness Trajectory (Strauss & Glaser, 1975; Corbin & Strauss, 1992), and the Shifting Perspectives Model (Paterson, 2001).

Chronic Illness Trajectory

The trajectory model, originally conceptualized by Anselm Strauss and Barney Glaser (1975) and later Corbin and Strauss (1992), has long aided health care providers to better understand the realities of chronic illness and its effect on individuals. According to this theoretical approach, chronic illness can be viewed from a life course perspective or along a trajectory trace. In this way, the course of a person's illness can be viewed as an integral part of their lives rather than an isolated event. The nurse's response is then holistic rather than isolated. Woog (1992) divided Glaser

and Strauss' model into eight phases for the purpose of identifying goals and developing interventions (Table 14-1). The shape and stability of the trajectory is influenced by the combined efforts, attitudes, and beliefs held by the older person, family members, and significant others, and the involved health care providers. Key points of the model are presented in Box 14-2.

The Shifting Perspectives Model of Chronic Illness

The chronic illness trajectory model described earlier views living with a chronic illness as a progression of phases in which the person follows a predictable trajectory. The Shifting Perspectives Model (Paterson, 2001), derived from a synthesis of qualitative research findings, views living with chronic illness as an ongoing, continually shifting process in which the person moves between the perspectives of wellness in the foreground or illness in the foreground.

This model is more reflective of an "insider" perspective on chronic illness as opposed to the more traditional "outsider" view. Further, this model provides a change in perspective from the traditional approach of patient-as-client to one of client-as-partner in care, and focuses on health within illness rather than loss and burden (Larsen et al., 2006, p. 40). People's perspective of the chronic illness is neither right nor wrong but is a reflection of their needs and situation. How people perceive the chronic illness at any given time influences how they interpret and respond

TABLE 14-1	The Chronic Illness Trajectory
Phase	**Definition**
1. Pre-trajectory	Before the illness course begins, the preventive phase, no signs or symptoms present
2. Trajectory Onset	Signs and symptoms are present, includes diagnostic period
3. Crisis	Life-threatening situation
4. Acute	Active illness or complications that require hospitalization for management
5. Stable	Controlled illness course/symptoms
6. Unstable	Illness course/symptoms not controlled by regimen but not requiring or desire hospitalization
7. Downward	Progressive decline in physical/mental status characterized by increasing disability/symptoms
8. Dying	Immediate weeks, days, hours preceding death

Examples of goals that nurses might establish include the following:
1. To assist a client in overcoming a plateau by increasing adherence to a regimen so that he or she might reach the highest level of functional ability possible within limits of the disability.
2. To assist a client in making the attitudinal and lifestyle changes that are needed to promote health and prevent disease.
3. To assist a client who is in a downward trajectory to be able to maintain sense of self and receive expert palliative care.
4. To assist with advance care planning to assure wishes are met.
5. To assist the client who is in an unstable phase to gain greater control over symptoms that are interfering with his or her ability to carry out everyday activities.

See Woog P: *The chronic illness trajectory framework: the Corbin and Strauss nursing model,* New York, 1992, Springer.

BOX 14-2 Key Points in the Chronic Illness Trajectory Framework

- The majority of health problems in late life are chronic.
- Chronic illnesses may be lifelong and entail lifetime adaptations.
- Chronic illness and its management often profoundly affect the lives and identities of both the individual and the family members or significant others.
- The acute phase of illness management is designed to stabilize physiological processes and promote a recovery (comeback) from the acute phase.
- Other phases of management are designed primarily to maximize and extend the period of stability in the home, with the help of family and augmented by visits to and from health care providers and other members of the rehabilitation and restoration team.
- Maintaining stable phases is central in the work of managing chronic illness.
- A primary care nurse is often in the role of coordinator of the multiple resources that may be needed to promote quality of life along the trajectory.

---

to the disease, themselves, caregivers, and situations affected by the illness (Paterson, 2001; Lindqvist et al., 2006).

Chronic illness contains elements of both illness and wellness, and people with chronic illness live in the "dual kingdoms of the well and the sick" (Donnelly, 1993, p. 6). The illness in the foreground perspective is characterized by a focus on sickness and the suffering, loss, and burden the illness causes. The illness in the foreground perspective occurs when people are newly diagnosed, when new disease-related symptoms appear, or during an acute phase of the illness. This perspective has a protective function, may assist in conserving energy, and helps a person learn more about the illness and try to adjust and come to terms with it (Paterson, 2001).

Shifts toward the illness in the foreground perspective occur when there are perceived threats to control (signs of disease progression, lack of skills to manage the symptoms, disease-related stigma, interactions with others that emphasize dependence and hopelessness). Return to the wellness perspective calls for courage and resilience as well as the development of strategies and resources to adjust to the changes. Nurses can assist by understanding the person's perspective and providing education and support. The shift from illness to wellness is an active process triggered by the need to return to the wellness perspective.

In the wellness in the foreground perspective, the focus is centered more on the self than the disease and its consequences. The illness becomes part of who a person is but it does not define the person. The illness is seen as an opportunity for growth and meaningful changes in relationships with the environment and others. This perspective is fostered by learning as much as possible about the illness, creating supportive environments, paying attention to one's own patterns of response to the illness, and sharing one's knowledge of the disease with others.

With this perspective, one is able to focus on the emotional, spiritual, and social aspects of life while still attending to disease management and the effects of the illness on one's life. Health care professionals who see the person with chronic illness as sick, focusing only on the disease and its symptoms, may not provide opportunities or support for wellness.

Paterson (2001) suggests that the shifting perspectives model calls for understanding the person's perspective and the reasons the person varies in his or her attention to symptoms; the nurse must support persons with either perspective. The person shifts between a wellness and an illness perspective depending on the moment and the needs and demands of living with a chronic illness. At any point in time, one may take precedence over the other, but the goal is to move toward the highest level of well-being even in the presence of illness through appropriate interventions.

Implications for Gerontological Nursing and Healthy Aging

Chronic illnesses are illnesses to live with, and nursing's response is one of long-term caring. The focus of treatment for chronic illness is seldom on cure, but rather on care for the person. This kind of nursing requires a different focus from acute care nursing, where the emphasis is on attention to immediate and life-threatening needs and attempts to cure. "Chronic health problems are not fixable with shiny new technology, and do not promise the suspense, exhilarating hope, and dramatic ending that acute medical crises often do. They simply continue day after day, often invisible or misunderstood" (Hodges et al., 2001, p. 390).

Assessment

Assessment of the elder with a chronic illness involves the selection of appropriate tools, ongoing evaluation of responses and outcomes, careful observation, periodic monitoring, alert watchfulness, and most importantly, discussion and collaboration with elders about their perceptions and the meaning their illness has for them. In the case of chronic illness and the great variability in presentation and impact on individual lifestyle, adequate assessment is critical. In chronic illness, assessment focuses on function and how the chronic illness affects function.

Functional assessments strive to identify the quantity and quality of disability in chronic illness. These assessments, although sometimes not specific to the medical treatment regimen, are often a good measure of the patient's response and adaptation to chronic health problems. Disability assessment helps identify the gap between the existing patient self-care abilities and needed self-care resources. The difference between these two (existing abilities and needed resources) identifies areas where nursing care should focus. In this approach to assessment we are embracing the idea of an illness as chronic; patients can achieve various degrees of adaptation, and as nurses we can help maximize their function and therefore their quality of life. Chapter 7 discusses comprehensive assessment and assessment instruments.

Because many people with chronic illness manage their conditions in a community setting and may need assistance from caregivers, assessment must also focus on the ability of family or significant others to assist and cope with caregiving. Chapter 24 presents a discussion of the caregiving role.

Interventions

Interventions in the care of chronically ill individuals must take into consideration the client's emotional responses, perspectives on the illness, individual needs, self-care ability, support from family and friends, and available resources, as well as the trajectory experience. Chronic illness affects all aspects of a person's life, and interventions must be holistic in focus. Eliopoulos (2001, p. 480) states, "The success to which a chronic condition is managed can make the difference between a satisfying lifestyle, in which control of the illness is but one routine component, and a life controlled by the demands of the illness."

Older adults with chronic illnesses are not seeking cure; rather, they need care of the highest quality. Nursing's response of caring brings this expertise to assist people in adapting, continuing to grow, and attaining a level of wellness and wholeness despite chronic illnesses and functional limitations. "The nurse-client relationship is integral to the care of people living with a chronic illness" (Giddings et al., 2007, p. 564). Gerontological nurses know that understanding and caring for older adults with chronic illnesses and long-term disabilities requires close caring relationships and accompanying the person on their journey, day after day, with hope, courage, and joy. Nursing roles in the care of persons with chronic illnesses are presented in Box 14-3.

Improving Care for Chronic Illness

Caring for patients with chronic illness is different than caring for patients with episodic illnesses. Individuals with chronic conditions "need care that is coordinated across time and centered on their needs, values and preferences. They need self-management skills to ensure the prevention of predictable complications, and they need providers who understand the fundamental difference between episodic illness that is identified and cured, and chronic conditions

---

BOX 14-3   Nursing Roles in Caring for Persons with Chronic Illness

- Listen to the story, and come to know the person and what gives him or her meaning in life.
- Provide education about the illness and its management.
- Provide ongoing assessment with a focus on prevention of complications.
- Relieve symptoms that interfere with function and quality of life.
- Help clients set realistic goals and expectations.
- Focus on potential rather than limitations.
- Teach the skills required for effective self-care.
- Ensure delivery of needed care and support for both the person and the family or significant others.

- Encourage verbalization of feelings.
- Provide support for losses and facilitate the grieving process.
- Provide access to resources.
- Refer appropriately and when needed.
- Assist in helping the chronically ill person balance the effects of treatment on quality of life.
- Maintain hope through development of caring, reciprocal relationships, and hopeful environments.
- Assist to die with dignity and comfort.

that require management across many years" (WHO, 2012, pps. 16-17). The traditional medical care model and models of public health have not been effective in dealing with the complexity of chronic illness. Additionally, the training, education, and skill of today's health care personnel is not adequate to provide evidence-based care to individuals with chronic illness (WHO, 2012). Enhanced content in care of older adults and other individuals with chronic illness is essential in health care education programs.

Although not all people with a chronic illness experience high care needs, the cost of care for those who do is rising exorbitantly, and funding is becoming increasingly limited. Almost half of Americans living with chronic illness reported that the cost of care is a financial burden; 89% have difficulty in obtaining adequate health insurance; and 72% report having difficulty getting necessary care from health care providers (Chin et al., 2006).

People with chronic illnesses often have to navigate a system that requires them to coordinate several disparate financing and delivery systems themselves, making it more difficult to obtain the full range of appropriate services. People who need access to different programs are likely to find that each program has different eligibility criteria and sets of providers, and that there is little communication or coordination between providers. As a result, the health care delivery system for those with chronic illnesses is complex and confusing, and care is often fragmented, less effective, and more costly. A summary of the challenges in care of the older person with a chronic illness is presented in Box 14-4.

BOX 14-4 Challenges in the Care of the Older Person with a Chronic Illness

- Long-term and uncertain nature of the illness
- Costs associated with care
- Little coordination of care across the continuum
- Inadequate funding for preventive and long-term care
- Lack of health care professionals with expertise in geriatrics and chronic care
- Acute and episodic focus in medical care and in reimbursement
- Growing numbers of uninsured and continued disparities in health care outcomes for racially and culturally diverse individuals
- Need for active partnership between the individual and family and significant others and the health care provider

---

To create a well-functioning health care system, reform is necessary at many levels. The World Health Organization (WHO) has provided a conceptual framework that addresses the components necessary to improve care for patients with chronic illness "across multiple levels of the health care system: the general policy environment, the health care organization and community, and the patient-care level" (2005, p. 17) (Box 14-5).

Model Chronic Illness Self-Management Programs

More research is needed to evaluate models of care for chronic illness that enhance self management and promote successful outcomes while decreasing costly hospitalizations. *Healthy People 2020* includes self-management of chronic diseases as an important individual behavior determinant of health. The Centers for Medicare & Medicaid Services is conducting and evaluating projects involving disease management, case management, and transitional care (see Chapter 3) designed to improve quality and outcomes of care for older adults with chronic illness (http://www.innovations.cms.gov/initiatives/index.html). The Affordable Health Care Act also includes several initiatives for chronic illness management.

Many of these models utilize registered and advanced practice nurses and there are many opportunities for the profession of nursing to assume a leadership role in improving care for individuals with chronic illness (see Chapter 3). Characteristics of successful models include some key features (Box 14-6). Several models, including Geriatric Resources for Assessment and Care of Elders Model (GRACE), Guided Care Results, and the Program of All Inclusive Care for the Elderly (PACE), are described by Boult and Wieland (2010).

Implications for Gerontological Nursing and Healthy Aging

In summary, management of chronic illness in late life is an issue for the individual, the family, the health care profession, and the world. Nurses work toward the achievement of the goals of *Healthy People 2020* to prepare individuals for a healthier old age and to enhance health and wellness for those already in later life. Nurses must work with older adults holistically to maximize their assets, minimize their limitations, and make the most of what they have. Nursing roles may include direct caregiver, resource person, advisor, teacher, and facilitator.

BOX 14-5   Competencies to Improve Care for Chronic Conditions

1. Patient-Centered Care
- Interviewing and communicating effectively
- Identifying, caring about, and respecting patient's preferences, values, differences, and expressed needs
- Understanding and incorporating the experience of living with chronic illness from the perspective of those living with the illness
- Assisting changes in health-related behaviors
- Providing education and information
- Promoting wellness and healthy lifestyles
- Coordinating continuous and timely care
- Supporting self-management
- Relieving pain and suffering; shift from acute to palliative care as needed
- Sharing decision making and management

2. Partnering
- Partnering with patients
- Partnering with other providers
- Partnering with communities

3. Quality Improvement
- Measuring care delivery and outcomes
- Learning and adapting to change
- Translating evidence into practice

4. Information and Communication Technology
- Designing and using patient registries
- Electronic patient records
- Using computer technologies
- Communicating with partners

5. Public Health Perspective
- Providing population-based care
- Systems thinking
- Working across the care continuum
- Working in primary health care–led systems

Modified from World Health Organization: *Preparing a health care workforce for the 21st century: the challenge of chronic conditions,* World Health Organization, 2005. Available at http://www.who.int/chp/knowledge/publications/workforce_report/en/.

BOX 14-6   Characteristics of Successful Chronic Illness Management Models

- Teams of health care professionals (always includes nursing)
- Comprehensive assessment (CGA)
- Development of a comprehensive care plan that incorporates evidence based protocols
- Implementation of the plan over time
- Promotion of patient and family caregivers active engagement in care
- Proactive monitoring of the patient's clinical status and adherence to the care plan
- Coordination of professionals in care of the patient
- Coordination of primary care, specialty care, hospitals, EDs, SNFs, other medical institutions, and community agencies
- Facilitation of transitions across settings and access to community resources
- Facilitation of the patient's access to community resources, such as meals programs, handicapped-accessible transportation, adult day centers, support groups, and exercise programs

Modified from Boult and Wieland, 2010

This kind of nursing requires a different focus than acute care nursing, where the emphasis is on attention to immediate and life-threatening needs and attempts to cure. Chronic illnesses, on the other hand, are illnesses to live with, and nursing's response is one of long-term caring. Progress is not measured in attempts to achieve cure, but rather in maintenance of a steady state or regression of the condition, all the while remembering that the condition does not define the person. Understanding the meaning of the experience of chronic illness from the person's perspective, a holistic approach, and working collaboratively with the person are of utmost importance.

Living with chronic and disabling conditions often puts a damper on all but the most robust individual. Because an illness limits an older person physically or cognitively, it does not have to limit the person's human potential. Healthy aging does not mean the absence of disease; rather, it means moving toward wellness in spite of disease. Someone once said that a chronic illness is like a grain of sand in an oyster; it irritates and creates a pearl, or the oyster just dies. Part of nursing intervention is aimed at helping create that pearl.

Application of Maslow's Hierarchy

Chronic illnesses and the consequences of treatment can affect an older adult's ability to fulfill basic physiological needs without assistance or adaptation. Nursing interventions are directed at enhancing self-care abilities as well as providing care to ensure that basic needs can be met with as much independence as possible. A wellness approach centers on assisting elders to meet as many of Maslow's defined needs as possible. Chronic illnesses and disabilities may impair physical function, but a sense of safety, security, belonging, self-esteem, and self-actualization can still be attained. Maintaining integrity and achieving one's maximal potential despite functional limitations and illness may be one of the greater accomplishments of many older people. Our care must support the potential for wellness at all stages in life.

KEY CONCEPTS

- Declines in mortality, a growing older adult population, increasing medical expertise, and sophisticated technological developments have resulted in a great increase in the survival of the very old with multiple chronic disorders.
- The effects of chronic illness range from mild to life-limiting, with each person responding to unique circumstances in a highly individualized manner.
- The Chronic Illness Trajectory and the Shifting Perspectives Model of Chronic Illness offer useful frameworks to understand chronic illness and design nursing interventions.
- People with chronic illnesses can achieve wellness, and the role of the nurse is critical in the promotion of wellness.
- The goals of healthy aging include minimizing risk for disease, encouraging health promotion, and in the presence of disease, alleviating symptoms, delaying or avoiding the development of complications, and maximizing function and quality of life.
- New models of cost-effective care are needed that increase access and improve outcomes and quality of

life for persons with chronic illness. Nurses are particularly well prepared to assume major roles in chronic illness care.

ACTIVITIES AND DISCUSSION QUESTIONS

1. What type of education and counseling might the nurse provide to a 30-year-old client to promote health and prevent chronic illness in later life?
2. What do you think would be the most devastating loss in activities of daily living?
4. What are some nursing interventions to assist a person with chronic illness to deal with loss? Practice or role-play various ways that these issues can be addressed.
5. How would you encourage an individual toward maximal participation in self-care?
6. What would be the measures of wellness during chronic illness?

REFERENCES

Boult C, Wieland G: Comprehensive primary care for older patients with multiple chronic conditions: "nobody rushes you through", *JAMA* 304(17): 1936–1943, 2010.

Centers for Disease Control and Prevention [CDC] (2012). *Chronic disease and health promotion*. Available at www.cdc.gov/chronicdiease/overview/index.htm.

Chin P, Papenhausen J, Burgess C: Nurse case management. In Lubkin I, P Larsen P, editors: *Chronic illness: impact and interventions*, Sudbury, MA, 2006, Jones & Bartlett.

Corbin JM, Strauss A: A nursing model for chronic illness management based upon the trajectory framework. In Woog P, editor: *The chronic illness framework: the Corbin and Strauss nursing model*, New York, 1992, Springer.

Curtin M, Lubkin I: What is chronicity? In Lubkin I, Larsen P, editors: *Chronic illness: impact and interventions*, Sudbury, MA, 2006, Jones & Bartlett.

Donnelly G: Chronicity: concepts and reality, *Holist Nurs Prac* 8(1):1–7, 2003.

Dunn HL: *High level wellness*, ed 2, Arlington, VA, 1972, Beatty.

Eliopoulos C: *Gerontological nursing*, ed 6, Philadelphia, 2001, Lippincott Williams & Wilkins.

Fries JF: Reducing disability in older age, *JAMA* 288:3164, 2002.

Giddings L, Roy D, Predeger E: Women's experience of ageing with a chronic condition, *J Adv Nurs* 58(6):557–565, 2007.

Hodges HF, Keeley AC, Grier EC: Masterworks of art and chronic illness experiences in the elderly, *J Adv Nurs* 36(3):389–398, 2001.

Hooyman N, Kiyak H: *Social gerontology*, ed 9, Boston, 2011, Pearson.

Hwang W, Weller W, Ireys H, et al: Out of pocket medical spending for care of chronic conditions, *Health Affairs* 20(6):268–269, 2001.

Jevne R: Enhancing hope in the chronically ill, *Hum Med* 9(2):121–130, 1993.

Larsen P, Lewis P, Lubkin I: Illness behavior and roles, In Lubkin I, Larsen P: *Chronic illness: impact and interventions,* Sudbury, MA, 2006, Jones & Bartlett.

Lindqvist O, Widmark A, Rasmussen B: Reclaiming wellness—living with bodily problems, as narrated by men with advanced prostate cancer, *Cancer Nurs* 29(4):327–337, 2006.

Lundman B, Jansson L: The meaning of living with a long-term disease: to revalue and be revalued, *J Nurs Chron Illness* in association with *J Clin Nurs* 16(7b):109–115, 2007.

Manton K, Gu X, Lowrimore G: Cohort changes in active life expectancy in the U.S. elderly population: experience from the 1982-2004 national long term care survey, *J Gerontol B Psychol Sci Soc Sci* 63B(5):S269–281, 2008.

Paterson BL: The shifting perspectives model of chronic illness, *J Nurs Scholarsh* 33(1):21–26, 2001.

Strauss A, Glaser B: *Chronic illness and the quality of life,* St. Louis, 1975, Mosby.

U.S. Department of Health and Human Services. Office of Disease Prevention and Health Promotion. *Healthy People 2020* (2012). Available at http://www.healthypeople.gov/2020.

Woog P: *The chronic illness trajectory framework: the Corbin and Strauss nursing model,* New York, 1992, Springer.

World Health Organization [WHO]: *Preparing a health care workforce for the 21st century: the challenge of chronic conditions* (2005). Available at www.who.int/chp/knowledge/publications/workforce_report/en/.

World Health Organization [WHO]: *Preventing chronic diseases: a vital investment* (2012). Available at www.who.int/chp/chronic_disease_report/en/.

Zauszniewski J, Bekhet A, Lai C, et al: Effects of teaching resourcefulness and acceptance on affect, behavior, and cognition of chronically ill elders, *Issues Mental Health Nurs* 28(6):575–592, 2007.

CHAPTER 15

Pain and Comfort

Kathleen F. Jett

evolve.elsevier.com/Ebersole/gerontological

LEARNING OBJECTIVES

Upon completion of this chapter, the reader will be able to:

- Define the concept of pain and how this may be interpreted by the older adult.
- Differentiate the various types of pain.
- Identify data to include in a pain assessment.
- Describe pharmacological and nonpharmacological measures to promote comfort for the person in pain.
- Discuss the goals of pain management in aging.
- Discuss the special circumstances of pain in the cognitively impaired or nonverbal person.
- Develop a nursing care plan for an elder in acute pain and chronic pain.

GLOSSARY

Adjuvant A drug that has a primary use other than pain (e.g., antidepressant, anticonvulsant) but also is used to enhance the effects of traditional pain medication.

Equianalgesic The dosage and route of administration of one drug that produces approximately the same degree of effect as the dosage of another drug.

Titration The adjustment of the dosage of a given medication until the desired effect is produced.

THE LIVED EXPERIENCE

Ms. S. had cancer of the stomach and was in moderate to severe pain most of the time. She was referred to the local hospice, and the nurse worked with her and her physician to make Ms. S. comfortable. First the nurse assessed potential causes for the pain, the level of pain, the type of pain, and what level of relief was desired. After a careful titration of her medications, it was found that only a long-acting morphine provided her with comfort and an improved quality of life. However, at the dose needed she also hallucinated, seeing several puppies in the room with her. When asked if she wanted to reduce the dosage to eliminate this side effect, she responded, "No—I'll keep the puppies, I know they are not real and they don't hurt anything. I'd rather have them with me than the pain."

Helen, age 93

Pain is a sensation of distress, be it physical, psychological, or spiritual; it occurs at the foundational level of Maslow's Hierarchy of Needs. Pain is a multidimensional phenomenon, and usually one type is intertwined with another. Pain is always a subjective experience; it is whatever a person says it is. When one is in pain it can result in reduced socialization, impaired mobility, or even a reconsideration of the meaning of one's life.

How pain is expressed is highly influenced by the unique history of the individual and the meaning he or she ascribes to the pain. Some are only able to express pain in terms of "not feeling well," others are highly articulate but controlled; still others are highly vocal and expressive. It is important for the nurse to realize that an individual responds to pain in a way that reflects his or her own cultural expectations and understanding of acceptable behavior. How we respond to pain is part of who we are—part of our very core. Even the words we use to describe it are personal and many. Pain may be referred to as an ache, a hurt, a pester, a nuisance, a bother and so forth, with the language and the willingness to express it a manifestation of the person's relationship to whom he or she is speaking.

The communication of pain is often not straightforward. Depression masks expression, as do sedating drugs (which do not necessarily ease pain). The nurse cannot assume that those individuals who do not, cannot, or will not verbalize their pain in ways that are standard practice in the medical model (see Chapter 4), for whatever reason, do not have pain or as much pain as others. Instead, the nurse must be alert to the cues that suggest that pain and discomfort are present. He or she must counter myths, stereotypes, and generalizations often held about aging and pain, such as that older adults, especially those with cognitive impairments, don't feel as much pain, or that they complain all the time (and are therefore ignored) (Box 15-1). The nurse can be instrumental in understanding the person and providing comfort.

This measurement of comfort provided to patients is a quality indicator, that is, a marker of the level of care that is being provided (Joint Commission, 2012; Schofield, 2010). As is pain, comfort is uniquely defined, experienced, and expressed by each person as members of a family, community, and culture. Comfort is a personal and intrinsic balance of the most basic physiological, emotional, social, and spiritual needs. Without the level of comfort sought by the individual, wellness is beyond reach.

Expert pain management is now part of evidence-based practice (see the Evidence-Based Practice box). Health care providers, including nurses, are expected to adequately address patients' pain; it is now considered the "fifth vital sign." Nonetheless, there remains inadequate assessment and undertreatment of pain, especially when the patient is an older adult, from a minority group, or residing in a nursing home (Inelman et al., 2011; Smith, 2005). The reasons for this undertreatment are many and include the nurses' own definitions and expectations of how pain is expressed. As are patients, nurses are influenced by the way we respond to pain—in this case, the pain of others. The influences come from the nurses' personal and professional experiences, culture, and so on. Yet we have a responsibility to let go of our own expectations and promote comfort for those who are suffering, regardless of the cause and manner of expression of this suffering. The best gerontological nursing care is that which is provided in a nonjudgmental manner with the goal of comfort always—not just to lessen pain but to relieve it and prevent its reoccurrence.

BOX 15-1   Fact and Fiction About Pain in Older Adults

MYTH: Pain is a normal part of aging.
FACT: Pain is not part of the normal changes with aging; however, its occurrence increases with age.
MYTH: Pain sensitivity and perception decrease with aging.
FACT: Not true; however, the older adult may appear to have a greater tolerance for pain due to adjustment to inadequate relief of long standing.
MYTH: If patients don't complain of pain, they do not have pain.
FACT: Persons may not report pain for a variety of reasons but nonetheless have pain. They may feel that it is culturally inappropriate to "complain" of pain or feel that they are burdensome to those around them, including nurses.
MYTH: A person who has no functional impairment, appears occupied, or is otherwise distracted from pain must not have significant pain.
FACT: Patients have a variety of reactions to pain. Many patients are stoic and refuse to "give in" to their pain.
MYTH: Narcotic medications are inappropriate unless used for short periods of time.
FACT: Opioid analgesics are often the best treatment for moderate to severe persistent pain in order to help restore the person's ability to function and have some quality of life.
MYTH: Potential side effects of narcotic medication make them too dangerous to use in older adults.
FACT: Narcotics may be used safely in older adults.

EVIDENCE-BASED PRACTICE

Pain Management

- Evidence-based recommendations from the International Association for the Study of Pain for the management of neuropathic pain (2007):
  http://www.rsds.org/pdfsall/Dworkin_OConner_Backonja.pdf
- Consensus Statement from an Expert Panel related to the use of WHO step III opioids (2008):
  http://onlinelibrary.wiley.com/doi/10.1111/j.1533-2500.2008.00204.x/pdf
- Clinical Practice Recommendations from the American Society of Pain Management Nurses (2006):
  http://www.painmanagementnursing.org/article/S1524-9042(06)00033-6/abstract
- Nursing Standard of Practice Protocol: Pain Management in Older Adults (2012):
  http://consultgerirn.org/topics/pain/want_to_know_more

Acute and Persistent Pain

Pain is first classified as that which is related to cancer or noncancer. It is either acute or persistent, otherwise known as chronic, and finally it is classified as nociceptive, neuropathic, or idiopathic. It also may be of mixed types (Box 15-2).

Acute Pain

Acute noncancer pain in late life, as in earlier life, is usually episodic in nature. Acute physical pain is temporary and includes postoperative, procedural, and traumatic pain. Acute physical pain is usually easily controlled by common analgesic medications. In the hospital setting an analgesic pump controlled by the patient is used for a restricted period. Acute pain at some point is a universal experience for older adults owing simply to the length of life lived, opportunities for traumatic injury, and the development of pain-producing illness. At the same time, the older one is, the more likely one will have an adverse reaction to a medication (see Chapter 8). For example, most analgesics cause sedation. Although use of the medication may be necessary, this side effect also increases the risk for falls, delirium, and any of the geriatric syndromes. In most cases acute pain in older adult is superimposed on a preexisting level of persistent pain, primarily because of the very high prevalence of osteoarthritis (see Chapter 18).

Acute pain may also be psychological or spiritual in nature, such as in early bereavement or in a major depressive episode. Because of the high number of losses in the lives of older adults (see Chapters 24 and 25), the risk for such acute pain is high.

Persistent Pain

Research has indicated that physical pain in late life tends to be persistent, moderate to severe, and present in about 50% of those over 65 years of age living in the community in the United States (Horgas & Yoon, 2008; Schofield, 2010) and includes those with long-standing cancer pain. For those living in long-term care facilities, the number of those in pain, largely untreated or undertreated, is thought to be much higher, perhaps 85% (Horgas & Yoon, 2008; Robinson, 2010). The barriers to adequate care are many (Box 15-3).

The most common type of pain in later life is persistent, noncancer, and musculoskeletal in nature, and from arthritis and degenerative spinal conditions (e.g., degenerative joint disease [DJD]) (American Geriatrics Society [AGS], 2009). Neuralgias occur frequently from long-standing diabetes, peripheral vascular disease, herpes zoster, and other syndromes such as stroke and iatrogenic side effects with treatment such as following chemotherapy.

Loneliness and emotional pain from loss (see Chapters 22 and 25) decrease the ability to cope with physical pain. The psychosocial aspects of an elder's pain experience are rarely or superficially assessed by the nurse or included in the plan of care. The current cohort of pre–baby boomers in pain may underreport pain and undertreat themselves because of the cost of the medications, belief in an associated stigma, attribution of the pain to normal burdens of "old age," or the fear of addiction.

Persistent pain may be a sequela to an episode of acute pain (e.g., herpes zoster for physical pain or the emotional pain of bereavement); it is not time-limited and may vary in

---

> ### BOX 15-2   Types of Physical Pain Sensations
>
> - **Nociceptive pain** is associated with injury to the skin, mucosa, muscle, or bone and is usually the result of stimulation of pain receptors. This type of pain arises from tissue inflammation, trauma, burns, infection, ischemia, arthropathies (rheumatoid arthritis, osteoarthritis, gout), nonarticular inflammatory disorders, skin and mucosal ulcerations, and internal organ and visceral pain from distention, obstruction, inflammation, compression, or ischemia of organs. Pancreatitis, appendicitis, and tumor infiltration are common causes of visceral pain. Nociceptive mechanisms usually respond well to common analgesic medications and nonpharmacological interventions.
> - **Neuropathic pain** involves a pathophysiological process of the peripheral or central nervous system and presents as altered sensation and discomfort. Conditions causing this type of pain include postherpetic or trigeminal neuralgia, poststroke or postamputation pain (phantom pain), diabetic neuropathy, or radiculopathies (e.g., spinal stenosis). This type of pain may be described as stabbing, tingling, burning, or shooting. Neuropathic pain is very difficult to treat and may occur at the same time as nociceptive and idiopathic (from an unknown cause) pain.
> - **Mixed or unspecified pain** usually has mixed or unknown causes. Examples include recurrent headaches and vasculitis. A compression fracture causing nerve root irritation, common in older people with osteoporosis, is an example of a mix of nociceptive and neuropathic pain.

intensity throughout the day or with changes in activity.
For example, persons with depression usually feel worse in
the morning with a lifting of mood as the day progresses
(see Chapter 22). Persons with rheumatoid arthritis also
have the most pain in the morning with slow but limited
improvement with movement. Herpes zoster presents a
unique situation in part due to a number of factors.

Herpes Zoster

Nearly 1 million cases of herpes zoster (HZ), or shingles,
occur each year, most often in persons between 60 and
79 years of age, most often after the age of 50. About 1 in
5 people who have had chickenpox will develop shingles
at some time in their lives (NINDS, 2011). HZ is a viral
infection which is dormant in the nerve cells only to erupt
decades later. It is characterized by the sensations of
itching, and what is often acute stinging, burning pain
along the pathway of the affected nerve (dermatome).
Finally serous vesicles erupt in the area where the pain was
felt. An acute episode or outbreak lasts from days to weeks.
When the eye is affected, it is a medical emergency with a
high risk of blindness and brain involvement.

A combination of antiviral medications, steroids, aspirin, and topical anesthetics may be the most effective for
the acute outbreaks. However, the most important aspect
of an HZ outbreak is in the risk for the development of a
chronic neuropathic pain syndrome after the resolution of
the acute infection and pain. The chronic pain condition is
known as postherpetic neuralgia (PHN) and can be quite
intense. Antiviral agents such as acyclovir and famciclovir
may shorten the duration of an outbreak and may prevent
PHN when given promptly. PHN is persistent pain from
the now damaged nerves following HZ and hard to treat
once established. Narcotics may be necessary for pain relief
but as the cause is neuropathic they are not always effective.
Low doses of tricyclic antidepressants (e.g., desipramine,
amitriptyline [Elavil]) have also been used but in most cases
considered inappropriate in older adults because of their
anticholinergic effects and the availability of safer alternatives (AGS, 2012) (see Chapter 8). Instead, anticonvulsants
especially gabapentin (Neurontin), and pregabalin (Lyrica)
have been found to be useful for some persons with fewer
side effects.

In promoting healthy aging the nurse can advocate
for and facilitate shingles vaccine campaigns. Research
has indicated that the number of expected cases can be
reduced by over 50% for those who receive the vaccine. It
cannot be used for those who have an acute infection or
are suffering from PHN (NINDS, 2011).

Pain in Elders with Cognitive Impairments

Persons with cognitive impairment are consistently untreated or undertreated for pain (Herr et al., 2006a, 2006b;
Kovach et al., 2006a, 2006b; Ware et al., 2006). Studies
have shown that older adults who are cognitively impaired
receive less pain medication, even though there is no
convincing evidence that peripheral transmission of the
sensation of pain to the brain is impaired in people with
dementia (Herr & Decker, 2004, pp. 47-48). However as
persons with dementia cannot always express their pain or
understand why or where they are feeling it, their expressions of pain may be different from those who can express
themselves. It is best to practice under the "assumption

that any condition that is painful to a cognitively intact person would also be painful to those with advanced dementia who cannot express themselves" (Herr, 2010, p. S1). Research has suggested that older people with mild to moderate cognitive impairment can provide valid reports of pain using self-report scales, but people with more severe impairment and loss of language skills may be unable to communicate the presence of pain in a manner that is easily understood.

For persons who are no longer able to express themselves verbally either due to dementia or other neurological conditions such as aphasia following a stroke, communication of pain usually occurs through changes in behavior, such as agitation, aggression, increased confusion, or passivity. Caregivers should be educated to be particularly alert for passive behaviors because they are less disruptive and may not be recognized as changes that may signal pain. Providing comfort to those who cannot express themselves requires careful observation of behavior and attention to caregiver reports, knowing when subtle changes have occurred, and a willingness to help (Box 15-4). In nursing homes, the certified nursing assistants (CMAs) play an important role in pain assessment.

BOX 15-4 Pain Cues in the Person with Communication Difficulties

Changes in Behavior
Restlessness and/or agitation or reduction in movement
Repetitive movements
Physical tension such as clenching teeth or hands
Unusually cautious movements, guarding

Activities of Daily Living
Sudden resistance to help from others
Decreased appetite
Decreased sleep

Vocalizations
Person groans, moans, or cries for unknown reasons
Person increases or decreases usual vocalizations

Physical Changes
Pleading expression
Grimacing
Pallor or flushing
Diaphoresis (sweating)
Increased pulse, respirations, or blood pressure

Implications for Gerontological Nursing and Healthy Aging

Care of the elder in pain begins with assessment and continues through to the evaluation of the effectiveness of the interventions. The nurse is usually the person most attuned to the needs of patients and working with other staff members such as nursing assistants can assure that pain interventions are effective; that the patient is comfortable and has the highest quality of life possible regardless of health status or disabling conditions.

Assessment

Pain management begins with a complete history and physical, as well as an assessment specific to pain. For those who are able to express themselves the assessment begins with a person's self-report of pain. The use of spoken, written or visual analog scales (Figure 15-1) has become the standard of care; most can be used cross-culturally or with a person with limited English proficiency. For example, the patient is asked to rate their pain on a scale of 1 to 10, with 1 being no pain and 10 being the worst they can imagine. A person who does not appear to be in pain may be comfortable indicating it on a scale, such as 8 out of 10, or pointing to a drawing of a grimacing or crying face. Visual analog scales have been clinically tested and meet best-practices guidelines for use with older adults (Taylor et al., 2005).

The use of the scale will help the person who would otherwise not report pain directly. Other direct questions include detailed descriptions of pain intensity, **o**nset, **l**ocation, **d**uration, **c**haracteristics, **a**ggravating and **r**elieving factors, and **t**reatment (OLD CART) such as "When did it start?" "Do you have pain [discomfort, etc. based on descriptors acceptable to the individual] now?" "Where is your pain?" "Do you have pain every day?" "How would you describe it?" "What makes it worse?" "What makes it better?" Patients are asked to rate their pain the worst it has ever been and as it is today, now, this week, etc. (Box 15-5). The assessment also includes how the pain is affecting function, sleep, appetite, activity, mood, relationships with others, and other factors particularly pertinent to older adults (Box 15-6). Medication history (especially for what treatments have been tried) includes prescribed medication, herbs and supplements, over-the-counter drugs, and street drugs. Regular, repeated assessments, use of standardized tools with consistent documentation, and communication are the most important components of pain assessment. This leads to the ability to adjust the plan of care promptly, consistently, and expertly in the promotion of comfort. For more information on pain assessment see the *Try This:*

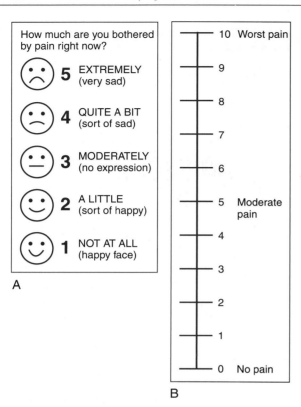

How much are you bothered by pain right now?

5 EXTREMELY (very sad)

4 QUITE A BIT (sort of sad)

3 MODERATELY (no expression)

2 A LITTLE (sort of happy)

1 NOT AT ALL (happy face)

A

10 Worst pain

9

8

7

6

5 Moderate pain

4

3

2

1

0 No pain

B

May be duplicated for use in clinical practice.

FIGURE 15-1 Examples of visual analog scales. **A,** Example of a visual analog scale (VAS) showing a series of faces with expressions of varying intensities. **B,** Example of a numeric rating scale.

BOX 15-5   **Basic Pain Assessment**

1. **Self-report of pain intensity (rating):** _____
2. OLD CART
   Onset: _____
   Location: _____
   Duration: _____

   Characteristics: _____
   Aggravating factors: _____
   Relieving factors: _____
   Treatment previously tried: _____

BOX 15-6   **Additional Factors to Consider When Assessing Pain in Older Adults**

Function: How is the pain affecting the ability to participate in usual activities and perform activities of daily living and instrumental activities of daily living?

Alternative expression of pain: Have there been recent changes in cognitive ability or behavior, such as increased pacing, grimacing, or irritability? Is there an increase in the number of complaints? Are they vague and difficult to respond to? Has there been a change in sleep-wake patterns? Is the person resisting certain activities, movements, or positions?

Social support: What are the resources available to help the person cope and tolerate treatment? How is pain affecting the person's usual role? How is pain affecting relationships with others?

Pain history: How have previous experiences with pain been managed? What is the perceived meaning of the past and the present pain? What are the cultural factors that affect the belief in the meaning of the pain and the ability to express pain and receive relief?

---

materials available at the website for the Hartford Institute for Geriatric Nursing (www.hartfordign.org).

Assessment of Pain in Cognitively Impaired or Nonverbal Older Adults

When the person has cognitive impairments or difficulties with communication, assessment is particularly challenging. When limitations are present due to dementia, delerium, or aphasia, an alternate approach is needed (Box 15-7). Indicators of discomfort most often include restlessness and increased confusion but are at the very best subtle (Box 15-8).

BOX 15-7   **Hierarchy of Pain Assessment in the Cognitively Impaired**

Patient report, even if "yes" or "no"
Evaluate and treat all potential causes of pain
Observe for behaviors that may indicate pain
Surrogate report of behavior change
Observe response to analgesic trial

From Hadjistavropoulos T, Herr K, Turk DC, et al: Interdisciplinary expert consensus statement of pain in older persons, *Clin J Pain* 23(1 Suppl): S1-S43, 2007.

BOX 15-8　"Did My Back Hurt?"

Ms. R. had moderate dementia; she mistook her son for her husband, and did not know that she was in a nursing home. She began moaning from time to time, grimacing and pacing and spending less time "visiting" with the other residents she believed were her guests. She began holding her back and refusing to get out of bed, and when up, to pace with more intensity of motion. An x-ray study of her back showed severe osteoporosis. She was started on calcitonin—a medication for osteoporosis with a side effect of pain relief for some. Over the course of about 6 weeks, Ms. R. began resuming her usual activities and was much cheerier than she had been in a long time. When asked if her back still hurt she responded, "Did my back hurt?" Her back pain was expressed in behavior change. Although she could not express the physical pain, she was nonetheless feeling it: she could only express it in her own way. It was up to the nurse to observe, interpret potential causes, and seek treatment on her behalf.

In 2008 and 2010, Dr. Herr and colleagues conducted reviews of pain assessment tools for use with nonverbal patients and for use in the nursing home setting. The Pain Assessment in Advanced Dementia Scale (PAINAD) and Pain Assessment Checklist for Seniors with Limited Ability to Communicate (PACSLAC) were recommended for use. They are complementary to the Minimum Data Set 3.0 (MDS 3.0) assessment, which is already required for use in the facilities (see Chapter 7). If the person cannot rate his or her pain on one of the pain scales (including pointing) described earlier, it has been recommended that both tools be used to determine the presence or absence of pain based on behavior at initial assessment and during monitoring.

The PAINAD is a simple, short, focused tool that has been found to demonstrate sensitivity to change in response to an intervention or over time (Warden et al., 2003). Four behaviors are rated by an observer on a scale of 0 to 2: breathing when not speaking, negative vocalizations, facial expression and body language, and if the person can be comforted. The tool is described in detail at a number of sites easily available online. It is in use in its original form internationally. The PACSLAC includes four domains of observation: facial expression, activity/body movement, social/personality/mood, and physiological/sleeping/eating/vocal. The PACSLAC can serve as a guide for the care provided by the CNA in a nursing facility (Fuchs-Lachelle & Hadjistavropoulos, 2004; Herr, 2010). Detailed instructions and downloads

of the PACSLAC are available online in various formats. Understanding what the person is trying to communicate through his or her behavior is an essential skill for all staff caring for older people with limitations in ability to communicate.

Interventions

The goals of pain management in the older adult are to promote comfort, maintain the highest level of functioning and self-care possible, and balance the risks and benefits of the various treatment options. Careful use of pharmacological and nonpharmacological approaches helps to achieve these goals. A holistic approach is necessary due to the complex and pervasive nature of pain, especially in later life. Yet achieving pain management is especially challenging.

To provide optimal care of the person in pain, attention is given to all types of pain as well as the spiritual, psychological, and social consequences of physical pain. Reducing suffering calls for first determining if there is a reversible cause, such as a urinary tract infection or a fracture and address these accordingly. If pain persists, the nurse intervenes with expert assessment, careful listening, unconditional positive regard, ongoing support, and mobilization of resources. Use of pillows for support or body positioning, appropriate and comfortable seating and mattresses, frequent rest periods, and pacing of activities to balance activity and rest are important aspects of providing comfort.

The nurse encourages elders and their significant others to have an active role in pain management. The patient can keep a personal journal or pain diary of levels of pain; this includes the times, types, and doses of medication taken, its effect, and the duration of its benefit; and which activities increase or decrease the pain regardless of the type. This information helps establish patterns that may be useful in improving comfort by adjusting activity, providing medications at the right times, and helping the patient feel in control of some aspect of their lives. A pain graph provides a visual picture of the highs and lows of the pain. The diary should be reviewed with the care provider and used to adjust dosages or timing for optimal relief. The website www.optimismonline.com provides an excellent tool for chronicling and recording the highs and lows of psychological pain.

The nurse also encourages patients to stay as active as is possible within their comfort range. When a person has pain with a needed specific activity (e.g., as in rehabilitation or psychotherapy), anticipation anxiety may decrease both the motivation and the ability to participate fully. In this case, the plan of care may include both pharmacological and nonpharmacological interventions such as relaxation before the recommended activity. Administering an effective short-acting medication 30 to 40 minutes before the specific activity may eventually lessen or eliminate the fear of discomfort and can greatly enhance the individual's capacity for that activity (see also Chapters 7 and 22). The nurse should learn the patient's ability to cope with pain and work within those parameters.

Pharmacological Interventions

A pharmacologic approach to pain relief is accomplished by medication aimed at altering sensory transmission to the cerebral cortex. This approach is most effective when implementation of the treatment regimen involves teamwork between the patient, the health care providers (nurses included), family members, and significant others. In some cultures the patient is not the decision maker regarding treatment. Instead the tribal elders, the oldest son, or others must be consulted first with permission of the patient (see Chapter 4).

In 2009, the American Geriatrics Society published an update of their original 1998 guidelines for the management of persistent physical pain. A panel of experts recognized the significant difficulties encountered when using pharmacological interventions in later life but nonetheless urged providers to use these in a manner consistent with the traditional World Health Organization (WHO) stepwise progression (Figure 15-2). Analgesics (nonopioid and opioid agents) and adjuvant medications (antidepressants, anticonvulsants, herbal preparations) have all been found to have a role in promoting comfort in older adults in pain;

however, several age-related changes and common conditions need to be considered. In addition, nonopioid nonsteroidal antiinflammatory drugs (NSAIDs) must be used with more caution than was previously thought (AGS, 2009; AGS, 2012) (Box 15-9).

To achieve the highest level of pain control of any type, it is best to erase the "memory of pain," especially for those whose persistent pain is intense (e.g., some psychological, neuropathic, or cancer-related pain). This means that it is necessary to both relieve and prevent the pain. The most effective way to do this is to provide around-the-clock (ATC) dosing, at the appropriate dosage (Portenoy et al., 2006). In gerontological nursing it is essential that medications are started at the lowest dose possible. However, it is equally as important for the dosages to be titrated to the level that pain is relieved to a point that is acceptable to the patient and the relief is continuous. Too often, while a low dose is started, increases are delayed and suffering is prolonged unnecessarily. The adage "Start low, go slow, but go!" is important to remember.

Nonopioid Analgesics. Acetaminophen (Tylenol) and NSAIDs are the non-narcotic analgesics most often used for relief of physical pain in older adults. Acetaminophen has been found to be effective for the most common causes of pain, such as osteoarthritis and back pain, and should always be considered a first-line approach unless contraindicated (AGS, 2009). If acetaminophen is used for persistent pain, ATC dosing may provide adequate relief. When used appropriately, it is not associated with gastrointestinal bleeding or adverse renal or cardiac effects.

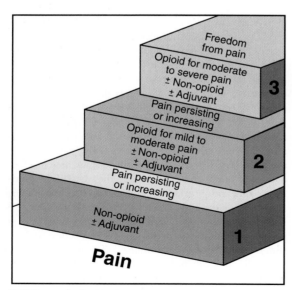

FIGURE 15-2 WHO's Pain Relief Ladder. (From World Health Organization: WHO's pain ladder. Available at www.who.int/cancer/palliative/painladder/en/.)

BOX 15-9   General Principles of Pharmacological Management of Pain in Older Adults

1. When pain is assessed, negotiate a pain relief or comfort goal with the patient.
2. Be aware of other conditions which may affect assessment and management of pain.
3. Anticipate age-associated, but unpredictable, differences in sensitivities and toxicities related to medication use.
4. Always start at a low dose and slowly titrate to relief.
5. Use the least-invasive route of administration possible first.
6. Plan timing of medication administration to meet the needs of the patient.
7. Never use placebos.
8. Consider complementary, nonpharmacological, and pharmacological approaches.

SAFETY ALERT

The maximum dose of acetaminophen is 4 g (4000 mg) in 24 hours from **all sources** and is reduced for people with renal or hepatic dysfunction or who drink alcohol; the dose is easily reached when "extra-strength" formulations are taken at 1000 mg per tablet.

When persistent pain is of an inflammatory nature or during a short arthritic flare, one of the NSAIDs are sometimes used. However, older adults have been found to be at a higher risk for adverse drug effects from NSAIDs than younger adults, especially in persons with heart or renal disease, preexisting gastric irritation, or in those with low albumin levels (AGS, 2012). In addition to the known potential for gastrointestinal distress, new findings indicate that NSAIDs may increase blood pressure, reduce renal function, and worsen heart failure. A significant number of NSAID-related hospitalizations for adverse drug reactions have occurred, especially when co-administered with aspirin (AGS, 2009; Papaleontiou et al., 2010). The use of NSAIDs has been found to increase the risk for cardiac events. As a result, the Food and Drug Administration in the United States issued a warning in 2006 alerting the public that, when taken together, ibuprofen reduces the cardioprotective effects of aspirin (i.e., there is less antiplatelet effect), and the person's risk for a cardiac event such as an acute myocardial infarction increases. The recent Beers Criteria list the NSAIDs as inappropriate for use in the older adult due to these reasons (AGS, 2012).

 SAFETY ALERT

In 2006, the Food and Drug Administration in the United States issued a warning regarding the use of aspirin (81 mg) and ibuprofen (Advil) at the same time. When taken together, the aspirin is less cardioprotective (i.e., there is less antiplatelet effect), and the person's risk for a cardiac event increases. For persons who take immediate-release aspirin with even a single dose of ibuprofen (400 mg), the ibuprofen should be taken at least 30 minutes after or 8 hours before the aspirin.

Data from Food and Drug Administration: *Information for healthcare professionals: concomitant use of ibuprofen and aspirin* (2006). Available at http://www.fda.gov/Drugs/DrugSafety/PostmarketDrugSafetyInformationforPatientsandProviders/ucm125222.htm.

An approach that has been used to address the potential adverse drug reactions to NSAIDs is to alternatively use cyclooxygenase-2 (COX-2) inhibitors. COX-2 selective inhibitors appear to be as effective and have fewer gastrointestinal (GI) side effects. Of particular note is the newest drug in this class, meloxicam (Mobic), which has been found to have even fewer GI side effects. However, other potential side effects do not differ from the other NSAIDs, cautions from the American Geriatrics Society remain, and renal function in particular must be monitored. Two of the three originally in this group have been taken off the market for their risk for adverse cardiac effects; only celecoxib (Celebrex) and the recently introduced Mobic remain. Co-administration of any of the gastric agents available (misoprostol, histamine-2 [H_2] antagonists, or proton pump inhibitors) may be helpful and reasonable, especially for persons at a higher risk for GI bleeding.

Opioid Analgesics. Opioid analgesics effectively treat both acute and persistent physical pain and have a very important role in the management of persistent severe pain in the older adult (Gianni et al., 2009). They do produce a greater analgesic effect, a higher peak, and a longer duration of effect in older adults when compared to younger adults due in part to prolonged half-lives (see Chapter 8). The recommendation to start with the lowest anticipated effective dose, monitor response frequently, and titrate slowly to desired effect is especially applicable with the use of opioid pain relievers.

Pain relief should be planned for the "around the clock" approach with a combination of long-acting or sustained-release analgesics and generous use of as-needed (prn) medications for "breakthrough" pain. The doses of the prn medications are monitored so that the long-acting doses can be adjusted to the point that breakthrough pain is at a minimum. If breakthrough medication is needed on a regular basis, this is an indication that the long-acting medication dosage needs adjustment. Breakthrough pain may occur occasionally during a stable regimen of long-acting medication, and additional medication should always be available. Opioids used long-term for chronic pain control should be convenient and easy to administer or take. As with all other medications, the simplest regimen is the one most likely to be effective, to be followed more consistently, and least likely to be misused (see Chapter 8).

Side effects should be expected and transient or treatable. These include gait disturbance, dizziness, sedation, falls, nausea, pruritus, and constipation. Side effects may be lessened or prevented when the prescribing provider works closely with the patient and the nurse to slowly titrate the dosage of the drug to a point where the best relief can be obtained with the fewest side effects. Sedation and impaired cognition do occur when opioid analgesics are started or dosages increased. This often causes great concern from patients, families, and nurses but is usually temporary. Patients and caregivers should be cautioned about the potential for falls, and appropriate safety precautions should be instituted.

The nurse provides close observation of the person's response and works to prevent and promptly treat side effects or adverse drug reactions. Since constipation is almost universal when opioids are used in older patients, the nurse can ensure that an appropriate bowel regimen is begun at the same time as the opioids. A daily dose of a combination stool softener and mild laxative may be very helpful, along with ensuring adequate fluid intake and exercise.

Although many of the opioid pain relievers can be used in the older adult, albeit with caution, *the use of meperidine (Demerol) is absolutely contraindicated.* The metabolites of meperidine can quickly produce confusion, psychotic behavior, and seizure activity. The same can be said for pentazocine (Talwin), and nonopioid methadone. The nurse can refer to the Agency for Healthcare Research and Quality guidelines for acute and chronic pain management as well as the latest equianalgesic charts if they are needed (www.ahrq.gov).

Adjuvant Drugs. There are a number of drugs developed for other purposes that have been found to be useful in the management of physical pain, sometimes alone, but more often in combination with an analgesic; these are referred to as *adjuvant drugs.*

Adjuvant drugs are thought to be most effective for neuropathic pain syndromes such as postherpetic neuralgia and diabetic nephropathy (pain described as sharp, shooting, piercing, or burning) (see Chapter 8). The tricyclic antidepressants such as amitriptyline had been used widely; however, due to their potential for adverse effects, they are now used less often. Although the mechanism is unknown, anticonvulsants (e.g., gabapentin [Neurontin]), the mixed serotonin and norepinephrine reuptake inhibitors (SNRIs) (e.g., duloxetine [Cymbalta] and venlafaxine [Effexor]) seem to be effective with fewer problems (AGS, 2009).

Other Agents. Topical agents (e.g., capsaicin, lidocaine patch) may have some mild to moderate local effect; skin must be intact and the area watched for signs of irritation.

Nonpharmacological Measures of Pain Relief

Nurses have a long history of comforting patients through nonpharmacological measures. This may be in the form of a caring and supportive relationship or through the use of specific techniques performed either by the nurse or at the recommendation of the nurse.

It has now been shown that a combination of pharmacological and nonpharmacological interventions appears to be most effective in the relief of both acute and chronic pain. In one study it was found that up to 50% of the older adults reported using at least three different strategies at the same time to control their pain (Barry et al., 2005). The basic approach to pain control is to encourage whatever strategies have been effective in the past without causing harm. This is particularly applicable for older adults with a lifetime of experience at managing their own pain and that of others. In some cases, what is now referred to as complementary and alternative medicine (CAM) is actually the formalization of approaches that people have used for years. More and more of what is considered CAM is gaining acceptance by insurers such as Medicare. Several methods that elders use are briefly reviewed here, but it must be acknowledged that this represents only a small sample of what is available (www.nccam.nih.gov).

Cutaneous Nerve Stimulation. Nurses have long provided massage, vibration, heat, cold, and ointments. Heat and cold temporarily interrupt the transmission of pain impulses to the cerebral pain center; however, caution must be used in consideration of the cause of the pain. Heat is effective for some things, for example, the deep pain of inflammatory musculoskeletal conditions such as rheumatoid arthritis. On the other hand, heat will increase the circulation to the area and therefore is contraindicated in occlusive vascular disease and in nonexpansive tissue such as bursae (some joints), where it may increase pain. At the same time, intermittent application of cold packs is helpful in low back pain and some situations of nerve irritation. Care must be taken when applying heat and cold to older skin to prevent skin damage due to normal age-related thinning (see Chapter 5).

Transcutaneous Electrical Nerve Stimulation. Another form of nerve stimulation known as TENS, or transcutaneous electrical nerve stimulation, has been used in a variety of settings to treat a range of conditions and become very popular with both patients and health professionals. Patients often anecdotally reported that at least they were doing "something" for their chronic pain. In 2001, the state of the science related to efficacy was examined and only inconclusive evidence was found, making it impossible to support or refute this approach (Carroll et al., 2001). In 2008, the efficacy of this approach was still in question (Nnoaham & Kumbang, 2008). In many cases Medicare will pay for the use of a prescribed TENS unit. The units are available from physical therapists and pain specialists.

Acupuncture and Acupressure. Pain is registered as impulses pass through the theoretical pain gate in the spine and register the sensation in the brain, which in turn signals the central mechanism of the brain to return counterimpulses, which close the gate. Acupuncture uses tiny needles inserted along specific meridians or pathways in the body (Mayo Clinic Staff, 2012). Acupressure is pressure applied with the thumbs or tip of the index finger at the same locations as those used in acupuncture. It is thought that acupuncture and acupressure stimulate nerve clusters that cause the gate to close more quickly or that trigger the release of the body's own opiate substances, enkephalins (endorphins). Acupuncture and acupressure have been used for thousands of years, and scientific evidence of their effectiveness in the treatment of persistent pain is growing (Vas et al., 2006; Vickers et al., 2012; Witt et al., 2006). In some cases Medicare and some private insurance companies will pay for the cost of acupuncture treatment from a licensed acupuncturist.

Touch. Some say the use of touch therapies is a legacy in nursing. Over the years, different kinds of touch have been formalized to include those referred to as Healing Touch, Therapeutic Touch, Reiki, and others. A review of all of the literature and experts available through 2008 was conducted and published in the Cochrane database. Only modest pain relief was found (So et al., 2008). However, when combined with purposeful relaxation, touch may decrease anxiety, reduce muscle tension, and help relieve pain. The acceptability of touch by individual and culture varies considerably. Some touch may never be acceptable, such as cross-gender touch in strict Muslim or Orthodox Jewish traditions (International Strategy and Policy Institute [ISPI], 1999). The culturally sensitive nurse always requests permission before touching a patient.

Biofeedback. Biofeedback is a cognitive-behavioral approach that has been applied to pain control. It is based on the theory that an individual can learn voluntary control over some body processes and alter them by changing the physiological correlates appropriate to them. Training and equipment of some type are needed to learn how to alter one's body response through biofeedback. It requires full cognitive functioning and manual dexterity for self-treatment.

Distraction. Distraction is a behavioral strategy that lessens the perception of pain by drawing the person's attention away from the pain. In some instances the individual is completely unaware of the pain; in other instances the intensity of pain is significantly diminished. Pain messages are more slowly transmitted to the pain center in the brain, and therefore less pain is felt.

Mild to moderate pain responds well to distraction. At times, if an individual concentrates intently on another subject, the acute pain may be relieved. The most common forms of distraction include slow rhythmical breathing, slow rhythmical massage, rhythmical singing or tapping, active listening, guided imagery, and humor (Steele & Steele, 2009).

Relaxation, Meditation, and Imagery. As a behavioral strategy, relaxation enables the quieting of the mind and the muscles, providing the release of tension and anxiety. Relaxation should be adjunctive to all pharmacological interventions and for all types of pain. Meditation and imagery are two methods of promoting relaxation. Imagery uses the client's imagination to focus on settings full of happiness and relaxation rather than on stressful situations. Several studies using guided imagery have shown that there was a decrease in pain perception in foot pain and abdominal pain. It was suggested that a strong image of a pain-free state effectively alters the autonomic nervous system's responses to pain (National Center of Alternative and Complementary Medicine [NCCAM], 2007).

Pain Clinics

Pain clinics provide a specialized, often comprehensive and multidisciplinary approach to the management of pain that has not responded to the usual, more standard approaches as described earlier. The use of pain clinics by elders has been limited. However, their use should be encouraged when appropriate. The number and types of pain clinics and programs have increased as a response to continued poor pain management by general health care practice. Pain center programs may be inpatient, outpatient, or both. Pain clinics are generally one of three types: syndrome-oriented, modality-oriented, or comprehensive. Syndrome-oriented centers focus on a specific chronic pain problem, such as headache or arthritis pain. Modality-oriented centers focus on a specific treatment technique, such as relaxation or acupuncture/acupressure. The comprehensive centers tend to be larger and associated with medical centers. These centers include many services and provide a thorough initial assessment (physical, mental, psychosocial) of the person in pain. A comprehensive treatment plan is developed utilizing multiple modalities and usually a multidisciplinary team of interventionists.

The goals of pain management centers are to decrease pain intensity to a tolerable limit or eliminate it, if possible; improve functionality and activities of daily living (ADLs); increase involvement in family and social activities; decrease depression; and improve mood. This is accomplished by improving quality and frequency of assessment, improving optimal use of analgesics, assisting in minimizing analgesic adverse reactions, selecting nonpharmacological interventions, and evaluating outcomes associated with treatment (Fine, 2012). Physiological and cognitive-behavioral modalities are used to reduce or alleviate pain. The nurse should be familiar with the types of pain management clinics available in their communities to provide the patient and family with necessary information to make a knowledgeable decision in selecting a reputable center.

Evaluation

The nurse, the patient, and the significant others work together to find comfort for the patient where pharmacological and nonpharmacological interventions work in harmony. Evaluation of pain relief strategies requires repeated reassessment of the patient's status and comfort level. Indicators of comfort include relaxation of skeletal muscles that were tense and rigid during pain, increased activity level and sense of self-worth, and the ability to better concentrate, focus, and increase attention span, regardless of cognitive status. The individual is better able to rest, relax, and sleep. Verbal indicators reflect the patient referring to the decrease in pain or the absence of pain during conversation.

The evaluation of pain management and relief is also measured with the same instruments used in the initial assessment for a means of comparison. Reevaluations of the frequency and intensity of pain and response to pharmacological and nonpharmacological interventions are done. Adjustments of treatment regimens and interventions are based on reassessment findings and continue until optimal comfort is produced and maintained and in doing so health is promoted at any stage of life and wellness.

KEY CONCEPTS

- The absence of expressed pain does not necessarily imply comfort. Comfort is a state of ease and satisfaction of body needs, self-worth, as well as freedom from pain and anxiety.
- The experience of pain is not limited to that which is of physical origin. Pain related to psychological or spiritual factors can have the same effect and is often combined with that arising from physical causes.
- Assessment of pain is influenced by many misconceptions, myths, and stereotypes about pain. Inadequate treatment of pain is a major concern for older adults in care settings today.
- Culture, ethnicity, family, and individual characteristics all influence one's tolerance and expression of pain as well as the acceptance of relief interventions.
- Older people with various degrees of cognitive impairment may demonstrate pain by increased levels of confusion, restlessness, or withdrawal.

- Although it is sometimes assumed, it has not been shown that pain sensitivity and perception decrease with age or changes in cognitive status.
- The nursing goal is to assist in pain relief. Some pain medications are more appropriate than others for use with elders.
- Acute pain and persistent pain necessitate different therapeutic approaches. Persistent pain predominates in the lives of many older adults.
- Various combinations of pharmacological and nonpharmacological pain control can be effective but must be individually designed with the elder and significant others involved in the decision making.

ACTIVITIES AND DISCUSSION QUESTIONS

1. What is pain?
2. Compare the features of acute and persistent pain.
3. List data necessary for an accurate pain assessment.
4. How might pain be expressed in cognitively impaired older people?
5. How does assessment of pain differ in cognitively impaired older people?
6. What pharmacological and nonpharmacological therapy is available, and how can each type work with the other to relieve pain?

REFERENCES

American Geriatrics Society [AGS]: Pharmacological management of persistent pain in older persons: American Geriatrics Society panel on the pharmacological management of persistent pain in older persons, *J Am Geriatr Soc* 57:1331, 2009.

American Geriatrics Society [AGS]: American Geriatrics updated Beers Criteria for potentially inappropriate medication use in older adults, *J Am Geriatr Soc* 60(4): 616–631, 2012.

Barry L, Gill T, Kerns R, et al: Identification of pain reduction strategies used by community-dwelling older persons, *J Gerontol A Biol Sci Med Sci* 60(12):1569–1575, 2005.

Carroll D, Moore RA, McQuay HJ, et al: Transcutaneous electrical nerve stimulation (TENS) for chronic pain, *Cochrane Database Syst Rev* 3:CD003222, 2001.

Fine PG: Treatment guidelines for the pharmacological management of pain in older persons, *Pain Med* 13(Suppl 2): S57–S66, 2012.

Fuchs-Lachelle S, Hadjistavropoulos T: Development and preliminary validation of the Pain Assessment Checklist for Seniors with Limited Ability to Communicate (PACSLAC), *Pain Manag Nurs* 5:37, 2004. Available at http://e-pacslac.com.

Gianni W, Ceci M, Bustacchini S, et al: Opioids for the treatment of chronic non-cancer pain in older people, *Drugs Aging* 26(Suppl 1): 63–73, 2009.

Herr K: Pain in the older adult: an imperative across all health care settings, *Pain Manag Nurs* 11(2 Suppl):S1, 2010.

Herr K, Decker S: Assessment of pain in older adults with severe cognitive impairment, *Ann Longterm Care* 12:46, 2004.

Herr K, Coyne PJ, Key T, et al: Pain assessment in the nonverbal patient: position statement with clinical practice recommendations, *Pain Manag Nurs* 7:44, 2006a.

Herr K, Bjoro K, Decker S: Tools for assessment of pain in nonverbal older adults with dementia: a state of the science review, *J Pain Symptom Manage* 31:170, 2006b.

Horgas A, Yoon SL: *Pain: Nursing standards of practice protocol: pain management in older adults* (2008). Available at http://consultgerirn.org/topics/pain/want_to_know_more.

Inelman EM, Mosele M, Sergi G, et al: Chronic pain in the elderly with advanced dementia. Are we doing our best for their suffering? *Aging Clin Exp Res*, 3 Oct 2011. [Epub ahead of print.]

International Strategy and Policy Institute [ISPI]: *Guidelines for health care providers interacting with Muslim patients and their families* (1999). Available at http://www.ispi-usa.org/guidelines.htm.

Joint Commission: *Health care issues: pain management* (2012). Available at http://www.jointcommission.org/pain_management/.

Kovach C, Logan BR, Noonan PE, et al: Effects of the Serial Trial Intervention on discomfort and behavior of nursing home residents with dementia, *Am J Alzheimers Dis Other Demen* 21:147, 2006a.

Kovach C, Noonan PE, Schlidt AM, et al: The Serial Trial Intervention: an innovative approach to meeting the needs of individuals with dementia, *J Gerontol Nurs* 32:18, 2006b.

Mayo Clinic Staff: *Acupuncture* (2012). Available at http://www.mayoclinic.com/health/acupuncture/MY00946.

National Center of Complementary and Alternative Medicine [NCCAM]: *An introduction to reiki* (2007). Available at http://nccam.nih.gov/health/reiki.

National Institute of Neurological Disorders and Stroke [NINDS]: *Shingles: hope through research* (2011). Available at http://www.ninds.nih.gov/disorders/shingles/detail_shingles.htm.

Nnoaham KE, Kumbang J: Transcutaneous electrical nerve stimulation (TENS) for chronic pain, *Cochrane Database Syst Rev* 16:CD003222, 2008.

Papaleontiou M, Henderson CR, Turner BJ, et al: Outcomes associated with opioid use in the treatment of chronic noncancer pain in older adults: a systematic review and meta-analysis, *J Am Geriatr Soc* 58:1353, 2010.

Portenoy RK, Bennett DS, Rauck R, et al: Prevalence and characteristics of breakthrough pain in opioid-treated patients with chronic cancer pain, *J Pain* 7:583, 2006.

Robinson P: Pharmacological management of pain in older persons, *Consult Pharm* 25(Suppl A):11, 2010.

Schofield P: "It's your age": The assessment and management of pain in older adults, *CEACCP* 10:93, 2010.

Smith M: Pain assessment in nonverbal older adults with advanced dementia, *Perspect Psychiatr Care* 41(3):99–113, 2005.

So PS, Jiang Y, Qin Y: Touch therapies for pain relief in adults. *Cochrane Database Syst Rev* Oct 8(4):CD006535, 2008.

Steele LL, Steele JR: Chronic pain. In Larsen PD, Lubkin IM, editors: *Chronic illness: impact and intervention*, 7th ed., 2009, pp. 395–412.

Taylor L, Harris J, Epps C, Herr K: Psychometric evaluation of selected pain-intensity scales for use with cognitively impaired and cognitively intact older adults, *Rehabil Nurs* 30:55–61, 2005.

Vas J, Perea-Milla E, Mendez C, et al: Efficacy and safety of acupuncture for chronic uncomplicated pain: a randomized controlled study, *Pain* 126:245, 2006.

Vickers AJ, Cronin AM, Maschino AC, et al: Acupuncture for chronic pain: individual patient data meta-analysis. *Arch Intern Med* Sept 10, 2012: 1–10. [Epub ahead of print.]

Warden V, Hurley AC, Volicer L: Development and psychometric evaluation of the Pain Assessment in Advanced Dementia (PAINAD) scale, *J Am Med Dir Assoc* 4:9, 2003. Available at http://www.amda.com/publications/caring/may2004/painad.cfm.

Ware LJ, Epps CD, Herr K, et al: Evaluation of the revised faces pain scale, verbal descriptor scale, numeric rating scale, and Iowa pain thermometer in older minority adults, *Pain Manag Nurs* 7:117, 2006.

Witt CM, Jena S, Brinkhaus B, et al: Acupuncture in patients with osteoarthritis of the knee or hip: a randomized, controlled trial with an additional nonrandomized arm, *Arthritis Rheum* 54:3485, 2006.

CHAPTER 16

Diseases Affecting Vision and Hearing

Theris A. Touhy

evolve   evolve.elsevier.com/Ebersole/gerontological

LEARNING OBJECTIVES

Upon completion of this chapter, the reader will be able to:

- Discuss the assessment and treatment of diseases of the eye and ear that may occur in older adults.
- Describe the importance of health education and screening for eye diseases to prevent unnecessary vision loss in older adults.
- Increase awareness of the resources available to assist elders with visual and hearing impairments.

GLOSSARY

Drusen Yellow deposits under the retina, often found in people over 60 years of age.
Funduscopy Opthalmoscopic examination of the fundus of the eye.
Keratoconjunctivitis sicca Diminished tear production with age.
Lipofuscin Fatty brown pigment found in the tissues related to aging.
Tonometry The procedure used by eye care professionals to determine the intraocular pressure of the eye.

THE LIVED EXPERIENCE

For quite a while now, I've been pretending. That it was just that I was tired. That the light was bad. But my eyes are really getting worse. I'm afraid to go to the doctor because I'm afraid of what he'll say. Which is silly. Either there is something to be done. Or there is not. If it's glasses, hallelujah, and help me find the money. If it's an operation, see me through. If I am going blind, hold me. Help me put down the terror that rises in my gut at the word. Blind. There. I've said it. The ghost word that has been haunting me. Help me remember, if I have to walk in the dark, that I have had a lot of years of seeing clean and clear. I know the slender shape of a birch tree. I have seen thousands and thousands of things in my life. I can conjure them in my mind's eye. No matter what happens, I shall not be without beautiful sights. It is just that I may have to settle for the ones I have already seen.
From Maclay E: *Green winter: celebrations of old age,* New York, 1977, Crowell. Copyright ©1977 Elise Maclay.

This chapter discusses diseases that affect vision and hearing in older adults and adaptations to enhance communication for those with vision and hearing impairments. *Healthy People 2020* (U.S. Department of Health and Human Services [USDHHS], 2012) has set goals for vision and hearing (see the Healthy People boxes). To help the student understand more about the eye diseases discussed in this chapter, the following website provides a simulation of glaucoma, cataracts, macular degeneration, and diabetic retinopathy: http://www.visionsimulations.com/.

HEALTHY PEOPLE 2020

Objectives Vision – Older Adults

- Increase the proportion of adults who have had a comprehensive eye examination, including dilation, within the past 2 years.
- Reduce visual impairment due to diabetic retinopathy.
- Reduce visual impairment due to glaucoma.
- Reduce visual impairment due to cataract.
- Reduce visual impairment due to age-related macular degeneration.
- Increase the use of vision rehabilitation services by persons with visual impairment.
- Increase the use of assistive and adaptive devices by persons with visual impairment.

From U.S. Department of Health and Human Services, Office of Disease Prevention and Health Promotion: *Healthy people 2020* (2012). Available at http://www.healthypeople.gov/2020.

 HEALTHY PEOPLE 2020

Objectives Hearing – Older Adults

- Increase the proportion of persons with hearing impairment who have ever used a hearing aid or assistive listening devices or who have cochlear implants.
- Increase the proportion of adults 70 years of age who have had a hearing examination in the past 5 years.
- Increase the number of persons who are referred by their primary care physician or other health care provider for hearing evaluation and treatment.
- Increase the proportion of adults bothered by tinnitus who have seen a doctor or other health care professional.
- Increase the proportion of persons with hearing loss and other sensory communication disorders who have used Internet resources for health care information, guidance, or advice in the past 12 months.

From U.S. Department of Health and Human Services, Office of Disease Prevention and Health Promotion: *Healthy people 2020* (2012). Available at http://www.healthypeople.gov/2020.

Vision

Blindness and visual impairment are among the 10 most common causes of disability in the United States and are associated with shorter life expectancy and lower quality of life. For older adults, visual problems have a negative impact on quality of life, equivalent to that of life-threatening conditions such as heart disease and cancer. The leading causes of visual impairment are diseases that are common in older adults: age-related macular degeneration (AMD), cataract, glaucoma, and diabetic retinopathy. Figure 16-1 shows the effect of vision loss from these diseases. Vision loss is becoming a major public health problem and is projected to increase substantially with the aging of the population (National Eye Institute, 2004). By the year 2020, the number of people who are blind or have low vision is projected to reach 5.5 million (USDHHS, 2012).

Older adults represent the vast majority of the visually impaired population. More than two thirds of those with visual impairment are over 65 years of age. Visual impairment among nursing home residents ranges anywhere from 3 to 15 times higher than for adults of the same age living in the community (Owsley et al., 2007). Racial and cultural disparities in vision impairment are significant. African Americans are twice as likely to be visually impaired than are white individuals of comparable socioeconomic status; Hispanics also have a higher risk of visual complications than the white population. A recent survey conducted in the United States reported that among all racial and ethnic groups participating in the survey, Hispanic respondents reported the lowest access to eye health information, knew the least about eye health, and were the least likely to have their eyes examined (National Eye Institute, 2008).

Clearly, prevention and treatment of eye diseases is an important priority for nurses and other health care professionals. The National Eye Health Education Program (NEHEP) of the National Eye Institute provides a program for health professionals with evidence-based tools and resources that can be used in community settings to educate older adults about eye health and maintaining healthy vision (www.nei.nih.gov/SeeWellToolkit). The program emphasizes the importance of annual dilated eye examinations for anyone over 50 years of age and stresses that eye diseases often have no warning signs or symptoms, so early detection is essential.

Diseases of the Eye

Glaucoma

Glaucoma is a leading cause of blindness and visual impairment in the United States, affecting as many as 2.2 million people. An additional 2 million are unaware they have the disease. There are no symptoms of glaucoma in the early stages of the disease. Types of glaucoma include congenital glaucoma, primary open-angle glaucoma, low tension or normal tension glaucoma, secondary glaucoma (complication of

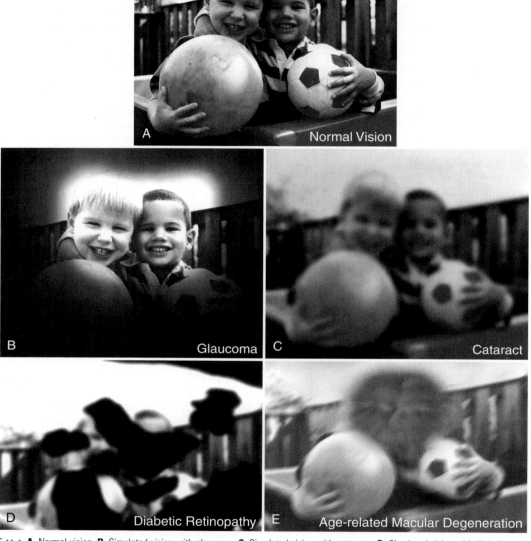

FIGURE 16-1 **A,** Normal vision. **B,** Simulated vision with glaucoma. **C,** Simulated vision with cataracts. **D,** Simulated vision with diabetic retinopathy. **E,** Simulated loss of vision with age-related macular degeneration (AMD). (From National Eye Institute, National Institutes of Health, 2010.)

other medical conditions), and acute angle-closure glaucoma, which is an emergency. The etiology of glaucoma is variable and often unknown. However, when the natural fluids of the eye are blocked by ciliary muscle rigidity and the buildup of pressure, damage to the optic nerve occurs. Glaucoma can be bilateral, but it more commonly occurs in one eye.

Open-angle glaucoma accounts for about 80% of cases and is asymptomatic until very late in the disease, when there is a noticeable loss in visual fields. However, if detected early, glaucoma can usually be controlled and serious vision loss prevented. Signs of glaucoma can include headaches, poor vision in dim lighting, increased sensitivity to glare, "tired eyes," impaired peripheral vision, a fixed and dilated pupil, and frequent changes in prescriptions for corrective lenses.

An acute attack of angle-closure glaucoma is characterized by a rapid rise in intraocular pressure (IOP) accompanied by redness and pain in and around the eye, severe headache, nausea and vomiting, and blurring of vision. It occurs when the path of the aqueous humor is blocked and intraocular pressure builds up to more than 50 mm Hg. If untreated, blindness can occur in 2 days. An iridectomy, however, can ease pressure. Many drugs with anticholinergic properties including antihistamines, stimulants, vasodilators, clonidine, and sympathomimetics, are particularly dangerous for patients predisposed to angle-closure glaucoma. Older people with glaucoma should be counseled to review all medications, both over-the-counter and prescribed, with their primary care provider.

Low tension or normal tension glaucoma is a type of glaucoma that also occurs in older adults. In this type, intraocular pressure is within normal range but there is damage to the optic nerve and narrowing of the visual fields. The cause is unknown, but risk factors include a family history of any kind of glaucoma, Japanese ancestry, and cardiovascular disease. Management consists of the same medications and surgical interventions that are used for chronic glaucoma (Glaucoma Research Foundation, 2008).

A family history of glaucoma, as well as diabetes, steroid use, and past eye injuries have been noted as risk factors for the development of glaucoma. Age is the single most important predictor of glaucoma, and older women are affected twice as frequently as older men. Among African Americans, glaucoma is the leading cause of blindness. African Americans develop glaucoma at younger ages, and the incidence of the disease is 5 times more common in African Americans than in whites and 15 times more likely to cause blindness. Factors contributing to this increased incidence include earlier onset of the disease as compared with other races, later detection of the disease, and economic and social barriers to treatment (National Eye Institute, 2010a). Research is ongoing to investigate the complex genetic and biological factors that cause glaucoma and to develop treatments that protect optic nerves from the damage that leads to vision loss (USDHHS, 2012).

Screening and Treatment. Adults over 65 years of age should have annual eye examinations, and those with medication-controlled glaucoma should be examined at least every 6 months. Annual screening is also recommended for African Americans and other individuals with a family history of glaucoma who are older than 40. A dilated eye examination and tonometry are necessary to diagnose glaucoma. These procedures can be performed by a primary care provider, optometrist, or a nurse practitioner, who will then refer the person to an ophthalmologist if glaucoma is suspected. Medicare pays for annual screening for glaucoma but only in high-risk patients.

Management of glaucoma involves medications (oral or topical eye drops) to decrease IOP and/or laser trabeculoplasty. Medications lower eye pressure either by decreasing the amount of aqueous fluid produced within the eye or by improving the flow through the drainage angle. Beta blockers are the first-line therapy for glaucoma, and the patient may need combinations of several types of eye drops. Usually medications can control glaucoma, but laser surgery treatments (trabeculoplasty) may be recommended for some types of glaucoma. Surgery is usually recommended only if necessary to prevent further damage to the optic nerve.

When caring for older adults in the hospital or long-term care settings, it is important to obtain a past medical history to determine if the person has glaucoma and to ensure that eye drops are given according to the person's treatment regimen. Without the eye drops, eye pressure can rise and cause an acute exacerbation of glaucoma (Capezuti et al., 2008).

Cataracts

Cataracts are a prevalent disorder among older adults caused by oxidative damage to lens protein and fatty deposits (lipofuscin) in the ocular lens. By 80 years of age, more than half of all Americans either have a cataract or have had cataract surgery. When lens opacity reduces visual acuity to 20/30 or less in the central axis of vision, it is considered a cataract. Cataracts are categorized according to their location within the lens and are usually bilateral.

Cataracts are recognized by the clouding of the ordinarily clear ocular lens; the red reflex may be absent or may appear as a black area. The cardinal sign of cataracts is the appearance of halos around objects as light is diffused. Other common symptoms include blurring, decreased perception of light and color (giving a yellow tint to most things), and sensitivity to glare.

The most common causes of cataracts are heredity and advancing age. They may occur more frequently and at earlier ages in individuals who have been exposed to excessive sunlight, have poor dietary habits, diabetes, hypertension, kidney disease, eye trauma, or history of alcohol intake and tobacco use. There is some evidence that a high dietary intake of lutein and zeaxanthin, compounds found in yellow or dark leafy vegetables, as well as intake of vitamin E from food and supplements, appears to lower the risk of cataracts in women. Further research is indicated (Moeller et al., 2008).

When visual acuity decreases to 20/50 and the cataract affects safety or quality of life, surgery is recommended. Cataract surgery is the most common surgical procedure performed in the United States. Most often, cataract surgery involves only local anesthesia and is one of the most successful surgical procedures, with 95% of patients reporting excellent vision after surgery. The surgery involves removal of the lens and placement of a plastic intraocular lens (IOL). Cataract surgery is performed with local anesthesia on an outpatient basis, and the procedure has greatly improved with advances in surgical techniques.

Nursing interventions when caring for the person experiencing cataract surgery include preparing the individual for significant changes in vision and adaptation to light and insuring that the individual has received adequate counseling regarding realistic postsurgical expectations. Postsurgical teaching includes covering the need to avoid heavy lifting, straining, and bending at the waist. Eye drops may be prescribed to aid healing and prevent infection. If the person has bilateral cataracts, surgery is performed first on one eye with the second surgery on the other eye a month or so later to ensure healing.

Although race is not a factor in cataract formation, racial disparities exist in cataract surgery in the United States, with African-American Medicare recipients only 60% as likely as whites to undergo cataract surgery (Miller, 2008; Wilson & Eezzuduemhoi, 2005). Unfortunately, cataracts and other related eye diseases such as maculopathy, diabetic retinopathy, or glaucoma often occur simultaneously, which complicates the management of each.

Diabetic Retinopathy

Diabetes has become an epidemic in the United States (see Chapter 17). Diabetic eye disease is a complication of diabetes and a leading cause of blindness. Diabetic retinopathy is a disease of the retinal microvasculature characterized by increased vessel permeability. Blood and lipid leakage leads to macular edema and hard exudates (composed of lipids). In advanced disease, new fragile blood vessels form that hemorrhage easily. Because of the vascular and cellular changes accompanying diabetes, there is often rapid worsening of other pathologic vision conditions as well.

There are no symptoms in the early stages of diabetic retinopathy. Estimates are that 40.8% of adults 40 years of age and older with diabetes have diabetic retinopathy, and the incidence increases with age. Most diabetic patients will develop diabetic retinopathy within 20 years of diagnosis. Prevalence rates for diabetes and diabetic retinopathy are higher among racially and culturally diverse individuals and among American Indian and Alaska Native populations (National Eye Institute, 2010b).

Screening and Treatment. There is little to no evidence of retinopathy until 3 to 5 years or more after the onset of diabetes. Early signs are seen in the funduscopic examination and include microaneurysms, flame-shaped hemorrhages, cotton wool spots, hard exudates, and dilated capillaries. Constant, strict control of blood glucose, cholesterol, and blood pressure and laser photocoagulation treatments can halt progression of the disease. Laser treatment can reduce vision loss in 50% of patients, and recent evidence suggests that treatment with various drugs may deliver a better outcome (USDHHS, 2012). Annual dilated funduscopic examination of the eye is recommended beginning 5 years after diagnosis of diabetes type 1 and at the time of diagnosis of diabetes type 2.

Macular Degeneration

Age-related macular degeneration (AMD) is the leading cause of vision loss in Americans 60 years of age and older. The prevalence of AMD increases drastically with age, with more than 15% of white women over 80 years of age having the disease. Whites and Asian Americans are more likely to lose vision from AMD than African Americans. With the number of affected older adults projected to increase over the next 20 years, AMD has been called a growing epidemic (National Eye Institute, 2010c).

AMD is a degenerative eye disease that affects the macula, the central part of the eye responsible for clear central vision. The disease causes the progressive loss of central vision, leaving only peripheral vision intact. Early signs of AMD include blurred vision, difficulty reading and driving, increased need for bright light, colors that appear dim or gray, and an awareness of a blurry spot in the middle of vision.

AMD results from systemic changes in circulation, accumulation of cellular waste products, tissue atrophy, and growth of abnormal blood vessels in the choroid layer beneath the retina. Fibrous scarring disrupts nourishment of photoreceptor cells, causing their death and loss of central vision. The greatest risk factor for AMD is age. Although etiology is unknown, risk factors are thought to include genetic predisposition, smoking, obesity, family history, and excessive sunlight exposure.

There are two forms of macular degeneration, the "dry" form and the "wet" form. Dry AMD accounts for the majority of cases and rarely causes severe visual impairment, but can lead to the more aggressive wet AMD. Dry AMD generally affects both eyes, but vision can be lost in one eye while the other eye seems unaffected. One of the most common early signs is drusen. Drusen are yellow deposits under the retina and are often found in people over 60 years of age. The relationship between drusen and AMD is not clear, but an increase in the size or number of drusen increases the risk of developing either advanced AMD or wet AMD (National Eye Institute, 2010c).

Wet AMD occurs when abnormal blood vessels behind the retina start to grow under the macula. These new blood vessels are fragile and often leak blood and fluid, which raise the macula from its normal place at the back of the eye. With wet AMD, the severe loss of central vision can be rapid, and many people will be legally blind within 2 years of diagnosis. Peripheral vision usually remains normal, but the person will have difficulty seeing at a distance or doing detailed work such as sewing or reading. Faces may begin to blur, and it may become harder to distinguish colors. An early sign may be distortion that causes edges or lines to appear wavy.

An Amsler grid is used to determine clarity of central vision (Figure 16-2). A perception of wavy lines is diagnostic of beginning macular degeneration, and vision loss can occur in days. In the advanced forms, the person may begin to see dark or empty spaces that block the center of vision. People with AMD are usually taught to test their eyes daily using the Amsler grid so that they will be aware of any changes.

Early diagnosis of AMD is the key, and individuals over 40 years of age should have a dilated eye examination at least every 2 years. The National Eye Institute's Age-Related Eye Disease Study (AREDS) (www.nei.nih.gov/) found that a high-dose formulation of antioxidants and zinc significantly reduces the risk of advanced AMD and associated vision loss (National Eye Institute, 2010c).

Treatment of wet AMD includes photodynamic therapy (PDT), laser photocoagulation (LPC), and anti-VEGF therapy. LPC uses a laser to destroy the fragile, leaky blood vessels, but it may also destroy healthy tissue and some vision so it is used in only a small number of people with wet AMD. Lucentis and Avastin (anti–vascular endothelial growth factor [VEGF] therapy), are biological drugs that are the most common form of treatment in advanced AMD. These drugs are injected into the eye as often as once a month and can help slow vision loss from AMD, and in some cases can improve sight.

Detached Retina

This condition can develop in persons with cataracts or recent cataract surgery or trauma, or can occur spontaneously.

It manifests as a curtain coming down over the person's line of vision. It necessitates immediate emergency treatment.

Dry Eye

Dry eye is not a disease of the eye but is a frequent complaint among older people. Tear production normally diminishes as we age. The condition is termed keratoconjunctivitis sicca. It occurs most commonly in women after menopause. There may be age-related changes in the mucin-secreting cells necessary for surface wetting, in the lacrimal glands, or in the meibomian glands that secrete surface oil, and all of these may occur at the same time. The older person will describe a dry, scratchy feeling in mild cases. There may be marked discomfort and decreased mucus production in severe situations.

Medications can cause dry eye, especially antihistamines, diuretics, beta blockers, and some sleeping pills. The problem is diagnosed by an ophthalmologist using a Schirmer tear test, in which filter paper strips are placed under the lower eyelid to measure the rate of tear production. A common treatment is artificial tears, but dry eyes may be sensitive to them because of preservatives, which can be irritating. The ophthalmologist may close the tear duct channel either temporarily or permanently. Other management methods include keeping the house air moist with humidifiers, avoiding wind and hair dryers, and the use of artificial tear ointments at bedtime. Vitamin A deficiency can be a cause of dry eye, and vitamin A ointments are available for treatment.

Interventions to Enhance Vision

General principles in caring for the older adult with visual impairment include the following: use warm incandescent

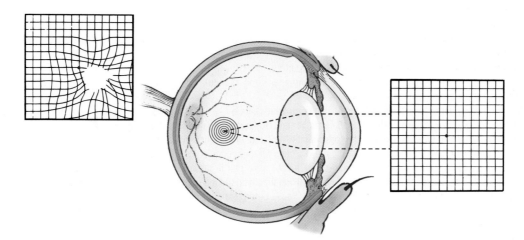

FIGURE 16-2 Macular degeneration distortion of central vision, normal peripheral vision. (Illustration by Harriet R. Greenfield, Newton, MA.)

lighting; increase intensity of lighting; control glare by using shades and blinds; suggest yellow or amber lenses to decrease glare and sunglasses that block all ultraviolet light; select colors with good contrast and intensity; and recommend reading materials that have large, dark, evenly spaced printing.

Use of Contrasting Colors

Color contrasts are used to facilitate location of items. Sharply contrasting colors assist the partially sighted. For instance, a bright towel is much easier to locate than a white towel hanging on a beige wall. When choosing color, it is best to use primary colors at the top end of the spectrum rather than those at the bottom. If you think of the colors of the rainbow, it is more likely that people will see reds and oranges better than blues and greens.

Low-Vision Assistive Devices

Technology advances in the past decade have produced some low-vision devices that may be used successfully in the care of the visually impaired elder. Persons with severe visual impairment may qualify for disability and financial and social services assistance through government and private programs including vision rehabilitation programs.

An array of low-vision assistive devices are now available, including insulin delivery systems, talking clocks and watches, large-print books, magnifiers, telescopes (handheld or mounted on eyeglasses), electronic magnification through closed circuit television or computer software, and software that converts text into artificial voice output. Because individual needs are unique, it is recommended that before investing in vision aids, the client consult with a low-vision center or low-vision specialist.

Implications for Gerontological Nurses and Healthy Aging

Vision impairment is common among older adults in connection with aging changes and eye diseases and can significantly affect communication, functional ability, safety, and quality of life. The issues of concern to nurses who care for older adults are appropriate assessment; adapting the environment to enhance vision and safety; communicating appropriately; and providing appropriate health teaching and referrals for prevention and treatment. Suggestions for communicating effectively with older adults with vision impairment are presented in Box 16-1.

BOX 16-1   Strategies for Communicating with Elders with Visual Impairment

- Make sure you have the person's attention before you start talking.
- Always speak promptly and clearly identify yourself and others with you. State when you are leaving to make sure the person is aware of your departure.
- Get down to the person's level and face them when speaking.
- Speak normally but not from a distance; do not raise or lower your voice and continue to use gestures if that is natural to your communication.
- When others are present, address the visually impaired person by prefacing remarks with his or her name or a light touch on the arm.
- Use the analogy of a clock face to help locate objects (e.g., describe positions of food on a plate in relation to clock positions such as meat at 3 o'clock, dessert at 6 o'clock).
- Ensure adequate lighting on your face and eliminate glare.
- Select colors for paint, furniture, pictures with rich intensity (red, orange).
- Use large, dark, evenly spaced printing.
- Use contrast in printed material (e.g., black marker on white paper).
- Do not change the room arrangement or the arrangement of personal items without explanation.
- Use some means to identify patients who are visually impaired, and include visual impairment in the plan of care.
- Screen for vision loss, and recommend annual eye exams for older people.
- If the person is institutionalized, label glasses and have a spare pair if possible.
- Be aware of low-vision assistive devices such as talking watches, talking books, and facilitate access to these resources.
- If the person is blind, offer your arm while walking. Pause before stairs or curbs and alert the person. When seating the person, place his or her hand on the back of the chair. Always let the person know his or her position in relation to objects. Never play with or distract a seeing-eye dog.

Hearing Impairment

Hearing loss is the third most prevalent chronic condition in older Americans and the foremost communicative disorder of older adults. The prevalence of hearing loss is 90% in those older than 80 years of age. Hearing loss is a common condition in middle-aged adults as well. Estimates are that 20.6% of adults 48 to 59 years of age have impaired hearing. Increases in blast exposure in combat situations have led to a dramatic rise in ear damage in military personnel. Noise-induced hearing loss may be reduced through the development of better ear-protection devices and emerging research into interventions that may protect or repair hair cells in the ear, which are key to the body's ability to hear (USDHHS, 2012).

Cardiovascular disease risk factors may also be important correlates of age-related auditory dysfunction, and hearing loss may be a largely unrecognized complication of diabetes. Hearing loss may not be an inevitable part of aging and if detected early, it may be a preventable chronic disease because the same healthy lifestyle changes that improve cardiovascular health may also prevent or delay hearing loss (University of Wisconsin School of Medicine and Public Health, 2011). In all age groups, men are more likely than women to be hearing-impaired.

Hearing loss diminishes quality of life and is associated with multiple negative outcomes including decreased function, miscommunication, depression, falls, loss of self-esteem, safety risks, and cognitive decline (Wallhagen & Pettengill, 2008). Hearing impairment increases feelings of isolation and may cause older adults to become suspicious or distrustful or to display feelings of paranoia. Because older persons with a hearing loss may not understand or respond appropriately to conversation, they may be inappropriately diagnosed with dementia. Older people may be initially unaware of hearing loss because of the gradual manner in which it develops (Box 16-2). The Better Hearing Institute (Washington, DC) provides an online hearing test for older adults who want to check their own hearing (http://www.betterhearing.org/hearing_loss/online_hearing_test/index.cfm).

Hearing impairment is underdiagnosed and undertreated in older people. Although screening for hearing impairment and appropriate treatment are considered an essential part of primary care for older adults, it is rarely done. Hearing loss is "an overlooked geriatric syndrome in primary care settings—an assessment gap that can have significant negative consequences" (Wallhagen & Pettengill, 2008, p. 41). A single question—Do you feel you have a hearing loss?—has been shown to have reasonable sensitivity and specificity for hearing impairment (Schumm et al., 2009).

BOX 16-2   Do I Have a Hearing Problem?

- Do I have a problem hearing on the telephone?
- Do I have trouble hearing when there is noise in the background?
- Is it hard for me to follow a conversation when two or more people talk at once?
- Do I have to strain to understand a conversation?
- Do many people I talk to seem to mumble (or not speak clearly)?
- Do I misunderstand what others are saying and respond inappropriately?
- Do I have trouble understanding the speech of women and children?
- Do people complain that I turn the TV volume up too high?
- Do I hear a ringing, roaring, or hissing sound a lot?
- Do some sounds seem too loud?

From National Institute on Deafness and Other Communication Disorders. Available at www.nidcd.gov/health/hearing/older.asp.

The screening rate for hearing impairment among older adults is estimated to be as low as 12.9%, and only about 20% of persons with hearing impairments receive hearing aids (Ham et al., 2007; Wallhagen & Pettengill, 2008). Factors associated with lack of hearing aid use include cost, perceived lack of benefit, and denial of hearing loss. Wallhagen (2009) also suggests that the perceived stigma associated with hearing loss and use of hearing aids is another factor that should be examined. The cost of hearing aids is not covered under Medicare and other health plans, but screening for hearing loss is recommended as part of the comprehensive physical for older adults joining Medicare for the first time.

Types of Hearing Loss

The two major forms of hearing loss are conductive and sensorineural. *Sensorineural hearing loss* results from damage to any part of the inner ear or the neural pathways to the brain. *Presbycusis* is a form of sensorineural hearing loss that is related to aging. It is the most common form of hearing loss in the United States. Presbycusis is a bilateral and symmetrical sensorineural hearing loss that also affects the ability to understand speech.

Changes in the middle and inner ear make many elders intolerant of loud noises and incapable of distinguishing among some of the sibilant consonants such as *z, s, sh, f, p, k, t,* and *g*. People often raise their voice when speaking to a hearing-impaired person. When this happens, more consonants drop out of speech, making hearing even more difficult. Without consonants, the high-frequency–pitched language becomes disjointed and misunderstood. Older people with presbycusis have difficulty filtering out background noise and often complain of difficulty understanding women's and children's speech and conversations in large groups.

The condition progressively worsens with age. Use of rapid speech when conversing with an older adult with a hearing impairment will make sounds garbled and unintelligible, and even though the problem is related to presbycusis, it is one that is easily remedied. Sensorineural hearing loss is treated with hearing aids and, in some cases, cochlear implants.

Conductive hearing loss usually involves abnormalities of the external and middle ear that reduce the ability of sound to be transmitted to the middle ear. Otosclerosis, infection, perforated eardrum, fluid in the middle ear, or cerumen accumulations cause conductive hearing loss. Cerumen impaction is the most common and easily corrected of all interferences in the hearing of older people. Cerumen impaction has been found to occur in 33% of nursing home residents (Hersh, 2010).

Cerumen interferes with the conduction of sound through air in the eardrum. The reduction in the number and activity of cerumen-producing glands results in a tendency toward cerumen impaction. Long-standing impactions become hard, dry, and dark brown. Individuals at particular risk of impaction are African Americans, individuals who wear hearing aids, and older men with large amounts of ear canal tragi (hairs in the ear) that tend to become entangled with the cerumen. When hearing loss is suspected, or a person with existing hearing loss experiences increasing difficulty, it is important first to check for cerumen impaction as a possible cause. If cerumen removal is indicated, it may be removed through irrigation, cerumenolytic products, or manual extraction (Hersh, 2010). Box 16-3 presents a protocol for cerumen removal.

Tinnitus

Tinnitus is defined as the perception of sound in one or both ears or in the head when no external sound is present. It is often referred to as "ringing in the ears" but may also manifest as buzzing, hissing, whistling, cricket chirping, bells, roaring, clicking, pulsating, humming, or swishing sounds. The sounds may be constant or intermittent and are more acute at night or in quiet surroundings. The most common type is high-pitched tinnitus with sensorineural

---

BOX 16-3   Protocol for Cerumen Removal

- Assess for ear pain, traumas, abnormalities, drainage, surgeries, or perforations. These or any other unusual findings should be referred to an otolaryngologist.
- When aural examination reveals cerumen impaction with no other abnormalities, the nurse may irrigate for cerumen removal using the following techniques.
  NOTE: Do not use a water pick for cerumen removal because water pressure is too high and may damage the ear.
1. Carefully clip and remove hairs in ear canal.
2. Instill a softening agent such as slightly warm mineral oil 0.5 to 1 mL twice daily or ear drops such as Cerumenex, Debrox, or Murine for several days until wax becomes softened. Allergic reactions to Cerumenex have been noted if used for longer than 24 hours.
3. Protect clothing and linens from drainage of oil or wax by placing small cotton ball in each external ear canal.
4. When irrigating the ear, use hand-held bulb syringe, 2- to 4-ounce plastic syringe, or otologic syringe (20- to 50-mL syringe equipped with an Angiocath or Jelso catheter rather than a needle) with emesis basin under ear to catch drainage; tip head to side being drained.
5. Use solution of 3 ounces of 3% hydrogen peroxide in quart of water warmed to 98° to 100° F; if client is sensitive to hydrogen peroxide, use sterile normal saline.
6. Place towels around neck; empty emesis basin frequently, observing for residue from ear; keep client dry and comfortable; do not inject air into client's ear or use high pressure when injecting fluid.
7. If the cerumen is not successfully washed out, begin the process again of instilling a softening agent for several days.

loss; less common is low-pitched tinnitus with conduction loss such as is seen in Meniere's disease.

Tinnitus generally increases over time. It is a condition that afflicts many older people and can interfere with hearing, as well as become extremely irritating. It is estimated to occur in nearly 11% of elders with presbycusis. Approximately 50 million people in the United States have tinnitus and about 2 million are so seriously debilitated that they cannot function on a "normal," day-to-day basis. The incidence of tinnitus peaks between 65 and 74 years of age and is higher in men than in women; in men, the incidence seems to decrease after this age. Tinnitus is a growing problem for America's military personnel and is the leading cause of service-connected disability of veterans returning from Iraq or Afganistan (American Tinnitus Association, 2010).

The exact physiological cause or causes of tinnitus are not known but there are several likely factors that are known to trigger or worsen tinnitus. Exposure to loud noises is the leading cause of tinnitus, and the exposure can damage and destroy cilia in the inner ear. When damaged, they cannot be renewed or replaced. See http://www.ata.org/for-patients/at-risk#Loud for a simulation of tinnitus and a video of ways to mitigate noise exposure. Other possible causes of tinnitus include head and neck trauma, certain types of tumors, cerumen build-up, jaw misalignment, cardiovascular disease, and ototoxicity from medications. More than 200 prescription and nonprescription medications list tinnitus as a potential side effect, aspirin being the most common.

Assessment

Tinnitus may be described as pulsatile (matching the beating of the heart) or nonpulsatile (unilateral, asymmetric, or symmetric).

Some persons with tinnitus will never find the cause; for others the problem may arbitrarily disappear. Hearing aids can be prescribed to amplify environmental sounds to obscure tinnitus, and there is a device that combines the features of a masker and a hearing aid, which emits a competitive but pleasant sound that distracts from head noise. Therapeutic modes of treating tinnitus include transtympanal electrostimulation, iontophoresis, biofeedback, tinnitus masking with alternative sound production (white noise), dental treatment, cochlear implants, and hearing aids. Some have found hypnosis, cognitive-behavioral therapy, acupuncture, chiropractic, naturopathic, allergy, or drug treatment to be effective.

Nursing actions include discussions with the client regarding times when the noises are most irritating and having the person keep a diary to identify patterns. There is some evidence that caffeine, alcohol, cigarettes, stress,

and fatigue may exacerbate the problem. Assess medications for possibly contributing to the problem. Discuss lifestyle changes and alternative methods that some have found effective. Also, refer clients to the American Tinnitus Association for research updates, education, and support groups.

Interventions to Enhance Hearing

Hearing Aids

A hearing aid is a personal amplifying system that includes a microphone, an amplifier, and a loudspeaker. There are numerous types of hearing aids and the appearance and effectiveness of hearing aids have greatly improved over the years. Many can be programmed to meet specific needs. Most individuals can obtain some hearing enhancement with a hearing aid.

Although hearing aids generally improve hearing by about 50%, they do not correct hearing deficits. It is important that hearing-impaired elders understand that the goal of hearing aid use is to improve communication and quality of life, not to restore normal hearing.

Hearing aids necessitate a period of adjustment and training in correct use. In most states, the purchase of a hearing aid comes with a 30-day trial during which the purchase price is totally refundable. The investment in a good hearing aid is considerable, and a good fit is critical. Before a hearing aid can be purchased, medical clearance must be obtained from a physician. Hearing aids can range in price from about $500 to several thousand dollars, depending on the technology. Batteries are changed every 1 to 2 weeks, adding to overall costs. The cost of hearing aids is not usually covered by health insurance or Medicare.

It is important for nurses in hospitals and nursing homes to be knowledgeable about the care and maintenance of hearing aids. Many older people experience unnecessary communication problems when in the hospital or nursing home because their hearing aids are not inserted and working properly, or are lost. Box 16-4 presents suggestions for the use and care of hearing aids.

Cochlear Implants

Cochlear implants are increasingly being used for older adults who are profoundly deaf as a result of sensorineural hearing loss. A cochlear implant is a small, complex electronic device that consists of an external portion that sits behind the ear and a second portion that is surgically placed under the skin. Unlike hearing aids that magnify sounds, the cochlear implant bypasses damaged portions of the ear and directly stimulates the auditory nerve. Hearing

---

BOX 16-4   The Use and Care of Hearing Aids

Hearing Aid Use
- Initially, wear the aid 15 to 20 minutes a day.
- Gradually increase wearing time to 10 to 12 hours.
- Be patient and realize that the process of adaptation is difficult but ultimately will be rewarding.
- Make sure fingers are dry and clean before handling hearing aids. Use a soft dry cloth to wipe your hearing aids.
- Each day, remove any earwax that has built up on the hearing aids. Use a soft brush to clean difficult-to-reach areas.
- Insert aid with the canal portion pointing into the ear; press and twist until snug.
- Turn aid slowly to one-third to one-half volume.
- A whistling sound indicates incorrect ear-mold insertion or that aid is in wrong ear.
- Adjust volume to a level for talking at a distance of 1 yard.
- Do not wear aid when using hair dryer or when swimming or taking a shower or bath.
- Note that fine particles of hair spray or make-up can obstruct the microphone component of the hearing aid.

Care of the Hearing Aid
- Insert and remove your hearing aid over a soft surface. When inserting or removing battery, work over a table or countertop or soft surface.
- Insert battery when hearing aid is turned off.
- Store hearing aid in a marked container in a safe place when not in use; remove batteries.
- Batteries last 1 week with daily wearing of 10 to 12 hours.
- Common problems include switch turned off, clogged ear mold, dislodged battery, twisted tubing between ear mold and aid.
- Ear molds need replacement every 2 or 3 years.
- Check ear molds for rough spots that will irritate ear.
- If sound is not loud enough, check for the following: need new battery? sound channel blocked? aid turned off? volume set too low? battery door not closed? hearing aid loose?
- Check the battery by turning the hearing aid on, turning up the volume, cupping your hand over the ear mold and listening. A constant whistling sound indicates that the battery is functioning. A weak sound may indicate that the battery is losing power and needs replacement.

Removing the Hearing Aid
- Turn the hearing aid off and lower the volume. The on/off switch may be marked by an O (off), M (microphone), T (telephone), or TM (telephone/microphone). If the aid is not turned off, the batteries will continue to run.
- Remove the ear mold by rotating it slightly forward and then pulling outward.
- Remove the battery if the hearing aid will not be used for several days. This will prevent corrosion from battery leakage.
- Store in a safe place, away from heat and moisture, to prevent loss or damage.

From Adams-Wendling L, Pimple C: Evidence-based guideline: Nursing management of hearing impairment in nursing facility residents, *J Gerontol Nurs* 34(11):9-16, 2008.

---

through a cochlear implant is different from normal hearing and takes time to learn or relearn. For persons whose hearing loss is so severe that amplification is of little or no benefit, the cochlear implant is a safe and effective method of auditory rehabilitation. Most insurance plans cover the cochlear implant procedure. The transplant carries some risk because the surgery destroys any residual hearing that remains. Therefore, cochlear implant users can never revert to using a hearing aid. Individuals with cochlear implants need to be advised not to undergo magnetic resonance imaging (MRI) since it may dislodge the implant or demagnetize its internal magnet.

Assistive Listening and Adaptive Devices
Assistive listening devices (also called personal listening systems) should be considered as an adjunct to hearing aids or used in place of hearing aids for people with hearing impairment. These devices are available commercially

and can be used to enhance face-to-face communication and to better understand speech in large rooms such as theaters, to use the telephone, and to listen to television. Examples of assistive listening and adaptive devices include text messaging devices for telephones and closed-caption television, now required on all televisions with screens 13 inches and larger. Alerting devices, such as vibrating alarm clocks that shake the bed or activate a flashing light, and sound lamps that respond with lights to sounds, such as doorbells and telephones, are also available. Assistive devices, such as personal amplifiers, that amplify sound and send it to the user's ears through earphones, clips, or headphones, are helpful in health care situations in which accurate communication and privacy are essential.

Any facility that receives financial aid from Medicare is required by the Americans with Disabilities Act to provide equal access to public accommodations. This includes access to sign language interpreters, telecommunication devices for the deaf (TDDs), and flashing alarm systems. Nurses working in these facilities should be able to obtain appropriate devices to improve communication with hearing-impaired individuals.

Implications for Gerontological Nursing and Healthy Aging

Hearing impairment is common among older adults and significantly affects communication, function, safety, and quality of life. Inadequate communication with older adults with hearing impairment can also lead to misdiagnosis and affect adherence to a medical regimen. The gerontological nurse must be able to assess hearing ability and use appropriate communication skills and devices to help older adults minimize or even avoid problems. The Hartford Institute for Geriatric Nursing (New York, NY) *Try This:* series provides guidelines for hearing screening (http://consultgerirn.org/uploads/File/trythis/try_this_12.pdf). An evidence-based guideline for nursing management of hearing impairment in nursing facility residents is also available (Adams-Wendling & Pimple, 2008). Box 16-5 presents communication strategies for elders with hearing impairment.

BOX 16-5   Communication Strategies for Elders with Hearing Impairment

- Never assume hearing loss is from age until other causes are ruled out (infection, cerumen buildup).
- Inappropriate responses, inattentiveness, and apathy may be symptoms of a hearing loss.
- Face the individual, and stand or sit on the same level; don't turn away while speaking (e.g., face a computer).
- Gain the individual's attention before beginning to speak. Look directly at the person at eye level before starting to speak.
- Determine if hearing is better in one ear than another, and position yourself appropriately.
- If hearing aid is used, make sure it is in place and batteries are functioning.
- Ask patient or family what helps the person to hear best.
- Keep hands away from your mouth and project voice by controlled diaphragmatic breathing.
- Avoid conversations in which the speaker's face is in glare or darkness; orient the light on the speaker's face.
- Careful articulation and moderate speed of speech are helpful.
- Lower your tone of voice, use a moderate speed of speech, and articulate clearly.
- Label the chart, note on the intercom button, and inform all caregivers that the patient has a hearing impairment.
- Use nonverbal approaches: gestures, demonstrations, visual aids, and written materials.
- Pause between sentences or phrases to confirm understanding.
- Restate with different words when you are not understood.
- When changing topics, preface the change by stating the topic.
- Reduce background noise (e.g., turn off television, close door).
- Utilize assistive listening devices such as pocket talker.
- Verify that the information being given has been clearly understood. Be aware that the person may agree to everything and appear to understand what you have said even when they did not hear you (listener bluffing).
- Share resources for the hearing-impaired and refer as appropriate.

From Adams-Wendling L, Pimple C: Evidence-based guideline: Nursing management of hearing impairment in nursing facility residents, *J Gerontol Nurs* 34(11):9-16, 2008.

Application of Maslow's Hierarchy

Hearing and vision impairments can contribute to challenges at all levels of the hierarchy from meeting biological integrity needs, such as activity, safety, and security needs to the higher-level needs such as a sense of belonging, feeling of self-esteem, and self-actualization. The consequences of these impairments severely affect quality of life and predispose the individual to potential negative health and quality-of-life outcomes. Whatever the age or the impairments experienced, continued growth and development toward self-actualization, the task of aging, requires interactions and environments in which the older adult is assured that basic needs are met, compensations are made for losses, and meaningful and satisfying experiences continue to be a part of life.

KEY CONCEPTS

- Vision and hearing impairment can significantly affect functional ability, safety, and quality of life among older adults.
- Vision loss from eye disease is a global concern and preventive interventions, early detection, and treatment of eye diseases is an important priority for nurses and other health care professionals.
- The major diseases affecting vision are glaucoma, cataracts, macular degeneration, and diabetic retinopathy. Many of these diseases can be identified and appropriately treated through proper screening. All adults over 65 years of age should have annual eye examinations.
- Ear damage and hearing impairment are increasing due to the aging of the population and increased exposure to loud noises such as blast exposure in combat situations among military personnel. The two types of hearing impairment are sensorineural and conductive.
- Tinnitus is a common condition among older people and can interfere with hearing, as well as become extremely irritating. It is characterized by ringing in the ear and may also manifest as buzzing, hissing, whistling, clicking, pulsating, or swishing sounds.

ACTIVITIES AND DISCUSSION QUESTIONS

1. How can nurses enhance awareness and education about vision and hearing disorders?
2. What is the role of a nurse in the acute care setting in screening and assessment for eye and ear diseases?
3. Develop a teaching plan for an older adult with glaucoma.
4. What type of resources could a nurse in any setting offer to an older adult who has vision and hearing loss?
5. Develop a plan of care for an older adult with diabetic retinopathy.

REFERENCES

Adams-Wendling L, Pimple C: Evidence-based guideline: nursing management of hearing impairment in nursing facility residents, *J Gerontol Nurs* 34:9, 2008.

American Tinnitus Association: *About tinnitus* (2010). Available at http://www.ata.org/for-patients/about-tinnitus.

Capezuti J, Swicker D, Mezey M, et al, editors: *Evidence-based geriatric nursing protocols for best practice*, New York, 2008, Springer.

Glaucoma Research Foundation: *Are you at risk for glaucoma?* (2008). Available at http://www.glaucoma.org/glaucoma/are-you-at-risk-for-glaucoma.php.

Ham R, Sloane P, Warshaw G: *Primary care geriatrics*, ed 5, St. Louis, 2007, Mosby.

Hersh S: Cerumen: insights and management, *Ann Longterm Care* 18:39, 2010.

Maclay E: *Green winter: celebrations of old age*, New York, 1977, Thomas W. Crowell.

Miller C: *Nursing for wellness in older adults*, ed 5, Philadelphia, 2008, Wolters Kluwer/Lippincott Williams & Wilkins.

Moeller S, Taylor A, Tucker K, et al: Associations between age-related nuclear cataract and lutein and zeaxanthin in the diet and serum in the carotenoids in the age-related eye disease study (CAREDS), an ancillary study of the Women's Health Initiative, *Arch Opthalmol* 126(3):354–364, 2008.

National Eye Institute, National Institutes of Health: *Vision loss from age will increase as Americans age* (2004). Available at http://www.nei.nih.gov/news/pressreleases/041204.asp#.

National Eye Institute, National Institutes of Health: *Survey of public knowledge, attitudes, and practices related to eye health and disease* (2008). Available at www.nei.nih.gov/news/pressreleases/031308.asp#.

National Eye Institute, National Institutes of Health: *About glaucoma* (2010a). Available at http://www.nei.nih.gov/health/glaucoma/glaucoma_facts.asp.

National Eye Institute, National Institutes of Health: *Diabetic eye disease* (2010b). Available at www.nei.nih.gov/nehep/programs/diabeticeyedisease/goals.asp.

National Eye Institute, National Institutes of Health: *Facts about macular degeneration*, (2010c). Available at www.nei.nih.gov/health/maculardegen/armd_facts.asp.

Owsley C, Ball K, McGwin G, et al: Effect of refractive error correction on health-related quality of life and depression in older nursing home residents, *Arch Ophthalmol* 125:1471, 2007.

Schumm L, McClintock M, Williams S, et al: Assessment of sensory function in the National Social Life, Health, and Aging Project, *J Gerontol B Psychol Sci Soc Sci* 64(Suppl 1): i76, 2009.

University of Wisconsin School of Medicine and Public Health: *Hearing loss common in middle age, but could be preventable*

(2011). Available at http://www.med.wisc.edu/news-events/news/hearing-loss-common-in-middle-age-but-could-be-preventable/30654.

U.S. Department of Health and Human Services [USDHHS]: *Healthy people 2020*. (2012). Available at http://www.healthy-people.gov/2020/default.aspx.

Wallhagen M: The stigma of hearing loss, *Gerontologist* 50:66, 2009.

Wallhagen M, Pettengill E: Hearing impairment significant but underassessed in primary care settings, *J Gerontol Nurs* 34:36, 2008.

Wilson MR, Eezzuduemhoi DR: Opthalmologic disorders in minority populations, *Med Clin North Am* 89(4):795–804, 2005.

CHAPTER 17

Metabolic Disorders

Kathleen F. Jett

evolve evolve.elsevier.com/Ebersole/gerontological

LEARNING OBJECTIVES

Upon completion of this chapter, the reader will be able to:
- Explain the risks for and complications of endocrine disorders in older adults.
- Describe the assessment necessary in the screening and monitoring of persons with diabetes.
- Identify the unique aspects of diabetes management in older adults.
- Explain the important components of diabetes management.
- Develop a nursing care plan for elders with endocrine disorders.
- Discuss the nurse's role in care for persons with endocrine disorders.
- Propose a reason for the significantly higher rate of diabetes among those over 75 years of age when compared to those over 50.

GLOSSARY

Autoimmune Term applied to the condition in which the body sees a part of itself as a foreign object and attempts to destroy itself.

Hgb A$_{1c}$ (Glycosylated hemoglobin) A blood test that measures the amount of glucose in the hemoglobin of red blood cells averaged over the 90-day life span of the cell.

Insulin resistance A condition in which body cells are less sensitive to the insulin produced by the pancreas, thus impairing normal glucose metabolism.

THE LIVED EXPERIENCE

I can see that Anna is going to need a lot of help learning to manage her diabetes. I know now that I have already overwhelmed her with brochures and information. She just looked frightened to death, and she really just has a mild elevation in blood sugar; it could probably be controlled with diet and exercise. I will call her tomorrow and see if she is less anxious.

Anna's gerontological clinical nurse specialist

Although the exact relationship between normal changes with aging and endocrine function is unknown, endocrine disorders, especially hypothyroidism and diabetes, most commonly occur in later life. It has been suggested that these are associated with the increase in autoimmune activity of the body as it ages (see Chapter 5) but the findings are inconclusive. Nonetheless, due to the large number of elders who are affected, the gerontological nurse should have a working knowledge of these conditions to provide the care needed to promote healthy aging.

Thyroid Disease

The thyroid is small gland in the neck which stores and secretes thyroid hormones, which regulate metabolism and affect nearly every organ in the body. It is estimated that about 5% of all Americans have overt hypothyroidism (National Institute of Diabetes and Digestive and Kidney Diseases [NIDDK], 2012c) and about 1% have hyperthyroidism (NIDDK, 2012b). Women are more likely to have both, affecting an estimated 5% to 10% of those over 65 years of age (Brashers & Jones, 2010). Usually easy to diagnose, many of the signs and symptoms in an older population are unfortunately non-specific, atypical, or absent. Signs such as decline in cognitive function or functional status or even an irregular heartbeat may be incorrectly attributed to normal aging, another disorder, or to side effects of medications when it is actually a thyroid disturbance.

Hypothyroidism

The most common thyroid disturbance in older adults is hypothyroidism, that is, the failure of the thyroid to produce an adequate amount of the hormone thyroxine. The onset is often subtle, developing slowly, and thought to be caused most frequently by chronic autoimmune thyroiditis or an inflamed thyroid. It may be iatrogenic, resulting from radioiodine treatment, a subtotal thyroidectomy, or medications. It can also be caused by a pituitary or hypothalamic abnormality (Jones et al., 2010).

The person may complain of heart palpitations, slowed thinking, gait disturbances, fatigue, weakness, or heat intolerance. These and other symptoms and signs are often evaluated for other causes before the possibility of hypothyroidism is considered. Blood tests to measure the amount of thyroid-stimulating hormone (TSH) and a free thyroxine (FT_4) are used for diagnosis. An elevated TSH combined with a low FT_4 indicates that the pituitary is working extra hard to get the thyroid to secrete when it may not be able to do so (Brashers & Jones, 2010). The treatment is to replace the missing thyroxine, usually in the form of the medication levothyroxine. However, it can only be done slowly due to the toxicity of the drug, beginning with doses of 0.025 mg/day (Shorr, 2007). To advance a dose rapidly could be life threatening. Most older adults never need to advance to a higher dose.

Hyperthyroidism

Hyperthyroidism is a disease of the secretion of an excess amount of thyroxine. Graves' disease is the most common cause in later life. Thyroid disease from multinodular toxic goiter and adenomas are also more common among older than younger adults. It can also result from ingestion of iodine or iodine-containing substances, such as those found in some seafood, radiocontrast agents, the medication amiodarone (a commonly prescribed antiarrhythmic agent), or too high a dose of levothyroxine. The same blood tests are done, this time the TSH would be very low and the FT_4 high. However, FT_4 is closely associated with protein levels in the blood. If protein is too low, the FT_4 will be artificially low making diagnosis difficult, especially in the large number of medically frail elders with hypoproteinemia (Pagana & Pagana, 2010).

Compared to hypothyroidism, the onset of hyperthyroidism may be quite sudden. The signs and symptoms in the older adult include unexplained atrial fibrillation, heart failure, constipation, anorexia, muscle weakness, and other vague complaints. Symptoms of heart failure or angina may cloud the clinical presentation and prevent the correct diagnosis. The person may be misdiagnosed as being depressed or having dementia. On examination, the person is likely to have tachycardia, tremors, and weight loss. In elders a condition known as apathetic thyrotoxicosis, rarely seen in younger persons, may occur in which usual hyperactivity is replaced with slowed movement and depressed affect. If left untreated it will increase the speed of bone loss and is as life threatening as hypothyroidism.

Complications

Complications occur both as the result of treatment and in the failure to diagnose and therefore failure to treat in a timely manner. Myxedema coma is a serious complication of untreated hypothyroidism in the older patient. Rapid replacement of the missing thyroxine is not possible due to risk of drug toxicity. If the disease is not detected until quite advanced, even with the best treatment, death may ensue.

Thyroxine increases myocardial oxygen consumption; therefore, the elevations found in hyperthyroidism produce a significant risk for atrial fibrillation and exacerbation of angina in persons with preexisting heart failure or may precipitate acute congestive heart failure (see Chapter 19).

Implications for Gerontological Nursing and Healthy Aging

The management of thyroid disturbances is largely one of careful pharmacological intervention and, in the case of hyperthyroidism, one of surgical or chemical ablation. As advocates, nurses can ensure that a thyroid screening test be done anytime there is a possibility of concern. The nurse caring for frail elders can be attentive to the possibility that the person who is diagnosed with atrial fibrillation, anxiety, dementia, or depression may instead have a thyroid disturbance. Although the nurse may see little that can be done to prevent thyroid disturbances in late life, organizations such as the Monterey Bay Aquarium have launched campaigns to inform consumers of the iodine and mercury found in seafood (www.seafoodwatch.org).

The nurse may be instrumental in working with the person and family to understand both the seriousness of the problem and the need for very careful adherence to the prescribed regimen. If the elder is hospitalized for acute management, the life-threatening nature of both the disorder and the treatment can be made clear so that advanced planning can be done that will account for all possible outcomes.

For the person in ongoing maintenance treatment, the nurse works with the person and significant others in the correct self-administration of medications and in the appropriate timing of monitoring blood levels and signs or symptoms which may indicate the need for a medication adjustment. Patient education includes instructions to always take the same brand, to take it at the same time every day and to not take any mineral products at the same time of the day, such as multivitamins, calcium, or some over-the-counter stomach preparations such as Tums (contain calcium) as these interfere with absorption (Shorr, 2007).

Diabetes

Diabetes mellitus (DM) is a syndrome of disorders of glucose metabolism resulting in hyperglycemia; that is, the body is unable to use the glucose that is both produced and ingested. Because glucose is necessary for life, DM is a life-threatening condition. The two main forms are type 1 (T1DM) and type 2 (T2DM). Additionally, gestational diabetes is that which happens for the first time when a woman is pregnant—usually with a very large fetus. Finally, of importance to older adults is steroid-induced diabetes, a unique circumstance caused by either long-term steroid use in persons with chronic obstructive pulmonary disease (COPD) or acute steroid use following an infection such as pneumonia.

T1DM (formerly called *insulin-dependent diabetes mellitus* [IDDM] and *juvenile onset*) develops early in life and is a result of autoimmune destruction of the insulin-producing beta cells in the pancreas. The absence of insulin is incompatible with life and without replacement of the insulin, the person will soon die. It has been rare that someone with T1DM lives to late life. Among U.S. residents at least 65 years of age in 2010, 10.9 million or 26.9% had diabetes, the majority of these with T2DM

(90% to 95%) (formerly called *non–insulin dependent diabetes mellitus* [NIDDM] or *adult onset*), making age alone a major risk factor (NIDDK, 2011). In this case, the pancreas makes insulin but either it does not make enough to keep up with the needs of the body and/or the tissues develop a resistance to naturally occurring insulin. The onset is usually insidious with few if any symptoms until end-organ damage has occurred. Older adults with T2DM often have other health problems, including problems with the metabolism of lipids and proteins. This considerably complicates providing care to them.

There are also a large number of persons of every age who have not yet been diagnosed or have conditions that may advance to DM if left untreated, specifically impaired glucose tolerance (IGT) or impaired fasting glucose (IFG) (Box 17-1). Who is likely to get DM or even die from DM varies by ethnicity, place of residence, and age (Figures 17-1 and 17-2, Box 17-2). DM affects African Americans the most, or about 18.7%, especially women between 65 and 75 years of age. American Indian and Alaskan Natives have an overall rate double that of non-Hispanic whites (14.2%) but this varies by group, from

---

BOX 17-1   Diagnosis of Disorders of Glucose Metabolism

Diagnosis of Diabetes Mellitus Requires Either:

ONE random plasma glucose ≥200 mg/dL when exhibiting symptoms

OR

TWO of any combination of positive tests on different days:

- Fasting plasma glucose (FPG) ≥126 mg/dL on separate occasions (NOTE: This is not blood glucose level that is obtained with a fingerstick.)
- Oral glucose tolerance test (OGTT) ≥200 mg/dL 2 hours after glucose
- Random plasma glucose ≥200 mg/dL without symptoms

Diagnosis of Impaired Fasting Glucose (IFG) Requires:

Fasting blood glucose between 110 and 125 mg/dL

Diagnosis of Impaired Glucose Tolerance Requires:

Glucose between 141 and 199 mg/dL 2 hours after a glucose challenge

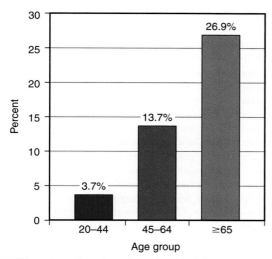

FIGURE 17-1 Comparison of prevalence of combined diagnosed and undiagnosed diabetes mellitus by age group. (From 2005-2008 National Health and Nutrition Examination Survey. Available at http://diabetes.niddk.nih.gov/dm/pubs/statistics/index.aspx#fast. Revised March 2011.)

5.5% for Alaskan Natives to 33.5% for those in southern Arizona. DM affects approximately 11.8% of all Hispanic adults again with a great amount of variability; Cubans with the lowest (7.6%) and those from Puerto Rico with the highest (13.8%) (Centers for Disease Control and Prevention [CDC], 2011).

Signs and Symptoms

The classic signs and symptoms of diabetes include thirst and excessive urinating as the body tries to reduce the relative concentration of glucose in the blood. Yet hyperglycemia appears to be well tolerated in later life and there may be no early warning symptoms until the person is found to be in a life-threatening (hyperosmolar nonketotic) coma. For unknown reasons diabetic coma is more common among African-American elders. It is not unusual to find asymptomatic older persons with fasting glucose levels of 300 mg/dL or higher or as low as 50 mg/dL. Early signs may instead be dehydration, confusion, or delirium and are very dangerous. Instead of urinary frequency, the high amount of glucose in the urine often causes incontinence. The catabolic state caused by lack of insulin causes polyphagia (excessive hunger) in younger persons but causes weight loss and anorexia in elders (lack of appetite). Other vague signs and symptoms include fatigue, nausea, delayed wound healing, and paresthesias; the later is a sign that the person has already had the disease for many years (Jones et al., 2010) (Box 17-3).

Complications

Complications of DM are serious and significantly affect both the person's morbidity (i.e., wellness) and mortality (i.e., length of life); they include heart disease, stroke, neuropathy, and periodontal disease. DM is the leading cause of end-stage renal disease and blindness and is especially prevalent among persons over 65 years of age. Adults with diabetes have two to four times the rate of heart disease and stroke. Nerve damage occurs in 60% to 70% of persons ranging from peripheral neuropathy (numbness in the extremities) to gastroparesis (delays in emptying of the stomach) (NIDDK, 2012a). The microvascular problems include loss of vision (diabetic retinopathy) and end-stage renal failure from diabetic nephropathy (kidney damage). Wound healing is delayed, which may lead to amputation when combined with peripheral neuropathy. Diabetes is associated with a high rate of depression; those with diabetes are twice as likely to be depressed and the combination leads to a higher rate of death (National Diabetes Education Program [NDEP], 2012).

Combined macrovascular and microvascular damage also leads to male sexual impotence, a result of reduction in vascular flow, peripheral neuropathy, and uncontrolled circulating blood glucose. Sexual dysfunction is two to five

Age-Adjusted Diabetes Death Rates per 100,000 (2006)			
	African Americans	**Non-Hispanic White**	**African Americans/Non-Hispanic White Ratio**
Male	50.6	24.7	2.0
Female	42.4	17.0	2.5
Total	45.9	20.4	2.3

FIGURE 17-2 Comparative death rate by racial group. (From Centers for Disease Control and Prevention: *National vital statistics report,* vol 57, no. 14, Table 17 (2009). Available at http://www.cdc.gov/nchs/data/nvsr/nvsr57/nvsr57_14.pdf.)

BOX 17-2   Risk Factors for Diabetes Mellitus

- Hispanic men*
- African-American men and women*
- Increasing age
- Blood pressure ≥140/90 mm Hg
- First-degree relative (parent, sibling, child) with DM
- History of impaired glucose tolerance or impaired fasting plasma glucose
- Obesity: >120% of desirable weight or body mass index (BMI) >30 kg/m^2
- Previous gestational DM or having had a child with a birth weight of >9 pounds
- History of vascular disease
- Undesirable lipid levels: high-density lipoproteins (HDLs) ≤35 mg/dL or triglycerides ≥250 mg/dL

* Data regarding other groups are less accurate.

BOX 17-3   Signs and Symptoms Suggestive of Diabetes in the Late Life

- Recurrent infections, particularly of bacterial or fungal origin, that involve the skin, intertriginous areas, or the genitourinary tract and sores or wounds that tend to heal slowly
- Neurological dysfunction, including paresthesia, dysesthesia, or hyperesthesia; muscle weakness and pain (amyotrophy); cranial nerve palsies; autonomic dysfunction of the gastrointestinal tract (diarrhea), cardiovascular system (orthostatic hypotension, dysrhythmias), reproductive system (impotence), or bladder (atony, overflow incontinence)
- Arterial disease (macroangiopathy) involving the cardiovascular, cerebrovascular, or peripheral vasculature structures
- Small-vessel disease (microangiopathy) involving the kidneys (proteinuria, glomerulopathy, uremia) and eyes (macular disease, exudates, hemorrhages)
- Lesions of the skin, such as Dupuytren's contractures, facial rubeosis, and diabetic dermopathy
- Endocrine-metabolic complications, including hyperlipidemia, obesity, and a history of thyroid or adrenal insufficiency (Schmidt's syndrome)
- A family history of type 1 or type 2 diabetes and a poor obstetrical history (miscarriages, stillbirths, large babies)

times greater in this group than in the general population, even though interest and desire are still present.

Persons with diabetes commonly have problems with their feet, which can have a considerable impact on their functional status (see Chapter 12). Although the problem may not be from DM in particular, they are often related. Common foot problems include cold feet and intermittent pain from claudication (vascular insufficiency); burning, tingling, hypersensitivity, or numbness (neuropathies); gradual change in shape or sudden, painless change without trauma (musculoskeletal changes); and infections, skin color and texture changes, and slow-healing, exquisitely painful or painless wounds (dermatological sensitivities) (NIDDK, 2012a).

Older adults who are receiving treatment, especially sulfonylureas (e.g., Glipizide) or sliding scale insulin, are at particular risk for hypoglycemia (blood glucose <60 mg/dL), both of which are on the Beers list of inappropriate medications (see Chapter 8) (American Geriatrics Society [AGS], 2012). Hypogycylemia can come from many causes, such as unusually intense exercise, alcohol intake, or medication mismanagement (Jones et al., 2010). Signs in the older adult include tachycardia, palpitations, diaphoresis, tremors, pallor, and anxiety. Later symptoms may include headache, dizziness, fatigue, irritability, confusion, hunger, visual changes, seizures, and coma. Immediate care involves giving the patient glucose either by mouth or intravenously.

Persons with diabetes most often die of heart disease. Since the national efforts to move toward goals established by *Healthy People 2000, 2010,* and now *2020* (U.S. Department of Health and Human Services [USDHHS], 2012), there has been a decrease in the number of deaths. However, death from heart disease remains very high among persons with diabetes; 68% die of heart disease, and the risk for stroke is two to four times that of those without diabetes (NDEP, 2012).

Implications for Gerontological Nursing and Healthy Aging

Diabetes is a chronic disease that, even in the best of circumstances, will likely damage the body's organs. When diabetes is untreated or undertreated, the complications develop more quickly and more severely in the older adult. Therefore, the goals are twofold: control the blood sugar and reduce the risk for complications.

Based on the results of several large studies, the American Diabetes Association modified their recommendations in 2011 for glycemic control in older adults (ADA, 2011). They now recommend that the degree of gylcemic control be based on the condition of the person rather than a universal number. For healthy elders with a reasonably long life expectancy, the same evidence-based practice as younger adults should be followed. However for those who are very medically fragile and whose life expectancy is limited, such as those in nursing homes, some flexibility may be more appropriate, with an emphasis on quality of life rather than length of life. Tight control of glucose levels in these circumstances may lead to life-threatening hypoglycemia. There is now some discussion that a goal of a Hemoglobin A_{1c} of greater than 8% for the very frail may be adequate (Zarowitz, 2011). Unfortunately this leads to an increase in urinary tract infections (UTIs) in the presence of glucosuria, especially *Klebsiella* and *E. coli*.

The goals of promoting healthy aging in persons with diabetes are to maintain the best health that is realistically possible and ensure that the care is received (see the Evidence-Based Practice box). Caring for the elder with diabetes centers on reducing modifiable risks of complications and their early identification. The nurse can participate in early detection through public screenings or pay attention to the need for screening of persons residing in communal settings such as nursing homes and assistive living centers. The nurse can also promote healthy aging by helping people do what they can to reduce their risk for diabetes, such as obtaining or maintaining an ideal body weight, eating a healthy diet that provides for adequate protein without excessive carbohydrates, exercising, and keeping their cholesterol levels and blood pressure under control.

For persons at higher risk for diabetes, especially those with pre-diabetes, attention should be directed at reducing the risk for both diabetes and heart disease. This means education and interventions to help the person reach the following goals:

- No smoking or smoking cessation
- Blood pressure ≤130/80 mm Hg
- Cholesterol <200 mg/dL
- Low-density lipoprotein (LDL) <100 mg/dL
- High-density lipoprotein (HDL) >40 mg/dL
- Triglycerides <150 mg/dL
- Fasting blood glucose <126 mg/dL

Annual screening of fasting plasma glucose measurements is recommended for all persons in high-risk groups, which includes all persons over 65 years of age.

Assessment

The nurse begins with the assessment for risk factors and a subjective report of signs and symptoms, including the evaluation of the presence or absence of hyperglycemia or hypoglycemia. When there are symptoms, the duration and character of these should be described. Nutrition, weight, and exercise history are important to identify eating patterns, an active or sedentary lifestyle, and weight control measures, all of which can provide clues for realistic

education and how to encourage better adherence to a therapy regimen if necessary, which promotes health and wellness. Assessing economic resources helps establish the person's ability to purchase equipment, materials, and foods that may be needed to maintain diabetes control. This is especially important for older adults, many of whom have very limited incomes. History of alcohol and tobacco use provides information related to the risk for complications, especially cardiovascular.

The nursing assessment also includes paying attention for the earliest signs and symptoms of complications. This includes careful measurement of blood pressure, visual acuity, and gross neurological function. Distant vision can be checked with a Snellen chart and near vision with a newspaper. The skin and feet should be thoroughly inspected for any injury, such as corns, calluses, blisters, cracks, or fungal infections. Use of the Semmes-Weinstein monofilament instrument is recommended to test for peripheral neuropathy. This is available to nurses and easy to use. It is a very helpful measure of the progression of peripheral neuropathy. The measurement of the hemoglobin A_{1c} is the best measure of ongoing glycemic control and can now be used as a diagnostic indicator as well (Figure 17-3).

Management

Promoting healthy aging in person with diabetes requires an array of interventions and usually involves persons from a number of disciplines working together with the patient and significant others. Management of such a disease requires expertise in medication use, diet, exercise, counseling, and giving support. The persons involved may include the usual care nurses as well as nutritionists, pharmacists, podiatrists, ophthalmologists, physicians or nurse practitioners, and counselors. If the person's disease is hard to control, endocrinologists are involved, and as

A_{1c} (%)	eAG (mg/dL)
6	126
7	154
8	183
9	212
10	240
11	269
12	298

FIGURE 17-3 Hemoglobin A_{1c} readings in comparison to the calculated estimated average glucose (eAG). (Adapted from American Diabetes Association: Standards of medical care in diabetes, Table 9, *Diabetes Care* 34[Suppl 1]: S11–S61, 2011. Available at http://www.diabetes.niddk.nih.gov/dm/pubs/A1CTest/.)

complications develop, more specialists, such as nephrologists, cardiologists, and wound care specialists, are called. Nurses with a special interest in diabetes can become certified diabetic educators.

The focus of management is now geared more toward life expectancy and the recognition of the importance of cardiovascular health promoting strategies. The benefits of better control of blood pressure and lipids can be seen in 2 to 3 years. Promoting health in this area has the potential to be the most efficacious in the minimization of complications (Auerhahn et al., 2007). In comparison, research has indicated that it may take 8 years of glycemic control before benefits are seen.

Diabetes self-management (DSM), diabetes self-management education (DSME), and patient empowerment are now the cornerstones of disease management (Funnell & Anderson, 2004; Mensing et al., 2007) (see the Evidence-Based Practice box). The skills needed for self-management include knowledge about nutrition, the development of an exercise plan, safe medication use, what to do during periods of other illness, and attention to the psychological aspects of dealing with a chronic illness. Other self-management skills include the use of personal glucose monitors, optimal care of the feet, and knowledge about the disease. The nurse is instrumental in the teaching of self-management skills, encouraging patient empowerment and supporting the person while he or she struggles with a complicated and very serious disease. Experiential teaching, encouragement, and mastery are important to successful self-management. However, there are multiple factors related to

aging that can affect this goal (see the Evidence-Based Practice box). Standards have now been established for DSME, and the cost is covered by many insurance companies including Medicare (Mensing et al., 2007). Medicare pays 100% of the costs of an initial 10 hours of education and 2 hours each year after that. Limited diabetic supplies are also now covered by Medicare (Centers for Medicare and Medicaid Services [CMS], 2012).

DSME includes self-monitoring blood glucose (SMBG) (see the Healthy People 2020 box). This includes teaching the patient how to obtain a blood sample, use the glucose monitoring equipment, troubleshoot when there are results indicating an error, and record the values from the machine. Older adults with arthritis, low vision, or peripheral neuropathy from whatever cause will have difficulties with the mechanics of SMBG and will require creative teaching, perhaps enlisting friends or neighbors in the tasks that are necessary; however, new technologies and drug delivery systems are being designed to make these tasks easier. The education plan includes the timing and frequency of the self-monitoring, the correct adjustment in the schedule when ill, and what to do with the results and the importance of bringing the results to each health care visit.

Daily foot care and foot examination should be discussed and demonstrated. Persons who are not particularly flexible will have difficulty reaching and inspecting their feet, and a family member or friend can be asked to do this. As long as vision is adequate, checking can also be done by placing a mirror on the floor to examine the sole. Attention

---

 EVIDENCE-BASED PRACTICE

Minimum Standards of Care for the Person with Diabetes

At Each Visit:
- Monitor weight and BP.
- Inspect feet.
- Review self-monitoring glucose record.
- Review/adjust medications as needed.
- Review self-management skills/goals.
- Assess mood.

Quarterly Visits:
- Obtain hemoglobin A_{1c} (biannually if stable).

Annual Visits:
- Obtain fasting lipid profile and serum creatinine.
- Obtain albumin-to-creatinine ratio.
- Refer for dilated eye exam.
- Perform comprehensive foot exam.
- Refer to dentist for comprehensive exam and cleaning.
- Administer influenza vaccination.

Once in Lifetime:
- Administer pneumococcal vaccination (consider repeat if over 5-10 years).

Modified from National Diabetes Education Program: *Guiding principles for diabetes care: for health care professionals* (2009). Available at http://ndep.nih.gov/publications/PublicationDetail.aspx?PubId=108.

EVIDENCE-BASED PRACTICE

Self-Care Skills Needed for the Person with Diabetes

Glucose Self-Monitoring
- Obtaining a blood sample correctly
- Using the glucose monitoring equipment correctly
- Troubleshooting when results indicate an error
- Recording the values from the machine
- Understanding the timing and frequency of the self-monitoring
- Understanding what to do with the results

Medication Self-Administration
Where Appropriate, Insulin Use
- Selecting appropriate injection site
- Using correct technique for injections

- Disposing of used needles and syringes correctly
- Storing and transporting insulin correctly

Oral Medication Use
- Knowing drug, dose, timing, and side effects
- Knowing drug-drug and drug-food interactions
- Recognizing side effects and knowing when to report

Foot Care and Examination
- Selecting and using appropriate and safe footwear

Handling Sick Days
- Recognizing the signs and symptoms of both hyperglycemia and hypoglycemia

---

 HEALTHY PEOPLE 2020

Examples of Goals Related to Diabetes

Objective D-13
Increase the proportion of adults with diabetes who perform self–blood glucose monitoring at least once daily.
- *Baseline:* 64.0% of adults aged 18 years and older with diagnosed diabetes performed self–blood glucose monitoring at least once daily in 2008.
- *Target:* 70.4%
- *Target-setting:* 10% improvement
- *Data source:* Behavioral Risk Factor Surveillance Survey, CDC, NCCDPHP

Objective D-14
Increase the proportion of persons with diagnosed diabetes who receive formal diabetes education.
- *Baseline:* 56.8% of adults aged 18 years and older with diagnosed diabetes received formal diabetes education in 2008.
- *Target:* 62.5%
- *Target-setting:* 10% improvement
- *Data source:* Behavioral Risk Factor Surveillance Survey, CDC, NCCDPHP

From U.S. Department of Health and Human Services, Office of Disease Prevention and Health Promotion: *Healthy people 2020* (2012). Available at http://www.healthypeople.gov/2020.

---

to foot care can reduce the risk of amputation. Awareness of the need for good shoes that fit well is essential. Those who have Medicare are eligible for one pair of specially made shoes annually.

Knowledge about the disease and its effects includes knowing what affects the blood sugar such as high carbohydrate foods and skipping meals. The elder should have a list of warning signs for high and low blood sugar levels, especially one that reflects the signs and symptoms he or she typically experiences (Box 17-4), and know that extra SMBG should be done any time the person feels clammy or cold, sweaty, shaky, or confused, all signs of low blood

sugar. An identification bracelet is highly recommended especially because of the quick misdiagnosis that can occur if the person is found to be confused and mistakenly believed to have dementia.

Nutrition

Adequate and appropriate nutrition is a key aspect in diabetes management. An initial nutrition assessment with a 24-hour recall will provide some clues to the patient's dietary habits, intake, and style of eating. It is always necessary to know who shops for and prepares the

BOX 17-4 Interaction Between Diabetes and the Aging Process

1. A decline in visual acuity can affect the individual's ability to see printed educational material, medication labels, markings on a syringe, and blood glucose monitoring devices.
2. Auditory impairments can lead to difficulty hearing instructions.
3. Altered taste can affect food choices and nutritional status.
4. Poor dentition or changes in the gastrointestinal system can lead to difficulties with food ingestion and digestion.
5. Altered ability to recognize hunger and thirst may lead to weight loss, dehydration, and increased risk for hyperosmolar nonketotic syndrome.
6. Changes in hepatic or renal function can affect ability to self-administer medications.
7. Arthritis or tremors can affect ability to self-administer medications and use monitoring devices.
8. Polypharmacy complicates medication choices.
9. Depression affects motivation for self-management.
10. Cognitive impairment and dementia decrease self-care ability.
11. Inadequate education and poor literacy call for modifications in the method of teaching about diabetes care.
12. The level of income can affect the level of care sought or obtained.
13. Living alone without a resource person for help with management can have a negative effect on the person with diabetes.
14. A sedentary lifestyle and obesity can result in decreased tissue sensitivity to insulin.

food. If the person is from an ethnic group different from the nurse, the nurse will need to learn more about the usual ingredients and methods of food preparation to be able to give reasonable instructions. Ideally, all persons with diabetes should have medical nutrition therapy by a registered dietitian who is a certified diabetic educator on an annual basis. At the time of this writing this service is covered by Medicare (CMS, 2012).

The ADA (2012) guidelines focus on a healthful diet with attention to an adequate variety of foods with portion control. Recommended daily caloric intake ranges from 1600 to 2000 calories for women and 2000 to 2600 calories for men over 60 years of age, depending on activity level. The goal is to keep the glucose level under control by balancing exercise with eating, weight loss if overweight, and limiting saturated fats in the diet. Carbohydrates are included, but these are restricted to those that are full-grain. It is part of the nurse's responsibility to learn if there is difficulty with access to food, including food preparation and shopping for food. Working with elders, whose dietary habits have been formed over a lifetime, can be difficult but is not impossible.

Exercise

Daily exercise is an important aspect of therapy for T2DM because it decreases blood sugar by increasing insulin production and decreasing insulin resistance. Walking is an inexpensive and beneficial way to exercise. Unfortunately, in some communities, environmental conditions prevent walking in one's neighborhood. This is most applicable to elders who live in warm climates or communities with high crime rates. Walking in a local mall, where it is climate controlled and safe, has proved to be a good alternative. Those who have limited mobility can still do chair exercises or if possible use exercise machines that permit sitting and holding on for support.

Exercise in conjunction with an appropriate diet may be sufficient to maintain blood glucose levels within normal limits in some cases. A more intensive exercise program should not be started until the person has had a physical examination, including a stress test and electrocardiogram (ECG). A physician or nurse practitioner and a diabetic educator will then have the information necessary to develop a safe and individualized exercise plan. If the person is using insulin, exercise must be done on a regular rather than an erratic basis, and blood glucose should be tested before and after exercise to avoid hypoglycemia. Resources about exercise and diabetes are available at the National Institute of Diabetes and Digestive and Kidney Disorders (http://diabetes.niddk.nih.gov/index.htm).

Medications

Antihyperglycemics include oral agents and insulin, including the new inhalant insulin. Oral medications are prescribed according to the insulin deficit identified: no secretion of insulin, insulin resistance, or inadequate secretion of insulin. The sulfonylureas (e.g., Glucotrol) and meglitinides (e.g., Starlix) increase insulin secretion. Biguanides (e.g., metformin) or thiazolidinediones (e.g., Actos) and the newer Januvia have been useful to enhance insulin sensitivity by decreasing insulin resistance.

The mainstay of treatment of T2DM in later life is oral medication; however, when the blood sugar is consistently over 200 and difficult to control, insulin may be necessary. It is important to note that the use of insulin by someone with T2DM does not "convert" them to a type 1 diabetic, because the diagnosis is made on the type of disorder rather than on the treatment. Diabinase and the other sulfonylureas should never be prescribed for the older adult or only with great caution due to a very high risk for hypoglycemia (AGS, 2012). Metformin (Glucophage) has been found to be very safe and effective but can only be used by people with good renal functioning (creatinine level no greater than 1.5 mg/dL for men and at or below 1.4 mg/dL for women) (Shah, 2010). Renal function must be monitored periodically and any time there is a dose change.

If other medications are prescribed, they must be carefully reviewed. The effect of drugs on blood glucose must be given serious consideration because a number of medications commonly used for elders adversely affect blood glucose levels, especially psychotropics, antibiotics, and steroids. Therefore older adults should be advised to ask if a particular drug prescribed affects their therapy and should check with their primary care provider or pharmacist before taking any over-the-counter medications.

Where appropriate, demonstration and return demonstration should be given for drawing up insulin, selecting the injection site, injecting and storing insulin, and disposing of the used needle and syringes. For those who can afford them, insulin pens require less manual dexterity. Finally, knowing how to safely transport insulin when traveling is also important.

Long-Term Care and the Elder with Diabetes

Many of the persons cared for by gerontological nurses in long-term care facilities have diabetes. In this setting the nurse may be responsible for many of the activities that would otherwise fall to the patient or a home caregiver to carry out. Nutritional status, intake and output, and exercise and activity are monitored. The nurse regularly assesses the person for signs of hypoglycemia and hyperglycemia as well as evidence of complications. The nurse ensures that evidence-based practice is followed. The nurse monitors the effect and side effects of diet, exercise, and medication use and encourages self-care whenever possible. The nurse administers or supervises the administration of medications.

If the person requires *sliding scale insulin,* in which the dosage depends on the current glucose reading, it is the nurse who must make the determination of the dosage under sliding scale guidelines. While this approach is commonly used, it is one of the newer drug regimens considered "inappropriate" at times for use in older adults due to the high risk for hypoglycemia, calling for utmost caution (AGS, 2012).

KEY CONCEPTS

- Signs and symptoms of endocrine disorders in the older adult may be vague or suggestive of other medical conditions or considered as part of "old age" rather than the usual and expected symptoms. For example, polyuria, polydipsia, and polyphagia in an older adult with hyperglycemia are unusual.
- Although thyroid disorders only affect a small number of persons, the incidence increases with age and is potentially life threatening.
- Consideration of the person's life expectancy and the risks and benefits of treatment are taken into account when determining the appropriate level of glycemic control in the older adult with DM.
- Management of diabetes is a comprehensive team effort and should include the elder as much as he or she can realistically participate. If this is not possible, the caregiver, if not the nurse, will need to ensure that the medical regimen is effective.
- Caring for persons with DM includes working with them to reduce their risk for cardiovascular diseases.
- Preventive foot care is essential for prevention of the possibility of future problems.
- Any time a person is being evaluated for depression, atrial fibrillation, dementia or confusion, the assessment should include consideration of a thyroid disturbance.
- Very low doses of thyroid replacement are usually adequate in older adults. When dose changes are necessary, they must be made very slowly.

ACTIVITIES AND DISCUSSION QUESTIONS

1. What are the risks and complications of DM for the older adult?
2. What are the risks of treatment of the older adult with DM?
3. State the components of diabetes management, and explain what each component entails.
4. Describe the nurse's role in the management of endocrine disorders in older adults.

REFERENCES

American Diabetes Association [ADA]: Standards of medical care in diabetes, *Diabetes Care* 34(Suppl 1):S11–S61, 2011.

American Geriatrics Society [AGS]: American Geriatrics updated Beers Criteria for potentially inappropriate medication use in older adults, *J Am Geriatr Soc* 60(4):616–631, 2012.

Auerhahn C, Capezuti E, Flaherty R, Resnick B, editors: *Geriatric nursing review syllabus: a core curriculum in advance geriatric nursing,* ed 2, New York 2007, American Geriatric Society.

Brashers VL, Jones RE: Mechanisms of hormonal regulation. In McCance K, Huether S, Brashers V, et al, editors: *Pathophysiology: the biological basis for disease in adults and children,* ed 6, St. Louis, 2010, Mosby.

Centers for Disease Control and Prevention [CDC]: *2011 National diabetes fact sheet* (2011). Available at http://www.cdc.gov/diabetes/pubs/estimates11.htm.

Centers for Medicare and Medicaid Services [CMS]: *Medicare preventive services: quick reference information* (2012). Available at http://www.cms.gov/PrevntionGenInfo.

Funnell MM, Anderson R: Empowerment and self-management of diabetes. *Clin Diabetes* 22:123–127, 2004.

Jones R, Brashers V, Huether S: Alterations of hormonal regulation. In McCance K, Huether S, Brashers V, et al, editors: *Pathophysiology: the biological basis for disease in adults and children,* ed 6, St. Louis, 2010, Mosby.

Mensing C, Boucher J, Cypress M, et al.: National standards for diabetes self-management education, *Diabetes Care* 30(Suppl 1): S96–S103, 2007.

National Diabetes Education Program [NDEP]: *Diabetes: the numbers* (2012). Available at http://www.ndep.nih.gov/resources/ResourceDetail.aspx?ResId=151.

National Institute of Diabetes and Digestive and Kidney Diseases [NIDDK]: *National Diabetes Statistics* (2011). Available at http://diabetes.niddk.nih.gov/dm/pubs/statistics/index.aspx.

National Institute of Diabetes and Digestive and Kidney Diseases [NIDDK]: *Complications of diabetes* (2012a). Available at http://diabetes.niddk.nih.gov/complications/index.aspx.

National Institute of Diabetes and Digestive and Kidney Diseases [NIDDK]: *Hyperthyroidism* (2012b). Available at http://endocrine.niddk.nih.gov/pubs/hyperthyroidism/index.aspx.

National Institute of Diabetes and Digestive and Kidney Diseases [NIDDK]: *Hypothyroidism* (2012c). Available at http://endocrine.niddk.nih.gov/pubs/hypothyroidism/index.aspx.

Pagana KD, Pagana TJ: *Mosby's manual of diagnostic and laboratory tests,* ed 4, St. Louis, 2010, Mosby.

Shah A: Endocrinology. In Durso SC, editor: *Oxford handbook of geriatric medicine,* New York, 2010, Oxford Press, pp. 433–465.

Shorr RI, editor: *Drugs for the geriatric patient, Philadelphia, 2007,* Saunders.

U.S. Department of Health and Human Services [USDHHS]: *Healthy people 2020* (2012). Available at www.healthypeople.gov.

Zarowitz B: The ADA focus on diabetes, *Geriatr Nurs* 32(2): 119–122, 2011.

CHAPTER 18

Bone and Joint Problems

Kathleen F. Jett

evolve evolve.elsevier.com/Ebersole/gerontological

LEARNING OBJECTIVES

Upon completion of this chapter, the reader will be able to:

- Describe the most common bone and joint problems affecting older adults.
- Discuss the potential dangers of osteoporosis.
- Recognize postural changes that suggest the presence of osteoporosis.
- Explain some effective ways of preventing or slowing the progression of osteoporosis.
- Compare the differences in common arthritic conditions.
- Describe the nurse's responsibility in care for the person with arthritic conditions.
- Name several methods of promoting healthy aging in the person with pain and disability from joint and bone disorders.

GLOSSARY

Bone mineral density (BMD) Mineral content of the bones.
Crepitus The sound or feel of bone rubbing on bone.
Osteopenia Loss of bone mineral density and structure at a mild to moderate level.
Osteophyte Excessive bone growth.
Osteoporosis Loss of bone mineral density and structure to a great degree.
Resorption The loss of a substance or bone by physiological or pathological processes.

THE LIVED EXPERIENCE

It is so discouraging to wake up feeling so stiff and sore every morning. Just getting out of bed seems like a real effort, but I usually feel better after I have moved around a bit. I was always so athletic, I can't understand how I have become so crippled up. And now I know that what my grandmother used to say about the weather affecting her rheumatism is really true. I can feel it when a storm is coming.

Mabel, age 80

I don't know how folks with arthritis can stand being uncomfortable so much of the time. I know Mabel takes medications, but she still seems to be in a lot of pain and has so much trouble moving about. I'll try to be as gentle as possible when I help her bathe.

Elva, student nurse

Musculoskeletal System

A healthy musculoskeletal system not only allows the body to be upright but also is necessary for comfortably carrying out the most basic activities of daily living (ADLs). For some, later life is an opportunity to explore the limits of their ability and become master athletes. For others, later life is a time of significant restriction in movement. However, both athletes and nonathletes have to deal with the challenges of one or more of the musculoskeletal problems commonly encountered in later life.

The gerontological nurse attends to the needs of older adults with musculoskeletal problems and works to promote healthy bones and joints. In this chapter we discuss osteoporosis and the different forms of arthritis, and their implications for nursing intervention and the promotion of healthy aging.

Osteoporosis

In the normal process of growth, known as bone turnover, the bones build up mass (formation) and strength at the same time they are losing both through resorption. Peak bone mass is reached at about 30 years of age. After that, the loss of bone mineral density (BMD) is quite minimal at first but speeds up with age. For women, the period of the fastest overall loss of BMD is in the 5 to 7 years immediately following menopause.

Osteoporosis means *porous bone*. Primary osteoporosis is sometimes thought to be part of the normal aging process, especially for women. Secondary osteoporosis is that which is caused by another disease state, such as Paget's disease, or by medications, such as long-term steroid use. Both are characterized by low BMD and subsequent deterioration of the bone structure and changes in posture (Figure 18-1). Low BMD affects about 44 million or 55% of people over 50 years of age. Eighty percent of those affected are women, especially thin white women. Ten million have osteoporosis and the rest have osteopenia or a lesser degree of the loss of BMD (National Osteoporosis Foundation [NOF], 2011).

Osteoporosis is a silent disorder; a person may never know she has osteoporosis until a fracture occurs. It is diagnosed through a dual energy x-ray absorptiometry (DEXA) scan but is presumed in older adults with non-traumatic fractures, a loss of 3 inches or more in height, and/or kyphosis (see Figure 18-1). The nurse may be the one to identify the changes that had not yet been medically diagnosed. Without a diagnosis the person cannot be treated.

The most serious complication of osteoporosis is the increased risk for a fracture and subsequent death or disability. Each year more than 1.6 million older adults go to

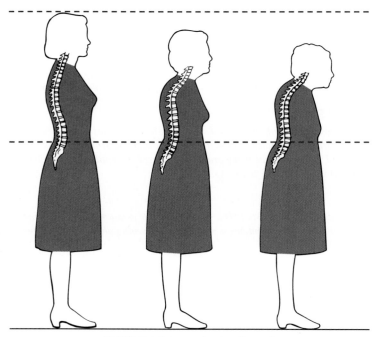

FIGURE 18-1 Osteoporosis spine alignment.

BOX 18-1   Risk Factors for Osteoporosis

Nonmodifiable Factors
Gender (female)
Race (Caucasian, Asian)
Age
Family history of osteoporosis

Modifiable Factors
Weight (underweight)
Diet (Low calcium, excessive caffeine, ethyl alcohol)
Hormonal deficiencies
Activity level (low)
Medications (steroids, anticonvulsants)
Cigarette smoking

emergency rooms for fall-related injuries, the number one cause of fracture, trauma admissions to hospitals and injury-related deaths (NIH, 2011). Fractures of the hip, pelvis, spine, arm, hand, or ankle are those most commonly associated with osteoporosis. It was estimated that there were about 2 million related fractures in 2005 and the number is expected to climb (NOF, 2011). Among persons over 50 years of age, who were healthy and active before the fracture usually go home, but those with other health problems may not ever be able to return to independent living (National Institutes of Health [NIH], 2011).

A number of factors increase or decrease a person's risk for both osteopenia and osteoporosis. Some of these cannot be changed (e.g., gender, race, family history, or ethnicity), but others (e.g., calcium intake, exercise) are amenable to change (Box 18-1). African-American women have the highest BMD but are still at risk. The U.S. Preventive Services Task Force recommends that all women 65 years of age or older and younger women with significant risk factors (e.g., family history) be screened for osteoporosis. There is currently insufficient evidence to make a recommendation about screening in men (USPSTF, 2011). If the screening is positive the nurse can advocate for the elder to receive appropriate treatment. The nurse can always recommend preventive measures such as adequate amounts of calcium and vitamin D and smoking cessation (see later).

Implications for Gerontological Nursing and Healthy Aging

With the treatments and interventions now available, some osteoporosis can be prevented or treated and stabilized to some extent. It is always possible to promote healthy aging for the person with osteoporosis. However, for those already with osteoporosis it becomes paramount to reduce osteoporosis-related injury.

Reducing Osteoporosis-Related Risk and Injury

Measures to prevent osteoporosis-related injury or progression of the disease include exercise, nutrition, and lifestyle changes to reduce known risk factors. As with many other diseases, smoking is one risk factor that can be changed. Home safety inspection and education regarding injury prevention strategies are essential (see Chapter 13). An assortment of print and interactive educational materials for both the lay and professional audience can be found at http://www.niams.nih.gov/Health_Info/Bone/Osteoporosis/default.asp.

Weight-bearing physical activity and exercises help to maintain bone mass (see the Evidence-Based Practice box). Brisk walking and working with light weights apply mechanical force to the spine and long bones (see Chapters 11 and 13). Muscle-building exercises help to maintain skeletal architecture by improving muscle strength and flexibility. The Asian art of T'ai Chi has been used successfully for strengthening of both ambulatory and nonambulatory elders (Wayne et al., 2007, 2010). T'ai Chi and exercise have the added advantage of improving balance and stamina, which may prevent falls or limit the damage if a fall should occur.

Patient teaching includes key aspects of the prevention and treatment of osteoporosis. Information about the sites most vulnerable to injury should be provided. Explanation should be given about changes in the upper spine that occur when vertebrae are weakened, and about the pain that results from strain on the lower spine that is caused by the effort to compensate for balance and height changes attributable to alteration of the upper spine. Education also includes the appropriate way to take medications and how to handle their side effects.

Fall prevention is especially important to decrease the morbidity and mortality associated with osteoporosis. Shoes with good support should be worn. Handrails should be used, and walking in poorly lighted areas should be avoided. Basic body mechanics, such as how to lift heavy objects, should be learned. Use of step stools or chairs for reaching things in high places should be discouraged; instead these things can be moved to a more reachable level. Attention must be paid to home safety and improvements should include good lighting, railings, and other aids as needed. Walkways should be kept free of obstacles; loose rugs and electrical cords

EVIDENCE-BASED PRACTICE

The Role of Arthritis and the Risk for Fractures

Purpose
The purpose of the study was to determine the relationship between the different forms of arthritis, osteoporosis, and fractures.

Sample
The study included almost 147,000 women who participated in the Women's Health Initiative supported by the National Institute of Arthritis and Musculoskeletal and Skin Diseases.

Method
Statistical comparison of reports of fractures occurring over an 8-year period.

Results
Those with either osteoarthritis (OA) or rheumatoid arthritis (RA) had significantly more fractures than those without. Those with RA had greater risk for all types of fractures, while those with OA had a modest overall risk and spine fractures, but not an increased risk for hip fractures.

Implications
The results indicate the importance of utilizing effective fall and injury preventive strategies which are particularly geared to persons who already have arthritis.

From National Institute of Arthritis and Musculoskeletal and Skin Diseases: *Spotlight on research: study further elucidates role of arthritis in fracture risk* (2011). Available at http://www.niams.nih.gov/News_and_Events/Spotlight_on_Research/2011/fracture_risk_arthritis.asp.

should be arranged so that they do not cause falls. Environmental safety and fall prevention is addressed in detail in Chapter 13.

Pharmacological Interventions
Considerable progress has been made in the last decade in the development of pharmacological treatments for both the prevention and the treatment of osteoporosis. Adequate intake of calcium and vitamin D is recommended for persons at all ages and must be taken with all of the prescribed treatments currently available (Ragucci & Shrader, 2011).

Ideally, optimal nutrition in late life has followed a lifetime of good eating habits (see Chapter 9). The diet during adolescence is probably a key to healthy bones later. A balanced diet that includes food sources of calcium is best (Box 18-2). Women over 50 years of age and men over 70 years of age should ingest 1200 mg of calcium per day; 1000 mg a day is recommended for men between 51 and 69 years of age and can come from combined dietary and supplementary sources (Kessenich, 2007; NIH, 2011). If using supplements, combination calcium–vitamin D supplements (e.g., Caltrate-D) are recommended. The doses are best spread over the course of the day; for example, 400 mg of calcium three times a day. The present recommendation includes the regular use of 600 to 800 international units of supplemental vitamin D to achieve blood levels of greater than or equal to 50 nmol/L and less than 125 nmol/L (Office of Dietary Supplements [ODS]/NIH, 2011). Older adults are at particularly high risk for vitamin D deficiencies due to changes in the skin that reduce the ability to synthesize vitamin D efficiently. For those living in institutional settings or northern climates, the reduced opportunities for sunlight exposure only increase the risk for deficiencies.

BOX 18-2 Sources of Calcium

Food Item

Dairy products (e.g., yogurt, milk, cheese)
Chinese cabbage or bok choy
Tofu (calcium fortified)
Soy milk (calcium fortified)
Orange juice (calcium fortified)
Dried figs
Cheese pizza

Green leafy vegetables (e.g., broccoli, brussels sprouts, mustard greens)
Beans/legumes
Tortillas
Cooked soybeans
Sardines or salmon with edible bones
Nuts (especially almonds)
Bread

From National Institutes of Health: *Sources of calcium* (2011). Available at http://www.niams.nih.gov/Health_Info/Bone/Bone_Health/bone_health_for_life.asp.

Patient teaching includes discussion of the factors that inhibit calcium absorption (e.g., excess alcohol, protein, or salt), excretion enhancers (e.g., caffeine; excess fiber; phosphorus in meats, sodas, and preserved foods); and the influence of the body's response to stress (decreased calcium absorption, increased excretion of calcium in the urine). Constipation, already a problem for many as they age, is worsened by calcium supplements and may reduce the person's willingness to take them. Good nursing care includes developing a preventive plan with the person, including the use of stool softeners and extra fluid intake if not contraindicated.

 SAFETY ALERT

Neither calcium nor calcium-enriched products can be taken at the same time as thyroid preparations.

For many years estrogen supplementation was given to postmenopausal women to treat hot flashes and prevent or treat osteoporosis. However, rigorous clinical trials had not been conducted on the effect of estrogen supplementation on women until the 1990s and early 2000s. As a result of a large study, the Women's Health Initiative, it was found that although it did increase BMD, it also increased the rate of breast cancer, colon cancer, and heart disease. As a result of these findings estrogen is no longer used for this purpose (Brucker & Youngkin, 2002; Women's Health Initiative [WHI], 2012).

The currently available medications include bisphosphonates, selective estrogen receptor modulators (SERMs), calcitonin, hormone therapy, and the new monoclonal antibody Xgeva. New formulations and medications continue to come on the market. All increase bone mass, reduce bone turnover, or both. The bisphosphonates (e.g., Fosamax, Actonel) are often prescribed in daily, weekly, or monthly formulations.

 SAFETY ALERT

Owing to the seriousness of the risk for esophageal erosion, bisphosphonates must be taken on an empty stomach, with a full glass of water, and with the person completely upright for a half hour after ingestion. They are not appropriate for the person with memory loss or anyone else who cannot be depended upon to comply with these directions.

The SERM raloxifene (Evista) is used as a substitute for estrogen, yet decreases the risk for breast cancer. It is approved for both the prevention and the treatment of bone loss, but it can cause hot flashes and coagulation disorders and is contraindicated for use by anyone with a history of a deep venous thrombosis (DVT) or who is taking blood thinners.

Another medication that is quite useful is calcitonin (Miacalcin). It is used to slow bone loss and increase spinal bone mineral density in women who are at least 5 years past menopause. It is not indicated for men. Calcitonin has been found to incidentally reduce back pain in some women. It is given either subcutaneously or as a nasal spray at this time.

The Arthritides

Arthritis is the term used to apply to a number of musculoskeletal conditions. It is the most common cause of disability in the United States, limiting the activities of nearly 21 million adults. This figure includes the 50 million who self-report a diagnosis of arthritis of some kind (CDC, 2010). It is significantly more common in women in all age groups and increases dramatically after about 45 years of age. The most common forms of the disease that the gerontological nurse will encounter are osteoarthritis (OA), polymyalgia rheumatica (PMR), rheumatoid arthritis (RA), and gout.

Osteoarthritis

OA, the most common type of arthritis (Zhang & Jordan, 2010), is a degenerative joint disorder (DJD) that affects at least 33.6% (12.4 million) of Americans at least 65 years of age and about 27 million over the age of 25 (Centers for Disease Control and Prevention [CDC], 2011). Risk factors include increased age, obesity, family history, and repetitive use of or trauma to the joint. After the age of 65 more women than men are affected and will have radiographic evidence of OA even if they are asymptomatic. Native Americans have the highest prevalence of OA, and Asians and Pacific Islanders have the lowest. However, for all, OA causes joint stiffening and pain and eventually impairs functioning.

The osteoarthritic joint is one in which the normal soft and resilient cartilaginous lining becomes thin and damaged. This causes the joint space to narrow and ultimately, the bones of the joint to rub together, causing destruction, pain, swelling, and loss of motion. Bone spurs (osteophytes) may develop in the spaces, causing deformation and deterioration (Figure 18-2). OA results from a complex interplay of many factors, including genetic predisposition, local inflammation, joint integrity, mechanical forces, and cellular and biochemical processes. Treatment is palliative, which is geared toward comfort.

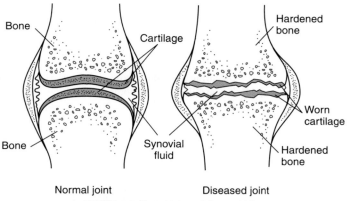

FIGURE 18-2 Normal joint and diseased joint.

In classic OA there is stiffness with inactivity which is relieved by activity. At the same time the activity may lead to pain which is relieved by rest. The stiffness is greatest in the morning after the disuse during sleep but should resolve within 30 minutes of arising. As the disease advances, there is pain at rest as well, and more joints become involved. There may be joint instability, and crepitus, a crunching or popping, may be felt or heard and is an indication of the deterioration of the joint. The joint will enlarge as osteophytes develop, and range of motion is reduced. OA of the cervical spine affects its curvature in a classic fashion (see Figure 18-1). The most common locations for symptomatic OA are the knees, hand, hip, and feet (CDC, 2011). The neck (cervical spine), the lower back (lumbar spine), the fingers, and the thumbs are also affected (Figure 18-3). Less often it is found in the shoulders. Depression, anxiety, and decreased functional status are all associated with OA.

At this time OA cannot be "cured" without a joint replacement (arthroplasty). These are often highly successful and restore the person to his or her previous level of functioning. Nearly twice as many women as men have joint replacements. African Americans and persons with low incomes have lower rates of replacements and higher rates of complications and mortality than whites (CDC, 2011). Surgical replacements are recommended for even the very old, in select cases. The nurse is involved in the preoperative and perioperative periods and rehabilitation while the person is learning to use the new joint.

Polymyalgia Rheumatica and Giant Cell Arteritis

Polymyalgia rheumatica (PMR) is one of the more common inflammatory diseases seen in older adults. It may

What Areas Does Osteoarthritis Affect?

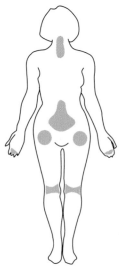

FIGURE 18-3 Common locations for osteoarthritis. (From National Institutes of Health: *Handout on health: osteoarthritis* (2010). Available at http://www.niams.nih.gov/health_info/osteoarthritis/default.asp.)

occur at the same time as OA, and the two may be difficult to distinguish from each other. The classic presentation of PMR is acute-onset (days) pain beginning in the neck and upper arms and possibly evolving to the pelvic and pectoral girdles. Fatigue and low-grade fever may occur. Pain is usually greatest at night and in the early morning, but usually no joint inflammation is present.

PMR causes stiffness, which occurs especially in the morning and lasts more than 1 hour, as well as severe stiffness and pain in the muscles of the neck, shoulders, lower back, buttocks, and thighs, rather than the joints. The onset may develop very suddenly or slowly. Unlike OA, PMR resolves in 1 to 2 years and necessitates different treatment. Symptoms may be quickly relieved by small doses of corticosteroids (Zimmerman-Górska, 2008).

PMR rarely occurs in people under 50 years of age. It occurs more often in whites in the United States and Europe with a fourfold increase in risk among women (Zimmerman-Górska, 2008). The cause is unknown, but is associated with immune disorders, genetic factors, and a recent infection (NIAMS, 2010a).

Giant cell arteritis (GCA) (also known as *temporal arteritis)* may occur at the same time as PMR. It does occur in those younger than 50 years of age. It is an acute inflammation of the arteries of the scalp and medium to large vessels, especially in the temporal area, which restricts blood flow. Sudden pain in the temporal area or changes in vision are always an emergency. If GCA is not treated early it can result in blindness. Treatment is with high-dose steroids.

Rheumatoid Arthritis

RA is a chronic, systemic, inflammatory joint disorder. It is considered an autoimmune disease in which products from the inflamed lining of the joint invade and destroy the cartilage and bone within the joint. The cause is unknown. RA affects more women than men; that is, about 1.3 million people, or 0.6% of the U.S. adult population. It most often starts in midlife between 40 and 60 years of age (NIAMS, 2009).

RA is characterized by pain and swelling in multiple joints in a symmetrical pattern; for example, both hands will be affected at the same time. It generally affects the small joints of the wrist, the knee, the ankle, and the hand,

although it can affect large joints as well. Whereas morning stiffness in OA lasts less than 30 minutes, in RA it lasts longer than 30 minutes. Since RA is a systemic disease, the person may feel generalized fatigue and malaise and have occasional unexplained fevers. The joints are warm and tender. Weight loss is common. The natural course of RA is highly variable, with good and bad days. The disease may last a few months or years or may become a chronic condition with progressive damage to the joints. Risk factors include environmental and genetic factors.

In the past, nonsteroidal antiinflammatory drugs (NSAIDs) were used for treatment early in the disease, and the use of the RA-specific drugs was "saved" for later. However, it has been found that prompt efforts may halt or slow the damage (Schreiber & Ling, 2010). Persons diagnosed with RA usually come under a rheumatologist's care, which involves aggressive therapy using a class of drugs called disease-modifying antirheumatic drugs (DMARDs). All the DMARDs are potentially toxic and are administered with care by a registered nurse, such as the charge nurse in a nursing home, or by a physician.

As with OA, care is palliative. It includes monitoring the progression of the disease and monitoring both the effectiveness and toxicity of treatment as well as providing comfort and support (Table 18-1). Support groups specific for persons with RA may help to empower, which in turn may improve their quality of life.

Gout

Gout is a common form of inflammatory arthritis in older adults. It appears to result from the accumulation of uric acid crystals in a joint. Uric acid is produced when purines found in food break down.

Gout typically starts with an acute attack. The person complains of exquisite pain in the affected joint, often

TABLE 18-1	Partial List of Signs and Symptoms of Toxicities Related to Common Disease-Modifying Anti-Rheumatic Drugs (DMARDs) for Rheumatoid Arthritis
Medication	**Signs and Symptoms of Potential Toxicity**
Methotrexate	Nausea, stomatitis (common), bone marrow suppression, liver disease, intestinal pneumonitis (rare)
Sulfasalazine	Nausea, rash, Stevens-Johnson syndrome (life-threatening), neutropenia, aplastic anemia
Hydroxychloroquine	Nausea, rash, bone marrow suppression, agranulocytosis, plastic anemia, corneal and retinal damage at higher doses
Biologicals (e.g., Enbrel, Humira, Kineret, Orencia)	Frequent infections, rash, pain, headache, cough, heart failure

From National Institute of Arthritis and Musculoskeletal and Skin Diseases: *Handout on health: rheumatoid arthritis* (2009). Available at http://www.niams.nih.gov/health_info/Rheumatic_Disease/default.asp; and Shorr, RI: *Drugs for the geriatric patient*, Philadelphia, 2008, Elsevier.

starting in the middle of the night during sleep. The joint is bright purple-red, hot, and too painful to touch. The most common treatments for an acute attack are NSAIDs (see Chapter 8); however, these can cause stomach irritation, affect the kidneys (rarely), or may interfere with the cardioprotective effects of aspirin if taken at the same time. For some, corticosteroids are necessary (NIAMS, 2010b).

After an acute attack, gout may become chronic with periodic acute "attacks." Risk factors include alcohol abuse, high blood pressure, a diet high in purines (Box 18-3), and certain medications especially thiazide diuretics, salicylates (e.g., aspirin), niacin, cyclosporines, and levodopa (Sinemet) (NIAMS, 2010b). The medical goal is to prevent another attack, systemic spread of the disease, and the development of chronic gout. This may be done with the avoidance of risk-elevating drugs, or of foods that are high in purine and alcohol, both of which increase uric acid levels; also, medications can be used to either decrease uric acid production (e.g., allopurinol, colchicine) or increase its excretion (e.g., probenecid) (Jett & Lester, 2004). The nurse ensures that the person takes in enough fluids to help flush the uric acid through the kidneys (2 L/day if not contraindicated).

The proximal joint of the great toe is the most typical site, although sometimes the ankle, the knee, the wrist, or the elbow is involved. The development of gout and the body's response to uric acid accumulation is highly individual. It is important to note that some people have elevated levels of uric acid and do not get gout, a clinical picture described as asymptomatic hyperuricemia, and others have gout and low levels of uric acid. The uric acid level itself does not result in a diagnosis.

The nurse's roles include teaching the person side effects of medications, how to decrease the likelihood of another attack, and care of the joint. In administering gout-related medications the nurse pays close attention to renal function and notifies the physician or nurse practitioner of any change so that the dosages can be adjusted promptly.

BOX **18-3**   **Examples of Foods High in Purines**

Asparagus	Sweetbread
Game meat	Mushrooms
Beef kidneys	Dried beans and seeds
Gravy	Scallops
Brain	
Herring, mackerel, and sardines	

Implications for Gerontological Nursing and Healthy Aging

Assessment

When assessing the musculoskeletal system, the nurse examines the joints and muscles for tenderness, swelling, warmth, and redness. The hands are examined for the presence or absence of osteophytes. If they appear in the distal joints as deformities of the fingers, they are called Heberden's nodes, and they are called Bouchard's nodes in the proximal joints (Figure 18-4). The nurse questions their effect on function. In GCA, the temporal arteries enlarge and become tender to touch.

Both passive and active range of motion are evaluated. How far can the person reach and bend all joints without assistance, and what are the flexion, and extension with assistance? The testing of passive range of motion must go only to the point of discomfort and never to that of inducing pain. Ask if there are any ADLs or instrumental activities of daily living (IADLs) which are limited or not possible because of musculoskeletal issues. Can the person comb the hair or tie a shoe, or can a woman fasten her bra?

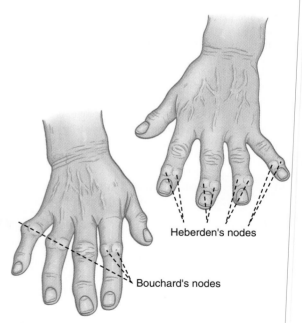

Heberden's nodes

Bouchard's nodes

FIGURE 18-4 Hand deformities in arthritis. (From McCance KL, Huether SE, Brashers VL, et al, editors: *Pathophysiology: the biologic basis for disease in adults and children*, ed 6, St. Louis, 2010, Mosby.)

Interventions

The goals of intervention and management of the different forms of arthritis are to obtain treatment as soon as possible for inflammatory conditions, control pain, and minimize disability. The nurse is very involved in advocacy for adequate and prompt treatment, pain control (see Chapter 15), medication administration, evaluation, and patient teaching. Pain management and the minimization of disability are interconnected. To minimize disability with OA and RA, the joint must be used carefully, strengthened, and protected.

It cannot be overstated that ongoing therapy from accredited physical therapists is necessary for persons with musculoskeletal problems to retain joint use. Weight loss, if necessary, and muscle building are highly recommended. In joint replacement, outcomes depend on the timing of surgery, the number of procedures that the surgeon has performed, the nursing care received, and the patient's medical status before the surgery and ability to participate in rehabilitation.

Exercise has been found to be the cornerstone to maintaining function with OA and RA. Regular exercise can improve flexibility and muscle strength, which in turn help to support the affected joints, reduce pain, and reduce falls. Walking, swimming, and water aerobics are preferred by many, and the latter is often available in senior centers, public pools, and YMCAs in many communities.

Attention should also be given to diet (see Chapter 9). With the decreases in activity associated with pain in all forms of arthritis, it is easy for the person to gain weight. Excess weight significantly increases the pressure and wear and tear on the joints, leading to less activity and more weight gain. Weight reduction should be considered for all persons who are overweight. The nurse and the registered dietitian can work with the person to identify realistic weight and caloric goals and develop meal plans that are personally and culturally acceptable but still balanced and healthy.

The use of heat and cold is well known in the management of pain in OA and RA. It should not be used in GCA. Patient preference is important, but cold usually works best for an acute process, for example the application of cold packs that decrease muscle spasm, decrease swelling, and relieve inflammatory pain. Heat may be applied superficially or deeply. Ultrasound provides deep heat and is usually provided by physical therapists. Hot packs, hydrotherapy, and radiant heat provide superficial heat. Liquid paraffin baths can be purchased in most drug stores for submerging the hands to provide deep heat and temporary relief (Wright, 2008).

Devices and techniques are available that relieve some of the pressure to the joints and protect the joints and muscles from further stress and, in doing so, to possibly decrease pain and improve balance and function. Canes, crutches, walkers, collars, shoe orthotics, and corsets are such devices in the case of OA and RA. A cane can relieve hip pressure and help support the person with the muscle weakness that accompanies PMR. A shoe lift can improve lumbar pain. A knee brace is useful, especially if there is lateral instability (the knee "gives out"). If the hands are affected the person can avoid carrying packages by the fingers or can use utensils and household equipment with larger rather than smaller grips. Preventing the exposure of the affected joints to cold temperatures may also help. The person is encouraged to wear leggings, gloves, or scarves as necessary while outside.

Complementary and Alternative Interventions

A number of complementary and alternative medicine (CAM) interventions are used by persons around the globe to attempt to treat the pain associated with musculoskeletal problems, especially osteoarthritis. Among these are the use of the dietary supplements glucosamine and chondroitin sulfate, along with acupuncture and massage. Following an in-depth review of the literature, the Osteoarthritis Research Society International found no difference in the effect of pharmacological and nonpharmacological interventions (Zhang et al., 2008). However, others disagree and find much promise in the use of an assortment of CAM (Pirotta, 2010; Vitetta et al., 2008). Further research is underway.

Application of Maslow's Hierarchy

The acute postsurgical nursing care is designed to restore the physiological functions to address the first level of Maslow's Hierarchy of Needs: maintaining fluids, movement, and nutritional adequacy. Effective pain management is critical to ensure that the individual is quickly able to participate in rehabilitation, which is essential for maximum recovery.

To provide care to the whole person with musculoskeletal disorders the nurse works with a number of approaches and teaches and empowers the person to participate fully in achieving the highest level of wellness possible at all levels of the Hierarchy.

KEY CONCEPTS

- Most people over 40 years of age will have osteoarthritis at some point in their lives.

- Osteoporosis is a crippling problem for many elders, especially women. Although it cannot be completely prevented, it can be minimized by early interventions: weight-bearing exercise, and calcium and vitamin D intake.
- The most serious outcomes of osteoporosis are fractures, which are associated with high mortality.
- Rheumatoid arthritis produces swelling, inflammation, intense pain, and distortion of the joints.
- Gout is both an acute and a chronic condition. One of the goals of treatment with gout is to minimize a future attack.
- Individuals have found certain types of complementary and alternative interventions very helpful for joint disorders and chronic discomfort.

ACTIVITIES AND DISCUSSION QUESTIONS

1. What are the most effective ways of preventing osteoporosis?
2. What lifestyle issues would you discuss with an individual with advanced osteoporosis?
3. What are the differences in appearance of osteoarthritis and rheumatoid arthritis?
4. What advice would you give someone who is experiencing joint pain and mobility limitations?
5. Activity: Which of your favorite activities would be difficult if you were afflicted with osteoarthritis?

REFERENCES

Brucker MC, Youngkin EQ: What's a woman to do? Exploring HRT questions raised by the Women's Health Initiative, *AWHONN Lifelines* 6(5):408–417, 2002.

Centers for Disease Control and Prevention [CDC]: *Arthritis data and statistics* (2010). Available at http://www.cdc.gov/arthritis/data_statistics.htm.

Centers for Disease Control and Prevention [CDC]: *Osteoarthritis* (2011). Available at http://www.cdc.gov/arthritis/basics/osteoarthritis.htm.

Jett KF, Lester PB: Musculoskeletal disorders. In Youngkin EQ, Sawin K, Israel D, editors: *Pharmcotherapeutics*, ed 2, Upper Saddle River, NJ, 2004, Prentice-Hall.

Kessenich CR: Calcium and vitamin D supplementation for post menopausal bone health, *J Nurs Pract* 3(3): 155–160, 2007.

National Institute of Arthritis and Musculoskeletal and Skin Diseases [NIAMS]: *Handout on health: Rheumatoid arthritis* (2009). Available at http://www.niams.nih.gov/Health_Info/Rheumatic_Disease/default.asp.

National Institute of Arthritis and Musculoskeletal and Skin Diseases [NIAMS]: *Questions and answers about polymyalgia rheumatica and giant cell arteritis* (2010a). Available at www.niams.nih.gov/Health_Info/Polymyalgia/default.asp.

National Institute of Arthritis and Musculoskeletal and Skin Diseases [NIAMS]: *Questions and answers about gout* (2010b). Available at http://www.niams.nih.gov/Health_Info/Gout/default.asp.

National Institutes of Health [NIH]: *Falls and older adults* (2011). Available at http://nihseniorhealth.gov/falls/aboutfalls/01.html.

National Osteoporosis Foundation [NOF]: *Fast facts* (2011). Available at http://www.nof.org/node/40.

Pirotta M: Arthritis disease–the use of complementary therapies, *Aust Fam Physician* 39(9):638–640, 2010.

Ragucci K, Shrader S: Osteoporosis treatment: an evidence-based approach, *J Gerontol Nurs* 37(7):17–22, 2011.

Schreiber C, Ling S: Musculoskeletal system. In Durso S, editor: *Oxford American handbook of geriatric medicine*, New York, 2010, Oxford, pp. 485–520.

U.S. Preventive Services Task Force [USPSTF]: *Screening for osteoporosis* (2011). Available at http://www.uspreventiveservicestaskforce.org/uspstf10/osteoporosis/osteors.htm.

Vitetta L, Cicuttini F, Sali A: Alternative therapies for musculoskeletal conditions, *Best Pract Clin Rheumatol* 22(3):499–522, 2008.

Wayne P, Kiel D, Krebs DE, et al: The effects of tai chi on bone mineral density in postmenopausal women: a systematic review, *Arch Phys Med Rehabil* 88(5):673–680, 2007.

Wayne P, Buring J, Davis R, et al: Tai chi for osteopenic women: design and rationale of a pragmatic randomized controlled trail, *BMC Musculoskelet Disord* 1:11–40, 2010.

Women's Health Initiative [WHI]: *Women's Health Initiative* (2012). Available at https://cleo.whi.org/SitePages/Home.aspx.

Wright W: Management of mild-to-moderate osteoarthritis: effective intervention by the nurse practitioner, *J Nurs Pract* 4(1):25–43, 2008.

Zhang W, Moskowitz R, Nuki M, et al: OARSI recommendations for the management of hip and knee osteoarthritis, part II: OARSI evidence-based, expert consensus, *Osteoarthritis Cartilage* 16:137–162, 2008.

Zhang Y, Jordan J: Epidemiology of osteoarthritis, *Clin Geriatr Med* 26(3):355–369, 2010.

Zimmerman-Górska I: Polymyalgia rheumatica: clinical picture and principles of treatment, *Pol J Intern Med* 118(6):377–389, 2008.

CHAPTER 19

Cardiovascular and Respiratory Disorders

Kathleen F. Jett

evolve   evolve.elsevier.com/Ebersole/gerontological

LEARNING OBJECTIVES

Upon completion of this chapter, the reader will be able to:

- Identify the most common types of cardiovascular and respiratory diseases occurring in late life.
- Discuss assessment of and intervention for cardiovascular and respiratory disease in the elder.
- Suggest ways to prevent cardiovascular and respiratory disease to the extent possible.
- Differentiate infectious, obstructive, and restrictive lung disease.
- Discuss the signs and symptoms of pneumonia in which rapid hospitalization may be recommended.
- Develop a tuberculosis surveillance plan for a long-term care facility.

GLOSSARY

Comorbidity More than one disease or health condition existing at the same time.
Dyspnea The subjective sensation of shortness of breath.
Morbidity Disability as the result of a health condition.
Mortality Death as a result of a health condition or event.
Nosocomial Pertaining to the institutional setting or treatment as the source (as in nosocomial infection).

THE LIVED EXPERIENCE

When I first had that heart attack, I was so frightened it seemed I would die just from the fear. It was the first time I realized how comforting, calm and efficient nurses could be. There was the one who came into the room a few days later and talked to me about the cardiac rehab program and that I could continue doing the things I had always done, except for changes in diet and more exercise. Even sex! I would never have asked that young thing, but she just told me it was OK.

Jerry, age 63

When Dad had that heart attack, it really scared us all, and I know we were afraid we would say or do something that would bring on another. I think he was also afraid of everything. I'm so grateful for the nurses at the hospital. They seem to give him lots of attention and information about the things he needed to know. He seems quite relaxed with himself now.

Ruth, Jerry's youngest daughter

Caring for older adults means caring for persons with cardiovascular disease (CVD), respiratory problems, or both. These two systems are interconnected. A problem in one is likely to cause or complicate a problem in the other. When the nurse is addressing a cardiac problem, such as heart failure, the respiratory system must be assessed as well. For example, pneumonia may trigger heart failure. Nursing interventions frequently overlap. One carefully planned action can address several systems at the same time and achieve goals meeting basic physiological needs and promoting healthy aging as much as possible.

Cardiovascular Disease

The American Heart Association identifies the major cardiovascular diseases as hypertension (HTN); coronary heart disease (CHD), including myocardial infarction (MI) and angina; and heart failure (HF). Although the numbers of deaths from heart disease have decreased, they remain the first and third cause of death and common causes of disability. It is the number one cause of death for African Americans, Caucasians, and Hispanics and second behind cancer for American Indians and Pacific Islanders (Centers for Disease Control and Prevention [CDC], 2012c). The rate of deaths per 100,000 increases dramatically with age from a combination of normal changes with aging and the presence of risk factors (Box 19-1). Older adults also undergo the majority of CVD-related procedures, but treatment approaches are highly variable by ethnicity and sex (Box 19-2).

BOX 19-1	**Risk Factors for Heart Disease**

- Age (>55 years of age for men; >65 years of age for women)
- Family history of premature CHD (<55 years of age for men; <65 years of age for women)
- Microalbuminuria or estimated GFR <60 mL/min
- Hypertension*
- Cigarette smoking
- Central obesity
- Physical inactivity
- Dyslipidemia*
- Diabetes, IGT, or IFG*

*Components of metabolic syndrome.
CHD, Coronary heart disease; *GFR,* glomerular filtration rate; *IFG,* impaired fasting glucose; *IGT,* impaired glucose tolerance.

BOX 19-2	**Treatment of Chest Pain Differs by Sex and Ethnicity**

The complaint of chest pain is often expressed by adult patients, especially in late life. When this chest pain is attributed to a cardiac origin, men are more likely than women to be diagnosed with angina (18% vs. 4%) and intermediate coronary syndrome (ICS) (21% vs. 10%), and women are more likely than men to be diagnosed with vague chest pain only (86% vs. 61%). African Americans receive more chest pain diagnoses than whites (71% vs. 62%) with similar angina and ICS diagnoses. However, both African Americans and women receive fewer cardiovascular medications than white men.

Data from Hendrix KH, Mayhan S, Lackland DT, et al: Prevalence, treatment, and control of chest pain syndromes and associated risk factors in hypertensive patients, *Am J Hypertens* 18(8):1026-1032, 2005.

Hypertension

Hypertension (HTN) is the most common chronic cardiovascular disease encountered by the gerontological nurse. It affects 70.34% of those over 65 years of age (Health Indicators Warehouse, 2005-2008a) but is only controlled in 45.64% of those persons (Health Indicators Warehouse, 2005-2008b). Both the definition of and the guidelines for treatment of HTN are provided by the Joint National Committee on the Detection, Evaluation, and Treatment of High Blood Pressure (JNC) (Box 19-3). HTN is diagnosed any time the diastolic blood pressure reading is 90 mm Hg or higher or the systolic reading is 140 mm Hg or higher on two separate occasions (JNC, 2003) (Table 19-1). More recently a joint consensus report of leading authorities in aging and cardiology recommended that three separate readings be used in older adults due to the variability inherent with the less compliant vasculature that is associated with aging (American College of Cardiology Foundation/American Heart Association [ACCF/AHA], 2011).

Blood pressure increases slightly with age, with a leveling off or decrease of the diastolic pressure for persons about 60 years of age and older. Older adults most often have isolated systolic hypertension, which is an elevation in only the systolic reading. This is quite different from the younger person, who is more likely to have an elevation in just the diastolic or in both. During the JNC's last review (#7) in 2003, it was noted that the definition for HTN does not change with age. The current blood pressure goal for all persons is 120/60 mm Hg (JNC, 2003).

BOX 19-3   Key Points of the JNC 7

- For persons older than 50 years of age, SBP is more important than DBP as a CVD risk factor.
- Starting at 115/75 mm Hg, CVD risk doubles with each increment of 20/10 mm Hg throughout the BP range.
- Persons who are normotensive at 55 years of age have a 90% lifetime risk for developing HTN.
- Those with SBP 120-139 mm Hg or DBP 80-89 mm Hg should be considered prehypertensive; they require health-promoting lifestyle modifications to prevent CVD.
- Thiazide type of diuretics should be the initial drug therapy either alone or combined with other drug classes unless compelling reasons are present.
- Certain high-risk conditions are compelling indications for other drug classes.
- Most patients will require two or more antihypertensive drugs to achieve goal BP.
- If BP is >20/10 mm Hg above goal, initiate therapy with two agents; one usually should be a diuretic of the thiazide type.

BP, Blood pressure; *CVD,* cardiovascular disease; *DBP,* diastolic blood pressure; *HTN,* hypertension; *JNC,* Joint National Committee on the Detection, Evaluation, and Treatment of High Blood Pressure; *SBP,* systolic blood pressure.
Adapted from JNC 7: *JNC 7 express: the seventh report of the Joint National Committee on the Prevention, Detection, Evaluation and Treatment of High Blood Pressure, USDHHS Pub No 03-5233,* 2003. Available at http://www.nhlbi.nih.gov/guidelines/hypertension/.

TABLE 19-1   Blood Pressure Classification

Classification	Blood Pressure
Normal	<120 systolic and <80 diastolic
Prehypertension	120-139 systolic or 80-89 diastolic
Stage 1 HTN	140-159 systolic or 90-99 diastolic
Stage 2 HTN	>160 systolic or >100 diastolic

HTN, Hypertension.

It is anticipated that the updated JNC 8 guidelines will be prepared soon.

Although often treatable, and in some cases preventable, the rate of HTN has increased in the last 15 or so years, especially for women (Table 19-2) and significant disparities between racial and ethnic groups persist. Although race, ethnicity, and a family history of hypertension

TABLE 19-2   Comparative Rates of Hypertension and Heart Disease

	Hypertension	Heart Disease
1995		
Men	41%	25%
Women	48%	19%
2008		
Men	53%	38%
Women	58%	27%

Adapted from Federal Interagency Forum on Aging-Related Statistics: *Older Americans 2000: key indicators of well-being* and *Older Americans 2010: key indicators of well-being.* Federal Interagency Forum on Aging-Related Statistics, Washington, DC, 2000 and 2010, U.S. Government Printing Office. Available at http://www.agingstats.gov/agingstatsdotnet.

BOX 19-4   Modifiable Factors That Increase the Risk for Essential Hypertension

- Cigarette smoking or tobacco use
- Excessive alcohol intake
- Sedentary lifestyle
- Inadequate stress and/or anger management
- Poor diet (high sodium, high saturated fat)

cannot be changed, a number of other factors are within control of the individual to reduce his or her risk for hypertension (Box 19-4).

Most HTN is discovered during health screening or examination for another problem, when related complications may have already developed (see the Evidence-Based Practice box). The most important complication of HTN is the long-term effects resulting in what is referred to as "end-organ damage," especially to the heart. Older persons with HTN have an absolute higher risk for cardiac disease such as CHD, atrial fibrillation, and heart failure, as well as acute cardiovascular and cerebrovascular events such as myocardial infarction, stroke, and sudden death. Poorly controlled HTN is also implicated in chronic renal insufficiency, end-stage renal disease, and peripheral vascular disease (ACCF/AHA, 2011).

Heart Disease

The beating heart, like other muscles, needs oxygen and other nutrients to provide energy for its work. However, the blood passing through the heart with each beat is not available to provide oxygen or nutrients to the organ itself.

🔍 EVIDENCE-BASED PRACTICE

Screening for Hypertension

The U.S. Preventive Services Task Force recommends blood pressure screening for all adults over 18 years of age a minimum of once every 2 years for persons with readings less than 120/80 and once a year for those with 120-139 mm Hg SBP or 80-89 mm HG DBP.

From U.S. Preventive Services Task Force: Screening for high blood pressure: U.S. Preventive Services Task Force recommendation statement. Reaffirmation recommendation statement, *Ann Intern Med* 147:783–786, 2007. Available at http://www.uspreventiveservicestaskforce.org/uspstf07/hbp/hbprs.htm.

Instead, like all other muscles, the heart receives its oxygen from arteries within it.

Heart disease (HD) is also referred to as coronary heart disease (CHD) and coronary artery disease (CAD). It develops from a number of causes, including stiffening of the blood vessels, referred to as *arteriosclerosis* or "hardening of the arteries," and when cholesterol and other fats are deposited in the layers of the arteries. Both of these reduce the blood flow through the heart vessels limiting the amount of oxygen reaching the tissue. HD is also a direct consequence of chronic, untreated or inadequately treated hypertension (Buttaro et al., 2008). The extent to which one suffers from HD is greatly affected by a personal history of exposure to smoke and pollutants and whether one also has diabetes or family history of such.

Heart disease can result in ischemia or when there is a sudden complete blockage of oxygen to the heart muscle. When the blockage is sudden but shortly resolves on its own it is called angina. A more serious and often permanent blockage is referred to as a myocardial infarction or acute MI (AMI). An AMI is seen as gripping chest pain, radiation to the shoulder, etc., in younger adults, but not always in the older adult. Instead the older adult is more likely to have what is called a *silent MI*. His or her discomfort may be mild and may be localized to the back, the abdomen, the shoulders, or either or both arms. Nausea and vomiting, or merely a sensation like heartburn, may be the only symptoms. More often there are no noticeable signs or symptoms at all, and the event is only noticed at the time of death or when an electrocardiogram (ECG) is performed for some other purpose. These vague symptoms often are not brought to the attention of a medical provider. Only about 45% of persons over 65 years of age are aware of even the usual symptoms and the appropriate response, making the risk for death associated with an AMI high (Health Indicators Warehouse, 2008).

Heart Failure

The damage to the heart from chronic HD or MI may lead to heart failure (HF), which is the most frequent discharge diagnoses for non-traumatic hospitalization of an older adult. Often this results in a transfer to a long-term care facility (Fang et al., 2008).

HF is a disease of the heart muscle in which the muscle is damaged, malfunctions, and can no longer pump enough blood to meet the needs of the body. In 2008 it affected over 5.7 million people in the United States, the majority of whom are over 65 years of age (CDC, 2012d). Causes of HF include hypertension, fever, hypoxia, anemia, metabolic disease, and infection (ACCF/AHA, 2011). Over time the heart is further damaged because of poor control of the underlying problem (e.g., hypertension) leading to more and more severe HF, known as congestive heart failure (CHF). An unhealthy diet, smoking, and lack of exercise aggravate the development of heart disease and the extent of damage, especially for those who have a family (genetic) history of heart disease. There is no cure for HF, only the management of symptoms and the attempt to prevent worsening. Fifty percent of persons with heart failure die within 5 years of diagnosis (CDC, 2012c).

Common signs and symptoms of heart failure in the elderly include fatigue or shortness of breath (dyspnea) with exertion, inability to lie flat without getting short of breath (orthopnea), waking up at night gasping for air, weight gain, and swelling in the lower extremities. Dyspnea may occur at rest or on exertion (DOE), or it may appear intermittently at night (paroxysmal nocturnal dyspnea). The dyspnea may be relieved by sitting up or sleeping on multiple pillows or with the head of the bed elevated. If a cough is present, it is worse at night. The New York Heart Association and the American College of Cardiology–American Heart Association provide us with convenient ways to classify the symptomatic experience of the HF, from symptom-free to severely disabled (Box 19-5).

In addition, the nurse should be alert for the atypical clinical presentation of exacerbations of HF in the elderly. The person may appear confused, or delirious; begin falling; or complain of insomnia or urinary frequency at night (nocturia). He or she may complain of dizziness or may have syncope (fainting). Or more often, the nurse will notice that the person has the "droops," or malaise and a subtle decline in activity tolerance or functional or cognitive abilities. The need for hospitalization is frequent. However, due to the added risks for the older adult in the acute care setting, a goal of *Healthy People 2020* (U.S. Department of Health and Human Services [USDHHS], 2012) is to reduce these and attempt to identify the need for more aggressive treatment earlier, thus potentially avoiding an inpatient stay (see the Healthy People box).

BOX 19-5   Classification of Heart Failure

Class I: Asymptomatic
Cardiac disease without resulting limitations of physical activity

Class II: Mild Heart Failure
Slight limitation of physical activity
Comfortable at rest
An increase in activity may cause fatigue, palpitations, dyspnea, or anginal pain

Class III: Moderate Heart Failure
Marked limitation in physical activity
Comfortable at rest
Ordinary walking or climbing of stairs can quickly bring on symptoms of fatigue, palpitations, dyspnea, or anginal pain
Substantial periods of bed rest required

Class IV: Severe Heart Failure
Almost permanently confined to bed
Inability to carry out any physical activity without discomfort or severe symptoms
Some symptoms occur at rest
Chronic shortness of breath is common

Developed by the New York Heart Association in 1928. Disseminated broadly. Available at http://www.abouthf.org/questions_stages.htm and http://www.americanheart.org/presenter.jhtml?identifier=4569.

HEALTHY PEOPLE 2020
Promoting Healthy Aging: Heart Disease

Reduce hospitalizations of older adults with heart failure as the principal diagnosis:
65-74 years of age
Baseline: 9.8 per 1000 in 2007
Target: 8.8 per 1000 in 2020
75-84 years of age
Baseline: 22.4 per 1000 in 2007
Target: 20.2 per 1000 in 2020
85 years of age and older
Baseline: 42.9 per 1000 in 2007
Target: 38.6 per 1000 in 2020

From U.S. Department of Health and Human Services, Office of Disease Prevention and Health Promotion: *Healthy people 2020* (2012). Available at http://www.healthypeople.gov/2020.

SAFETY ALERT

One of the major ways that cardiac conditions differ from other chronic problems in the older adult is that when they become acute problems, they can do so very rapidly, and often necessitate acute hospitalization and intensive treatment followed by rehabilitation. Many other chronic disorders are managed at home.

Implications for Gerontological Nursing and Healthy Aging

Assessment

As with any assessment, obtaining a pertinent history of the events leading up to and including the presentation of cardiovascular problems is essential, whether the history is from the patient or a friend or family member. Monitoring of vital signs, laboratory results, and kidney function, and assessing the cardiac and respiratory function and conducting a mental status exam are essential. An auscultatory gap, or time when the second heart sound ceases, begins again, and then finally is not heard, is common in the older adult (ACCF/AHA, 2011). The results of home monitoring may be particularly useful. Members of the University of Iowa Gerontological Nursing Intervention Center offer an evidence-based assessment tool that can be used as a basic assessment measure as well as one that indicates change in long-term care patients with heart failure (Harrington, 2008). The tool can be used to document status in three categories: activities of daily living, quality of sleep, and dyspnea. It is available for purchase at www.nursing.uiowa.edu/excellence/nursing_interventions/index.htm.

Interventions

For the person with CVD, the goals of therapy are to provide relief of symptoms, improve the quality of life, reduce mortality and morbidity, and slow or stop progression of dysfunction through the use of aggressive drug therapy. A key intervention to reduce heart attack–related disability and death is to teach all persons the warning signs and what to do if these are experienced. Additional goals are to maximize the elder's function and quality of life and, when appropriate, provide expert palliative care. Concurrent and supportive therapies include modifying the diet by decreasing fat, cholesterol, and sodium; exercise; education; and family and social supports (ACCF/AHA, 2011).

Nursing interventions assist the person to accomplish these goals and have been found to be highly effective (Sisk et al., 2006). What specific interventions are used will depend on the severity of the disease, the person, and the desire for either palliative or aggressive care. Nursing actions range from teaching the older adult about lifestyle changes in diet, activity, and rest (see Chapter 11), to acute measures, such as the administration of oxygen. Interventions about which the nurse should be knowledgeable are related to those assessed (Box 19-6).

The goal of the management of HTN is to minimize the risk of complications and reduce or eliminate modifiable risk factors. This means keeping the blood pressure less than 140/90 mm Hg for otherwise healthy adults and less than 130/80 mm Hg for persons with diabetes. By doing so, many of the long-term complications (e.g., heart disease) can be avoided, minimized, or delayed (Box 19-7) (see the Evidence-Based Practice box). To accomplish this, the nurse has a responsibility to work with the elder and his or her family comprehensively to promote healthy aging. Fortunately, the work of the American Heart Association working with the American Geriatrics Society and the JNC provides detailed evidence-based treatment guidelines for most children and adults. Unfortunately, less is known about the appropriate treatment of fragile older adults with CVD who are residing in long-term care facilities. A more careful risk-benefit analysis must be done related to treatment and outcomes in this setting. For someone with a limited life expectancy,

---

BOX 19-7 Minimizing Risk for Heart Disease

Maintain:
 Blood pressure ≤130/80
 Total cholesterol <200 mg/dL
 LDL <100 mg/dL
 HDL >40 mg/dL
 Triglycerides <150 mg/dL

HDL, High-density lipoprotein; *LDL,* low-density lipoprotein.

 EVIDENCE-BASED PRACTICE

Benefits of Controlling Blood Pressure

Average Percent Reduction in Risk for New Events
- 30% fewer strokes
- 64% less heart failure
- 23% fewer fatal cardiovascular events
- 21% fewer overall deaths

---

the significant side effects of some medications and limitations in food choices may result in an unnecessary decrease in quality of life. When aggressive treatment is no longer effective, a change of focus to palliative care is appropriate and may include a referral to a hospice agency or palliative care service (see Chapter 25).

The potential for wellness after a major cardiac event or procedure is increased when elders participate fully in a cardiac rehabilitation program, if available. Otherwise disability can progress rapidly, especially if the person believes that any exertion overtaxes the heart and will cause acute CHF, another heart attack, or death. To prevent this, cardiac exercise rehabilitation programs are designed to address the physical, mental, and spiritual needs and overall health of the person and his or her family. Reductions in mortality are reported from 18% to 45% (Franklin & Vanhecke, 2007). Typical programs are prescribed by the physician or nurse practitioner and begin with self-management education and light activity progressing to moderate activity under the supervision of a rehabilitation nurse and physical therapist. For those who are more physically compromised, it is necessary to identify energy-conserving measures applicable to their daily tasks.

BOX 19-6 Skills Required for Promoting Healthy Aging in the Person with Cardiovascular Disease

- Knowing appropriate technique for obtaining a blood pressure
- Monitoring response to prescribed exercise
- Administering medications and evaluating their effects correctly
- Monitoring for signs and symptoms of changes in cardiovascular condition
- Monitoring fluid intake and output and diet
- Monitoring weight (either daily, biweekly, or weekly)
- Auscultating heart and lung sounds
- Monitoring laboratory values
- Educating patient and caregivers related to all of the above
- Providing palliative care (see Chapter 25)

The nurse and the person with CVD must be cautious about exercise. For those who have had an AMI, exercise-related orthostatic hypotension is more likely to occur as a result of age-related decreases in baroreceptor responsiveness, which controls the body's ability to respond to the need for changes in blood pressure (see Chapter 5). Because thermoregulation is also impaired, exercise intensity must be reduced in hot, humid climates (see Chapter 11). A healthy alternative is to encourage "mall walking" in local covered and climate-controlled shopping centers. In some locations this has become a social event as well as a safe way to exercise.

Risk reduction programs should be instituted with a clear understanding of the difficulties involved in attempts to alter harmful lifestyle practices such as smoking, overeating, habitual anger or irritation, and a sedentary lifestyle. These practices may have been going on for a lifetime and are not easily changed by "education." The nurse's role in these instances is to discuss these practices in a nonjudgmental manner, providing acceptance, encouragement, resources, knowledge, and affirmation of both the difficulty of making lifestyle changes and the person's right to choose. The LEARN Model of communication (see Chapter 4) may be particularly useful for persons from any culture or background.

Respiratory Disorders

The normal physical changes with aging (see Chapter 5) result in a greater risk for respiratory problems, and when they occur, there is a higher risk for death than in younger persons. Diseases of the respiratory system are identified as infectious, as acute or chronic, and as involving the upper or lower respiratory tract. They are further defined as either *obstructive*—preventing airflow out as a result of obstruction or narrowing of the respiratory structures; or *restrictive*—causing a decrease in total lung capacity as a result of limited expansion. Other than asthma, almost all chronic obstructive pulmonary disease in late life arise from tobacco use or exposure to tobacco and other pollutants earlier in life. Although asthma may be triggered by environmental factors, there are strong genetic and allergic factors that contribute to its occurrence. The nurse's focus is on helping the person maintain function and quality of life, while being vigilant for signs of infection.

Chronic Obstructive Pulmonary Disease

Chronic obstructive pulmonary disease (COPD) is a catch-all term used to encompass those conditions that affect airflow. It includes asthma, bronchitis, and emphysema, and as a group remains the third leading cause of

death for both older men and women (Hoyert & Xu, 2012). Although the overall death rate from COPD has not increased, this is primarily due to a significant increase in COPD in women and closely tied to cigarette smoking (USDHHS, 2008).

The signs and symptoms seen varies with the type of COPD. For example, persons with emphysema have little sputum production and appear pink because they are actually able to get enough oxygen into the lungs. On the other hand, persons with chronic bronchitis have chronic sputum production, frequent cough, and are pale and somewhat cyanotic indicating low oxygen levels associated with getting oxygen into the lungs. In asthma, constrictions of the bronchial tubes keep air from exiting the lungs. Thorough discussions of these symptoms can be found in medical-surgical nursing and pathophysiology texts. What is crucial to gerontological nursing is the need to watch the person with COPD very closely for signs of worsening infection and of aggravation of any underlying heart disease.

When respirations exceed 30 per minute, the person with COPD is having a worsening of his or her illness and prompt response by the nurse is necessary, such as obtaining a measure of oxygen saturation rate and alerting the patient's prescribing practitioner. An acute episode of emphysema or bronchitis is characterized by significantly worsened dyspnea and increased volume and change in the color of sputum (Esherick, 2010). An acute episode of asthma is characterized by shortness of breath and wheezing. A number of factors including viral or bacterial infections, air pollution or other environmental exposures, or changes in the weather may trigger a change in the person's respiratory health.

Persons with advanced COPD, as seen in most of the older adults with the disease, can expect to have periods of worsening of symptoms and functioning between periods of control. During periods of illness, medication changes are usually needed. Persons who have well-developed skills in self-management often will begin to deal with the changes before consulting a health care provider. Hospitalization is always a possibility with COPD exacerbations, especially when one has or is suspected of having an infection.

Pneumonia

Pneumonia is a bacterial or viral lower respiratory tract infection that causes inflammation of the lung tissue. Pneumonia and influenza are ninth leading causes of death for persons over 65 years of age with some variation based on race and ethnicity (CDC, 2012a). Particularly susceptible are elders with comorbid conditions such as alcoholism, asthma, COPD, or heart disease, or those who live in institutional settings. Other factors that increase the risk of acquiring pneumonia relate to normal changes of aging of the respiratory system, such as a diminished cough reflex, increased residual volume, and decreased chest compliance (see Chapter 5). However, many cases of pneumonia can be either prevented by immunization or treated effectively by prompt interventions.

Pneumonia is classified as either community-acquired or nosocomial, including what is now referred to as a HAC or hospital-acquired condition. That is, it is either acquired as a consequence of living in the community or as a result of medical treatment or institutionalization. In the nursing home the most frequent causes of aspiration pneumonia are reflux of colonized oral secretions, from a feeding tube, or simply eating.

The usual signs and symptoms of pneumonia such as cough, fatigue, and dyspnea may easily be attributed initially to something else, such as the underlying COPD or medications. In older adults, the signs may be incorrectly attributed to associated geriatric syndromes seen such as falling, mental status changes or signs of confusion, general deterioration, weakness, or anorexia (loss of appetite). When one appears to have pneumonia, an abnormal chest x-ray, fever, and elevated white blood count are expected. However, these signs may be delayed in an older adult, and if treatment is not started until they are present, it may be too late and the result may be death due to sepsis. For the best possibility of survival of a frail elder with pneumonia, very prompt interventions are necessary as soon as an infection is determined to be a reasonable explanation for a sudden change (Jett, 2006).

One of the most important questions a nurse needs to consider is if a recommendation and advocacy for hospitalization is appropriate. Fortunately there are several evidence-based guidelines to help the nurse make this decision (see the Evidence-Based Practice box). However, the ultimate decision regarding hospitalization and aggressive treatment, such as the use of ventilators, is always up to the patient or the health care surrogate consistent with the known wishes of the patient (see Chapters 23 and 25). It is always imperative to make sure that the patient and the significant others realize the severity of the situation and that there are always options. In this case, the options are "as aggressive as possible" care in a long-term care facility equipped to provide this (e.g., intravenous [IV] antibiotics, oxygen), "comfort measures," or "acute treatment," which will most likely include an emergency room visit and artificial ventilation in an intensive care unit (Gulick & Jett, 2006). The decision will always be a personal one.

 EVIDENCE-BASED PRACTICE

Risk for Death in the Person with Pneumonia

The indicators of an increased likelihood of pneumonia-related death for persons in the community are as follows: (1) aggravation of another health condition at the same time; (2) respiratory rate >25; and (3) elevated C-reactive protein, if known. The indicators for an increased risk for death within 30 days for those in nursing homes are respiratory rate >30, pulse >125, altered mental status, and history of dementia. Studies have found that the death rate increases with even one risk factor, with greater risk for each additional factor (Ladenfield et al., 2004).

Implications for Gerontological Nursing and Healthy Aging

Assessment

The nursing assessment of the person with respiratory problems focuses on the objective observations of oxygen saturation, sputum production, and respiratory rate, and the subjective reports of dyspnea or shortness of breath, its effect on functional status, and quality of life. Only persons experiencing a problem can really tell us what it is like for them. Visual analog scales and numeric rating scales, similar to those used to assess pain, may be helpful (see Chapter 15). Persons can be asked how they would rate their breathing, from 1 (no dyspnea) to 10 (the worst dyspnea they can imagine), and so on.

When an infection is suspected and treatment is desired, it is never appropriate to use a "wait and see" approach; elevations in temperature or in white blood cell count may not occur until the person is in a septic state, and chest x-ray exams in debilitated persons are often falsely negative at the beginning of the infection or with dehydration. Patients and their families should be told the seriousness of this or any infection in older adults. More timely diagnosis calls for sensitive clinical assessments by both the nurse and the other health care providers.

Assessment includes detailed information about cough. When did it start? How long are the episodes of coughing? Is there any associated pain? What seems to make it better, and what makes it worse? Is the person using anything to treat the cough? Is the person smoking (and how much) or exposed to smoke or other respiratory irritants? If the cough is productive, what is the color, texture, and odor of the mucus? Does the color change according to the time of the day?

The remaining physical examination is the same as that used for persons with cardiac disease, since it is not always clear whether symptoms such as fatigue and shortness of breath are cardiac or respiratory in nature. Observations of airway clearance, breathing patterns, and mobility; the measurement of pulse oximetry; a mental status examination; and a functional assessment provides a clearer picture of the person's health status. Pulmonary function testing is most definitive in terms of lung capacity, and along with a chest x-ray examination, can show the extent of respiratory damage from acute or chronic conditions. Box 19-8 presents the key aspects of a respiratory assessment.

Interventions

As with CVD, many respiratory diseases in late life cannot be cured. Nursing interventions are based on palliative goals, namely, stabilizing the disease, reducing the risk of exacerbations and hospitalizations, promoting maximal functional capacity, and preventing premature disability. Education always includes smoking cessation, secretion clearance techniques, identification and management of exacerbations, breathing retraining, management of depression and anxiety,

nutritional support, the proper use and administration of medications, and dealing with supplemental oxygen therapy if and when it is necessary (Esherick, 2010). Except in severe cases, treatment can occur at home with home health or in a skilled nursing facility, as long as oxygen therapy, parenteral fluids, and antibiotics can be administered.

If the elder fails to improve or deteriorates in either setting, then hospitalization is often necessary, unless this is against the wishes of the patient. A change to active palliative care may be appropriate at any time (see Chapter 25). If the person is hospitalized, a prolonged rehabilitation may be necessary, most often in a skilled nursing facility. Pharmacological and mechanical interventions for the treatment of infection are individually tailored based on the health status of the person before the infection, other health problems, expected outcomes of treatment, where treatment will be provided, and wishes of the patient.

Interdisciplinary Care

Education is a part of every aspect of pulmonary care (Box 19-9). The person is taught to recognize the signs and symptoms of respiratory infection; how to maintain adequate nutrition; how to use an inhaler, nebulizer, and a peak flow meter, how to clean them and the importance of good oral care afterward. Patients and caregivers are taught the safe use of oxygen; the type of exercise that is beneficial; how to pace activities; coping strategies; and about other issues, such as sexual function. Each of these areas calls for teaching and indicates specific interventions that will help older adults to engage in self-care management.

Diet education should address the reason for monitoring weight and the signs of malnutrition. Weight loss can occur rapidly because of the energy expenditure needed to breathe while eating. A sense of being full early in the meal (early satiation) is caused by congestion in the abdomen due to a flattened diaphragm. Anorexia occurs as a result of sputum production and gastric irritation from the use of bronchodilators and steroids.

Activity and exercise tolerance should be assessed by the occupational and respiratory therapist, and activities should be prescribed to increase endurance and improve respiratory status. Exercise may be done with or without oxygen as a supplement to control symptoms so that the older adult can spend enough time in exercise to benefit from it. The person should be informed that sexual activity is still possible, and education and counseling information should be provided, either by the rehabilitation nurse or a professional medical counselor.

Medications are used to treat infection and control dyspnea, cough, and sputum production. As with any

---

BOX 19-8   Respiratory Assessment

Obtain the Following History:
Family
Past medical
Symptoms

Perform Assessment of the Following:
Overall body configuration (e.g., posture, chest symmetry, shape, etc.)
Respirations, including ease of ventilation, use of accessory muscles, etc.
Detailed description of level of dyspnea per activity
Oxygenation (pulse oximetry, skin color, capillary refill, pallor)
Sputum (color, amount, consistency)
Palpation, percussion, and auscultation
Functional status
Cognitive status if indicated
Mood if indicated
Discussion of wishes for treatment and advance planning
Presence or absence of a living will and designated health care surrogate

BOX 19-9   **Instructions for Persons with Chronic Obstructive Pulmonary Disease**

Nutrition

Eat small, frequent meals with high protein and caloric content.*

Select foods that do not require a lot of chewing or cut in bite-size pieces to conserve energy.

Drink 2 to 3 L of fluid daily.*

Weigh self at least twice each week.

Activity Pacing to Conserve Energy

Plan exertion during the best periods of the day.

Arrange regular rest periods.

Allow plenty of time to complete activities.

Schedule sex around best breathing time of day.

> Use prescribed bronchodilators 20 to 30 minutes before.
>
> Use a position that does not call for pressure on the chest or support of the arms.

General Instructions

Participate in regular exercise.*

Select and wear clothing and shoes that are easy to put on and remove.

Avoid indoor and outdoor pollutants.

Avoid exposure to others with illness.

Obtain an annual flu shot if not allergic.

Obtain pneumococcal immunization as appropriate.

Notify health care provider of changes:

> Temperature elevation
>
> Sputum color or amount produced
>
> Increased shortness of breath

*As prescribed.

medication teaching, the nurse can make sure that the person knows the purpose and the correct dosage and regimen of any medication he or she is taking, its side effects, and what to do if these occur (see Chapter 8). Inhalers are difficult for those with limited manual dexterity and/or strength, as with arthritis in the hands. However, special adaptive devices or nebulizers are available.

Rehabilitation is an important aspect of maximizing quality of life for the person with respiratory problems, as it is for those with cardiovascular problems. An older adult with COPD would be considered a candidate for pulmonary rehabilitation as long as he or she has pulmonary reserve and stable heart disease. Rehabilitation programs for the older adult with COPD consist of drug therapy, reconditioning exercises, and counseling. A multidisciplinary team of health professionals works collectively to help the older adult achieve the following goals:

Increase the level of independence

Maintain individuality and autonomy

Improve function in his or her environment

Decrease the number of hospitalizations and need for hospitalization

Increase exercise tolerance

Increase self-esteem and self-care skills

Improve the quality of life and comfort

The number of goals achieved depends on many factors, including extent of illness and coexisting conditions. For those recovering from pneumonia, the rehabilitative period may be prolonged.

Economic issues are always a concern for persons with chronic disease (see Chapter 23). A number of medications are used and can be very expensive, especially when needed for an indefinite period of time. Medicare coverage for oxygen and equipment such as nebulizers is limited to those persons with a moderate to severe level of disease as determined by their oxygen saturation rates, and oxygen is never covered by insurance for comfort only. The expense of therapy for persons with a limited income or no insurance (see Chapter 23) will interfere with the adequacy of therapy and result in feelings of anxiety and a focus on the lowest level of Maslow's Hierarchy of Needs (see Chapter 1).

Mouth care is very important, especially for the person receiving supplemental oxygen and all who are medically or physically debilitated. Inadequate mouth care leads to the propagation of bacteria, which compounds an already serious situation. Inadequate oral care may lead to aspiration pneumonia or an oral thrush infection. Sputum is considered potentially infectious and must be handled appropriately.

Monitoring nutrition and obtaining nutritional consultation as necessary is the responsibility of the nurse in all settings. The nurse will also ensure that the person recovering from pneumonia is adequately nourished and hydrated while monitoring fluid volume. Overload is a risk for persons with coexisting heart disease. Mobilizing the older person and referring him or her for physical and occupational therapy to prevent or stop functional decline should occur as soon as the person's condition allows.

The nurse also has a role in the prevention of complications and infections. Adults older than 65 years of age and those with chronic conditions should be encouraged to receive the pneumococcal vaccine (Pneumovax) unless it is contraindicated. While it is most often a one-time dose, their health care providers may recommend a second dose after about 5 years. Influenza-related pneumonias may be avoided or ameliorated with yearly (October to December) flu vaccinations. In years when there is a particularly intense infection outbreak in the fall, an additional immunization may be recommended by public health officials. Yearly dental cleanings and examinations should be encouraged as well, since dental caries and periodontal disease are common and predispose one to develop pneumonia as a secondary infection (Karnath et al., 2003). Finally, the nurse can be aware of the pertinent goals of *Healthy People 2020* and play a part in helping the nation to achieve them (see the Healthy People box).

 HEALTHY PEOPLE 2020

Chronic Obstructive Pulmonary Disease (COPD)

Reduce the number of persons 45 years of age and older with activity limitation related to COPD.
Baseline: 23.2% in 2008
Target: 18.7% in 2020
Reduce the number of COPD-related deaths in persons 45 years of age and older.
Baseline: 112.4 per 100,000 persons in 2007
Target: 98.5 per 100,000 persons by 2020
Reduce COPD-related hospitalizations in persons 45 years of age and older.
Baseline: 56 per 10,000 persons in 2007
Target: 50.1 per 10,000 persons by 2020

From U.S. Department of Health and Human Services, Office of Disease Prevention and Health Promotion: *Healthy people 2020* (2012). Available at http://www.healthypeople.gov/2020.

Applicaton of Maslow's Hierarchy

For persons with cardiovascular or respiratory disorders, all efforts of professionals, family caregivers, and the older adult are directed toward creating a safe and comfortable environment that will maximize function and attainment of the highest level of functioning and wellness, with or without direct assistance. Although Maslow's lowest level of basic needs is often the priority, efforts can be made for the person to be able to reach for satisfaction of higher level needs as well.

Tuberculosis (TB)

Tuberculosis (*Mycobacterium tuberculosis*) is one of the most deadly communicable bacterial infections affecting about one third of the world's population (CDC, 2012b). Although both the incidence of and related deaths have steadily declined in the last 10 years, in 2011 it still affected a little over 10,000 persons in the United States. The majority of those affected are foreign-born persons especially from Asian countries, men (Figure 19-1), and those who are immune compromised (CDC, 2012b). In 2009 there were 113 cases of multi-drug resistant TB (MDR-TB) (Pratt et al., 2010).

The term *tuberculosis infection* refers to a positive TB skin test with no evidence of active disease. *Tuberculosis disease* refers to persons who have a positive acid-fast smear or culture for *M. tuberculosis* or positive x-rays and clinical presentation of TB. Symptoms include unexplained weight loss or fever and a cough lasting more than 3 weeks, regardless of age group. Night sweats and generalized anxiety may be present. In more advanced stages, the person will also have dyspnea, chest pain, and hemoptysis (sputum with blood in it). Laboratory results in persons with TB may show an increased sedimentation rate and lymphocytopenia. Because these signs and symptoms are associated with many disorders common in older adults, diagnosis often is made during a health screening (Tierney et al., 2011). For persons with positive skin tests (Table 19-3), it is necessary to confirm a diagnosis with a chest x-ray and sputum culture (National Library of Medicine [NLM], 2012a). Many of our present elders were treated following infections during World War II. Many others were infected as children. As they become immune compromised as a result of chemotherapy, extreme old age, or human immunodeficiency virus (HIV) infection, the bacterium could be reactivated.

The rate among elders overall is low; 2230 persons at least 65 years of age in 2010 (CDC, 2011). Gerontological nurses working in areas with higher TB rates must be particularly knowledgeable about this potentially life-threatening disease and protect themselves and others (Figure 19-2). Persons who are immunosuppressed, who are from areas with high infection rates, or who live in group settings are at particular risk. Older residents of congregate living settings are between two and seven times more likely to acquire the disease than those who live in the community (Ferebee, 2006).

Implications for Gerontological Nursing in Long-Term Care Settings

In promoting healthy aging in the context of TB, the nurse has a responsibility to both the public and the individual. The nurse must be proactive in the prevention of contagious disease and in the prompt treatment of those who are or become ill. This is especially important in the

TB Case Rates by Age Group and Sex, United States, 2010

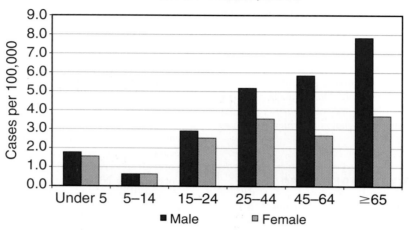

■ Male   ▫ Female

TB Case Rates by Age Group and Race/Ethnicity,* United States, 2010

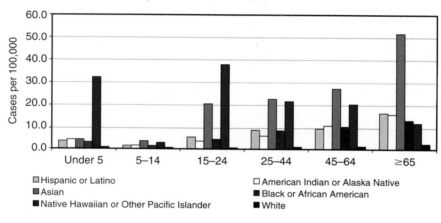

▫ Hispanic or Latino   ▫ American Indian or Alaska Native
■ Asian   ■ Black or African American
■ Native Hawaiian or Other Pacific Islander   ■ White

*All races are Non-Hispanic. Persons reporting two or more races
accounted for less than 1% of all cases.

FIGURE 19-1 TB case rates by age group and sex, United States, 2010; TB case rates by age group and ethnicity, United States, 2010. (From Centers for Disease Control and Prevention: *National Tuberculosis Surveillance System highlights from 2010.* Available at http://www.cdc.gov/tb/statistics/surv/surv2010/default.htm).

long-term care setting or when working with the homeless or in shelters. Elders in these settings are at higher risk because of communal living situations and the high rate of medical frailty and untreated medical conditions. In 1990 the Centers for Disease Control and Prevention (CDC) recommended that every person entering a long-term care facility as a resident or an employee undergo annual testing for TB (CDC, 2010). In 2005 the guidelines were updated considerably to reflect the changes in both incidence and prevalence in different geographical areas. To ensure prompt identification of persons with TB and limit its spread, especially in extended-care facilities, nurses should develop

TABLE **19-3**	Understanding the PPD Skin Test for TB Screening*	
Size of Reaction	**Affected Persons**	**Meaning of Result**
5 mm diameter	In persons who have HIV, have received an organ transplant, are immune-compromised, taking steroids of 15 mg/day for at least 1 month.	Positive results[†]; all else likely negative.[‡]
10 mm diameter	In health care workers; in persons with diabetes or renal failure; those with negative test in the last 2 years; injection drug users; children <4 years old; infants, children, and teens exposed to infected others; homeless; students, employees, and residents in group living settings such as nursing homes and prisons.	Positive results[†]; in all others likely to be negative.[‡]
≥15 mm diameter	For those with no known risks.	Positive results.[†]

*Area is examined for presence or absence of firmness and inflammation 48-72 hours after inoculation.
[†]All positive results require a chest x-ray and sputum culture to confirm diagnosis.
[‡]Up to 1 in 5 persons have false-negative results, especially those who are immune-compromised.
From National Library of Medicine: *PPD skin test* (2012). Available at http://www.nlm.nih.gov/medlineplus/ency/article/003839.htm.

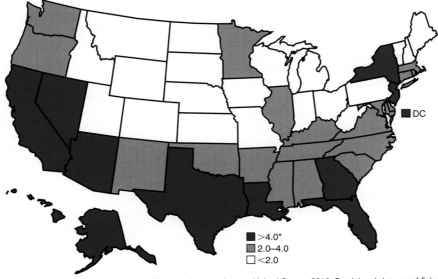

FIGURE 19-2 Rate (per 100,000 population) of tuberculosis cases, by state/area—United States, 2010. Provisional data as of February 26, 2011.
*20 states had TB case rates <2.0 (range: 0.61-1.88) per 100,000 population, 19 states had TB case rates of 2.0 to 4.0 (range: 2.07-3.92), and 11 states and the District of Columbia had TB case rates >4.0 (range: 4.15-8.77).
(Source: National TB Surveillance System. From Centers for Disease Control and Prevention: Trends in Tuberculosis—United States, 2010. *MMWR* 60(11):333-337. Available at http://www.cdc.gov/mmwr/preview/mmwrhtml/mm6011a2.htm?s_cid5mm6011a2_e%0d%0a.)

and implement an appropriate surveillance plan. If such a plan is not already in place, the CDC and the state health departments are excellent sources of guidance and assistance.

TB is a reportable condition, which means that all suspected and confirmed cases are reported to the local or state health authorities (NLM, 2012b). The local public

health nurses usually conduct investigations to ensure that all potentially infected people have been tested and that all persons with the disease receive treatment. The nurse actively participates in community health screenings that may include TB testing. As a health care provider, the nurse is also at risk for acquiring the infection

---

As a young public health nurse, it was my responsibility to periodically check on all persons in my assigned district who were undergoing treatment for tuberculosis (TB). A new person had moved into one of the many boarding houses of this inner-city neighborhood. Mr. Jones was a pleasant, robust 60-year-old who expressed pleasure in the visit and reported that he was doing well, that he had plenty of medications, and that they were not causing him any problems. He dashed out of the room, returned with a small suitcase, and opened it to assure me of his supply, and there before me were dozens of unopened bottles of isoniazid (INH), one of the staples of TB treatment. I called the medical director, who recommended that Mr. Jones be sent to the local hospital and, to make sure he got there, to deliver him forthwith. So I loaded him and his suitcase into my car and away we went; thinking of what Florence Nightingale would say, I left the windows open wide. When I returned to the health department, my first stop was for a TB test for myself and the plans for a follow-up after the incubation period. All for the sake of community well-being!

Kathleen Jett

and needs to be screened regularly to prevent becoming a carrier.

Nurses have a role in monitoring laboratory values, assessing for adverse drug reactions, and monitoring drug compliance in persons with TB, all of which are crucial to treatment effectiveness and the patient's well-being. The gerontological nurse participates in educating regarding the seriousness of the infection, and helping persons obtain the appropriate treatment as needed (Box 19-10).

KEY CONCEPTS

- Heart disease is the most common cause of death for persons in the United States.
- The underlying cause for the majority of cardiovascular and pulmonary disease is smoking; therefore, assisting persons in smoking cessation can have a significant impact on improving their health.
- Pneumonia and influenza are particularly important health problems for those over 65 years of age and significantly more so for those who are frail, immunocompromised, have HIV, or are otherwise decompensated.

- The mortality associated with pneumonia can be minimized through the use of pneumonia and influenza vaccinations and excellent oral hygiene.
- The goal of therapy for cardiac and respiratory disorders is to relieve symptoms, improve the quality of life, reduce mortality, stabilize and slow the progression of the disease, reduce the risk of exacerbation, and maximize functional capacity.
- Careful attention to the early detection and prompt treatment of tuberculosis is necessary to continue in the attempt to completely eradicate this communicable disease.

ACTIVITIES AND DISCUSSION QUESTIONS

1. What is heart failure, what is congestive heart failure, and how are they different from one another?
2. Discuss assessment and interventions for elders with a diagnosis of congestive heart failure.
3. Discuss assessment of elders with respiratory problems.
4. Why is pneumonia so dangerous to the older adult?
5. What preventive measures can be instituted to prevent or lessen the severity of pneumonia?

REFERENCES

American College of Cardiology Foundation/American Heart Association [ACCF/AHA]: 2011 Expert Consensus Document on Hypertension in the Elderly, *J Am Coll Cardiol* 57(20):2037–2114, 2011.

Buttaro TM, Trybulski J, Bailey PP, et al: *Primary Care: A Collaborative Approach*, ed 3, St. Louis, 2008, Mosby.

Centers for Disease Control and Prevention [CDC]: *People at high risk for becoming infected with Mycobacterium tuberculosis* (2010). Available at http://www.cdc.gov/tb/publications/slidesets/selfstudymodules/module2/highrisk_infected.htm.

Centers for Disease Control and Prevention [CDC]: *Reported tuberculosis in the United States, 2010* (2011). Available at http://www.cdc.gov/tb/statistics/reports/2010/table4.htm.

Centers for Disease Control and Prevention [CDC]: *National Vital Statistics Reports: Death: preliminary data for 2010* (2012a). Available at http://www.cdc.gov/nchs/data/nvsr/nvsr60/nvsr60_04.pdf.

Centers for Disease Control and Prevention [CDC]: *Tuberculosis (TB): data and statistics* (2012b). Available at http://www.cdc.gov/tb/statistics/default.htm.

Centers for Disease Control and Prevention [CDC]: *Heart disease facts* (2012c). Available at http://www.cdc.gov/heartdisease/facts.htm.

Centers for Disease Control and Prevention [CDC]: *Heart failure facts* (2012d). Available at http://www.cdc.gov/dhdsp/data_statistics/fact_sheets/fs_heart_failure.htm.

Esherick JS: *Tarascon Primary Care Pocketbook*, Sudbury, MA, 2010, Jones & Bartlett.

Fang J, Mensah GA, Croft JB, et al: Heart failure-related hospitalization in the U.S., 1979-2004, *J Am Coll Cardiol* 52(6):428–434, 2008.

Ferebee L: Respiratory function. In Meiner SE, Luecknotte AG, editors: *Gerontologic nursing,* ed 3, St. Louis, 2006, Mosby.

Franklin BA, Vanhecke TE: Preventing reinfarction: changing behavior after the MI: part 1, *Consultant* 47(6):517–522, 2007.

Gulick G, Jett KF: Applying evidence-based findings to practice: caring for older adults in subacute units, *Geriatr Nurs* 27(5):280–283, 2006.

Harrington CC: Evidence-based guideline: assessing heart failure in long-term care facilities, *J Gerontol Nurs* 34(2):9–14, 2008.

Health Indicators Warehouse: *Hypertension* (2005–2008a). Available at http://www.healthindicators.gov/Indicators/Hypertension2 cadults_897/Profile/Data.

Health Indicators Warehouse: *High blood pressure control among adults (%)* (2005–2008b). Available at http://www.healthindicators.gov/Indicators/Highbloodpressurecontrol_882/Profile/Data.

Health Indicators Warehouse: *Awareness of early symptoms and response to a heart attack* (2008). Available at http://www.healthindicators.gov/Indicators/Awarenessofandresponsetoearlywarningsymptomsofheartattack_894/Profile/Data.

Hoyert DL, Xu J: Deaths: preliminary data for 2011, *Natl Vital Stat Rep* 61(6):6, 2012.

Jett KF: Examining the evidence: knowing if and when to transfer a resident with pneumonia from the nursing home to the hospital or subacute unit, *Geriatr Nurs* 27(5):280, 2006.

Joint National Committee of the Detection, Evaluation, and Treatment of High Blood Pressure [JNC]: *JNC 7 express: the seventh report of the Joint National Commission of the prevention, detection, evaluation and treatment of high blood pressure* (2003). Available at www.nhlbi.nih.gov.

Karnath B, Agyeman A, Lai A: Pneumococcal pneumonia: update on therapy in the era of antibiotic resistance, *Consultant* 42(3):321–326, 2003.

Ladenfield CS, Palmer RM, Johnson MA, et al: *Current geriatric diagnosis and treatment,* New York, 2004, McGraw-Hill.

National Library of Medicine: *PPD skin test* (2012a). Available at http://www.nlm.nih.gov/medlineplus/ency/article/003839.htm.

National Library of Medicine: *Pulmonary tuberculosis* (2012b). Available at http://www.nlm.nih.gov/medlineplus/ency/article/000077.htm.

Pratt R, Price S, Miramontes R, et al: Trends in tuberculosis—United States, *MMWR* 60(11):333–337, 2010. Available at http://www.cdc.gov/mmwr/preview/mmwrhtml/mm6011a2.htm?s_cid=mm6011a2_e%0d%0a.

Sisk J, Herbert P, Horowitz C, et al: Effects of nurse management on the quality of heart failure care in minority communities: a randomized clinical trial, *Ann Intern Med* 145(4):273–283, 2006.

Tierney LM, Saint S, Whooley MA: *Current essentials of medicine,* ed 4, New York, 2011, Lange.

U.S. Department of Health and Human Services [USDHHS]: *Respiratory diseases: objectives* (2008). Available at http://www.healthypeople.gov/2020/topicsobjectives2020/objectiveslist.aspx?topicId=36.

U.S. Department of Health and Human Services [USDHHS], Office of Disease Prevention and Health Promotion: *Healthy people 2020* (2012). Available at http://www.healthypeople.gov/2020.

CHAPTER 20

Neurological Disorders

Kathleen F. Jett

ⓔvolve evolve.elsevier.com/Ebersole/gerontological

LEARNING OBJECTIVES

Upon completion of this chapter, the reader will be able to:

- Differentiate a transient ischemic attack from a stroke.
- Differentiate the hemorrhagic stroke from an embolic stroke and understand the care implications of the differences.
- Identify strategies to decrease the likelihood of a stroke.
- Contribute to the early recognition of Parkinson's disease.
- Develop a strategy to promote safety in persons with neurological disorders.
- Suggest ways to optimize communication with persons with communication difficulties due to a neurological impairment.

GLOSSARY

Aphasia A communication disorder that affects the ability to use and understand spoken or written words or both.

Bradykinesia Abnormally slowed movements of the body.

Dysarthria A speech disorder caused by weakness or incoordination of the muscles used for speech.

Dyskinesia The impaired ability to control movements resulting in involuntary movements which may be spasmodic or repetitive.

Dystonia Movements that are often sudden and the result of prolonged contraction of one or more muscles, resulting in twisting body motions, tremor, and abnormal posture.

THE LIVED EXPERIENCE

You know I lived a hard life – I smoked since I was a kid, didn't take care of myself, but somehow I never thought I might have a stroke. Now I have had one and life will never be the same.

Henry at 72

I just don't understand what she is trying to tell me. I know it must be very frustrating for her to feel kind of trapped inside and not being able to speak, but I am frustrated too, not knowing what she needs!

Angela, a new nurse

I n this chapter we review two of the most common neurological disorders seen in older adults, cerebrovascular disease and Parkinson's disease. Each of these has the potential to significantly impair a person's function and indeed affect every aspect of life. In as much, the role of the nurse is broad. In both of these the nurse plays an active role in helping the patient and the family navigate the rehabilitative process and minimize loss of function; this may include home visits to determine the safety measures needed in the environment. In case of cerebrovascular disease, the nurse is active in health promotion and disease prevention by ensuring prompt diagnosis and treatment at the time of the acute event (see the Healthy People box). Last, the gerontological nurse helps the elder and his or her significant others cope with the changes inherent in these disorders including grief support (see Chapter 25).

 HEALTHY PEOPLE 2020
Goal in Development: Signs of Stroke

HDS 17.1 Increase the proportion of adults who are aware of the early warning symptoms and signs of a stroke and the importance of accessing rapid emergency care by calling 911 or another emergency number.

From U.S. Department of Health and Human Services, Office of Disease Prevention and Health Promotion: *Healthy people 2020* (2012). Available at http://www.healthypeople.gov/2020.

Cerebrovascular Disease

Cerebrovascular disease is the most commonly occurring neurological disorder, and it is caused by an interruption of blood supply to the brain. Cerebrovascular disease is either ischemic or hemorrhagic in nature and it is manifested as either a stroke (the term *cerebrovascular accident* [CVA] is now discouraged) or a transient ischemic attach (TIA). Because the initial signs and symptoms are similar but the outcomes are different, diagnosis is geared toward identifying the specific cause and the location of the brain injury. Only when the cause is known can appropriate therapy be implemented.

More than 75% of all strokes occur in persons older than 65 years of age. Strokes are twice as common among African Americans as whites, and Hispanics have the lowest rate of all. Hispanics and African Americans are significantly more likely to die as a result of the stroke (Centers for Disease Control and Prevention [CDC], 2011) (Figure 20-1). The age-adjusted death rate is about equal in men and women. However, there are also significant regional differences (Figure 20-2).

Although the rate of strokes is decreasing, it remains the third most common cause of death behind heart disease and cancer for whites, African Americans, and Hispanics and the fifth leading cause of death for American Indians and Alaskan Natives (CDC, 2012). Each year about 795,000 people in the United States have a stroke, or one stroke every 40 seconds. For most people (610,000) this is a first-time event but for many others (185,000) it is a repeat event. Once every 4 minutes someone dies of a stroke (CDC, 2011).

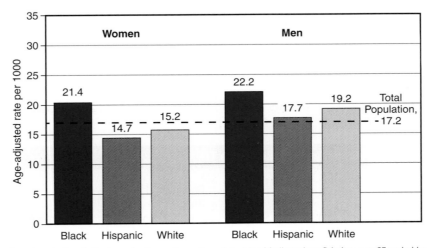

FIGURE 20-1 Age-adjusted stroke hospitalization rates by gender and race/ethnicity–Medicare beneficiaries ages 65 and older, 1995-2002. Average annual stroke hospitalization rates per 1000 Medicare beneficiaries are directly age-adjusted using the 2000 U.S. standard population aged ≥65 years. (From Casper ML, Nwaise IA, Croft JB, Nilasena DS: *Atlas of stroke hospitalizations among medicare beneficiaries.* Atlanta, 2008, U.S. Department of Health and Human Services, Centers for Disease Control and Prevention. Available at http://www.cdc.gov/dhdsp/atlas/2008_stroke_atlas/.)

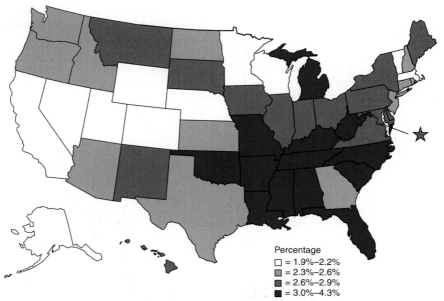

Percentage
□ = 1.9%–2.2%
▨ = 2.3%–2.6%
▦ = 2.6%–2.9%
■ = 3.0%–4.3%

FIGURE 20-2 Percentage of people who were ever told they had a stroke, 2008. (From CDC Behavioral Risk Factor Surveillance System (BRFSS). Available at http://www.cdc.gov/dhdsp/data_statistics/fact_sheets/fs_stroke.htm.)

Etiology

Ischemic Events

The majority (87%) of all cerebrovascular events are ischemic in nature (CDC, 2011). The four main types and causes are (1) arterial disease, (2) cardioembolism, (3) hematological disorders, and (4) systemic hypoperfusion. Cardioembolism includes those caused by an arrhythmia such as atrial fibrillation, which is frequently seen in coronary heart disease (see Chapter 19). The use of antithrombotics (e.g., aspirin, warfarin) in persons with heart disease is an attempt to reduce the risk for stroke. Hematological disorders include coagulation disorders and hyperviscosity syndromes. Hypoperfusion leading to a stroke can occur from dehydration, hypotension (including overtreatment of hypertension), cardiac arrest, or fainting (syncope) (Graykowski, 2008).

A TIA is ischemic but clinically different from an ischemic stroke in that the symptoms of a TIA begin to resolve within minutes and all neurological deficits caused by it resolve within 24 hours. In some cases a TIA is followed by a stroke, but most strokes are not preceded by TIAs (Box 20-1).

Approximately 24% to 29% of those who have a TIA will have a stroke in the 5 years following the event (Goldstein, 2011). Up to 500,000 TIAs are diagnosed each year in the United States. More men than women have TIAs, with 101 cases per 100,000 men and 70 cases per 100,000 women. However, the most significant difference is by age, with

---

BOX 20-1   Relative Risk for a Major Stroke After a TIA

Age >60 = 1 point
BP >140/90 = 1 point
Resulting unilateral weakness = 2 points
Speech impairment, no weakness = 1 point
Duration of deficit 10-59 minutes = 1 point
Duration >1 hour = 2 points

Diabetes = 1 point
Risk:
Score 6-7: High risk (8.1% chance of a major stroke in 2 days)
Score 4-5: Moderate risk (4.1% chance)
Score 0-3: Low risk (1% chance)

From Llinas R: Stroke. In Durso SC, editor: *Oxford American handbook of geriatric medicine,* New York, 2010, Oxford Press, p.168.

1 to 3 per 100,000 persons in those under 35 years of age but 1500 per 100,000 in those over 85 years of age.

Hemorrhagic Events

Hemorrhagic strokes are less frequent than ischemic strokes but more life threatening. They are primarily caused by uncontrolled hypertension and less often by malformations of the blood vessels (e.g., aneurysms). Although the exact mechanism is not fully understood, it appears that the chronic hypertension causes thickening of the vessel wall, microaneurysms, and necrosis. When enough damage to the vessel accumulates, it is at risk for rupture. The spontaneous rupture may be large and acute or small with a slow leaking of blood into the adjacent brain tissue. In many cases, there is a rupture or seepage of blood into the ventricular system of the brain with damage to the affected tissue through necrosis or death of brain tissue (Boss, 2010a). Resolution of the event can occur only with the resorption of excess blood and damaged tissue.

Signs and Symptoms of Cerebrovascular Disease

The first signs of both strokes and TIAs are acute neurological deficits consistent with the part of the brain affected. They are often preceded by a severe headache. In subarachnoid hemorrhages, the headache is not only sudden but also explosive, very severe, and without other neurological manifestations (Graykowski, 2008).

Some of the clinical signs and symptoms are suggestive of either ischemia or hemorrhage (Box 20-2). Persons with hemorrhage have more specific neurological changes, including seizures and more depressed level of consciousness than those with an ischemic stroke. If a person is deeply unresponsive following a stroke he or she is unlikely to survive (Boss, 2010a). Nausea and vomiting are suggestive

---

BOX 20-2	Early Signs and Symptoms of Stroke

- Sudden numbness or weakness of the face, arm, or leg—especially on one side of the body.
- Sudden confusion or trouble speaking or understanding.
- Sudden trouble seeing in one or both eyes.
- Sudden trouble walking, dizziness, or loss of balance or coordination.
- Sudden severe headache with no known cause.

From Centers for Disease Control and Prevention: *Stroke fact sheet* (2012). Available at http://www.cdc.gov/dhdsp/data_statistics/fact_sheets/fs_stroke.htm.

---

of increased cerebral edema in response to an event of either type. Neurological changes may include alterations in motor, sensory, and visual function; coordination; cognition; and language and depend on the area of damage.

Diagnosis includes the determination and correction of possible extra-cerebral causes, if any (e.g., infection or hypoglycemia), confirmation of the type of stroke and identifying exactly where in the brain the damage has occurred. This is done through the use of a computed tomography (CT) scan or magnetic resonance imaging (MRI).

Complications

After a TIA resolves, there should be no residual effect other than an increased chance of recurrence and the possible increased risk for stroke as noted earlier. Early complications of a simple stroke include extension of the amount of damage and recurrence. Brain edema is always a problem, and could result in obstructive hydrocephalus (Graykowski, 2008).

The potential long-term effects of a stroke may be minimal but also may include paralysis and hemiparesis limiting movement, and dysarthrias, dysphagias, and aphasias limiting speech. Post-stroke depression has been found to negatively affect rehabilitation. Whenever paralysis or hemiparesis occurs, the development of spasticity or unusually tight muscles in the affected limb(s) is a risk. Spasticity can lead to contractures if it is not managed well and even sometimes when it is. Pain in the affected side is not uncommon and may be treated with muscle relaxants or medications specific for neuropathic pain (see Chapter 8). The medications, added to the potential limitations of the stroke, significantly increase the risk for falls. Other complications include blood clots (deep vein thrombosis [DVT]) in the affected limb, pressure ulcers, aspiration pneumonia, and urinary tract infections (Llinas, 2010).

Management

All actual or potential cerebrovascular events are considered emergencies and should be treated as such. However, because TIAs are highly transient they often resolve on their own before the person is even seen by a health care provider. Instead, the person reports "I think I had a small stroke last week" or they do not seek care at all. If the deficits and symptoms were fleeting, the diagnosis is made through the clinical interview. Management is considered preventive—to prevent recurrences and to decrease any possible risk factors for strokes (see the Healthy People box). The person and family are also instructed in the appropriate emergency response to the return of any signs or symptoms of a stroke or another TIA (see Box 20-1). Anticoagulant therapy has been proven to prevent recurrent cardioembolic strokes and TIAs. Aspirin, 81 to 325 mg/day, is the mainstay of therapy for elders with TIAs. However, for those who are aspirin sensitive, clopidogrel (Plavix) may be used (Llinas, 2010). Warfarin therapy or one of the newer related medications is usually used in persons to prevent another stroke and in those with atrial fibrillation to prevent the occurrence of the first stroke (Graykowski, 2008).

 HEALTHY PEOPLE 2020

Goal in Development: Reduce Risk

HDS 20.2 (Developmental) Increase the proportion of adults who have had a stroke who have their low-density lipoprotein (LDL) cholesterol at or below recommended levels.

From U.S. Department of Health and Human Services, Office of Disease Prevention and Health Promotion: *Healthy people 2020* (2012). Available at http://www.healthypeople.gov/2020.

Acute management is accomplished in emergency departments and intensive care units. The acute management of the stroke requires careful attention to the accuracy of the diagnosis. For ischemic strokes caused by an embolism, the compromised circulation to the brain must be restored rapidly. This is done in emergency rooms and is called *reperfusion therapy* using recombinant tissue plasminogen activator (rt-PA) if the facility is equipped to do so (see the Healthy People box).

 SAFETY ALERT

Reperfusion therapy (using recombinant tissue plasminogen activator [rt-PA]) can only be used for ischemic occlusive (usually embolic) strokes and only if a CT scan confirms the absence of hemorrhage and is within 3 hours of the onset of the event (Llinas, 2010).

 HEALTHY PEOPLE 2020

Goal in Development: Prompt Treatment

HDS 19.3 (Developmental) Acute reperfusion therapy within 3 hours from symptom onset for patients with strokes.

From U.S. Department of Health and Human Services, Office of Disease Prevention and Health Promotion: *Healthy people 2020* (2012). Available at http://www.healthypeople.gov/2020.

If the person has had a hemorrhagic stroke and it is misdiagnosed, the bleeding will be rapidly accelerated by the rt-PA, and the person will die. The initial response to the hemorrhagic stroke is to find a means to stop the bleeding if possible.

About 90% of neurological recovery occurs within 3 months of the stroke; 10% occurs more slowly, especially after a hemorrhagic stroke (Porter & Kaplan, 2010-2011). At 18 months after the stroke, there tends to be a small decline. The inverse relationship between functional improvement and advanced age, social isolation, and emotional distress is clear. Recovery from stroke is affected by the location and extent of the brain damage. Difficulties and handicaps after stroke often involve neurological and functional deficits. Post–ischemic stroke management begins immediately with anticoagulants or antiplatelets and rehabilitation (see the Healthy People box).

 HEALTHY PEOPLE 2020

Goal in Development: Reduce Complications

HDS 23 (Developmental) Increase the proportion of adult stroke survivors who are referred to a stroke rehabilitation program at discharge.

From U.S. Department of Health and Human Services, Office of Disease Prevention and Health Promotion: *Healthy people 2020* (2012). Available at http://www.healthypeople.gov/2020.

Nowhere in the care of elders is the multidisciplinary team more essential than in the care of persons after a stroke. The assessment of needs is extremely complex; it requires evaluation by a team often coordinated by a rehabilitation nurse and includes a neurologist; a physiatrist; speech, occupational, and physical therapists; an ophthalmologist; a rehabilitation specialist; and a psychologist. It also may include a spiritual advisor. It always includes the person's significant other, who may be involved with the day-to-day life. Acute support services are now available in specialized stroke centers. These have been found to improve outcomes in persons with ischemic strokes (Llinas, 2010).

Implications for Gerontological Nursing and Healthy Aging

The best approach to stroke, despite new therapies and medications, is prevention and prompt intervention. Identifying high-risk or stroke-prone elders is something nurses can do in the elders' homes, in the community, or at the health facilities where the nurses work. In a quick assessment of risk factors (Box 20-3), the nurse can work with individuals to reduce their risk for stroke and teach them how to respond to any signs or symptoms (see the Healthy People box).

BOX 20-3   **Risk Factors for Stroke**

Heart disease (and risk factors for)
Hypertension
Arrhythmias
Hypercholesterolemia
Diabetes
Smoking
Coagulopathies
Brain tumors
Family history

TABLE 20-1	**Assessment of the Person Following a Stroke or TIA**
General	**Neurological**
Vital signs	Level of arousal, orientation, attention
Cardiovascular	Speech (dysarthria, dysphasia)
Respiratory	Cranial nerves
Abdominal	Motor strength
	Coordination
	Sensation
	Gait (if possible)
	Reflexes

⚫ **HEALTHY PEOPLE 2020**

Objectives Related to Strokes: Reduce Stroke-Related Deaths

Baseline (2007): 42.2 per 100,000 persons
Target (2020): 33.8 per 100,000 persons

From U.S. Department of Health and Human Services, Office of Disease Prevention and Health Promotion: *Healthy people 2020* (2012). Available at http://www.healthypeople.gov/2020.

Smoking cessation and tight control of blood pressure may be the most important of the strategies in approaching modifiable risk factors. Reducing the blood pressure 5 mm Hg in a hypertensive person reduces risk of death from a stroke 14% (National Heart, Lung and Blood Institute [NHLBI], 2003). Maintaining the blood pressure equal to or less than 130/85 mm Hg is recommended. Additional primary prevention includes a healthful diet, limited salt and alcohol, and aspirin therapy unless contraindicated. Controlling lipids and diabetes and preventing atrial fibrillation have been found to be helpful, as well as regular exercise and weight-management programs.

In the acute period the nurse participates in patient assessment (Table 20-1). The nurse works to prevent aspiration and the development of DVTs. Pneumatic stocking devices, compression stockings, and low-weight heparin may be used (if ischemic). Early mobilization is also necessary and physical therapists are often involved even before the patient leaves the acute care setting. Eating may be a problem and a nasogastric (NG) tube may be required. If this is anticipated to be a persistent problem, the patient and family may elect to have a semipermanent percutaneous endoscopic gastrostomy (PEG) tube inserted directly into the stomach.

The nurse has an active role in the prevention and minimization of disability, that is, the promotion of healthy aging in persons with significant functional limitations

following a stroke. A period of intense rehabilitation often takes place in a rehabilitation or skilled nursing facility setting and continues long after the person returns home or to an assisted living setting. An important role for the nurse is documenting clearly and in detail the functional capacities that are retained and those that are impaired. The assessment must be redone routinely to carefully evaluate and document areas of progress, areas of need, and signs of depression, a common sequela.

The nurse works to prevent iatrogenic complications such as skin breakdown, falls, and increased confusion from medications. The nurse monitors the patient for changes in mental status, respiratory functioning, and ensures and maximizes the capacity for self-care, especially related to mobility, activity, eating, maintaining adequate fluid intake, and continence. The nurse is alert for problems with sleep, constipation, and depression. The nurse acts as an advocate in the recommendation to or participation in support groups for both the persons after a stroke and their significant others or caregivers. The gerontological nurse is challenged to take an active role in improving the quality of life of elders with cerebrovascular disorders, especially those with functional limitations.

Parkinson's Disease

Parkinson's disease (PD) is the most common neurodegenerative disorder (Shapira, 2010). It is a slowly progressing disease that is the result of a destruction of the cells in a portion of the brain called the substantia nigra. As the tract deteriorates it is no longer able to produce the neurotransmitter dopamine. Dopamine is a brain chemical that plays a major part in regulating movement; thus PD is considered a movement disorder. By the time the first symptoms are seen, 80% of the specific brain cells have been lost and 70% to 80% of the dopamine needed for the control of involuntary movement and the initiation of voluntary, smooth movement has been lost

(Boss, 2010b). Although not true PD, older adults are especially prone to the development of PD-like symptoms as a side effect of antipsychotic medications, and any older adult receiving these medications should be routinely screened for extrapyramidal symptoms (EPSs), which look like PD (see Chapter 8). The exact cause of PD is unknown. It is thought to be a combination of genetics and environmental factors such as smoking and exposure to viruses and toxins (such as pollutants) (Boss, 2010a; Jordan, 2008; Tanner et al., 2009).

PD was first described in 1817 in a paper by Dr. James Parkinson, a British physician, who described "the shaking palsy" and presented its major symptoms. It affects more than half a million people in the United States and is most often diagnosed when the person is 60 years of age or more (National Institute of Neurological Disorders and Stroke [NINDS], 2012a). Only about one third of those with PD appear to have a familial component, leaving the vast majority with no clear inheritance pattern (Shapira, 2010). PD appears to be slightly more common in men than in women; those of Ashkenazi Jewish heritage may be at particular risk (Shapira, 2010). The median time between diagnosis and death is 9 years (Boss, 2010b).

Signs and Symptoms

PD usually starts very slowly, making it difficult to diagnose, particularly in the early stages. Diagnosis is one of exclusion, ruling out other possible causes of symptoms. When there is no other explanation, a diagnosis is made on the presence of two of the four classic symptoms (Box 20-4). One of these must be either a resting tremor or bradykinesia (or "paucity of movement") (Boss, 2010b). Diagnosis is supported by a challenge test in which a person with symptoms is given a dose of levodopa. If there is a significant and rapid improvement, the diagnosis is thought to be confirmed. Early falls, poor response to levodopa, symmetry of motor symptoms, lack of tremor, and early autonomic dysfunction (e.g., incontinence) may be useful in distinguishing other movement disorders from PD (Boss, 2010b).

The symptoms of PD are many. Although tremor is the most conspicuous, especially in the early stages, bradykinesia is seen most often, is most disabling, and is often overlooked. There are fewer overall movements of the body; this may be a reduction in facial muscle movement or arms that hang at the sides instead of swing while walking. There is also a "freezing" that occurs when the person is moving but suddenly appears to "get stuck" and then has difficulty starting again.

When a person has a tremor it is asymmetrical, pin-rolling, regular, rhythmic, of a low-amplitude and occurs at rest. It disappears briefly during voluntary movement. It

---

BOX 20-4 Signs and Symptoms of Parkinson's Disease

Classic Signs and Symptoms
Bradykinesia (slowness of movement)
Tremor, at rest (trembling in hands, arms, legs, jaw, or face)
Cogwheel rigidity (resistance of the limbs and trunk in a jerking manner)
Postural instability (impaired balance and coordination)

Other Signs
Disordered sleep
Constipation
Fatigue
Excessive salivation
Pain
Depression
Visual disturbances
Psychosis
Seborrhea
Excessive sweating
Hypotension
Soft-spoken voice
Little facial animation
Infrequent blinking
Restless legs

---

can occur in the leg, but more often affects the arm. Rarely is the head involved. All tremors increase with stress and anxiety. They are not present during sleep.

Other causes of disability include rigidity and postural instability. The characteristic gait is called *festination* and consists of very short steps and minimal arm movements. Turning is difficult and may require many steps. Postural reflexes are lost. The elder will have involuntary flexion of the head and neck, a stooped posture, and a tendency to fall backward. If off balance, correction is very slow, so falls are common. For the person with moderately advanced PD the nurse will typically see a person who is bent forward from the waist but with head up, standing still and then suddenly moving forward relatively rapidly but with a shuffling manner and small steps. The person may come to a sudden halt, only to start all over again, clearly with effort. The necessity of high-back wheelchairs is not uncommon sometime in the course of the illness.

Rigidity impedes both passive and active movement. It is a state of involuntary contractions of all striated muscles.

Severe muscle cramps may occur in the toes or hands. When examined, a limb may exhibit either "lead pipe" or "cogwheel" (intermittent) resistance during passive movement. Muscles in the extremities, trunk, ocular area, and face may be affected, including the muscles of mastication (chewing), deglutition (swallowing), and articulation (speaking). Handwriting is small (micrographia). The person with PD will sit for long periods or lie motionless with few shifts in position and few changes in facial expression (Boss, 2010b). This lack of movement makes the person at high risk for pressure ulcers.

There are also a number of cognitive and affective symptoms. A full 50% of persons with PD show signs of depression, sometimes severe. It is believed that this is associated with the disease and not necessarily with the situation. About 30% of those persons with PD living in the community have dementia as well and up to 80% of those who require nursing home care. The depression may vary from day to day but in all cases it worsens over time (Boss, 2010b).

The severity of the symptoms of PD is based on the degree of neuron damage and how much dopamine is lost. PD is progressive, and symptoms worsen over time. However, the symptoms and their intensity vary from person to person; some become severely disabled, and others experience only minor disturbances in movement. The progression of symptoms may take 20 years or more. In late stages of the disease, complications (e.g., pressure ulcers, pneumonia, aspiration, and falls) can lead to death.

Management

Drug therapy focuses on replacement, mimicking, or slowing dopamine breakdown. First-line approaches include the combination of carbidopa and levodopa (Sinemet), other dopamine agonists pramipexole (Miraplex) or ropinirole (Requip). The monoamine oxidase (MAO) inhibitors selegiline (Eldepryl) and rasagiline (Azilect) are also used in initial treatment (Douglas, 2011). Sinemet loses effectiveness as the amino acid L-*dopa*. competes with other amino acids for absorption at both the intestinal wall and the blood-brain barrier. It also has a high risk of dyskinesia as a side effect (see Chapter 8).

 SAFETY ALERT

Sinemet must be taken 1 hour before or 2 hours after a meal to minimize GI side effects, and it must also be given routinely and on time to prevent fluctuations in symptoms.

 SAFETY ALERT

MAO inhibitors, sometimes used to control PD symptoms have significant drug-drug and drug-food interactions and must be used with caution. The nurse must monitor the patient carefully.

Other medications useful in management include the catechol *O*-methyltransferase (COMT) inhibitors; antihistamines; and anticholinergics (for tremor relief). Although anticholinergics are not usually recommended for use in older adults due to their high association with falls but are sometimes necessary for the person with PD. Many of these medications may be used in combination for specific effects.

Persons who are stable on Sinemet are often followed by their primary care providers. However, when this is no longer effective they are more often cared for by neurologists specializing in PD. Medication therapy is complicated and must be closely supervised. Hypotension, dyskinesias (involuntary movements), dystonia (lack of control of movement), hallucinations, sleep disorders, and depression are common side effects of both the disease and the medications used to treat it. Currently, selective serotonin reuptake inhibitors (SSRIs) such as venlafaxine are used. Bupropion, sertraline, paroxetine, trazodone, and mirtazapine also are used. For patients with PD and psychosis, antipsychotics may be required and should be those with the least anticholinergic effects (see Chapter 8).

Deep brain stimulation (DBS) may be used in patients who have not responded to drug therapy or have intractable motor fluctuations, dyskinesias, or tremor (NINDS, 2012b). Exercise therapy and speech therapy for patients with dysarthria should be considered.

Implications for Gerontological Nursing and Healthy Aging

Ongoing nursing care focuses on making sure the person gets good care, increasing functional ability, preventing excess disability, and decreasing risk of injury (see the Evidence-Based Practice box). Persons with PD experience significant functional problems in mobility, communication, and activities of daily living. Nursing interventions can contribute greatly to quality of life and functional ability. Comprehensive functional assessments with attention to self-care abilities and nutritional assessment (see Chapter 9) are important, as well as fall assessment and risk reduction interventions (see Chapter 13).

EVIDENCE-BASED PRACTICE

Components of an Annual Medical Exam for the Person with Parkinson's Disease

- Review of current medications
- Assessment of mental health (evidence of psychosis, depression, anxiety, impulse control disorders)
- Cognitive status
- Evidence of autonomic dysfunction: orthostatic hypotension, constipation, urinary or fecal incontinence or urinary retention, erectile dysfunction
- Sleep quality
- History of falls
- Outcome of rehabilitation if used
- Safety issues relative to the stage of the disease
- Compliance with current medications

Nurses caring for people with PD in the acute care setting must be knowledgeable about functional abilities and interventions to maintain function during episodes of acute illness. The goal of treatment is to preserve self-care abilities and prevent complications. Encouragement to persons in the support system and information about the disease are essential if the family and the person are to cope with the losses associated with PD (see Chapter 25). The Sickness Impact Profile (SIP) is a useful tool that can be used by nurses to determine problems most troublesome from the person's perspective.

Exercise—including walking, moving all of the joints, and improving balance—needs to be included early in the course of PD treatment; physical therapy evaluation and treatment are important. Rigidity of facial muscles and bradykinesia affect eating ability, nutrition, swallowing, and communication. Occupational therapy can assist with adaptive equipment such as weighted utensils, non-slip dinnerware, and other self-care aids. Speech therapy is beneficial for dysarthria and dysphagia (see later in this chapter). Patients can be taught facial exercises and swallowing techniques. Regular pain assessments and appropriate management (see Chapter 15) are also essential to address the often unnoticed problem of pain related to rigidity, contractures, dystonias, and central-pain syndromes of the disease itself, which may cause unexplained uncomfortable sensations. Other important interventions are assessment and treatment of postural hypotension, incontinence (see Chapter 10), gastrointestinal (GI) distress, depression and anxiety (see Chapter 22), sleep disturbances (see Chapter 11), and constipation (see Chapter 10).

Because of the usually slow progression of the disease and the disability that accompanies PD, individuals experience a change in roles, activities, and social participation. Tremors may produce embarrassing moments. The expressionless face, slowed movement, and soft, monotone speech may give the impression of apathy, depression, or disinterest, and might discourage others from socializing with affected individuals. Observing these symptoms, others may feel that the person is unable to participate in activities and relationships and may even think the person is cognitively impaired. A sensitive nurse is aware that the visible symptoms produce an undesired façade that may hide an alert and responsive individual who wishes to interact but is trapped in a body that no longer responds. It is important to see beyond the disease to the person within and provide nursing interventions that enhance hope and promote the highest quality of life despite disease. In an analysis of the stories of older adults with PD, Whitney (2004) found that learning what gives persons purpose and meaning in life and helping them understand what is happening to their bodies can assist in coping with their losses. Listening to stories is a wonderful way to come to know the person and individualize interventions to meet expressed needs.

Many resources are available for people with PD to provide practical information about living with the disease and a means to learn about new developments and treatments. The Evolve website for this book provides further information that the nurse can use for referral.

Communication and Elders with Neurological Disorders

Three major categories of impaired verbal communication arise from neurological disturbances: (1) reception, (2) perception, and (3) articulation. Reception is impaired by anxiety or is related to a specific disorder, hearing deficits, or altered level of consciousness. Perception is distorted by stroke, dementia, and delirium (see Chapter 21). Articulation is hampered by mechanical difficulties such as dysarthria, respiratory disease, destruction of the larynx, and strokes. Specific difficulties may include the following:

- *Anomia:* Word retrieval difficulties during spontaneous speech and naming tasks.
- *Aphasia:* A communication disorder that can affect a person's ability to use and understand spoken or written words. It results from damage to the side of the brain dominant for language. For most people, this is the left side. Aphasia usually occurs suddenly and often results from a stroke or head injury, but it can also develop slowly because of a brain tumor, an infection, or dementia.

- *Dysarthria:* Impairment in the ability to articulate words as the result of damage to the central or peripheral nervous system that affects the speech mechanism.

Aphasia

The most common language disorder after a stroke is aphasia. In varying degrees, it affects a person's ability to communicate in one or more ways, including speaking, understanding, reading, writing, or gesturing. Depending on the type and severity of the aphasia, there may be little or no speech, speech that is fragmented or broken, or speech that is fluent but empty in content. When the event affects the dominant half of the brain, some disruption will occur in the "word factories," which are the Broca's and Wernicke's areas in the cerebral cortex. The National Aphasia Association categorizes the two major types of aphasia as fluent and nonfluent. Following is a description of several types of aphasia that the nurse may encounter:

- *Fluent aphasia* is the result of a lesion in the part of the brain adjacent to the primary auditory cortex (Wernicke's area). This type is also known as sensory, posterior, or Wernicke's aphasia. The person speaks easily with many long runs of words, but the content does not make sense. They have problems finding the correct word and often substitute an incorrect word. The speech sounds like what is sometimes referred to as "jabberwocky," with unrelated words strung together or syllables repeated. The person may be unaware of their speech difficulties and cannot understand why others do not understand them. In some cases there is also difficulty understanding spoken language.
- *Nonfluent aphasia* typically involves damage to the Broca's area. This type is also called motor, anterior, or Broca's aphasia. Persons with nonfluent aphasia usually understand others but speak very slowly and use minimal numbers of words. They often struggle to articulate a word and seem to have lost the ability to voluntarily control the movements of speech. Difficulties are experienced in communicating orally and in writing.
- *Verbal apraxia or apraxia of speech* is a motor speech disorder that affects the ability to plan and sequence voluntary muscle movements. The muscles of speech are not paralyzed; instead there is a disruption in the brain's transmission of signals to the muscles. When thinking about what to say, the person may be unable to speak at all or may struggle to say words. In contrast, the person may be able to say many words or sentences correctly when not thinking about the words. Apraxia frequently occurs with aphasia.

- *Anomic aphasia* is associated with lesions of the dominant temporoparietal regions of the brain, although no single location has been identified. Persons with anomic aphasia understand and speak readily but may have severe word-finding difficulty. They may be unable to remember crucial content words. This is a frequent form of aphasia characterized by the inability to name objects. The individual struggles to come forth with the correct noun and often becomes frustrated at his or her inability to do so.
- *Global aphasia* is the result of large left hemisphere lesions and affects most of the language areas of the brain. Persons with global aphasia cannot understand words or speak intelligibly. They may use meaningless syllables repetitiously.

A speech language pathologist (SLP) should be consulted for each type of aphasia to develop appropriate rehabilitative plans as soon as the individual is physiologically stabilized. SLPs bring expertise in all types of communication disorders and are an essential member of the interdisciplinary team. The SLP can identify the areas of language that remain relatively unimpaired and can capitalize on the potential strengths. Much can be done in aggressive speech-retraining programs to regain intelligible conversational ability. For those who do not regain meaningful speech, assistive and augmentative communication devices can be helpful. Happ and Paull (2008) note the importance of consulting with the SLP in acute and critical care settings, as well as in rehabilitation and long-term care, and describe a program to improve communication with patients in the intensive care unit who are unable to speak (the Study of Patient-Nurse Effectiveness with Assisted Communication Strategies [SPEACS]).

Dysarthria

Dysarthria is a speech disorder caused by a weakness or incoordination of the speech muscles. It occurs as a result of central or peripheral neuromuscular disorders that interfere with the clarity of speech and pronunciation. Dysarthria is second in incidence only to aphasia as a communication disorder of older adults and may be the result of stroke, head injury, PD, multiple sclerosis, and other neurological conditions. Dysarthria is characterized by weakness, slow movement, and a lack of coordination of the muscles associated with speech. Speech may be slow, jerky, slurred, quiet, lacking in expression, and difficult to understand. It may involve several mechanisms of speech, such as respiration, phonation, resonance, articulation, and prosody (the meter, or rhythm of speech). A weakness or lack of coordination in any one of the systems can result in dysarthria. If the respiratory system is weak, then speech may be too quiet and be produced one word at a time. If the laryngeal system is weak, speech may be breathy, quiet, and slow. If the articulatory system is affected, speech may sound slurred and be slow and labored.

Treatment of dysarthria depends on the cause, type, and severity of the symptoms. An SLP works with the individual to improve communication abilities. Therapy for dysarthria focuses on maximizing the function of all systems. In progressive neurological disease it is important to begin treatment early and continue throughout the course of the disease, with the goal of maintaining speech as long as possible.

Alternative and Augmentative Speech Aids

Alternative or augmentative systems are frequently used, and communication tools exist for every imaginable type of language disability. These can be low tech or high tech. An example of a low-tech system would be an alphabet or picture board that the individual uses to point to letters to spell out messages or point to pictures of common objects and situations. High-tech systems include electronic boards and computers. Studies have shown that computer-assisted therapy can help people with aphasia improve speech. An example is speech-therapy software that displays a word or picture, speaks the word (using prerecorded human speech), records the user speaking it, and plays back the user's speech. Murphy and colleagues (2005) report on research with frail elders experiencing communication difficulties using a "talking mat" to enhance communication and sharing of ideas and feelings. The "talking mat" is a visual framework using picture symbols to aid in expression of feelings about activities, the environment, people in their lives, and their own personal views and interests.

For individuals with hemiplegic or paraplegic conditions, electronic devices and computers can be voice-activated or have specially designed switches that can be activated by just one finger or by slight contact with the ear, nose, or chin.

Implications for Gerontological Nursing and Healthy Aging

Communication with the older adult experiencing aphasia and dysarthria can be frustrating for affected persons and all others involved in their lives as they struggle to understand each other. It is important to remember that in most cases of aphasia, the person retains normal intellectual ability. Therefore communication must always occur at an adult level but with special modifications. Sensitivity and patience are essential to promote effective communication.

The gerontological nurse needs to be familiar with techniques that facilitate communication with persons with communication difficulties, as well as strategies that can be taught to the person to improve communication (Boxes 20-5 and 20-6). This includes working closely with the speech and language pathologist.

The nurse may encounter persons with communication difficulties across the continuum of care and illness. It is most helpful if staff caring for the person remain consistent so that they can come to know and understand the needs of the person and how these needs are communicated. It is exhausting for the person to have to continually try to communicate needs and desires to an array of different people.

In addition to being knowledgeable about appropriate communication techniques, it is important for the nurse to be aware of equipment and resources available to the person with aphasia or dysarthria so that hope can be offered. Teaching families and significant others effective communication strategies is an important nursing role. Plans of care should include individualized communication strategies so that caregiving staff, health care providers, families, and significant others know the most effective way to enhance communication with persons with neurological disorders.

BOX 20-5   Tips for the Person with Dysarthria

Explain to people that you have difficulty with your speech.

Try to limit conversations when you feel tired.

Speak slowly and loudly and in a quiet place.

Pace out one word at a time while speaking.

Take a deep breath before speaking so that there is enough breath for speech.

Speak out as soon as you breathe out to make full use of the breaths.

Open the mouth more when speaking; exaggerate tongue movements.

Make sure you are sitting or standing in an upright posture. This will improve your breathing and speech.

If you become frustrated, try to use other methods, such as pointing, gesturing, or writing, or take a rest and try again later.

Practice facial exercises (blowing kisses, frowning, smiling), and massage your facial muscles.

Adapted from information about coping with dysarthria from the American Speech-Language-Hearing Association and the Royal College of Speech and Language Therapists. Available at www.asha.org and www.rcslt.org.

BOX 20-6   Tips for Communicating with Individuals Experiencing Dysarthria

Pay attention to the speaker; watch the speaker as he or she talks.

Allow more time for conversation, and conduct conversations in a quiet place.

Be honest, and let the speaker know when you have difficulty understanding.

If speech is very difficult to understand, repeat back what the person has said to make sure you understand.

Repeat the part of the message you did not understand so that the speaker does not have to repeat the entire message.

Remember that dysarthria does not affect a person's intelligence.

Check with the person for ways in which you can help, such as guessing or finishing sentences or writing.

Adapted from information about coping with dysarthria from the American Speech-Language-Hearing Association and the Royal College of Speech and Language Therapists. Available at www.asha.org and www.rcslt.org.

Application of Maslow's Hierarchy

When working with a person with neurological disorders and their sequelae, the nurse initially works at the most basic level of needs: bowel and bladder care; nutrition; ensuring oxygenation; ambulation; and communication. Once strategies have been developed to meet these needs, there is no reason why persons cannot be encouraged to move toward actualization of their new selves (see Chapters 1 and 25).

KEY CONCEPTS

- There are a number of things that an individual can do to reduce his or her risk for cerebrovascular disease.
- Ischemic strokes are the result of temporary loss of oxygen to the brain resulting in damage to the tissue
- Hemorrhagic strokes are less common than ischemic strokes but much more deadly and result from a rupture in a blood vessel in the brain.
- For the best possible outcomes, immediate treatment is required for the person with a stroke; persons need to learn the signs and symptoms and how to activate the emergency response system.
- Correct diagnosis of the type of stroke is necessary before treatment can begin.

- Parkinson's disease is progressive and incurable at this time.
- Parkinson's disease is a disorder that affects voluntary control of movement.
- The signs and symptoms of Parkinson's disease initially may be mistaken for other common disorders seen in older adults.
- Neurological disorders frequently affect one's ability to speak in a way that is understandable to others.
- Working with persons with neurological disorders requires a team approach that includes professionals, the patient, and significant others.

ACTIVITIES AND DISCUSSION QUESTIONS

1. What would you say to a person who tells you, "I thought I had a 'mini-stroke' the other day, but it did not last long and is not a problem today"?
2. You are teaching a class in the community on the signs of a stroke and what to do in response to them. What is the most important message you want to give?
3. Consider the things you can do in your life to reduce your risk for a stroke. Write them out on a piece of paper and then share them with a friend or family member. When you do so, discuss which strategies you can commit to doing to reduce your risk (e.g., stop smoking, eat more vegetables, etc.).
4. How do the symptoms of Parkinson's disease affect functional status?
5. Suggest strategies to optimize communication with persons who have communication difficulties as a result of a neurological problem.

REFERENCES

Boss B: Disorders of the central and peripheral nervous system and the neuromuscular junction. In McCance SE, Huether SE, Brashers VL, et al, editors: *Pathophysiology: the biological basis for disease in adults and children,* ed 6, Maryland Heights, MO, 2010a, Mosby.

Boss B: Alterations in cognitive systems, cerebral hemodynamics and motor function. In McCance SE, Huether SE, Brashers VL, et al, editors: *Pathophysiology: the biological basis for disease in adults and children,* ed 6, Maryland Heights, MO, 2010b, Mosby.

Centers for Disease Control and Prevention [CDC]: *Stroke fact sheet* (2011). Available at http://www.cdc.gov/dhdsp/data_statistics/fact_sheets/fs_stroke.htm.

Centers for Disease Control and Prevention [CDC]: *American Indian and Native Alaskan heart disease and stroke fact sheet* (2012). Available at http://www.cdc.gov/dhdsp/data_statistics/fact_sheets/fs_aian.htm.

Douglas V: Neurological disorders. In Tierney LM, Saint S, Whooley MA: *Current essentials of medicine,* ed 4, New York, 2011, McGraw-Hill.

Goldstein J: *Transient ischemic attack* (2011). Available at http://emedicine.medscape.com/article/1910519-overview.

Graykowski JJ: Cerebrovascular events. In Buttaro R, Trybulski J, Bailey JP, et al., editors: *Primary care: a collaborative practice,* ed 3, St. Louis, 2008, Mosby, pp. 1031–1036.

Happ M, Paull B: Silence is not golden, *Geriatr Nurs* 29(3): 166–167, 2008.

Jordan BL: Parkinson's disease. In Buttaro TM, Trybulski J, Bailey PB, et al, editors: *Primary care: a collaborative approach,* ed 3, St. Louis, 2008, Mosby, pp. 1072–1076.

Llinas R: Stroke. In Durso SC: *Oxford handbook of geriatric medicine,* New York, 2010, Oxford Press, pp. 165–194.

Murphy J, Tester S, Hubbard G, et al: Enabling frail older people with communication difficulties to express views: the use of talking mats as an intervention tool, *Health Soc Care Community* 13(2):95–107, 2005.

National Heart, Lung and Blood Institute [NHLBI]: *The seventh report of the Joint National Committee on Prevention, Detection, Evaluation, and Treatment of High Blood Pressure (JNC 7)* (2003). Available at http://www.nhlbi.nih.gov/guidelines/hypertension/index.htm.

National Institute of Neurological Disorders and Stroke [NINDS]: *Parkinson's disease research web overview* (2012a). Available at http://www.ninds.nih.gov/research/parkinsonsweb/index.htm.

National Institute of Neurological Disorders and Stroke [NINDS]: *NINDS deep brain stimulation for Parkinson's disease information page* (2012b). Available at http://www.ninds.nih.gov/disorders/deep_brain_stimulation/deep_brain_stimulation.htm.

Porter RS, Kaplan JL, editors: *The Merck manual online* (2010-2011). Available at http://www.merckmanuals.com/professional/index.html.

Shapira SK: *Glucocerebrosidase gene mutations and Parkinson's disease objectives* (2010). Available at http://www.cdc.gov/genomics/hugenet/CaseStudy/PARKINSON/PARKview.htm.

Tanner CM, Ross GW, Jewell SA, et al: Occupation and risk of parkinsonism: a multicenter case-control study. *Arch Neurol* 66:1106–13, 2009.

U.S. Department of Health and Human Services [USDHHS], Office of Disease Prevention and Health Promotion: *Healthy people 2020* (2012). Available at http://www.healthypeople.gov/2020.

Whitney CM: Managing the square: how older adults with Parkinson's disease sustain quality in their lives, *J Gerontol Nurs* 30(1): 28–35, 2004.

CHAPTER 21

Cognitive Impairment

Theris A. Touhy

Ⓔvolve evolve.elsevier.com/Ebersole/gerontological

LEARNING OBJECTIVES

Upon completion of this chapter, the reader will be able to:

- Differentiate between dementia, delirium, and depression.
- Discuss the different types of dementia and appropriate diagnosis.
- Describe nursing models of care for persons with dementia.
- Discuss common concerns in care of persons with dementia and nursing responses.
- Develop a nursing care plan for an individual with delirium.
- Develop a nursing care plan for an individual with dementia.

GLOSSARY

Excess disability A reversible deficit that is more disabling than the primary disability. Examples would be a patient with dementia who is kept in a wheelchair and therefore loses the ability to walk or a patient with a stroke who experiences a contracture or pressure ulcer on the affected side as a result of poor positioning or pressure relief.

Milieu The environment or setting.

THE LIVED EXPERIENCE

"The Alzheimer's patient asks nothing more than a hand to hold, a heart to care, and a mind to think for them when they cannot; someone to protect them as they travel through the dangerous twists and turns of the labyrinth. These thoughts must be put on paper now. Tomorrow they may be gone, as fleeting as the bloom of night jasmine beside my front door."

Diana Friel McGowin, who was diagnosed with Alzheimer's disease when she was 45 years old
(McGowin, 1993, p. viii)

This chapter focuses on cognitive impairment and the diseases that affect cognition. Included in the chapter is a discussion of delirium, Alzheimer's disease (AD), and other dementias. The chapter also presents nursing interventions for people experiencing delirium and dementia as well as caregiving for persons with dementia. Cognitive function in aging is discussed in Chapter 6 and cognitive screening instruments in Chapter 7.

Cognitive Impairment

Cognitive impairment (CI) is a term that describes a range of disturbances in cognitive functioning, including disturbances in memory, orientation, attention, and concentration. Other disturbances of cognition may affect intelligence, judgment, learning ability, perception, problem solving, psychomotor ability, reaction time, and social intactness. Dementia, delirium, and depression have been called the *three Ds of cognitive impairment* because they occur frequently in older adults. These important geriatric syndromes are not a normal consequence of aging, although incidence increases with age.

The Three D's

Because cognitive and behavioral changes characterize all three D's, it can be difficult to diagnose delirium, delirium superimposed on dementia (DSD), or depression. Inability to concentrate, with resulting memory impairment and other cognitive dysfunction, can occur in late-life depression. The term *pseudodementia* has been used to describe the cognitive impairment that may accompany depression in older adults (see Chapter 22).

Delirium is characterized by an acute or subacute onset, with symptoms developing over a short period of time (usually hours to days). Symptoms tend to fluctuate over the course of the day, often worsening at night. Symptoms include disturbances in consciousness and attention and changes in cognition (memory deficits, perceptual disturbances). Perceptual disturbances are often accompanied by delusional (paranoid) thoughts and behavior. In contrast, dementia typically has a gradual onset and a slow, steady pattern of decline without alterations in consciousness (Voyer et al., 2010).

Dementia, delirium, and depression represent serious pathology and require urgent assessment and intervention (Fletcher, 2012). However, changes in cognitive function in older adults are often seen as "normal" and not investigated. Any change in mental status in an older person requires appropriate assessment. Knowledge about cognitive function in aging and appropriate assessment and evaluation are keys to differentiating these three syndromes. Table 21-1 presents the clinical features and the differences in cognitive and behavioral characteristics in delirium, dementia, and depression.

TABLE 21-1	Differentiating Delirium, Depression, and Dementia		
Characteristic	**Delirium**	**Depression**	**Dementia**
Onset	Sudden, abrupt	Recent, may relate to life change	Insidious, slow, over years and often unrecognized until deficits are obvious
Course over 24 hr	Fluctuating, often worse at night	Fairly stable, may be worse in the morning	Fairly stable, may see changes with stress
Consciousness	Reduced	Clear	Clear
Alertness	Increased, decreased, or variable	Normal	Generally normal
Psychomotor activity	Increased, decreased, or mixed Sometimes increased, other times decreased	Variable, agitation or retardation	Normal, may have apraxia or agnosia
Duration	Hours to weeks	Variable and may be chronic	Years
Attention	Disordered, fluctuates	Little impairment	Generally normal but may have trouble focusing
Orientation	Usually impaired, fluctuates	Usually normal, may answer "I don't know" to questions or may not try to answer	Often impaired, may make up answers or answer close to the right thing or may confabulate but tries to answer
Speech	Often incoherent, slow or rapid, may call out repeatedly or repeat the same phrase	May be slow	Difficulty finding word, perseveration
Affect	Variable but may look disturbed, frightened	Flat	Slowed response, may be labile

Modified from Sendelbach S, Guthrie PF, Schoenfelder DP: Acute confusion/delirium, *J Gerontol Nurs* 35 (11):11-18, 2009.

Cognitive Assessment

An older person with a change in cognitive function needs a thorough assessment to identify the presence of specific pathological conditions as well as to rule out potentially reversible causes of cognitive impairment. Screening is used to determine if cognitive impairment exists, but basic screening methods do not diagnose specific pathological conditions. If impairment is identified through screening, the person should be referred for a more comprehensive evaluation to confirm a diagnosis of dementia, delirium, or depression, or some other health problem (Braes et al., 2008).

A comprehensive evaluation includes a complete assessment, including laboratory workup, to rule out any medical causes of cognitive impairment. Formal cognitive testing, neuropsychological examination, screening for depression and delirium, interview (family and patient), observation, and functional assessment are additional components of a comprehensive assessment. Computerized tomography (CT), magnetic resonance imaging (MRI), and an electroencephalogram (EEG) may be indicated in the diagnostic process. Several evidence-based guidelines are available for assessment of changes in mental status and diagnosis of dementia (www.guidelines.gov), and Fletcher (2012) presents a "Nursing Standard of Practice Protocol: Recognition and Management of Dementia."

Considerations in Cognitive Assessment

Most older adults worry about developing memory problems or getting AD. Cognitive testing or poor performance on tests of memory is often the cause of great anxiety. Too often, assessments are done when a person is not wearing hearing aids or glasses, or he or she is rushed through a series of questions in a noisy, distracting environment without any preparation or explanation.

It is important to attend to these concerns by establishing rapport and developing a therapeutic relationship, ensuring comfort, accommodating for physical impairments such as hearing and vision loss, creating an environment free of distractions, and putting the person in the best environment to ensure that performance is truly reflective of ability. The challenge is to stress the importance of the assessment without creating undue anxiety. Timing is also important, and cognitive assessments should not be conducted immediately upon awakening from sleep, or immediately before and after meals or medical diagnostic and therapeutic procedures (Braes et al., 2008). It is wise to remember that what seems to be a routine procedure to health professionals can be very intimidating for an older person, especially one who is ill or frail.

Delirium

Etiology

The development of delirium is a result of complex interactions among multiple causes. Delirium results from the interaction of predisposing factors (e.g., vulnerability on the part of the individual due to predisposing conditions, such as cognitive impairment, severe illness, and sensory impairment) and precipitating factors/insults (e.g., medications, procedures, restraints, iatrogenic events). Although a single factor, such as an infection, can trigger an episode of delirium, several coexisting factors are also likely to be present. A highly vulnerable older individual requires a lesser amount of precipitating factors to develop delirium (Inouye et al., 1999; Voyer et al., 2010).

The exact pathophysiological mechanisms involved in the development and progression of delirium remain uncertain, and further research is needed to understand its neuropathogenesis. Delirium is thought to be related to disturbances in the neurotransmitters in the brain that modulate the control of cognitive function, behavior, and mood. The causes of delirium are potentially reversible; therefore accurate assessment and diagnosis are critical. Delirium is given many labels: acute confusional state, acute brain syndrome, confusion, reversible dementia, metabolic encephalopathy, and toxic psychosis. The correct terminology is *delirium*.

Incidence and Prevalence

Delirium is a prevalent and serious disorder that occurs in elders across the continuum of care. Estimates are that delirium may affect up to 42% of hospitalized older adults and as many as 87% of older adults in intensive care units (ICUs) (Marcantonio et al., 2010; Sweeny et al., 2008). Older people who have undergone surgery and those with dementia are particularly vulnerable to delirium. The prevalence of delirium is as high as 65% after orthopedic surgery, particularly hip fracture repair (Rigney, 2006). Among older people experiencing cardiac surgery, as many as 20% to 25% experience delirium, affecting even those without any documented preoperative cognitive impairments (Clarke et al., 2010). A 16% delirium rate in patients newly admitted to subacute care has been reported (Marcantonio et al., 2010).

The incidence of DSD ranges from 22% to 89% (Tullmann et al., 2008). Older patients with dementia are three to five times more likely to develop delirium, and it is less likely to be recognized and treated than is delirium without dementia. DSD is associated with high mortality among hospitalized older people (Bellelli et al., 2008). Changes in the mental status of older people with dementia are often attributed to underlying dementia, or "sundowning," and not investigated. This is particularly significant because about 25% of all older hospitalized patients may have AD or another dementia (Voelker, 2008). Delirium can accelerate the trajectory of cognitive decline in individuals with AD. Despite its prevalence, DSD has not been well investigated, and there are only a few relevant studies in either the hospital or community setting.

Recognition of Delirium

Delirium is a medical emergency and one of the most significant geriatric syndromes (Waszynski & Petrovic, 2008). However, it is often not recognized by physicians or nurses. Studies indicate that delirium is unrecognized in 66% to 84% of patients (Pisani et al., 2006; Balas et al., 2007). A comprehensive review of the literature suggested that "nurses are missing key symptoms of delirium and appear to be doing superficial mental status assessments" (Steis & Fick, 2008, p. 47). Cognitive changes in older people are often labeled confusion by nurses and physicians, are frequently accepted as part of normal aging, and are rarely questioned. Confusion in a child or younger adult would be recognized as a medical emergency, but confusion in older adults may be accepted as a natural occurrence, "part of the older person's personality" (Dahlke & Phinney, 2008, p. 46).

Factors contributing to the lack of recognition of delirium among health care professionals include inadequate education about delirium, a lack of formal assessment methods, a view that delirium is not as essential to the patient's well-being in light of more serious medical problems, and ageist attitudes (Kuehn, 2010a; Waszynski & Petrovic, 2008). Failure to recognize delirium, identify the underlying causes, and implement timely interventions contributes to the negative sequelae associated with the condition (Tullmann et al., 2008; Kuehn, 2010a). Clearly, education and attitudes about older people must be addressed if we want to improve care outcomes for the growing number of older adults who will need care.

Risk Factors for Delirium

The risk of delirium increases with the number of risk factors present. Identification of high-risk patients, risk factors, prompt and appropriate assessment, and continued surveillance are the cornerstones of delirium prevention. More than 35 potential risk factors have been identified for delirium. Among the most predictive are immobility, functional deficits, use of restraints or catheters, medications, acute illness, infections, alcohol or drug abuse, sensory impairments, malnutrition, dehydration, respiratory

insufficiency, surgery, and cognitive impairment. Unrelieved or inadequately treated pain significantly increases the risk of delirium (Irving & Foreman, 2006). Medications account for 22% to 39% of all delirium, and all medications, particularly those with anticholinergic effects and any new medications, should be considered suspect. Invasive equipment, such as nasogastric tubes, intravenous (IV) lines, catheters, and restraints, also contribute to delirium by interfering with normal feedback mechanisms of the body (Box 21-1).

Clinical Subtypes of Delirium

Delirium is categorized according to the level of alertness and psychomotor activity. The clinical subtypes are hyperactive, hypoactive, and mixed. Box 21-2 presents the characteristics of each of these clinical subtypes. In non-ICU settings, approximately 30% of delirium is hyperactive, 24% hypoactive, and 46% is mixed. Because of the increased severity of illness and the use of psychoactive medications, hypoactive delirium may be more prevalent in the ICU. Although the negative consequences of hyperactive delirium are serious, the hypoactive subtype may be missed more often and is associated with a worse prognosis because of the development of complications such as aspiration, pulmonary embolism, pressure ulcers, and pneumonia. Increased hospital stays, longer duration of delirium, and higher mortality have been associated with hypoactive delirium.

Consequences of Delirium

Delirium has serious consequences and is a "high priority nursing challenge for all nurses who care for older adults" (Tullmann et al., 2008, p. 113). Delirium results in significant distress for the patient, his or her family and significant others, and nurses. Delirium is associated with increased length of hospital stay and hospital readmissions, increased services after discharge, and increased morbidity, mortality, and institutionalization, independent of age, coexisting illnesses, or illness severity (Witlox et al., 2010).

Recent research indicates that older adults are vulnerable to the development of accelerated cognitive decline irrespective of the severity of their illness or the length of their hospital stay, making accurate cognitive assessment and prevention and treatment of delirium a priority (Wilson et al., 2012). Delirium is also associated with lasting cognitive impairment and psychiatric problems that may persist after discharge and interfere with the ability to manage chronic conditions (Cole & McCusker, 2009; Hain et al., 2012; Lindquist et al., 2011). Screening all older adults before they leave the

BOX **21-1**   **Precipitating Factors for Delirium**

1. Total number of medications >6
2. Pharmacological agents, especially narcotics, anticon-vulsants, psychotropics, anticholinergics, hypnotics, anxiolytics
3. Hypoxemia and metabolic disturbances
4. Infection, especially respiratory and urinary tract
5. Dehydration, with and without electrolyte disturbances
6. Electrolyte imbalances
7. Volume overload
8. Intravenous catheter complications
9. Prolonged bleeding
10. Transfusion reaction
11. New pressure ulcer
12. Prolonged emergency room stay (>12 hours)
13. Emergency admission or admission from a long-term care facility
14. Prolonged emergency room stay (>12 hours)
15. Withdrawal syndromes (alcohol and sedative-hypnotic agents)
16. Major medical and surgical treatments (especially hip fracture and repair)
17. Nutritional deficiencies
18. Dementia
19. Circulatory disturbances (congestive heart failure [CHF], myocardial infarction [MI], cerebrovascular accident [CVA])
20. Anemia
21. Pain (either unrelieved or inadequately treated)
22. Sensory deficits
23. Social isolation, lack of family contact
24. Retention of urine and feces
25. Use of invasive equipment
26. Use of restraint or immobilizing device
27. Prolonged immobility
28. Functional deficits
29. Depression
30. Sensory overstimulation or understimulation
31. Abrupt loss of significant person
32. Multiple losses in short span of time
33. Move to radically different environment (hospitalization, nursing home)

BOX **21-2**   **Clinical Subtypes of Delirium**

Hypoactive Delirium
Quiet or pleasantly confused
Reduced activity
Lack of facial expression
Passive demeanor
Lethargy
Inactivity
Withdrawn and sluggish state
Limited, slow, and wavering vocalizations

Hyperactive Delirium
Excessive alertness
Easy distractibility

Increased psychomotor activity
Hallucinations, delusions
Agitation and aggressive actions
Fast or loud speech
Wandering, nonpurposeful repetitive movement
Verbal behaviors (yelling, calling out)
Removing tubes
Attempting to get out of bed

Mixed
Unpredictable fluctuations between hypoactivity and hyperactivity

hospital may help to identify those in need of specific transitional care (see Chapter 3) with more frequent follow-up after hospitalization (Lindquist et al., 2011). Further research is needed to determine the reasons for the long-term poor outcomes, whether characteristics of the delirium itself (subtype or duration) influence prognosis, and how the long-term effects might be decreased.

Implications for Gerontological Nursing and Healthy Aging

Assessment

Several instruments can be used to assess the presence and severity of delirium. To detect changes, it is very important to determine the person's usual mental status. If the person cannot tell you this, family members or other caregivers who are with the patient can be asked to provide this information. If the patient is alone, the responsible party or the institution transferring the patient can provide this information by phone. Do not assume the person's current mental status represents his or her usual state, and do not attribute altered mental status to age alone or assume that dementia is present. All older patients, regardless of their current cognitive function, should have a formal assessment to identify possible delirium when admitted to the hospital (see the Evidence-Based Practice box).

🔍 EVIDENCE-BASED PRACTICE

Delirium and Dementia
- Delerium:
  http://consultgerirn.org/topics/delirium/want_to_know_more
- Dementia series:
  http://consultgerirn.org/resources/#issues_on_dementia

Other Resources
- Braes T, Millisen K, Foreman M, et al: Nursing standard of practice protocol: assessing cognitive functioning. In Boltz M, Capezuti E, Fulmer T, et al, editors: *Evidence-based geriatric nursing protocols for best practice*, ed 4, New York, 2012, Springer.
- Hospital Elder Life Program (HELP):
  http://www.hospitalelderlifeprogram.org/public/public-main.php.

The Mini-Mental State Examination, 2nd Edition (MMSE-2) is considered a general test of cognitive status that helps identify mental status impairment. Although the MMSE-2 alone is not adequate for diagnosing delirium, it represents a brief, standardized method to assess mental status and can provide a baseline from which to track changes (see Chapter 7). Several delirium-specific assessment instruments are available, such as the Confusion Assessment Method (CAM) (Inouye et al., 1990), NEECHAM Confusion Scale (Neelon et al., 1996), and the CAM-ICU (Ely et al., 2001), an instrument specifically designed to assess delirium in an intensive care population.

Assessment using the MMSE-2, CAM, and NEECHAM should be conducted on admission to the hospital, throughout the hospitalization for all patients identified at risk for delirium, and for all patients who exhibit signs and symptoms of delirium or develop additional risk factors (Steis & Fick, 2008). Results of a study (Waszynski &

Petrovic, 2008) suggested that the CAM was useful in identifying delirium in hospitalized adults, and nurses found it very helpful in identifying changes in cognitive functioning. As a result of these findings, the CAM was made a customary part of the daily flow sheet.

When a patient is identified as having delirium, reassessment should be conducted every shift. Documenting specific objective indicators of alterations in mental status rather than using the global, nonspecific term *confusion* will lead to more appropriate prevention, detection, and management of delirium and its negative consequences. Findings from assessment using a validated instrument are combined with nursing observation, chart review, and physiological findings. Delirium often has a fluctuating course and can be difficult to recognize, so assessment must be ongoing and include multiple data sources.

Interventions

Nonpharmacological

Intervention begins with prevention. An awareness and identification of the risk factors for delirium and a formal assessment of mental status are the first-line interventions for prevention. Because the etiology of delirium is multifactorial, "for an intervention strategy to be effective, it should target the multifactorial origins of delirium with multicomponent interventions that address more than one risk factor" (Rosenbloom-Brunton et al., 2010, p. 23). Multidisciplinary approaches to prevention of delirium seem to show the most promising results, but continued research is needed to evaluate what type of approach has the most beneficial effect in specific clinical settings.

A well-researched multidisciplinary program of delirium prevention in the acute care setting, the Hospital Elder Life Program (HELP) (Inouye et al., 1999; Bradley et al., 2005; Rubin et al., 2006), focuses on managing six risk factors for delirium: cognitive impairment, sleep deprivation, immobility, visual impairments, hearing impairments, and dehydration. The program is used in more than 60 hospitals in the United States and internationally. Patient outcomes with the use of this model include a 40% reduction in the incidence of delirium, a 67% reduction in rates of functional decline, and significant cost savings in both hospitals and long-term care facilities. Most of the interventions can be considered quite simple and part of good nursing care.

Examples of interventions in the HELP program include the following: offering herbal tea or warm milk instead of sleeping medications, keeping the ward quiet at night by using vibrating beepers instead of paging systems, using silent pill crushers, removing catheters and other devices that hamper movement as soon as possible, encouraging mobilization, assessing and managing pain, and correcting hearing and vision deficits. Fall risk reduction interventions, such as bed and chair alarms, low beds, reclining chairs, volunteers to sit with restless patients, and keeping routines as normal as possible with consistent caregivers, are other examples of interventions.

The Family-HELP program, an adaptation and extension of the original HELP program, trains family caregivers in selected protocols (e.g., orientation, therapeutic activities, vision and hearing). Initial research demonstrates that active engagement of family caregivers in preventive interventions for delirium is feasible and supports a culture of family-oriented care (Rosenbloom-Brunton et al., 2010). Further information on HELP can be found at http://www.hospitalelderlifeprogram.org/public/public-main.php. Box 21-3 presents suggested interventions for delirium.

A commonly used intervention for patients with delirium in acute care is the use of "sitters" or "constant observers" (COs). Costs associated with this practice can be very high, and data indicate that the use of COs does not consistently decrease the incidence of unsafe patient behavior in the patient with delirium. Nor do they assist in identifying causes of delirium or identifying appropriate interventions (Sweeny et al., 2008). More effective and less costly interventions for patients with delirium include programs of fall risk–reduction strategies, assessment of delirium using the CAM, and protocols for intervention.

Pharmacological

Pharmacological interventions to treat the symptoms of delirium may be necessary if patients are in danger of harming themselves or others, or if nonpharmacological interventions are not effective. However, pharmacological interventions should not replace thoughtful and careful evaluation and management of the underlying causes of delirium. Pharmacological treatment should be one approach in a multicomponent program of prevention and treatment. Research on the pharmacological management of delirium is limited, but it has been suggested that "with increased understanding of the neuropathogenesis of delirium, drug therapy could become primary to the treatment of delirium" (Irving & Foreman, 2006, p. 122). A few studies have suggested that use of dexmedetomidine

---

BOX 21-3   Suggested Interventions to Prevent Delirium

- Know baseline mental status, functional abilities, living conditions, medications taken, alcohol use.
- Assess mental status using MMSE-2, CAM, NEECHAM, and document.
- Correct underlying physiological alterations.
- Compensate for sensory deficits (hearing aids, glasses, dentures).
- Encourage fluid intake (make sure fluids are accessible).
- Avoid long periods of giving nothing orally.
- Explain all actions with clear and consistent communication.
- Avoid multiple medications, and avoid problematic medications.
- Be vigilant for drug reactions or interactions; consider onset of new symptoms as an adverse reaction to medications.
- Avoid use of sleeping medications—use music, warm milk, noncaffeinated herbal tea to alleviate discomfort.
- Attempt to find out why behavior is occurring rather than simply medicating for it (e.g., need to toilet, pain, fear, hunger, thirst).
- Avoid excessive bed rest; institute early mobilization.
- Encourage participation in care for activities of daily living (ADLs).

- Minimize the use of catheters, restraints, or immobilizing devices.
- Use least restrictive devices (mitts instead of wrist restraints, reclining geri-chairs with tray instead of vest restraints).
- Hide tubes (stockinette over intravenous [IV] line), or use intermittent fluid administration.
- Activate bed and chair alarms.
- Place the patient near the nursing station for close observation.
- Assess fall risk and institute appropriate safety measures.
- Assess and treat pain.
- Pay attention to environmental noise.
- Normalize the environment (provide familiar items, routines, clocks, calendars).
- Minimize the number of room changes and interfacility transfers.
- Do not place a delirious patient in the room with another delirious patient.
- Have family, volunteer, or paid caregiver stay with the patient.

as a sedative or analgesic may reduce the incidence or duration of delirium (Kuehn, 2010b).

Ozbolt and colleagues (2008) conducted a literature review of the use of antipsychotics for treatment of delirious elders and concluded that the atypical antipsychotics demonstrate similar rates of efficacy to haloperidol for the treatment of delirium and have a lower rate of extrapyramidal side effects. Further research is needed since no double-blind placebo trials exist. Short-acting benzodiazepines are often used to control agitation but may worsen mental status. Psychoactive medications, if used, should be given at the lowest effective dose, monitored closely, and reduced or eliminated as soon as possible so that recovery can be assessed.

Caring for patients with delirium can be a challenging experience. Patients with delirium can be difficult to communicate with, and disturbing behaviors such as pulling out IV lines or attempting to get out of bed disrupt medical treatment and compromise safety. It is important for nurses to realize that behavior is an attempt to communicate something and express needs. The patient with delirium feels frightened and out of control. The calmer and more reassuring the nurse is, the safer the patient will feel. Box 21-4 presents some communication strategies that are helpful in caring for people experiencing delirium.

Dementia

In contrast to delirium, dementia is an irreversible state that progresses over years and causes memory impairment and loss of other intellectual abilities severe enough to cause interference with daily life. Degenerative dementias include AD, Parkinson's disease dementia (PDD), dementia with Lewy bodies (DLB), and frontotemporal lobe dementias (FTDs). AD accounts for 50% to 70% of all dementia cases. Vascular cognitive impairment (VCI) encompasses several syndromes: vascular dementia; mixed primary neurodegenerative disease and vascular dementia; and cognitive impairment of vascular origin that does not meet the dementia criteria. Increasing evidence suggests that most dementias have neurodegenerative (most commonly AD) and vascular features, and these seem to act synergistically (Desai et al., 2010).

Other less commonly occurring dementias are Creutzfeldt-Jakob disease (CJD) (subacute spongiform encephalopathy) and human immunodeficiency virus (HIV)–related dementia. Normal-pressure hydrocephalus (NPH) causes a dementia characterized by ataxic gait, incontinence, and memory impairment. This disease is reversible and treated with a shunt that diverts cerebrospinal fluid away from the brain (Table 21-2).

Different types of dementia have different symptom patterns and distinguishing microscopic brain abnormalities. The symptoms of dementia also overlap and can be further complicated by comorbid medical conditions. Accurate diagnosis is important, since treatment and prognosis vary. The rate of diagnosis of dementia is quite low despite advances in technology and knowledge about the different types and causes of dementia. In some studies, as many as 75% of patients with moderate to severe dementia and more than 95% of those with mild impairment escape diagnosis in the primary care setting. Clearly, education of both professionals and the community is needed so that more timely diagnosis and treatment can be initiated (Stefanacci, 2008). The diagnosis of dementia is complex, and it is essential that older people with symptoms of cognitive impairment receive specialized assessment to determine the causes so that treatment can be tailored appropriately.

BOX 21-4   Communicating with a Person Experiencing Delirium

- Know the person's past patterns.
- Look at nonverbal signs, such as tone of voice, facial expressions, gestures.
- Speak slowly.
- Be calm and patient.
- Face the person and keep eye contact—get to the level of the person rather than standing over him or her.
- Explain all actions.
- Smile.
- Use simple, familiar words.
- Allow adequate time for response.
- Repeat if needed.
- Tell the person what you want him or her to do rather than what you don't want him or her to do.
- Give one-step directions; use gestures and demonstration to augment words.
- Reassure of safety.
- Keep caregivers consistent.
- Assume that communication and behavior are meaningful and an attempt to tell us something or express needs.
- Do not assume the person is unable to understand or is demented.

TABLE 21-2	Types of Dementia and Typical Characteristics
Type of Dementia	**Characteristics**
Alzheimer's disease (AD)	Most common type of dementia, accounting for 60%-80% of cases. Hallmark abnormalities are deposits of the protein fragment beta-amyloid (plaques) and twisted strands of the protein tau (tangles). Difficulty remembering names and recent events, difficulty expressing oneself with words, spatial cognition problems, and impaired reasoning and judgment, apathy, depression are often early symptoms. Language disturbances may also be a presenting symptom. Later symptoms include impaired judgment, disorientation, behavior changes, and difficulty speaking, swallowing, and walking.
Vascular dementia, also known as multi-infarct or post-stroke dementia or vascular cognitive impairment (VCI)	Second most common type of dementia. Impairment is caused by decreased blood flow to parts of the brain due to a series of small strokes that block arteries. Symptoms often overlap with AD although memory may not be as seriously affected.
Mixed dementia	Characterized by the hallmark abnormalities of AD and another type of dementia, most commonly vascular dementia but also other types such as dementia with Lewy bodies. Mixed dementia is more common than previously thought. Neurodegenerative changes occur along with vascular changes.
Parkinson's disease dementia (PDD)	Later onset of dementia, at least 1 year after onset of parkinsonian features. Hallmark abnormality is Lewy bodies (abnormal deposits of the protein alpha-synuclein) that forms inside the nerve cells of the brain.
Dementia with Lewy bodies	Pattern of decline similar to AD including problems wih memory and judgment as well as behavior changes. Alertness and severity of cognitive symptoms may fluctuate daily. Visual hallucinations, muscle rigidity, and tremors are common. Exhibit a sensitivity to neuroleptic drugs, so these medications should be avoided.
Creutzfeldt-Jakob disease (CJD) and vCJD (transmissible spongiform encephalopathy)	A rapidly fatal and rare form of dementia characterized by tiny holes that give the brain a "spongy" appearance under microscope. May be hereditary, occur sporadically, or be transmitted from infected individuals. Failing memory, behavioral changes, lack of coordination, visual disturbances. vCJD (bovine spongiform encephalopathy/mad cow disease) occurs in younger patients and may be caused by contaminated feed.
Frontotemporal dementia	Involves damage to brain cells, especially in the front and side regions of the brain. Symptoms include change in personality and behavior and difficulty with language. Pick's disease, characterized by Pick's bodies in the brain, is one form of frontotemporal dementia.
Normal-pressure hydrocephalus	Caused by buildup of fluid in the brain without corresponding increase in cerebrospinal fluid (CSF) pressure. Symptoms include difficulty walking (ataxic gait), memory loss, incontinence. Can sometimes be corrected with surgical installation of a shunt to drain excess fluid.

Data from Alzheimer's Association: 2010 Alzheimer's disease facts and figures, *Alzheimer Dement* 6(2):158-194, 2010.

Incidence and Prevalence

Dementia is one of the most disabling and burdensome of chronic health conditions. The growing worldwide epidemic of dementia has frightening implications for the health of older people and their families as well as the health and societal costs associated with the disease. *Healthy People 2020* has added a new topic on dementia with the goal of reducing the morbidity and costs associated with the condition and of maintaining and enhancing the quality of life for persons with dementia, including AD (see the Healthy People box) (U.S. Department of Health and Human Services, 2012). The cost of care for someone with dementia is three times more than for those who do not have the disease (Alzheimer's Association, 2012).

 HEALTHY PEOPLE 2020

Dementias, Including Alzheimer's Disease

1. Increase the proportion of persons with diagnosed Alzheimer's disease and other dementias, or their caregivers, who are aware of the diagnosis.
2. Reduce the proportion of preventable hospitalizations in persons with diagnosed Alzheimer's disease and other dementias.

From U.S. Department of Health and Human Services, Office of Disease Prevention and Health Promotion: *Healthy people 2020* (2012). Available at http://www.healthypeople.gov/2020.

Alzheimer's Disease

AD, the most common form of dementia, was first described by Dr. Alois Alzheimer in 1906. In the United States, about 5.4 million people 65 years of age and older and 200,000 individuals younger than 65 years of age have AD. Of Americans 65 years of age and over, 1 in 8 has Alzheimer's; nearly half of people 85 years of age and older have the disease (Alzheimer's Association, 2012). If current trends continue, by the year 2050, the prevalence of AD is expected to quadruple unless medical breakthroughs identify ways to prevent or more effectively treat the disease. AD is the sixth leading cause of death and the nation's third most expensive medical condition.

Unless something is done, the care cost of AD and other dementias is projected to be $1.1 trillion by 2050. These costs include a 600% increase in Medicare costs and a 400% increase in Medicaid costs. One factor contributing to the soaring cost projections is that nearly half of the

individuals with AD would be in the later stages of the disease when more expensive around-the-clock care is often necessary (Alzheimer's Association, 2010). Although the ultimate goal is to discover a treatment that can prevent or cure AD, even modest improvements in treatment can have a huge impact.

Types of Alzheimer's Disease

AD is characterized by the development of neuronal intracellular neurofibrillary tangles consisting of the protein tau and extracellular deposits of amyloid-β (Aβ) peptides in fibril structures, the loss of connections between nerve cells in the brain, and the death of these nerve cells. These changes in the brain develop slowly over many years of pathology accumulation. At the same time, some people have the brain changes associated with AD and yet do not show symptoms of dementia.

AD has two types: early-onset dementia (EO-D) and late-onset dementia. EO-D is a rare form, affecting only about 5% of all people who have AD. It develops between 30 and 60 years of age. This form of AD can result from gene mutations on chromosomes 21, 14, and 1, and each of these mutations causes abnormal proteins to be formed. These mutations cause an increased amount of beta-amyloid protein, the major component of AD plaques, to be formed (National Institute on Aging [NIA], 2010).

The autosomal dominant inheritance pattern means that offspring in the same generation have a 50/50 chance of developing EO-D if one of their parents had it. Even if only one of these mutated genes is inherited from a parent, the person will almost always develop EO-D. Predictive genetic testing, with appropriate precounseling and postcounseling, may be offered to at-risk individuals with an apparent autosomal dominant inheritance of AD (Desai et al., 2010).

Most cases of AD are the late-onset form, developing after 60 years of age. The mutations seen in EO-D are not involved in this form of the disease. This disorder does not clearly run in families, and late-onset AD is probably related to variations in one or more genes in combination with lifestyle and environmental factors. The apolipoprotein E (APOE) gene, found on chromosome 19, has been extensively studied as a risk factor, and a particular variant of this gene, the e4 allele, seems to increase a person's risk for developing late-onset AD.

The inheritance pattern of late-onset AD is uncertain. People who inherit one copy of the APOE e4 allele have an increased risk of developing the disease; those who inherit two copies are at even greater risk. However, not all people with AD have the e4 allele, and not all people who have the e4 allele will develop the disease. A blood test is available that can identify which APOE alleles a person has, but screening for APOE e4 in asymptomatic individuals in the general population is not recommended. Using an approach called a genome-wide association study, four to seven other AD risk-factor genes have been identified (Desai et al., 2010; NIA, 2010).

Research

The focus of research on AD is on the interaction between risk-factor genes and lifestyle or environmental factors. Increasing evidence strongly points to the potential risk roles of vascular risk factors (VRFs) and disorders (e.g., midlife obesity, dyslipidemia, hypertension, cigarette smoking, obstructive sleep apnea, diabetes, and cerebrovascular lesions) and the potential protective roles of psychosocial factors (e.g., higher education, regular exercise, healthy diet, intellectually challenging leisure

activity, and active socially integrated lifestyle) in the pathogenesis and clinical manifestations of dementia (especially AD and VCI). Head trauma is also considered a risk factor (Table 21-3) (Ghetu et al., 2010). Addressing modifiable risk factors throughout life may delay or decrease the risks of developing dementias such as AD. "Prevention is the wave of the future in the dementia arena" (Kamat et al., 2010, p. 20).

Diagnosis of Alzheimer's Disease

In 2011, new diagnostic criteria for AD were published by the National Institute on Aging and the Alzheimer's Association (Hyman et al., 2012). The original diagnostic guidelines for AD were developed in 1984 and have not been revised since that time. These original guidelines were the first to address the disease and described only later stages, when symptoms of dementia are already evident.

TABLE **21-3**   **Risk Factors and Protective Factors for Alzheimer's Disease: Potential Mechanisms**

Factor	Risk	Potential Mechanisms
Advanced age	Increased risk	Possible decreased brain reserves
Sex	Females have increased risk	Living longer and loss of neuroprotective effects of estrogen
Family history	Increased risk	APP, presenilin-1, presenilin-2 mutations may result in oversecretion of amyloid-β (Aβ) in familial AD. APOE e4 allele increases risk of sporadic (late-onset) AD
Depression	Increased risk	May decrease brain reserves/transmitters
High-fat and cholesterol diet	Increased risk	Increased neuroinflammation; possible increased substrate for APP
CRP	Increased risk	Increased neuroinflammation
Homocysteine	Increased risk	Increased oxidative stress, free radical toxicity, increased atherosclerotic sequelae
Smoking	Increased risk	Accelerated cerebral atrophy, perfusional decline, and white matter lesions
Diabetes mellitus	Increased risk	Impaired glucose uptake in neuronal cells, decreased blood supply due to small-vessel disease
Hyperlipidemia	Increased risk	Increased Aβ accumulation
Genetic	Increased risk	Mutations of presenilin-1, presenilin-2, APP
Hypertension	Increased risk	Decreased cerebral blood flow/cerebral ischemia, white matter lesions
Head trauma	Increased risk	Not fully understood—possible blood-brain barrier disruption
Obesity	Increased risk	Hyperlipidemia and hypertension and via their mechanisms described earlier
Mediterranean diet	Decreased risk	Decreased neuroinflammation, decreased oxidative stress, decreased Aβ$_{42}$ toxicity
Increased education	Decreased risk	Education may increase neural connections
Increased mental activity	Decreased risk	Cognitive reserve model in which people cope better and can generate more neurons during their lifetime
Increased physical activity	Decreased risk	Increased cerebral blood flow, increased brain-derived neurotrophic factor

From Kamat S, Kamat A, Grossberg G: Dementia risk prediction: are we there yet? *Clin Geriatr Med* 26:113-123, 2010.
AD, Alzheimer's disease; *APP,* amyloid precursor protein; *CRP,* C-reactive protein.

The new guidelines describe three distinct stages of Alzheimer's: preclinical, mild cognitive impairment (MCI), and dementia due to Alzheimer's pathology. The new guidelines also address the use of imaging and biomarkers in blood and spinal fluid that may help determine whether changes in the brain and those in body fluids are due to AD. At this time, biomarkers are increasingly being used in the research setting to detect onset of the disease and to track progression, but cannot yet be used routinely in clinical diagnosis without further testing and validation. The overall goal of the new guidelines is to provide standards for research and practice that advance the field farther in the direction of early detection and treatment.

Preclinical. In this stage, individuals have measurable changes in the brain, cerebrospinal fluid and/or blood markers that indicate the earliest signs of disease, but they have not yet developed symptoms such as memory loss. This preclinical or presymptomatic stage reflects current thinking that Alzheimer's begins creating changes in the brain as many as 20 years before symptoms. With further research on biomarkers, as set forth in the new guidelines, it may be possible to predict who is at risk for the development of MCI and AD, and who would benefit most as interventions are developed (Alzheimer's Association, 2012).

Mild Cognitive Impairment (MCI). The guidelines for MCI are also largely for research, although they clarify existing guidelines for MCI for use in a clinical setting. In MCI, there would be evidence of concern about a change in cognition, in comparison to the person's prior level. The cognitive changes are more than would be expected for the patient's age and educational background. Memory problems are enough to be noticed and measured, but do not compromise a person's function. People with MCI may or may not progress to AD.

Alzheimer's Dementia. These criteria apply to the final stage of the disease, and are most relevant for health care providers and patients. They outline ways clinicians should approach evaluation of the cause and progression of cognitive decline. In addition to memory loss, the guidelines note that declines in other aspects of cognition, such as word-finding, vision/spatial issues, and impaired reasoning or judgment, may be the first symptom to be noticed. At this stage, biomarker test results may be used in some cases to increase or decrease the level of certainty about a diagnosis of AD and to distinguish AD from other dementias.

Cultural Differences

African Americans are about twice as likely to have AD as whites, and Hispanics are about 1.5 times more likely than whites. There does not appear to be any known genetic factor for these differences. The higher incidence of hypertension and diabetes in these populations may increase the risk of AD (Alzheimer's Association, 2010). Research is limited on cultural disparities in the incidence of dementia, as well as the influence of culture and ethnicity on the recognition and interpretation of cognitive changes and the assessment, diagnosis, and treatment of AD and other dementias (Tappen et al., 2010).

Further research is needed to understand how individuals from racially and culturally diverse groups view dementia and how cultural beliefs about disease etiology and symptoms influence diagnosis, treatment, and help-seeking behaviors (Williams et al., 2010). Development of culturally and linguistically appropriate sources of information about dementia is important. The Alzheimer's Association provides information on culturally appropriate education and outreach to diverse populations (http://www.alz.org/professionals_and_researchers_general_resources.asp).

Treatment

Individuals with cognitive impairment require ongoing monitoring of disease progression and response to therapy as well as regular health maintenance and health promotion interventions. "Successful treatment of AD and its symptoms is likely to be just as complex as its etiology" (Kolanowski et al., 2010, p. 215). Despite the lack of disease-modifying therapies, studies have consistently shown that active medical management of AD and other dementias can significantly improve quality of life through all stages of the disease for individuals and their caregivers. Active management includes (1) appropriate use of available treatment options; (2) effective management of coexisting conditions; (3) coordination of care among medical providers, other health care professionals, and lay caregivers; (4) participation in activities and adult day programs; and (5) taking part in support groups and supportive services such as counseling (Alzheimer's Association, 2012).

Assessment should occur at least every 6 months after diagnosis or any time there is a change in behavior or increase in the rate of decline. Assessment should include daily functioning, cognitive status, comorbid medical conditions, behavioral symptoms, medications, living arrangement, and safety. Beginning at the time of diagnosis and continuing through the course of the disease, ongoing assessment of the individual's decision-making capacity is essential. Health care surrogates should be determined and wishes for palliative and end-of-life care determined. In early stages, individuals usually retain their decision-making capacity and should be involved in all discussions.

Caregivers of individuals with dementia also need ongoing assessment, attention to physical and emotional health, support, and education, and this should begin with the diagnosis. Access to a knowledgeable provider who can follow them throughout the course of the illness is essential and leads to improved outcomes and less distress (Hain et al., 2010). Issues related to caregiving are discussed later in this chapter. Collaborative care management programs for the treatment of AD, often led by advanced practice nurses, have been shown to improve quality of care, decrease the incidence of behavioral and psychological symptoms of dementia, and decrease caregiver stress (Callahan et al., 2006; Duru et al., 2009). Chodosh and colleagues (2007) reported that adherence to guideline-recommended dementia care was less than 40%, so continued attention to effective care models is important. Nurses can play a significant role in the development and implementation of such models.

Medications. Current treatment guidelines recommend cholinesterase inhibitor (CI) therapy as first-line treatment in patients with mild to moderate AD, and these medications may also be prescribed for MCI and the vascular dementias. The currently available CIs are donepezil, galantamine, and rivastigmine. These medications work by blocking acetylcholinesterase. They have similar efficacy and side effects. The most common side effects with the CIs are nausea and diarrhea. Recommendations should start at low doses with slow titration to decrease side effects. Rivastigmine (Exelon) is now available in a patch that may be more convenient to use, has fewer side effects, and provides a consistent day-long dose.

No published study directly compares these drugs. Because they work in a similar way, it is not expected that switching from one of these drugs to another will produce significantly different results. However, a person may respond better to one drug than another. Treatment with these drugs should be started on diagnosis or after 6 months of AD symptoms with effectiveness reassessed every 6 months. Dosage of these medications should be reduced gradually when discontinuing to prevent rapid decompensation (Hall et al., 2009).

Memantine, an *N*-methyl-D-aspartate receptor antagonist, is also approved for moderate AD and may be used either alone or in conjunction with a CI. Further trials are needed to assess the potential for memantine either alone, or added to CIs, in mild and moderate AD (Howard et al., 2012). At this time, there is insufficient evidence to support the use of antioxidant therapy with vitamin E, gingko biloba, estrogen, or nonsteroidal anti-inflammatory drugs (NSAIDs) (Desai et al., 2010).

Medication therapy is directed toward the symptoms of AD and does not affect the neuronal decline that will eventually produce severe disability. The medications are aimed at slowing, not reversing, cognitive decline. Data from clinical trials and meta-analyses indicate that there is a small, statistically significant benefit on cognition, activities of daily living, and behavior with the use of these medications. Patients and family members must be provided with realistic expectations from pharmacological therapy (Segal-Gidan, 2010).

Delaying both disease onset and progression would significantly reduce the burden of AD, particularly in the late stages of the disease. Positive effects on the behavioral manifestations of AD have also been shown with CI therapy, suggesting that cholinergic mechanisms, among other neurotransmitters, are involved in the manifestation of some behavioral and psychological symptoms of dementia (Figiel & Sadowsky, 2008). A number of drugs are being investigated for treatment and prevention of AD. A major area of focus is on drugs that prevent or reduce beta-amyloid buildup (NIA, 2010).

Implications for Gerontological Nursing and Healthy Aging

Nurses provide direct care for people with dementia in the community, hospitals, and long-term care facilities. They also work with families and staff, teaching best practice approaches to care and providing education and support. With the rising incidence of dementia, nurses will play an even larger role in the design and implementation of evidence-based practice and provision of education, counseling, and supportive services to individuals with dementia and their caregivers (Teri et al., 2008).

Person-Centered Care

Irreversible dementias such as AD have no cure, and although new medications offer hope for improved function, the most important treatment for the disease is competent and compassionate person-centered care. Person-centered care looks beyond the disease and the tasks we must perform to the person within and our relationship with them. The focus is not on what we need to do to the person but on the person himself or herself and how to enhance well-being and quality of life.

Gerontological nurses know that the person, not the disease, is always the focus of care, and they practice from a belief that the person with dementia is still a whole person, someone who can think, feel, learn, grow, and be in a relationship (Touhy, 2004). "The person with dementia is not an object, not a vegetable, not an empty body, not a child, but an adult, who, given support, might exercise choices and respond to a respectful approach" (Woods, 1999, p. 35). Person-centered care fosters abilities, supports limitations, ensures safety, enhances quality of life, prevents excess disability, and offers hope. The culture change movement in the nation's nursing homes is grounded in the concept of person-centered care and quality of life (Kolanowski et al., 2010) (see Chapter 3).

Despite a growing body of evidence on the importance of person-centered care and therapeutic work with people with dementia, the emphasis in the literature and in practice continues to be on the care of the body (bathing, feeding) and the management of aggressive and problematic behavior. "Despite the emphasis on individualized care and culture change, for many staff, the goal of care hasn't changed: control of behavior is still a priority" (Kolanowski et al., 2010, p. 216).

Nutrition, activities of daily living (ADLs), maintenance of health and function, safety, communication, behavioral changes, caregiver needs and support, and quality of life are the major care concerns for patients, families, and staff who care for people with dementia. Mary Opal Wolanin, a gerontological nursing pioneer, suggested that nurses are not as interested in the neurofibrillary tangles in the brain as they are in trying to smooth out the environmental and relational tangles the person experiences. Special skills and attitudes are required to nurse the person with dementia, and caring is paramount. It is not an area of nursing that "just anyone can do" (Splete, 2008, p. 11).

The overriding goals in caring for older adults with dementia are to maintain function and prevent excess disability, structure the environment and relationships to maintain stability, compensate for the losses associated with the disease, and create a therapeutic milieu that nurtures the personhood of the individual and maintains quality of life. Box 21-5 presents an overview of general

nursing intervention principles in the care of persons with dementia. The Evidence-Based Practice box on page 316 presents evidence-based resources that nurses will find helpful in designing care for persons with dementia.

Four common care concerns for people with moderate to late-stage dementia are discussed in the remainder of this chapter: communication, behavior concerns, ADL care, and wandering. Nutrition is discussed in Chapter 9.

Communication

The experience of losing cognitive and expressive abilities is both frightening and frustrating. Older adults experiencing dementia have difficulty expressing their personhood in ways easily understood by others. However, the need to communicate and the need to be treated as a person remain despite memory and communication impairments. No group of patients is more in need of supportive relationships with skilled, caring health care providers. People with cognitive and communication impairments "depend on their relationship with and trust of others to provide emotional support, solve problems, and coordinate complex activities" (Buckwalter et al., 1995, p. 15).

Communication with elders experiencing cognitive impairment requires special skills and patience. "Caregivers are subject to frustration and anxiety when their attempts to communicate with the person who has cognitive limitations are unsuccessful" (Williams & Tappen, 2008, p. 92). Dementia affects both receptive and expressive communication components and alters the way people speak. Early in the disease, word-finding is difficult (anomia), and remembering the exact facts of a conversation is challenging. The following quote from an older adult with dementia illustrates:

> "I'm aware that I'm losing larger and larger chunks of memory . . . I lose one word and then I can't come up with the rest of the sentence. I just stop talking and people think something is really wrong with me. For awhile, I'll search for a word and I can see it walking away from me. It just gets littler and littler. It always comes back, but at the wrong time. You just can't be spontaneous." (Snyder, 2001, pp. 8, 11, 16)

People with dementia often use nonsensical or "made-up" words such as calling an electric razor a "whisker grinder." Automatic language skills (e.g., saying hello) are retained for the longest time. The person may wander from the topic of conversation and bring up seemingly unrelated topics. The person with dementia may fail to pick up on humor or sarcasm or abstract ideas in conversation. Nonverbal and behavioral responses become especially

---

| BOX 21-5 | **General Nursing Interventions in Care of Persons with Dementia** |

- Address safety.
- Structure daily living to maximize remaining abilities.
- Monitor general health and impact of dementia on management of other medical conditions.
- Support advance care planning and advanced directives.
- Educate caregivers in the areas of problem-solving, resources access, long range planning, emotional support, and respite.

From Evans L: *Complex care needs in older adults with common cognitive disorders.* Available at www.hartfording.org/uploads/file/gnec_state_of_science_papers/gnec_dementia.pdf.

important as a way of communication as verbal skills become more limited. As the disease progresses, verbal output may become less frequent although the grammar and sounds of the language being spoken remain relatively intact.

Williams and Tappen (2008) remind us that even in the later stages of dementia, the person may understand more than you realize and still needs opportunities for interaction and caring communication, both verbal and nonverbal. Often, health care providers do not communicate with older adults with cognitive impairment, or they limit communication only to task-focused topics or yes-or-no answers. Opportunities to express thoughts and feelings are just as important to a person with dementia as they are to each of you reading this book.

To effectively communicate with a person experiencing cognitive impairment, it is essential to believe that the person is trying to communicate something. It is just as essential for nurses to believe that what the person is trying to communicate is important enough to make the effort to understand. The best thing we can do is to treat everything the person says, however jumbled it may seem, as important and an attempt to tell us something. It is our responsibility as professionals to know how to understand and respond. The person with cognitive impairment cannot change his or her communication; we must change ours (Box 21-6).

Communication strategies differ depending on the purpose of communication (e.g., performing activities of daily living [ADLs], encouraging expression of feelings)

BOX 21-6 Communicating Effectively with Persons with Dementia

Envision a tennis game: the caregiver is like the tennis coach, and whenever the coach plays the ball, he or she seems to be able to put the ball where the person on the other side of the net can return it. The coach also returns the ball in such a way as to keep the rally going; he or she does not return it to score a point or win the match, but rather returns the ball so that the other player is able to reach it and, with encouragement, hit it back over the net again. Similarly, in our communication with people with dementia, our conversation and words must be put into play in a way such that the person can respond effectively and share thoughts and feelings.

From Kitwood T: *Dementia reconsidered: the person comes first,* Bristol, PA, 1999, Open University Press.

---

and the person's ability to understand (Box 21-7). One strategy may be best in an assessment situation but this same strategy may be a barrier to conversation designed to facilitate expression of concerns and feelings (Williams & Tappen, 2008, p. 93).

In the past, structured programs of reality orientation (RO) (orienting the person to the day, date, time, year,

---

BOX 21-7 Four Useful Strategies for Communicating with Individuals Experiencing Cognitive Impairment

Simplification Strategies (Useful with ADLs)
- Give one-step directions.
- Speak slowly.
- Allow time for response.
- Reduce distractions.
- Interact with one person at a time.
- Give clues and cues as to what you want the person to do. Use gestures or pantomime to demonstrate what it is you want the person to do—for example, put the chair in front of the person, point to it, pat the seat, and say, "Sit here."

Facilitation Strategies (Useful in Encouraging Expression of Thoughts and Feelings)
- Establish commonalities.
- Share self.
- Allow the person to choose subjects to discuss.
- Speak as if to an equal.
- Use broad openings, such as "How are you today?"
- Employ appropriate use of humor.
- Follow the person's lead.

Comprehension Strategies (Useful in Assisting with Understanding of Communication)
- Identify time confusion (*in what time frame is the person operating at the moment?*).
- Find the theme (*what connection is there between apparently disparate topics?*). Recognize an important theme, such as fear, loss, or happiness.
- Recognize the hidden meanings (*what did the person mean to say?*).

Continued

BOX 21-7 **Four Useful Strategies for Communicating with Individuals Experiencing Cognitive Impairment—cont'd**

Supportive Strategies (Useful in Encouraging Continued Communication and Supporting Personhood)

- Introduce yourself, and explain why you are there. Reach out to shake hands, and note the response to touch.
- If the person does not want to talk, go away and return later. Do not push or force.
- Sit closely, and face the person at eye level.
- Limit corrections.
- Use multiple ways of communicating (gestures, touch).
- Search for meaning.
- Know the person's past life history as well as daily life experiences and events.
- Remember there is a person behind the disease.

- Recognize feelings, and respond.
- Treat the person with respect and dignity.
- Show interest through body posture, facial expression, nodding, and eye contact. Assume a pleasant, relaxed attitude.
- Attend to vision and hearing losses.
- Do not try to bring the person to the present or use reality orientation. Go to where the person is, and enjoy the conversation.
- When leaving, thank the person for his or her time and attention as well as information.
- Remember that the quality, not the content or quantity, of the interaction is basic to therapeutic communication.

ADLs, Activities of daily living.

---

weather, upcoming holidays) were often used in long-term care facilities and chronic psychiatric units as a way to stimulate interaction and enhance memory. This intervention is still often noted as being of benefit to persons with dementia. However, it has been found that structured RO may place unrealistic expectations on persons with middle- to late-stage dementia and may be distressing when they cannot remember these things. Families, and professional caregivers, can often be heard asking people with dementia to name relatives, state their birth year, and remember other current facts. One can imagine how upsetting and demoralizing this might be to a person unable to remember. Students reading this book may liken the feeling to being told they are taking a pop quiz on content not yet assigned for study, and that this will constitute their final course grade. This is not to say that we should not orient the person to daily activities, time of day, and other important events, but it should be offered without the expectation that they will remember.

Caregivers can provide orienting information as part of general conversation (e.g., "It's quite warm for April 20, but it will be a beautiful day for our lunch date"). Rather than structured RO, a better approach is to go where the person is in their world rather than trying to bring them into yours. Identifying with elements of the individual's past and helping them and their caregivers appreciate the connections and feelings are more therapeutic approaches. Validation

therapy, developed by Naomi Feil in the 1980s, involves following the person's lead and responding to feelings expressed rather than interrupting to supply factual data.

Implications for Gerontological Nursing and Healthy Aging

Care and communication that respect and value the dignity and worth of every person nursed, including those with cognitive impairment, and use of research-based communication techniques, will enhance communication and personhood. "Gerontological nurses who are sensitive to communication and interaction patterns can assist both formal and informal caregivers in using more personal verbal and nonverbal communication strategies that are humanizing and show respect for the person. Similarly, they can monitor and try to change object-oriented communication approaches, which are not only insensitive and dehumanizing, but also often lead to diminished self-image and angry, agitated responses on the part of the patient with cognitive impairment" (Buckwalter et al., 1995, p. 15).

Behavior Concerns and Nursing Models of Care

Behavior and psychological symptoms of dementia (BPSD) may present in as many as 90% of individuals at some point in the disease trajectory. BPSD are symptoms of disturbed perception, thought content, mood, and behavior and may include anxiety, depression, hallucinations, delusions, aggression, screaming, restlessness, agitation, and resistance to care (Dettmore et al., 2009; Kolanowski et al., 2010). BPSD symptoms cause a great deal of distress to the person and the caregivers and often precipitate institutionalization (Miyamoto et al., 2010).

Several nursing models of care are helpful in recognizing and understanding the behavior of individuals with dementia and can be used to guide practice and assist families and staff in providing care from a more person-centered framework. The Progressively Lowered Stress Threshold model (PLST) and the Need-Driven Dementia-compromised Behavior model (NDDB) emphasize the interaction between person, context, and environment. "These models propose that behavior is used to communicate or express, in the best way the person has available, unmet needs (physiological, psychosocial, disturbing environment, uncomfortable social surroundings) and/or difficulty managing stress as the disease progresses" (Evans, 2007, p. 7).

Progressively Lowered Stress Threshold Model

The PLST model (Hall & Buckwalter, 1987; Hall, 1994) was one of the first models used to plan and evaluate care for people with dementia. Symptoms such as agitation are a result of a progressive loss of the person's ability to cope with demands and stimuli when the person's stress threshold is exceeded. Five common stressors that may trigger these symptoms are fatigue; change of environment, routine, or caregiver; misleading stimuli or inappropriate stimulus levels; internal or external demands to perform beyond abilities; and physical stressors such as pain, discomfort, acute illness, and depression.

Using this model, care is structured to decrease the stressors and provide a safe and predictable environment. Positive outcomes from use of the model include improved sleep; decreased sedative and tranquilizer use; increased food intake and weight; increased socialization; decreased episodes of aggressive, agitated, and disruptive behaviors; increased caregiver satisfaction with care; and increased functional level (DeYoung et al., 2003; Hall & Buckwalter, 1987). Box 21-8 presents the principles of care derived from the PLST model.

Need-Driven Dementia-compromised Behavior Model

The NDDB model (Kolanowski, 1999; Richards et al., 2000; Algase et al., 2003) is a framework for the study and understanding of behavioral symptoms of dementia.

BOX 21-8   Principles of Care Derived from the PLST Model

- Maximize functional abilities by supporting all losses in a prosthetic manner.
- Establish caring relationship, and provide person with unconditional positive regard.
- Use behaviors indicating anxiety and avoidance to determine appropriate limits of activity and stimuli.
- Teach caregivers to try to find out causes of behavior and to observe and evaluate verbal and nonverbal responses.
- Identify triggers related to discomfort or stress reactions (factors in the environment, caregiver communication).
- Modify the environment to support losses and promote safe function.
- Evaluate care routines and responses on a 24-hour basis, and adjust plan of care accordingly.
- Provide as much control as possible—encourage self-care, offer choices, explain all actions, do not push or force the person to do something.
- Keep environment stable and predictable.
- Provide ongoing education, support, care, and problem solving for caregivers.

Adapted from Hall GR, Buckwalter KC: Progressively lowered stress threshold: a conceptual model for care of adults with Alzheimer's disease, *Arch Psychiatr Nurs* 1(6):399-406, 1987.

The NDDB model proposes that the behavior of persons with dementia carries a message of need that can be addressed appropriately if the person's history and habits, physiological status, and physical and social environment are carefully evaluated (Kolanowski, 1999). Rather than behavior being viewed as disruptive, it is viewed as having meaning and expressing needs. Behavior reflects the interaction of background factors (cognitive changes as a result of dementia, gender, ethnicity, culture, education, personality, responses to stress) and proximal factors (physiological needs such as hunger or pain, mood, physical environment [e.g., light, noise]) with social environment (e.g., staff stability and mix, presence of others) (Richards et al., 2000).

Optimal care is provided by manipulating the proximal factors that precipitate behavior and by maximizing strengths and minimizing the limitations of the background factors. For instance, sleep disruptions are common in people with dementia. If the person is not getting adequate sleep at night, agitated or aggressive behavior during the day may signal the need for more rest. Interventions to modify proximal factors interfering with sleep, such as noise, frequent awakenings during the night, and daytime boredom, can help meet the need for rest and sleep and decrease agitation or aggression.

Implications for Gerontological Nursing and Healthy Aging

Assessment

It is essential to view all behavior as meaningful and an expression of needs. The focus must be on understanding that behavioral expressions communicate distress, and the response is to investigate the possible sources of distress and intervene appropriately. There are many possible reasons for BPSD. After ruling out medical problems (e.g., pneumonia, dehydration, impaction, infection/sepsis, fractures, pain, or depression) as a cause of behavior, continued assessment to identify why distressing symptoms are occurring is important (Evans, 2007). Conditions such as constipation or urinary tract infections can cause great distress for cognitively impaired older people and may lead to marked changes in behavior (e.g., agitation, falls, refusal of care), so careful assessment is important. Pain is a frequent cause of aggressive behavior (striking out, resistance to care), and, after careful assessment of other possible causes, treatment with a trial of analgesics should be considered (Hall et al., 2009) (see Chapter 15).

Fear, discomfort, unfamiliar surroundings and people, illness, fatigue, depression, need for autonomy and control, caregiver approaches, communication strategies, and environmental stressors are frequent precipitants of behavioral symptoms. "For the individual with late-stage dementia, a good deal of their discomfort comes from non-physiological sources, for example, from difficulty sorting out and negotiating everyday life activities" (Kovach et al., 1999, p. 412). Hall and colleagues suggest that "caregivers may not understand that behaviors are a symptom of the disease, much as pain would be expected with a malignancy. Understanding what triggers behavior is important. What may appear as hallucinations or delusions to the caregiver might be misinterpretations by the person of a television program, family photographs, or images reflected in a mirror. In these cases, it is much safer to turn off the television, remove photographs from the area, or cover a mirror than to place the patient on an antipsychotic medication" (Hall et al., 2009, pp. 40, 41). Box 21-9 presents precipitating factors for BPSD.

BOX 21-9   Conditions Precipitating Behavioral Symptoms in Persons with Dementia

- Communication deficits
- Pain or discomfort
- Acute medical problems
- Sleep disturbances
- Perceptual deficits
- Depression
- Need for social contact
- Hunger, thirst, need to toilet
- Loss of control
- Misinterpretation of the situation or environment
- Crowded conditions
- Changes in environment or people
- Noise, disruption
- Being forced to do something
- Fear
- Loneliness
- Psychotic symptoms
- Fatigue
- Environmental overstimulation or understimulation
- Depersonalized, rushed care
- Restraints
- Psychoactive drugs

Putting yourself in the place of the person with dementia and trying to see the world from his or her eyes will help you understand their behavior. Questions of what, where, why, when, who, and what now are important components of the assessment of behavior. Box 21-10 presents a framework for asking questions about the possible meanings and messages behind observed behavior. Use of a behavioral log over a 2- to 3-day period to track when the behavior occurs, the circumstances, and the response to interventions is recommended and required in skilled nursing facilities.

Interventions

All evidence-based guidelines endorse an approach that begins with comprehensive assessment of the behavior and possible causes followed by the use of nonpharmacological interventions as a first line of treatment. Despite these recommendations, psychotropic medications to treat BPSD are often the first-line response. This is of serious concern in light of the side effects of such medications. None of these medications are approved for use in treatment of behavioral responses in dementia (Kuehn, 2010b; Schneider et al., 2006).

BOX 21-10   Framework for Asking Questions About the Meaning of Behavior

What?
What is being sought? What is happening? Does the behavior have a physical or emotional component or both? What are the person's responses? What would be done if the person was 20 years old instead of 80? What is the behavior saying? What is the emotion being expressed?

Where?
Where is the behavior occurring? Environmental triggers?

When?
When does the behavior most frequently occur? After what (e.g., activities of daily living [ADLs], family visits, mealtimes)?

Who?
Who is involved? Other residents, caregivers, family?

Why?
What happened before? Poor communication? Tasks too complicated? Physical or medical problem? Person being rushed or forced to do something? Has this happened before and why?

What Now?
Approaches and interventions (physical, psychosocial)? Changes needed and by whom? Who else might know something about the person or the behavior or approaches? Communicate to all and include in plan of care.

Adapted from Hellen C: Can you provide care for residents with difficult behaviors? *Alzheimers Care Q* 1(4):4, 2000; Ortigara A: Understanding the language of behaviors, *Alzheimers Care Q* 1(4):91, 2000.

In nursing homes, Kolanowski and colleagues (2010) suggest that "nurses continue to request and physicians continue to prescribe psychotropic drugs for the majority of residents with BPSD" (p. 215). Several authors suggest that insufficient staffing in nursing homes; time; emphasis on controlling residents rather than understanding; lack of interdisciplinary team approaches and family involvement; and inadequate education and research about behavior and use of nonpharmacologic interventions contribute to less than optimal practice (Dettmore et al., 2009; Kolanowski et al., 2010). Often these drugs are prescribed in response to frustration and helplessness on the parts of both caretakers and loved ones alike (Dettmore et al., 2009, p. 14).

Pharmacological approaches may be considered in addition to nonpharmacological approaches if there has been a comprehensive assessment of reversible causes of behavior; the person presents a danger to self or others; nonpharmacological interventions have not been effective; and the risk/benefit profiles of the medications have been considered (Dettmore et al., 2009; Kolanowski et al., 2010). If psychotropic medications are used, the person must be monitored closely for extrapyramidal signs, orthostasis, somnolence, and neuroleptic malignant syndrome. Strict federal regulations monitor the use of psychotropic medications in skilled nursing facilities (see Chapter 8).

Nonpharmacological Approaches

Nonpharmacological approaches are resident-centered and include interventions such as meaningful activities,

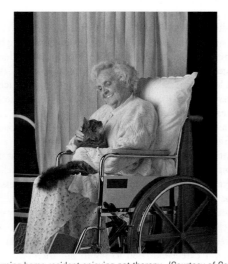
A nursing home resident enjoying pet therapy. (Courtesy of Corbis.)

validation therapy, social contact (real or simulated), animal-assisted therapy, exercise, sensory stimulation, reminiscence, Montessori-based activities, environmental design (e.g., special care units, homelike environments, gardens, safe walking areas), changes in mealtime and bathing environments, consistent staffing assignments, bright light therapy, aromatherapy, massage, music, relaxation, distraction, and nonconfrontational interaction (Dettmore et al., 2009; Evans, 2007; Edgerton & Richie, 2010; Kolanowski et al., 2010; Holliday-Welsh et al., 2009; Smith et al., 2009).

There is a large amount of literature on nonpharmacological interventions, and these approaches are recommended in the culture change movement. In general, these interventions have shown promise for improving quality of life for persons with dementia despite a lack of rigorous evaluation. Sensory enhancement/relaxation methods, such as bright light therapy, music therapy, Snoezelen (a relaxation technique popular in Europe), and massage, have been studied most extensively, and there is good evidence for their effectiveness.

Activities of Daily Living

The losses associated with dementia interfere with the person's communication patterns and ability to understand and express thoughts and feelings. Perceptual disturbances and misinterpretations of reality contribute to fear and misunderstanding. Often, bathing and the provision of other ADL care, such as dressing, grooming, and toileting, are the cause of much distress for both the person with dementia and the caregiver.

Bathing

Bathing and care for ADLs, particularly in nursing homes, can be perceived as an attack by persons with dementia who may respond by screaming or striking out. A rigid focus on tasks or institutional care routines, such as a shower three mornings each week, can contribute to the distress and precipitate distressing behaviors. Being touched or bathed against one's will violates the trust in caregiver relationships and can be considered a major affront (Rader & Barrick, 2000). The behaviors that may be exhibited by the person with dementia are not deliberate attacks on caregivers by a violent person. The message is, in the words of Rader and Barrick (2000, p. 49), "Please find another way to keep me clean, because the way you are doing it now is intolerable."

To care effectively for older adults with dementia, nurses and other caregivers need to try to put themselves in the place of the person with dementia and try to see the world from his or her eyes. The following paragraph will illustrate:

You are asleep in the chair at home when suddenly you are awakened by a person you have never seen before trying to undress you. Then he or she puts you naked into a hard, cold chair and wheels you down a hallway. Suddenly cold water hits you in the face and the person is touching your private areas. You don't understand why the person is trying to do this to you. You are embarrassed, frightened, cold, and angry. You hit and scream at this person and try to get away.

Family members and nurses caring for people with dementia must understand that they are the ones who must change their behavior, reactions, and approaches because the person with dementia cannot do this. Using appropriate communication strategies, explaining all actions before doing, not pushing or forcing people who are resistant, providing positive feedback, paying attention to body posture and facial expressions, using gestures, demonstration, one-step directions, staying calm and pleasant, providing warmth and comfort, and allowing appropriate time for response are some general suggested techniques to enhance ADL care interactions.

In research in nursing homes, Rader and Barrick (2000) have provided comprehensive guidelines for bathing people with dementia in ways that are pleasurable and decrease distress. Asking the question "What is the easiest, most comfortable, least frightening way for me to clean the person right now?" guides the choice of interventions (Rader & Barrick, 2000, p. 42). Suggested interventions to make bath time more pleasurable and safer include knowing the person's lifetime bathing routines and preferences; providing care only when the person is receptive; respecting refusals to participate in care; explaining all actions; realizing that a bath is not an essential intervention; encouraging self-care to the extent possible; making bathrooms and shower areas warm, comfortable, and safe; being attentive to pain and discomfort; and using alternative bathing methods, such as a towel bath or sponge bath (Rader et al., 2006).

Another innovative approach being investigated in Sweden is caregiver singing and the use of background music during ADL care in nursing homes. Caregivers play and sing familiar songs during care routines. When compared to usual care practices, this approach enhanced the expression of positive moods and emotions, increased the mutuality of communication, and reduced aggression and resistive care behaviors (Hammar et al., 2011; http://www.dementiacaresinging.com).

Wandering

Wandering associated with dementia is one of the most difficult management problems encountered in home and institutional settings. One in five people with dementia wander (Lester et al., 2012). Wandering is a complex behavior and is not well understood. Risk factors for wandering include visuospatial impairments, anxiety and depression, poor sleep patterns, unmet needs, and a more socially active and outgoing premorbid lifestyle (Lester et al., 2012). There is a need for more research on wandering as well as interventions for this behavior.

Wandering presents safety concerns in all settings. Wandering behavior affects sleep, eating, safety, the caregiver's ability to provide care, and interferes with the privacy of others. The behavior can lead to falls, elopement (leaving the home or facility), injury, and death (Futrell et al., 2010; Rowe et al., 2010). The stimulus for wandering arises from many internal and external sources. Wandering can be considered a rhythm, intrinsically and extrinsically driven. The following excerpt about wandering from an article by Laurenhue (2001) provides a great deal of insight into this concern from the person's perspective:

> *"Very often, I wander around looking for something which I know is very pertinent, but then after awhile I forget all about what it was I was looking for. When I'm wandering around, I'm trying to touch base with—anything, actually. If anything appeared I'd probably enjoy it, or look at it or examine it and wonder how it got there. I feel very foolish when I'm wandering around not knowing what I'm doing and I'm not always quite sure how to do any better. It's not easy to figure out what the heck I'm looking for."* (Henderson, 1998, p. 24)

Wandering behaviors can be predicted through careful observation and knowing the person's patterns. For example, if the person with dementia starts wandering or trying to leave the home around dinnertime every day, meaningful activities such as music, exercise, and refreshments can be provided at this time. Research suggests that wandering may be less likely to occur when the person is involved in social interaction. There are also several instruments to assess risk for wandering, and Futrell and colleagues (2010) developed an evidence-based protocol for wandering. Environmental interventions, such as camouflaging doorways, providing enclosed outdoor gardens and paths for walking, and electronic bracelets that activate alarms at exits, are also used. There are a number of assistive technology devices and programs that can enhance the safety of persons who wander. Box 21-11 presents other suggested interventions.

Wandering behavior may also result in people with dementia going outside and getting lost, a phenomenon studied by Rowe (2003). The Alzheimer's Association estimates that 60% of people with dementia will wander and become lost in the community at some point (www.alz.org/living_with_alzheimers_wandering_behaviors.asp). Caregivers must prevent people with dementia from leaving homes or care facilities unaccompanied, register the person in the Safe Return program, and have a plan of action in case the person does become lost. Rowe also suggests that police must respond rapidly to requests for searches, and the general public should be informed about how to recognize and assist people with dementia who may be lost (2003). Box 21-12 presents specific recommendations from this study.

BOX 21-11 · Interventions for Wandering or Exiting Behaviors

- Face the person, and make direct eye contact (unless this is interpreted as threatening).
- Gently touch the person's arm, shoulders, back, or waist if he or she does not move away.
- Call the person by his or her formal name (e.g., Mr. Jones).
- Listen to what the person is communicating verbally and nonverbally; listen to the feelings being expressed.
- Identify the agenda, plan of action, and the emotional needs the agenda is expressing.
- Respond to the feelings expressed, staying calm.
- Repeat specific words or phrases, or state the need or emotion (e.g., "You need to go home, you're worried about your husband.").
- If such repetition fails to distract the person, accompany him or her and continue talking calmly, repeating phrases and the emotion you identify.

- Provide orienting information only if it calms the person. If it increases distress, stop talking about the present situations. Do not "correct" the person or belittle his or her agenda.
- At intervals, redirect the person toward the facility or the home by suggesting, "Let's walk this way now" or "I'm so tired, let's turn around."
- If orientation and redirection fail, continue to walk, allowing the person control but ensuring safety.
- Make sure you have a backup person, but he or she should stay out of eyesight of the person.
- Have someone call for help if you are unable to redirect. Usually the behavior is time limited because of the person's attention span and the security and trust between you and the person.

Adapted from Rader J, et al: How to decrease wandering, a form of agenda behavior, *Geriatr Nurs* 6(4):196-199, 1985.

BOX 21-12   Recommendations to Avoid People with Dementia Getting Lost

- Do not leave the person with dementia alone in the home.
- Secure the environment so that the person cannot leave by himself or herself while the caregiver is asleep or busy.
- If the person lives in a nursing facility, keep in supervised area; do frequent checks; use bed, chair, and door alarms and Wanderguard bracelets; identify potential wanderers by special arm bands; disguise doorways.
- Place locks out of reach, hide keys, and lock windows.
- Consider motion detectors or home security systems that alert when doors are opened.
- Register the person in the Safe Return program of the Alzheimer's Association, and ensure that the person wears the Safe Return jewelry or clothing tags at all times.
- Register with the Silver Alert system if available.
- Let neighbors know that a person with dementia lives in the neighborhood.
- Prepare a search and rescue plan in case the person becomes lost.
- Keep copies of up-to-date photos ready for distribution to searchers, police, hospital, and the media.
- Conduct a search immediately if the person becomes lost.
- Call the local law enforcement agency and the Safe Return program to report the missing person.
- If the person is not found within 6 to 12 hours (or sooner depending on weather conditions), search any wooded areas or fields near where the person was last seen. People with dementia may not seek help or respond to calls and may try to hide from searchers; search in an organized manner with as many searchers as possible.

Adapted from Rowe M: People with dementia who become lost, *Am J Nurs* 103(7): 32-39, 2003.

Caregiving for Persons with Dementia

More than 70% of persons with dementia live at home, and family and friends provide nearly 75% of their care. Nearly 15 million people provide care for a loved one with AD or another form of dementia, amounting to 17 billion hours or more than $202 billion in unpaid care (Alzheimer's Association, 2012). These caregivers provide more hours of help than caregivers of other older people and experience more adverse consequences to their physical and mental health.

Caregivers of persons with dementia have lower self-rated health scores; display fewer health-promoting behaviors; and have higher depression and anxiety rates, higher morbidity and mortality rates, sleep problems, and higher numbers of illness-related symptoms (Alzheimer's Association, 2012; Elliott et al., 2010). Factors that influence the stress of caregiving include grief over the multiple losses that occur, the physical demands and duration of caregiving (up to 20 years), and resource availability. The deleterious effects of caregiving in dementia are intensified when the care recipient demonstrates behavioral disturbances and impairments in ADLs and instrumental activities of daily living (IADLs).

Most research has focused on caregiving in the late stages of dementia and on the "burden" of caregiving. Many authors suggest that the "concept of burden alone does not adequately explain the complexities of caregiving for an older person with dementia" (Suwa, 2002, p. 5). Warmth, pleasure, comfort, spiritual growth, self-transcendence, and other positive dimensions of caregiving have also emerged in qualitative studies (Acton, 2002; Farran et al., 2004). Further research is needed to help us understand how we can extend caring to both the caregiver and the person with dementia in ways that maintain personhood, enhance relationships, promote quality of life, and balance the stresses with the joys.

Caregiver intervention programs that include bundled interventions, such as individual and group modalities for both the person with dementia and the caregiver as well as combined groups, education, counseling, support group participation, care management, and the continuous availability of telephone support may be the most effective. Active skills training interventions to teach caregivers about AD and the skills to manage troublesome behaviors, maintain social support, reframe negative emotions, manage stress, and enhance their own healthy behaviors appear to be the most effective in reducing depression and burden and improving quality of life (Elliott et al., 2010; Mittelman et al., 2007). The importance of a proactive approach, with interventions offered at the beginning of the care trajectory, rather than a reactive approach, is being noted in the literature and treatment guidelines (Ducharme et al., 2009).

To date, the preponderance of research with caregivers has been directed toward those living with later stages of dementia. More research is needed to develop interventions for the growing numbers of individuals and their families experiencing EO-D, MCI, and early to mild stages of dementia whose needs are quite different from those in later stages.

Implications for Gerontological Nursing and Healthy Aging

Caregiving for someone with dementia by family members, or formal caregivers, requires exquisite skills, knowledge of evidence-based practice, and a deep knowing of the person. Rader and Tornquist (1995) reflect on the knowledge required and provide a view of caregiving roles that is quite useful and understandable for all caregivers. The author has found that nursing assistants and family caregivers can truly relate to the practical wisdom in these words.

- **Magician role:** To understand what the person is trying to communicate both verbally and nonverbally, we must be a magician who can use our magical abilities to see the world through the eyes, the ears, and the feelings of the person. We know how to use tricks to turn an individual's behavior around or prevent it from occurring and causing distress.
- **Detective role:** The detective looks for clues and cues about what might be causing distress and how it might be changed. We have to investigate and know as much about the person as possible to be a good detective.
- **Carpenter role:** By having a wide variety of tools and selecting the right tools for the job, we build individualized plans of care for each person.
- **Jester role:** Many people with dementia retain their sense of humor and respond well to the appropriate use of humor. This does not mean making fun of but rather sharing laughter and fun. "Those who love their work and do it well employ good doses of humor as part of the care of others as well as for self-care" (Rader & Barrick, 2000, p. 42). The jester spreads joy, is creative, energizes, and lightens the burdens (Rader & Barrick, 2000; Laurenhue, 2001).

Figure 21-1 presents a nursing situation that one nurse experienced in caring for a patient with dementia who was being admitted to a nursing home. Written from the perspective of the nurse and his knowing of the patient, the story provides insight into important nursing responses, such as person-centered care, therapeutic communication, and establishing meaningful relationships. It is a lovely example of expert gerontological nursing for older adults with dementia and a fitting way to end this chapter.

Application of Maslow's Hierarchy

Consistent with the philosophy of this book, the nursing care of older adults with dementia presented in this chapter is focused not only on meeting basic needs, but also on creating environments and relationships that promote growth, self-actualization, and quality of life. Despite their inability to express their thoughts and feelings in ways with which we are familiar, people with cognitive impairment still have higher-order needs, such as those for belonging, self-esteem, and a meaningful life. "The relationship between the caregiver and care recipient is the central determinant of quality of life and quality of care" (Rader & Barrick, 2000, p. 36). The care relationships and the environment must support the meeting of all their needs. Surely we would want the same for ourselves.

KEY CONCEPTS

- Nurses must advocate for thorough assessment of any elder who appears to be experiencing cognitive decline and inability to function in important aspects of life.
- Delirium sometimes is the result of physiological imbalances and may be caused by a variety of biological disturbances. Delirium is characterized by fluctuating levels of consciousness, sometimes in a diurnal pattern, and frequent misperceptions and illusions. It often goes unrecognized and is attributed to age or dementia. People with dementia are more susceptible to delirium. Knowledge of risk factors, preventive measures, and treatment of underlying medical problems is essential to prevent serious consequences.
- Medications and pain are frequently the causes of delirious states in older people.
- Irreversible dementias follow a pattern of inevitable decline accompanied by decreased intellectual function, personality changes, and impaired judgment. The most common of these is AD.
- AD has been the subject of enormous research in attempts to understand the causes. There is growing evidence that the disease starts many years before symptoms appear. Research is continuing in attempts to discover ways to protect against or halt the progress of the disease. There is no known cure, although some medications seem to slow the progress of the dementia for a time.
- Individuals with cognitive impairment respond best to calmness and patience, adaptations of communication techniques, and environments and relationships that enhance function, support limitations, ensure safety, and provide opportunities for a meaningful quality of life. Because cognitively impaired persons may be

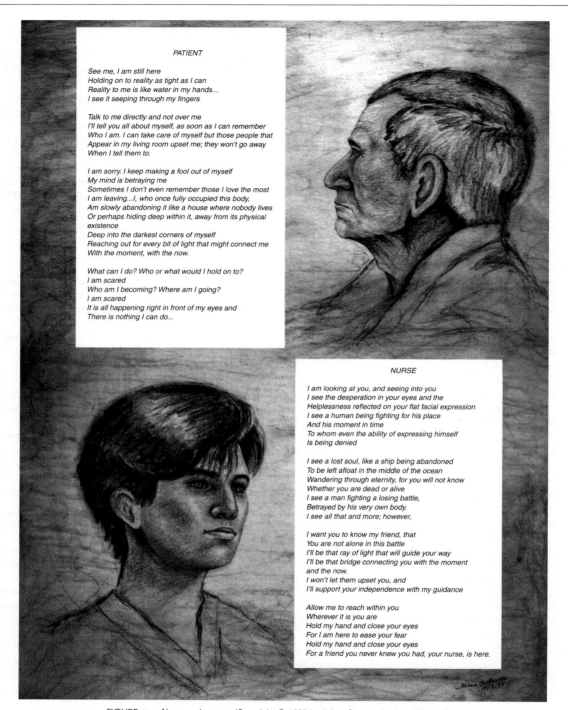

PATIENT

See me, I am still here
Holding on to reality as tight as I can
Reality to me is like water in my hands...
I see it seeping through my fingers

Talk to me directly and not over me
I'll tell you all about myself, as soon as I can remember
Who I am. I can take care of myself but those people that
Appear in my living room upset me; they won't go away
When I tell them to.

I am sorry. I keep making a fool out of myself
My mind is betraying me
Sometimes I don't even remember those I love the most
I am leaving...I, who once fully occupied this body,
Am slowly abandoning it like a house where nobody lives
Or perhaps hiding deep within it, away from its physical
existence
Deep into the darkest corners of myself
Reaching out for every bit of light that might connect me
With the moment, with the now.

What can I do? Who or what would I hold on to?
I am scared
Who am I becoming? Where am I going?
I am scared
It is all happening right in front of my eyes and
There is nothing I can do...

NURSE

I am looking at you, and seeing into you
I see the desperation in your eyes and the
Helplessness reflected on your flat facial expression
I see a human being fighting for his place
And his moment in time
To whom even the ability of expressing himself
Is being denied

I see a lost soul, like a ship being abandoned
To be left afloat in the middle of the ocean
Wandering through eternity, for you will not know
Whether you are dead or alive
I see a man fighting a losing battle,
Betrayed by his very own body.
I see all that and more; however,

I want you to know my friend, that
You are not alone in this battle
I'll be that ray of light that will guide your way
I'll be that bridge connecting you with the moment
and the now.
I won't let them upset you, and
I'll support your independence with my guidance

Allow me to reach within you
Wherever it is you are
Hold my hand and close your eyes
For I am here to ease your fear
Hold my hand and close your eyes
For a friend you never knew you had, your nurse, is here.

FIGURE 21-1 Nurse and person. (Copyright © 1998 by Jaime Castaneda, Lake Worth, Fla.)

unable to express their feelings and needs in ways that are easily understood, the gerontological nurse must always try to understand the world from their perspective.

- Families provide most of the care for persons with dementia, and while many gain satisfaction from this, they experience more adverse consequences than caregivers of other older adults. Comprehensive interventions for both the person with dementia and the caregiver should begin early in the disease and continue throughout the trajectory.

ACTIVITIES AND DISCUSSION QUESTIONS

1. What are the differences between delirium, dementia, and depression?
2. What are some of the risk factors for development of delirium?
3. Discuss communication strategies useful for the person experiencing delirium.
4. Why is it important to ensure that the person experiencing any change in mental status receives a thorough assessment and evaluation?
5. Brainstorm with fellow students how it would feel to be bathed by a total stranger.
6. The nursing assistants in a nursing home complain to you that Mr. G. hit them when they were trying to give him his required twice-weekly shower. How might you assist them in meeting Mr. G's need for bathing?
7. Describe how you would design a special care unit for individuals with dementia.
8. A family caregiver tells you that his or her loved one keeps trying to leave the house to find the children. What are some strategies you might share with the caregiver to deal with this situation?

REFERENCES

Acton G: Self-transcendent views and behaviors: exploring growth in caregivers of adults with dementia, *J Gerontol Nurs* 28(12):22–30, 2002.

Algase D, Beel-Bates C, Beattie E: Wandering in long-term care, *Ann Longterm Care* 11(1):33–39, 2003.

Alzheimer's Association: *World Alzheimer report 2010. the global economic impact of dementia* (2010). Available at http://www.alz.org/documents/national/World_Alzheimer_Report_2010.pdf.

Alzheimer's Association: 2012 Alzheimer's disease facts and figures, Alzheimer's and dementia, *Alzheimers Dement* 8:131-168, 2012. Available at http://www.alz.org/alzheimers_disease_facts_and_figures.asp#quickfacts.

Balas B, Gale M, Kagan S: Delirium in older patients in surgical intensive care units, *J Nurs Scholarsh* 39(2):47–154, 2007.

Bellelli G, Frisoni GB, Turco R, et al: Delirium superimposed on dementia predicts 12-month survival in elderly patients discharged from a postacute rehabilitation facility, *J Gerontol A Biol Sci Med Sci* 63(10):1124–1125, 2008.

Bradley E, Webster T, Baker D, et al: After adoption: sustaining the innovation: a case study of disseminating the Hospital Elder Life Program, *J Am Geriatr Soc* 53(9):1455–1461, 2005.

Braes T, Milisen K, Foreman M: Assessing cognitive function. In Capezuti E, Swicker D, Mezey M, et al, editors: *Evidence-based geriatric nursing protocols for best practice*, ed 3, New York, 2008, Springer.

Buckwalter KC, Gerdner LA, Hall GR, et al: Shining through: the humor and individuality of persons with Alzheimer's disease, *J Gerontol Nurs* 21:11, 1995.

Callahan C, Boustani M, Unverzagt F, et al: Effectiveness of collaborative care for older adults with Alzheimer's disease in primary care: a randomized clinical trial, *JAMA* 295(18):2148–2157, 2006.

Chodosh J, Mittman B, Connor K, et al: Caring for patients with dementia: how good is the quality of care? Results from three health systems, *J Am Geriatr Soc* 55:1260, 2007.

Clarke SP, McRae ME, Del Signore S, et al: Delirium in older cardiac surgery patients: directions for practice, *J Gerontol Nurs* 36(11):34–45, 2010.

Cole M, McCusker J: Improving the outcomes of delirium in older hospital inpatients, *Int Psychogeriatr* 21:613, 2009.

Dahlke S, Phinney A: Caring for hospitalized older adults at risk for delirium: the silent, unspoken piece of nursing practice, *J Gerontol Nurs* 34(6):41–47, 2008.

Desai A, Grossberg G, Chibnall J: Healthy brain aging: A road map, *Clin Geriatr Med* 26:1, 2010.

Dettmore D, Kolanowski A, Boustani M: Aggression in persons with dementia: use of nursing theory to guide clinical practice, *Geriatr Nurs* 30:8, 2009.

DeYoung S, Just G, Harrison R: Decreasing aggressive, agitated, or disruptive behavior participation in a behavior management unit, *J Gerontol Nurs* 28(6):22–30, 2003.

Ducharme F, Beaudet L, Legault A, et al: Development of an intervention program for Alzheimer's family caregivers following diagnostic disclosure, *Clin Nurs Res* 18:44, 2009.

Duru O, Etther S, Vassar S, et al: Cost evaluation of a coordinated care management intervention for dementia, *Am J Manag Care* 15:521, 2009.

Edgerton E, Richie L: Improving physical environments for dementia care: making minimal changes for maximum effect, *Ann Longterm Care* 18:43, 2010.

Elliott A, Burgio L, DeCoster J: Enhancing caregiver health: findings from the resources for enhancing Alzheimer's caregiver health II intervention, *J Am Geriatr Soc* 58:30, 2010.

Ely EW, Margolin R, Francis J, et al: Evaluation of delirium in critically ill patients: validation of the Confusion Assessment Method for the intensive care unit (CAM-ICU), *Crit Care Med* 29(7):1370–1379, 2001.

Evans L: *Complex care needs in older adults with common cognitive disorders, section A: assessment and management of dementia* (2007). Available at http://hartfordign.org/uploads/File/gnec_state_of_science_papers/gnec_dementia.pdf.

Farran C, Loukissa D, Lindeman D, et al: Caring for self while caring for others: the two-track life of coping with Alzheimer's disease, *J Gerontol Nurs* 30(5):38–46, 2004.

Figiel G, Sadowsky C: A systematic review of the effectiveness of rivastigmine for the treatment of behavioral disturbances in dementia and other neurological disorders, *Curr Med Res Opin* 24(1):157–166, 2008.

Fletcher K: Dementia. In Boltz M, Capezuti E, Fulmer T, et al, editors: *Evidence-based geriatric nursing protocols for best practice*, ed 4, New York, 2012, Springer.

Futrell M, Mellilo K, Remington R: Evidence-based guideline: wandering, *J Gerontol Nurs* 36:6, 2010.

Ghetu M, Bordelon P, Langan R: Diagnosis and treatment of mild cognitive impairment, *Clin Geriatr* 18:30–36, 2010.

Hain D, Tappen R, Diaz S, Ouslander J: Cognitive impairment and medication self-management errors in older adults discharged home from a community hospital, *Home Healthc Nurse* 30(4):246–254, 2012.

Hain D, Touhy T, Engstrom G: What matters most to carers of people with mild to moderate dementia as evidence for transforming care, *Alzheimer's Care Today* 11:162, 2010.

Hall GR: Caring for people with Alzheimer's disease using the conceptual model of progressively lowered stress threshold in the clinical setting, *Nurs Clin North Am* 29(1):129–141, 1994.

Hall GR, Buckwalter KC: Progressively lowered stress threshold: a conceptual model for care of adults with Alzheimer's disease, *Arch Psychiatr Nurs* 1(6):399–406, 1987.

Hammar L, Emami A, Engstrom G, Gotell E: Communicating through caregiver singing during morning care situations in dementia care. *Scand J Caring Sci* 25(1):160–168, 2011.

Henderson C: *Partial view: an Alzheimer's journal*, Dallas, 1998, Southern Methodist Press.

Holliday-Welsh D, Gessert C, Renier C: Massage in the management of agitation in nursing home residents with cognitive impairment, *Geriatr Nurs* 30:108, 2009.

Howard R, McShane R, Lindesay J, et al: Donazepil and memantine for moderate-to-severe Alzheimer's disease, *N Engl J Med* 366:893–903, 2012.

Hyman BT, Phelps CH, Beach TG, et al: National Institute on Aging–Alzheimer's Association guidelines for the neuropathologic assessment of Alzheimer's disease, *Alzheimers Dement* 8(1):1–13, 2012.

Inouye SK, Bogardus ST Jr, Charpentier PA, et al: A multicomponent intervention to prevent delirium in hospitalized older patients, *N Engl J Med* 340(9):669–676, 1999.

Inouye SK, van Dyck CH, Alessi CA, et al: Clarifying confusion: the Confusion Assessment Method: a new method for detection of delirium, *Ann Intern Med* 113(12):941–948, 1990.

Irving K, Foreman M: Delirium, nursing practice and the future, *Int J Older People Nurs* 1(2):121–127, 2006.

Kamat S, Kamat A, Grossberg G: Dementia risk prediction: are we there yet? *Clin Geriatr Med* 26:113, 2010.

Kolanowski A, Fick D, Frazer C, et al: It's about time: use of nonpharmacological interventions in the nursing home, *J Nurs Scholarsh* 42:214, 2010.

Kolanowski AM: An overview of the Need-Driven Dementia–Compromised Behavior Model, *J Gerontol Nurs* 25(9):7–9, 1999.

Kovach C, Weissman D, Griffie J, et al: Assessment and treatment of discomfort for people with late-stage dementia, *J Pain Symptom Manage* 18(6):412-419, 1999.

Kuehn B: Delirium often not recognized or treated despite serious long-term consequences, *JAMA* 304:389, 2010a.

Kuehn B: Questionable antipsychotic prescribing remains despite serious risks, *JAMA* 303:1582, 2010b.

Laurenhue K: Each person's journey is unique, *Alzheimers Care Q* 2(2):79–83, 2001.

Lester P, Garite A, Kohen I: Wandering and elopement in nursing homes, *Ann Longterm Care* 20(3):32–36, 2012.

Lindquist LA, Go L, Fleisher J, et al: Improvements in cognition following hospital discharge of community dwelling seniors, *J Gen Intern Med* 26(7):765–770, 2011.

Marcantonio E, Bergmann M, Kiely D, et al: Randomized trial of a delirium abatement program for postacute skilled nursing facilities, *J Am Geriatr Soc* 58(6):1019, 2010.

McGowin DF: *Living in the labyrinth: a personal journey through the maze of Alzheimer's*, New York, 1993, Dell.

Mittelman MS, Roth DL, Clay OJ, et al: Preserving health of Alzheimer caregivers: impact of a spouse caregiver intervention, *Am J Geriatr Psychiatry* 15(9):780, 2007.

Miyamoto Y, Tachimori H, Ito H: Formal caregiver burden in dementia: impact of behavioral and psychological symptoms of dementia and activities of daily living, *Geriatr Nurs* 31(4):246–253, 2010.

National Institute on Aging: *Alzheimer's disease progress report: a deeper understanding* (2010). Available at http://www.nia.nih.gov/alzheimers/publication/2-discovering-genes-behind-alzheimers-disease/large-studies-revealing.

Neelon VJ, Champagne M, Carlson J, et al: The NEECHAM confusion scale: construction, validation and clinical testing, *Nurs Res* 45(6):324–330, 1996.

Ozbolt L, Paniagua M, Kaiser R: Atypical antipsychotics for the treatment of delirious elders, *J Am Med Dir Assoc* 9(1):19–28, 2008.

Pisani M, Araujo K, Van Ness P, et al: A research algorithm to improve detection of delirium in the intensive care unit, *Crit Care* 10(4): R121, 2006. Available at http://ccforum.com/content/10/4/R121/abstract.

Rader J, Barrick A: Ways that work: bathing without a battle, *Alzheimer Care Q* 1(4):35–49, 2000.

Rader J, Barrick A, Hoeffer B, et al: The bathing of older adults with dementia, *Am J Nurs* 106:40, 2006.

Rader J, Doan J, Schwab M: How to decrease wandering, a form of agenda behavior, *Geriatr Nurs* 6(4):196–199, 1985.

Rader J, Tornquist E: *Individualized dementia care*, New York, 1995, Springer.

Richards K, Lambert C, Beck C: Deriving interventions for challenging behaviors from the need-driven, dementia-compromised behavior model, *Alzheimer Care Q* 1(4):62–76, 2000.

Rigney T: Delirium in the hospitalized elder and recommendations for practice, *Geriatr Nurs* 27(3):151–157, 2006.

Rosenbloom-Brunton D, Henneman E, et al: Feasibility of family participation in a delirium prevention program for hospitalized older adults, *J Gerontol Nurs* 36:22, 2010.

Rowe MA: People with dementia who become lost, *Am J Nurs* 103(7):32–39, 2003.

Rowe MA, Kairalla JA, McCrae CS: Sleep in dementia caregivers and the effects of a nighttime monitoring system, *J Nurs Scholarsh* 42:338, 2010.

Rubin FH, Williams J, Lescisin D, et al: Replicating the Hospital Elder Life Program in a community hospital and demonstrating effectiveness using quality improvement methodology, *J Am Geriatr Soc* 54(6):969–974, 2006.

Schneider LS, Tariot P, Dagerman K, et al: Effectiveness of atypical antipsychotic drugs in patients with Alzheimer's disease, *N Engl J Med* 355(15):1525–1538, 2006.

Segal-Gidan F: *Alzheimer's management from diagnosis to late stage* (2010). Available at www.clinicaladvisor.com/alzheimer's-management-from-diagnosis-to-late-stage/printarticle/173456.

Smith M, Kolanowski A, Buettner L, et al: Beyond bingo: meaningful activities for persons with dementia in nursing homes, *Ann Longterm Care* 17:22, 2009.

Snyder L: The lived experience of Alzheimer's—understanding the feeling and subjective accounts of persons with the disease, *Alzheimers Care Q* 2:8, 2001.

Splete H: Nurses have special strategies for dementia, *Caring for the Ages* 9(6):11, 2008.

Stefanacci R: Evidence-based treatment of behavioral problems in patients with dementia, *Ann Longterm Care* 16(4):33–35, 2008.

Steis M, Fick D: Are nurses recognizing delirium? *J Gerontol Nurs* 34(9):40–48, 2008.

Suwa S: Assessment scale for caregiver experience with dementia, *J Gerontol Nurs* 28 (12):5–12, 2002.

Sweeny S, Bridges S, Wild L, et al: Care of the patient with delirium, *Am J Nurs* 108(5):72CC–72FF, 2008.

Tappen R, Rosselli M, Engstrom G: Evaluation of the functional activities questionnaire (FAQ) in cognitive screening across four American ethnic groups, *Clin Neuropsychol* 24:646, 2010.

Teri L, McKenzie G, LaFazia D, et al: Improving dementia care in assisted living residences: addressing staff reactions to training, *Geriatr Nurs* 30:153, 2008.

Touhy T: Dementia, personhood and nursing: learning from a nursing situation, *Nurs Sci Q* 17(1):43–49, 2004.

Tullmann D, Mion LC, Fletcher K, et al: Delirium: prevention, early recognition, and treatment. In Capezuti E, Swicker D, Mezey M et al, editors: *Evidence-based geriatric nursing protocols for best practice*, ed 3, New York, 2008, Springer.

U.S. Department of Health and Human Services. Office of Disease Prevention and Health Promotion: *Healthy people 2020.* (2012). Available at http://www.healthypeople.gov/2020.

Voelker R: Programs ease hospitalization experience for patients with dementia, *CNS Senior Care* 7(1):3, 17–18, 2008.

Voyer P, Richard S, Doucet L, et al: Examination of the multifactorial model of delirium among long-term care residents with dementia, *Geriatr Nurs* 31:105, 2010.

Waszynski C, Petrovic K: Nurses' evaluation of the confusion assessment method: a pilot study, *J Gerontol Nurs* 34(4):49–56, 2008.

Williams C, Tappen R: Communicating with cognitively impaired persons. In Williams C, editor: *Therapeutic interaction in nursing*, ed 2, Boston, 2008, Jones and Bartlett.

Williams C, Tappen R, Rosselli M, et al: Willingness to be screened and tested for cognitive impairment: cross-cultural comparison, *Am J Alzheimers Dis Other Demen* 26(2):160–166, 2010.

Wilson RS, Hebert LE, Evans DA, et al: Cognitive decline after hospitalization in a community of older persons, *Neurology* Mar 2012. [Epub.]

Witlox J, Eurelings L, deJonghe J, et al: Delirium in elderly patients and the risk of postdischarge mortality, institutionalization, and dementia: a meta-analysis, *JAMA* 304:443, 2010.

Woods B: Dementia challenges assumptions about what it means to be a person, *Generations* 13(3):39, 1999.

CHAPTER 22

Mental Health

Theris A. Touhy

evolve evolve.elsevier.com/Ebersole/gerontological

LEARNING OBJECTIVES

Upon completion of this chapter, the reader will be able to:

- Discuss factors contributing to mental health and wellness in late life.
- List symptoms of late-life anxiety and depression, and discuss assessment, treatment, and nursing responses.
- Recognize elders who are at risk for suicide, and utilize appropriate techniques for suicide assessment and interventions.
- Specify several indications of substance abuse in elders, and discuss appropriate nursing responses.
- Evaluate interventions aimed at promoting mental health and wellness in older adults.

GLOSSARY

Dysthymia At least 2 years of depressed mood for more days than not, accompanied by additional depressive symptoms, but symptoms do not meet the criteria for a major depressive episode.

Hallucination A false sensory perception in the absence of a real stimulus (e.g., hearing voices that no one else can hear).

Idiosyncratic A peculiarity of constitution or temperament: an individualizing characteristic or quality; individual hypersensitivity (as to a drug or food)

Illusion Misinterpretation of a real experience (e.g., thinking a curled rope is a snake).

THE LIVED EXPERIENCE

An older man wrote his philosophy succinctly:

"I have no ideas about what would constitute happiness for anyone else, considering the differences in taste and prefer-ences, and no spate of ideas about improving the lot of the aged. But I am sure that among other things, a calm acceptance of the facts of life is a great help. I consider serenity and peace of mind two of the greatest gifts I have, although I cannot tell you where they come from or how to get them."

(Burnside, 1975)

Mental Health

Mental health is not different in later life, but the level of challenge may be greater. Developmental transitions, life events, physical illness, cognitive impairment, and situations calling for psychic energy may interfere with mental health in older adults. These factors, though not unique to older adults, often influence adaptation. However, anyone who has survived 80 or so years has been exposed to many stressors and crises and has developed tremendous resistance. Most older people face life's challenges with equanimity, good humor, and courage. It is our task to discover the strengths and adaptive mechanisms that will assist them to cope with the challenges.

Evans (2008) notes that most older adults manage the transitions and stresses that may accompany aging with "resilience, hardiness and resourcefulness but those with specific vulnerabilities may develop maladaptive responses and mental illness" (p. 2). Older adults who lack adequate social support or have accumulated stressors, unresolved grief, preexisting psychiatric illness, cognitive impairment, or inadequate coping resources are most vulnerable to mental health problems. Particularly at risk are older adults who have dual risk factors of life transition and loss of social support.

What it means to be mentally healthy is subject to many interpretations and familial and cultural influences (see Chapter 4). Mental health, as with physical health, can be thought of as being on a fluctuating continuum from wellness to illness. Mental health in late life is difficult to define because a lifetime of living results in many variations of personality, coping, and life patterns. One can say what 5-year-olds or 15-year-olds in general are like, but the same is not true for older people. Each individual becomes, the older he or she gets, more uniquely himself or herself.

Autonomy, intimacy, generativity, and integrity are all aspects of mentally healthy adult adaptation (Erikson et al., 1986) (see Chapter 6). Well-being in late life can be predicted by cognitive and affective functioning earlier in life. Thus, it is very important to know the older person's past patterns and life history. Using Maslow's Hierarchy of Needs model (see Chapter 1), the higher one rises in terms of needs met, the more likely one is to be emotionally healthy (self-actualization).

Qualls (2002) offered the following comprehensive definition of mental health in aging: A mentally healthy person is "one who accepts the aging self as an active being, engaging available strengths to compensate for weaknesses in order to create personal meaning, maintain maximum autonomy by mastering the environment, and sustain positive relationships with others" (p. 12).

Including older adults with dementia, nearly 20% of people older than 55 years of age experience mental health disorders that are not part of normal aging, and these figures are expected to rise significantly in the next 25 years with the aging of the population. "The long-term consequences of military conflict and the twentieth century drug culture will add to the burden of psychiatric illnesses" (Kolanowski & Piven, 2006). Prevalence of mental health disorders may be even higher because these disorders are both underreported and not well researched, especially among racially and culturally diverse older people. The numbers of older people with mental illness will soon overwhelm the mental health system.

Mental disorders are associated with increased use of health care resources and overall costs of care (Evans, 2008) and are the leading cause of disability in the United States and Canada (U.S. Department of Health and Human Services [USDHHS], 2012). *Healthy People 2020* (USDHHS, 2012) includes mental health and mental health disorders as a topic area (see the Healthy People box).

 HEALTHY PEOPLE 2020

Mental Health and Mental Disorders (Older Adults)
- Reduce the suicide rate.
- Reduce the proportion of persons who experience major depressive episodes.
- Increase the proportion of primary care facilities that provide mental health treatment onsite or by paid referral.
- Increase the proportion of adults with mental disorders who receive treatment.
- Increase the proportion of persons with co-occurring substance abuse and mental disorders who receive treatment for both disorders.
- Increase depression screening by primary care providers.
- Increase the proportion of homeless adults with mental health problems who receive mental health services.

From U.S. Department of Health and Human Services, Office of Disease Prevention and Health Promotion: *Healthy people 2020* (2012). Available at http://www.healthypeople.gov/2020.

The focus of this chapter is on the differing presentation of mental health disturbances that may occur in older adults, alcohol and substance abuse problems, and the nursing responses important in maintaining the mental health of older adults at the optimum of their capacity. Readers should refer to a comprehensive psychiatric–mental health text for more in-depth discussion of mental health disorders. A discussion of cognitive impairment and the behavioral symptoms that may accompany this disorder is found in Chapter 21.

Factors Influencing Mental Health Care

Attitudes and Beliefs

The rate of utilization of mental health services for elders, even when available, is less than that of any other age group. Estimates are that 63% of older adults with a mental health disorder do not receive the services they need, and only about 3% report seeing mental and behavioral health professionals for treatment (American Psychological Association, 2012). Some of the reasons for this include reluctance on the part of older people to seek help because of pride of independence, stoic acceptance of difficulty, unawareness of resources, and fear of being "put away." Stigma about having a mental health disorder ("being crazy"), particularly for older people, discourages many from seeking treatment. Ageism also affects identification and treatment of mental health disorders in older people.

Symptoms of mental health problems may be looked at as a normal consequence of aging or blamed on dementia by both older people and health care professionals. In older people, the presence of comorbid medical conditions complicates the recognition and diagnosis of mental health disorders. Also, the myth that older people do not respond well to treatment is still prevalent. Other factors—including the lack of knowledge on the part of health care professionals about mental health in late life; inadequate numbers of geropsychiatrists, geropsychologists, and geropsychiatric nurses; and limited availability of geropsychiatric services—present barriers to appropriate diagnosis and treatment.

Settings of Care

Older people receive psychiatric services across a wide range of settings, including acute and long-term inpatient psychiatric units, primary care, and community and institutional settings. Nurses will encounter older adults with mental health disorders in emergency departments or in general medical-surgical units. Admissions for medical problems are often exacerbated by depression, anxiety, cognitive impairment, substance abuse, or chronic mental illness. Medical patients present with psychiatric disorders in 25% to 33% of cases, although they are often unrecognized by primary care providers. Evans (2008) suggests that nurses who can identify mental health problems early and seek consultation and treatment will enhance timely recovery.

Nursing homes and, increasingly, residential care/assisted living facilities (RC/ALs), although not licensed as psychiatric facilities, are providing the majority of care given to older adults with psychiatric conditions. Estimates of the proportion of nursing home residents with a significant mental health disorder range from 65% to 91%, and only about 20% receive treatment from a mental health clinician (Grabowski et al., 2010). Nursing homes are also caring for younger individuals with mental illness, and the number of individuals with mental illness other than dementia has surpassed the number of dementia admissions

(Splete, 2009). It is often difficult to find placement for an older adult with a mental health problem in these types of facilities, and few are structured to provide best practice care to individuals with mental illness. Older adults in home and community settings also experience mental health concerns and inadequate treatment.

Along a range of different measures of quality, the treatment of mental illness in nursing homes and residential care facilities is substandard (Grabowski et al., 2010). Some of the obstacles to mental health care in nursing homes and RC/AL facilities include (1) shortage of trained personnel; (2) limited availability and access for psychiatric services; (3) lack of staff training related to mental health and mental illness; and (4) inadequate Medicaid and Medicare reimbursement for mental health services. An insufficient number of trained personnel affects the quality of mental health care in nursing homes and often causes great stress for staff.

New models of mental health care and services are needed for nursing homes and RC/AL facilities to address the growing needs of older adults in these settings. Suggestions for optimal mental health services in nursing homes include the routine presence of qualified mental health clinicians; an interdisciplinary and multidimensional approach that addresses neuropsychiatric, medical, environmental, and staff issues; and innovative approaches to training and education with consultation and feedback on clinical practices (Grabowski et al., 2010). Training and education of frontline staff who provide basic care to residents is essential. There is an urgent need for well-designed controlled studies to examine mental health concerns in both nursing homes and RC/ALs and the effectiveness of mental health services in improving clinical outcomes.

Cultural and Ethnic Disparities

Lack of knowledge and awareness of cultural differences about the meaning of mental health, differences in the way concerns may become apparent, the lack of culturally sensitive instruments for measuring behavioral outcomes, the lack of culturally competent mental health treatment, and limited research in this area must all be addressed in light of the rapidly increasing numbers of culturally and ethnically diverse older adults (see Chapter 4) (Kolanowski & Piven, 2006). More data are needed on the mental health needs of geriatric and ethnic minority populations, and, in recognition of this need, a follow-up study to the Institute of Medicine's study (IOM, 2008), *Retooling for an Aging America: Building the Health Care Workforce,* will be conducted.

Gerontological nurses must advocate for better and more appropriate treatment of mental health needs for older people and should closely monitor proposals for federal and state revisions to services and budget cuts in this area. Increased attention to the preparation of mental health professionals specializing in geriatric care is important to improve mental health care delivery to older adults (Mellilo et al., 2005). Geropsychiatric nursing is the master's level subspecialty within the adult-psychiatric mental health nursing field. The Geropsychiatric Nursing Collaborative, a project of the American Academy of Nursing funded by the John A. Hartford Foundation, has developed geropsychiatric nursing competency enhancements for entry and advanced practice level education and will be developing a range of training materials and learning tools to improve the current knowledge and skills of nurses in mental health care for older adults (http://hartfordign.org/education/geropsych_nursing_comp/).

Mental Health Disorders

Anxiety Disorders

A general definition of anxiety is unpleasant and unwarranted feelings of apprehension, which may be accompanied by physical symptoms. Anxiety itself is a normal human reaction and part of a fear response; it is rational, within reason. Anxiety becomes problematic when it is prolonged, is exaggerated, and interferes with function.

Anxiety disorders are not considered part of the normal aging process, but the changes and challenges that older adults often face (e.g., chronic illness, cognitive impairment, emotional losses) may contribute to the development of anxiety symptoms and disorders. Many anxious older people have had anxiety disorders earlier in their lives, but late-onset anxiety is not a rare phenomenon. Anxiety disorders that occur in older people include generalized anxiety disorder (GAD), phobic disorder, obsessive-compulsive disorder, panic disorder, and post-traumatic stress disorder (PTSD). Additionally, the high prevalence of comorbid mood-anxiety disorders suggests the importance of further investigation of the modifying influence of anxiety on depression treatment outcomes (Byers et al., 2010).

Prevalence

Epidemiological studies indicate that anxiety disorders are common in older adults; however, relatively few patients are diagnosed with these disorders in clinical practice. The occurrence of anxiety meeting the criteria for a diagnosable disorder ranges from 3.5% to 12% of older people (Flood & Buckwalter, 2009). Anxiety symptoms that may not meet the *Diagnostic and Statistical Manual of Mental Disorders (DSM-IV)* (American Psychiatric Association, 2000) criteria (subthreshold symptoms) are even more prevalent, with estimated rates from 15% to 20% in community samples, with even higher rates in medically ill populations (Ayers et al., 2006).

Older people are less likely to report psychiatric symptoms or acknowledge anxiety, and often attribute their symptoms to physical health problems. Separating a medical condition from the physical symptoms of an anxiety disorder may be difficult. The presence of cognitive impairment also makes diagnosis complicated. It is estimated that 40% to 80% of older people with Alzheimer's disease or related dementias experience anxiety-related symptoms that may be expressed with behavior, such as agitation, irritability, pacing, crying, and repetitive verbalizations (Smith, 2005) (see Chapter 21).

Anxiety is frequently the presenting symptom of depression in older adults, and up to 60% of patients with a major depressive disorder also suffer from an anxiety disorder (Seekles et al., 2009). Anxiety disorders without comorbid depression are also common (Kolanowski & Piven, 2006). Risk factors for anxiety disorders in older people include the following: female, urban living, history of worrying or rumination, poor physical health, low socioeconomic status, high-stress life events, and depression and alcoholism.

Geriatric anxiety is associated with more visits to primary care providers and increased average length of visit. Anxiety symptoms and disorders are associated with many negative consequences including decreased physical activity and functional status, substance abuse, decreased life satisfaction, and increased mortality rates (Ayers et al., 2006; Kolanowski & Piven, 2006; Wetherell et al., 2005). Unidentified or untreated anxiety disorders in older people adversely affect well-being and quality of life.

Implications for Gerontological Nursing and Healthy Aging

Assessment

Data suggest that approximately 70% of all primary care visits are driven by psychological factors (e.g., panic, generalized anxiety, stress, somatization) (American Psychological Association, 2012). This means that nurses often encounter anxious older people and can identify anxiety-related symptoms and initiate assessments that will lead to appropriate treatment and management.

The general and pervasive nature of anxiety may make diagnosis difficult in older adults. In addition, older adults tend to deny the psychological symptoms, attribute anxiety-related symptoms to physical illness, and have coexistent medical conditions that mimic symptoms of anxiety. Some of the medical disorders that cause anxiety include cardiac arrhythmias, delirium, dementia, chronic obstructive pulmonary disease (COPD), heart failure, hyperthyroidism, hypoglycemia, postural hypotension, pulmonary edema, and pulmonary embolism.

Anxiety is also a common side effect of many drugs including anticholinergics, digitalis, theophylline, antihypertensives, beta-blockers, beta-adrenergic stimulators, corticosteroids, and over-the-counter (OTC) medications such as appetite suppressants and cough and cold preparations. Caffeine, nicotine, and withdrawal from alcohol, sedatives, and hypnotics will cause symptoms of anxiety.

Assessment of anxiety in older people focuses on physical, social, and environmental factors, as well as past life history, long-standing personality, coping, and recent events. Older people more often report somatic complaints rather than cognitive symptoms such as excessive worrying. It is important to remember that expressed fears and worries may be realistic or unrealistic, so the nurse must investigate and obtain collateral information from family or caregivers. For example, fear of leaving the home may be related to frequent falling or crime in the neighborhood. Worries about financial stability may be related to the current economic situation or financial abuse by other people.

It is important to investigate other possible causes of anxiety, such as medical conditions and depression. Diagnostic and laboratory tests may be ordered as indicated to rule out medical problems. Cognitive assessment, brain imaging, and neuropsychological evaluation are included if cognitive impairment is suspected (see Chapter 21). When comorbid conditions are present, they must be treated. A review of medications, including OTC and herbal or home remedies, is essential, with elimination of those that cause anxiety.

Interventions

Although further research is needed to provide evidence to guide treatment, existing studies suggest that anxiety disorders in older people can be treated effectively. Treatment choices depend on the symptoms, the specific anxiety diagnosis, comorbid medical conditions, and any current medication regimen. Nonpharmacological interventions are preferred and are often used in conjunction with medication (Smith, 2005).

Pharmacological

Research on the effectiveness of medication in treating anxiety in older people is limited. Age-related changes in pharmacodynamics and issues of polypharmacy make prescribing and monitoring in older people a complex undertaking. Antidepressants in the form of selective serotonin reuptake inhibitors (SSRIs) are usually the first-line treatment. Within this class of drugs, those with sedating rather than stimulating properties are preferred (e.g., citalopram, paroxetine, sertraline, venlafaxine).

Second-line treatment may include short-acting benzodiazepines (alprazolam, lorazepam) or mirtazapine. Treatment with benzodiazepines should be used for short-term therapy only (less than 6 months) and relief of immediate symptoms, but must be used carefully in older adults. Use of older drugs, such as diazepam or chlordiazepoxide, should be avoided because of their long half-lives and the increased risk of accumulation and toxicity in older people. All these medications can have problematic side effects, such as sedation, falls, cognitive impairment, and dependence. Nonbenzodiazepine anxiolytic agents (buspirone) may also be used. Buspirone has fewer side effects but requires a longer period of administration (up to 4 weeks) for effectiveness.

Nonpharmacological

Cognitive behavioral therapy (CBT), psychoeducation, skills training, and relaxation training are modalities utilized for older adults with anxiety disorders or symptoms. CBT is designed to modify thought patterns, improve skills, and alter the environmental states that contribute to anxiety. CBT may involve relaxation training and cognitive restructuring (replacing anxiety-producing thoughts with more realistic, less catastrophic ones), and education about signs and symptoms of anxiety. CBT is effective for older people but may have a lower efficacy than in younger people. Further research is needed to investigate other treatment approaches that may be used to substitute or augment this therapy for older people (Gould et al., 2012; Smith, 2005; Thorp et al., 2009). Interventions for stress management including meditation, yoga, and other therapies are also important in the treatment and management of anxiety in older people.

The therapeutic relationship between the patient and the health care provider is the foundation for any intervention. Family support, referral to community resources, support groups, and sources of educational materials, are other important interventions.

Posttraumatic Stress Disorder

According to the *DSM-IV* (American Psychiatric Association, 2000), PTSD was recognized over 20 years ago as a syndrome characterized by the development of symptoms after an extremely traumatic event that involves witnessing, or unexpectedly hearing about, an actual or threatened death or serious injury to oneself or another closely affiliated person. Individuals often reexperience the traumatic event in episodes of fear and experience symptoms such as helplessness, flashbacks, intrusive thoughts, memories, images, emotional numbing, loss of interest, avoidance of any place that reminds of the traumatic event, poor concentration, irritability, startle reactions, jumpiness, and hypervigilance.

Individuals with PTSD may have ongoing sleep problems, somatic disturbances, anxiety, depression, and restlessness. Older adults with PTSD have high rates of several physical health conditions and poorer physical functioning (Pietrzak et al., 2012). PTSD is fairly common with a lifetime prevalence of 7% to 12% of adults, but prevalence rates among older adults have not been adequately investigated.

In the cohort of Vietnam veterans (now in the "baby boomer" cohort), PTSD prevalence is 15%. The probability of significant increases in future prevalence of PTSD is likely (Kolanowski & Piven, 2006). It occurs increasingly in women. Rape is the most likely specific trauma that will result in PTSD in women, followed by child abuse, being threatened with a weapon, being molested, being neglected as a child, and physical violence. For men, the greatest trauma is also rape, followed by abuse as a child, combat, and being molested.

PTSD has become a part of our national vocabulary and reminds us of the deep and lasting toll that war and natural disasters take. PTSD was first recognized as an outcome of overwhelmingly stressful experiences of individuals in the war in Vietnam and is now a growing concern among Gulf War and Iraq War veterans. Only recently realized is the fact that many World War II veterans have lived most of their lives under the shadow of PTSD without it being recognized.

Seniors in our care now have also experienced the Great Depression, the Holocaust, racism, and the Korean conflict—events that also may precipitate PTSD. Although they may have managed to keep symptoms under control, a person who becomes cognitively impaired may no longer be able to control thoughts, flashbacks, or images. This can be the cause of great distress that may be exhibited by aggressive or hostile behavior. There may be some association between PTSD and a greater incidence and prevalence of dementia, but further research is needed (Qureshi et al., 2010).

Older individuals who are Holocaust survivors may experience PTSD symptoms when they are placed in group settings in institutions. Bludau (2002) described this as the concept of second institutionalization. Older women with a history of rape or abuse as a child may also experience symptoms of PTSD when institutionalized, particularly during the provision of intimate bodily care activities, such as bathing. Box 22-1 provides some clinical examples of PTSD.

BOX 22-1   Clinical Examples of PTSD in Older Adults

Ernie's Story

Ernie may have had PTSD, although it was only speculative after his suicide. On his eighteenth birthday, Ernie joined the U.S. Army Air Corps (precedent to our present U.S. Air Force) in 1941. He was quickly trained and sent to Burma, China, and India. During his 3-year stint, Ernie survived two airplane crashes, saw several of his companions mutilated in crashes, watched the torture of captured Japanese, and witnessed the capture of some of his friends. When Ernie returned to the United States, his hair had turned from deep auburn to pure white. He retired from the service after 20 years but was never really able to work after his retirement.

Ernie's life was filled with episodes of alcoholic binges, outbursts of anger, and episodes of abusing others, all seemingly quite out of his control. One friend remained from his service days and visited him periodically until his death in 1996. Other relationships seemed to have been superficial and to have had little meaning for Ernie. On his seventy-eighth birthday, which he spent alone, Ernie shot himself. One must wonder how many of the elderly veterans of World War II (WWII), the

most highly suicidal group in the United States, are suffering from PTSD.

Jack's Story

An 80-year-old WWII veteran resident with dementia was admitted to a large Veterans Administration (VA) nursing home. Jack's wife told the staff that he had been a high school principal who was very successful in his position. He had recurring frightening dreams throughout his life related to his war experiences and he would always turn off the radio or TV when there were programs about WWII. Now, due to his dementia, he was unable to control his thoughts and feelings. While in the nursing home, he would became very agitated and attempt to hit other residents around him when placed in the large day room. The staff recognized this as a PTSD reaction from his years as a prisoner of war. They always placed him in a smaller day room near the nursing station away from other residents, where he remained calm and pleasant. The aggression stopped without the need for medication.

PTSD, Posttraumatic stress disorder.

Implications for Gerontological Nursing and Healthy Aging

Assessment

PTSD prevention and treatment are only now getting the research attention that other illnesses have received over the years. The care of the individual with PTSD involves awareness that certain events may trigger inappropriate reactions, and the pattern of these reactions should be identified when possible. Knowing the person's history and life experiences is essential in understanding behavior and implementing appropriate interventions. An instrument to assess PTSD can be found in the Evidence-Based Practice box.

Interventions

Effective coping with traumatic events seems to be associated with secure and supportive relationships; the ability to freely express or fully suppress the experience; favorable circumstances immediately following the trauma; productive and active lifestyles; strong faith, religion, and hope; a sense of humor; and biological integrity. Interventions such as CBT, cognitive restructuring, trauma confrontation, prolonged exposure therapy, and age-specific narrative life review approach have produced promising results for individuals with PTSD. However, further research is needed to understand the various presentations of PTSD in late life and validate and improve the effectiveness of available treatment approaches (Bottche et al., 2012; Thorp, 2009). Evidence-based psycho-spiritual interventions may also be effective in the treatment of veterans with PTSD and may be more acceptable among those who have a fear of mental illness–related stigma (Bormann et al., 2008). Medication therapy is also used, and sertraline and paroxetine have U.S. Food and Drug Administration (FDA) approval to treat PTSD.

Obsessive-Compulsive Disorder

Obsessive-compulsive disorder (OCD) is characterized by recurrent and persistent thoughts, impulses, or images (obsessions) that are repetitive and purposeful, and intentional urges of ritualistic behaviors (compulsions) that improve comfort level but are recognized as excessive and unreasonable. OCD is an anxiety disorder that significantly impairs function and consumes more than 1 hour each day (American Psychiatric Association, 2000). Among older adults, symptoms are often not sufficient to seriously disrupt function and thus may not be considered a true disorder but rather a coping strategy. If symptoms progress to a point at which they disrupt function, the elder will need clinical attention. Recommended treatments include exercise and CBT in combination with pharmacological treatment (SSRIs), if indicated.

Psychiatric Symptoms in Older Adults

Paranoid Symptoms

The onset of true psychiatric disorders is low among older adults, but psychotic manifestations may occur as a secondary syndrome in a variety of disorders, the most common being Alzheimer's disease and other dementias, as well as Parkinson's disease. New-onset paranoid symptoms are common among older adults and can present in a number of conditions in late life. Paranoid symptoms can signify an acute change in mental status as a result of a medical illness or delirium, or they can be caused by an underlying affective or primary psychotic mental disorder.

These symptoms can also manifest as a result of behavioral and psychological symptoms of dementia. Paranoia is also an early symptom of Alzheimer's disease, appearing approximately 20 months before diagnosis. Medications,

---

 EVIDENCE-BASED PRACTICE

Mental Health Disorders in Older Adults

Assessment of PTSD:
http://consultgerirn.org/uploads/File/trythis/try_this_19.pdf
Assessment of depression:
http://consultgerirn.org/topics/depression/want_to_know_more
Assessment of suicide risk:
http://consultgerirn.org/topics/depression/need_help_stat/

Assessment of alcohol use:
http://consultgerirn.org/uploads/File/trythis/try_this_17.pdf
Detection of depression in older adults with dementia:
www.guideline.gov/summary.aspx?doc_id=11054&nbr=005833&string=depression+and+dementia

vision and hearing loss, social isolation, alcoholism, depression, the presence of negative life events, financial strain, and PTSD can also be precipitating factors in paranoid symptoms (Chaudhary & Rabheru, 2008).

Delusions

Delusions are beliefs that guide one's interpretation of events and help make sense out of disorder, even though they are inconsistent with reality. The delusions may be comforting or threatening, but they always form a structure for understanding situations that otherwise might seem unmanageable. A delusional disorder is one in which conceivable ideas, without foundation in fact, persist for more than 1 month.

Common delusions of older adults are of being poisoned, of children taking their assets, of being held prisoner, or of being deceived by a spouse or lover. In older adults, delusions often incorporate significant persons rather than the global grandiose or persecutory delusions of younger persons. Fear and a lack of trust originating from a basis in reality may become magnified, especially when one is isolated from others and does not receive reality feedback. Many delusions related to family members and their actions or intentions occur among institutionalized older people. Some may aid in coping, whereas others may be troubling to the person. One study found that 21% of 125 new nursing home residents had delusions (Grossberg, 2000). It is always important to determine if what "appears" to be delusional ideation is, in fact, based in reality.

Hallucinations

Hallucinations are best described as sensory perceptions of a nonexistent object and may be spurred by the internal stimulation of any of the five senses. Although not attributable to environmental stimuli, hallucinations may occur as a combined result of environmental factors. Hallucinations arising from psychotic disorders (e.g., schizophrenia) are less common among older adults, and those that are generated are thought to begin in situations in which one is feeling alone, abandoned, isolated, or alienated.

The character and stages of hallucinatory experiences in late life have not been adequately defined. Many hallucinations are in response to physical disorders, such as dementia, Parkinson's disease, sensory disorders, and medications. Hallucinations of older adults most often seem mixed with disorientation, illusions, intense grief, and immersion in retrospection, the origins being difficult to separate. Older people with hearing and vision deficits may also hear voices or see people and objects that are not actually present (illusions). Some have explained this as the brain's attempt to create stimulation in the absence of adequate sensory input. If illusions or hallucinations are not disturbing to the person, they do not necessitate treatment.

Implications for Gerontological Nursing and Healthy Aging

Assessment

The assessment dilemma is often one of determining if paranoia, delusions, and hallucinations are the result of medical illnesses, medications, dementia, psychoses, deprivation, or overload because the treatment will vary accordingly. Treatment must be based on a comprehensive assessment and a determination of the nature of the psychotic behavior (primary or secondary psychosis) and the time of onset of first symptoms (early or late). Treating the underlying cause of a secondary psychosis caused by medical illnesses, dementia, substance abuse, or delirium is a priority (Mentes & Bail, 2005).

Assessment of vision and hearing is also important since these impairments may predispose the older person to paranoia or suspiciousness. Psychotic symptoms and/or paranoid ideation also present with depression, so depression screening should also be conducted. Assessment of suicide potential is also indicated because individuals experiencing paranoid symptoms are at significant risk for harm to self.

It is never safe to conclude that someone is delusional or paranoid or experiencing hallucinations unless you have thoroughly investigated his or her claims, evaluated physical and cognitive status, and assessed the environment for contributing factors to the behaviors.

Interventions

Frightening hallucinations or delusions, such as feeling that one is being poisoned, usually arise in response to anxiety-provoking situations and are best managed by reducing situational stress, being available to the person, providing a safe, nonjudgmental environment, and attending to the fears more than to the content of the delusion or hallucination. Direct confrontation and arguing is never a useful approach and is likely to increase anxiety and agitation and the sense of vulnerability; it also may disrupt the relationship. A more useful approach is to establish a trusting relationship that is nondemanding and not too intense.

It is important to identify the client's strengths and build on them. Demonstrating respect and a willingness to listen to complaints and fears is important and the basis for a caring nurse-patient relationship. It is important that the nurse be trustworthy, give clear information, and present clear choices. Do not pretend to agree with paranoid beliefs or delusions, but rather ask what is troubling to the person and provide reassurance of safety. It is important to try to understand the person's level of distress as well as how he or she is experiencing what is troubling. For institutionalized older people, other suggestions are to avoid television, which can be confusing, especially if the person awakens and finds it on or has a hearing or vision impairment. In addition, reduce clutter in the person's room and eliminate shadows that can appear threatening. Provide glasses and hearing aids to maximize sensory input and decrease misinterpretations.

If symptoms are interfering with function and interpersonal and environmental strategies are not effective, antipsychotic drugs may be used. The newer atypical antipsychotics (risperidone, olanzapine) are preferred but must be used judiciously, with careful attention to side effects and monitoring of response. In the case of depression with psychotic features, combination therapy with an antidepressant and an atypical antipsychotic agent may be useful.

In cognitively impaired individuals with paranoid ideation, there is some evidence suggesting that treatment with cognitive enhancer medications (cholinesterase inhibitors and memantine) may be of benefit. If symptoms interfere with function and safety, and nonpharmacological interventions are not effective, antipsychotic medications may be used. However, none of the antipsychotic medications are approved for use in treatment of behavioral responses in dementia. The benefits are uncertain, and adverse effects offset any advantages (Schneider et al., 2006).

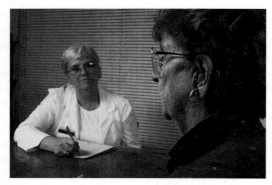

Demonstrating respect and a willingness to listen is the foundation for a caring nurse-patient relationship. (From Harkreader H, Hogan MA: *Fundamentals of nursing: caring and clinical judgment*, ed 3, St. Louis, 2007, Saunders.)

Psychoeducation, individual or group therapy, environmental and behavioral modification strategies, and supportive environments are also important treatment considerations. The presence of these symptoms contributes to caregiver burden and stress, and they are often precipitating factors to institutionalization, so caregiver support and utilization of community resources is important. See Chapter 21 for further discussion of behavior and psychological symptoms in dementia and nonpharmacological interventions.

Schizophrenia

Schizophrenia is a severe mental disorder characterized by two or more of the following symptoms: delusions, hallucinations, disorganized thinking, disorganized or catatonic behavior (called positive symptoms) and affective flattening, poverty of speech, or apathy (called negative symptoms) that cause significant social or occupational dysfunction, and are not accompanied by prominent mood symptoms or substance abuse or can be attributed to medical causes (American Psychiatric Association, 2000). The diagnostic criteria for schizophrenia are the same across the life span.

People with schizophrenia are the largest group of older people with severe mental health problems, and the numbers are expected to grow over the next decade with the increased longevity of the population. As Evans (2008) notes: "Persons living with mental illness also grow old and the changes associated with aging may further compromise a lifetime of challenged coping, thus exacerbating symptomatology and well-being" (p. 2). Although the onset of schizophrenia usually occurs between adolescence and the mid-30s, it can extend into and first appear in late life. However, 85% of older people with schizophrenia were diagnosed before age 45 (Berry & Barrowclough, 2009).

Prevalence of schizophrenia in older people is estimated to be approximately 0.6%—about half of the prevalence in younger adults. Distinction is made between early-onset schizophrenia (EOS), occurring before age 40; midlife onset (MOS), between ages 40 and 60; and late onset schizophrenia (LOS), after age 60. There is some suggestion that there may be neurobiologic differences between EOS and LOS, and further investigation is needed.

Patients with LOS are more likely to be women, and paranoia is the dominant feature of the illness. They tend to have a greater prevalence of visual hallucinations, less prevalence of a formal thought disorder, fewer negative symptoms, and less family history of schizophrenia. Women with LOS are also at greater risk for tardive dyskinesia, have less impairment in the areas of learning and abstraction, and require lower doses of neuroleptic medications for symptom management (Smith, 2005). Individuals with EOS who have grown older may experience fewer hallucinations, delusions, and bizarre behavior as well as inappropriate affect. Positive symptoms may wane, whereas negative symptoms tend to persist into late life (Mentes & Bail, 2005).

Implications for Gerontological Nursing and Healthy Aging

Interventions

Treatment for schizophrenia includes both medications and environmental interventions. Conventional neuroleptic medications (e.g., haloperidol) have been effective in managing the positive symptoms but are problematic in older people and carry a high risk of disabling and persistent side effects, such as tardive dyskinesia (TD). The Abnormal Involuntary Movement Scale (AIMS) is useful for evaluating early symptoms of TD. The newer atypical antipsychotic medications (e.g., risperidone, olanzapine, quetiapine), given in low doses, are associated with a lower risk of extrapyramidal symptoms (EPS) and TD. Federal guidelines for the use of antipsychotic medications in nursing homes provide the indications for use of these medications in schizophrenia. Other important interventions include a combination of support, education, physical activity, and CBT.

Families of older people with schizophrenia experience the burden of caring for a family member with a chronic disability as well as dealing with their own personal aging. Community-based support services are needed that include assistance with housing, medical care, recreation services, and services that help the family plan for the future of their relative. There are relatively few services in the community for older persons with schizophrenia. The National Alliance for the Mentally Ill (NAMI) (www.nami.org) is an important resource for clients and their families (Mentes & Bail, 2005).

Individuals with severe persistent mental illnesses such as schizophrenia form a disenfranchised group whose access to medical care has been limited, leading to greater functional declines, morbidity, and mortality (Davis, 2004). Schizophrenia is a costly disease both in terms of personal suffering and medical care costs. An estimated 41% of older people with schizophrenia now reside in nursing homes

(Leutwyler & Wallhagen, 2010). Interventions to improve independent functioning irrespective of age and in conjunction with community services would decrease the expenses associated with institutionalization (Madhusoodanan & Brenner, 2007, p. 30).

Bipolar Disorder

Bipolar disorder is not common in late life, but recurrence of remitted disease does occur. It is anticipated that with the growing number of older people, more cases will be seen. Ten percent of inpatient psychiatric admissions among older adults are for bipolar disorder. The disease occurs more often among individuals 60 to 64 years of age, with a declining incidence in older cohorts (Sherrod et al., 2010). Bipolar disorders, characterized by periods of mania and depression, often level out in late life, and individuals tend to have longer periods of depression. Mania is a more frequent cause of hospitalization than depression, but depression may account for more disability. Similar to other psychiatric disorders in older adults, comorbidities often mask the presence of the disorder and it is frequently misdiagnosed, underdiagnosed, and undertreated (Kennedy, 2008).

Implications for Gerontological Nursing and Healthy Aging

Assessment

Assessment includes a thorough physical examination and laboratory and radiological testing to rule out physical causes of the symptoms and identify comorbidities. A medication review should be conducted since symptoms can be a side effect of medications such as antidepressants, benzodiazepines, amphetamines, prednisone, and captopril. Obtaining an accurate history from the individual, as well as the family, is important and should include assessment of symptoms associated with depression, mania, hypomania, and a family history of bipolar disorder.

The genetic basis of the disease is being investigated, and two genes that influence the activity of nerve cells in the brain may play a key role in an individual's risk for bipolar disorder. Sherrod and colleagues (2010) provide two algorithms for the appropriate diagnosis and management of bipolar disorder, and the National Institute of Mental Health (NIMH) provides comprehensive information on the diagnosis and treatment of bipolar disorder (www.nimh.nih.gov/health/publications/bipolar-disorder/complete-index.shtml).

Interventions

Lithium, the most commonly used substance for individuals with bipolar disorders, has neurological effects that make it difficult for older people to tolerate; it also has a long half-life (more than 36 hours). Careful monitoring of blood levels and patient response is important. Recommended treatment consists of a combination of one or more mood stabilizers (e.g., lithium, valproic acid, carbamazepine, lamotrigine). If the patient does not respond to these medications, atypical antipsychotic drugs are possible alternative treatments, but with the same safety warnings discussed earlier and are not to be used if dementia is suspected. Olanzapine, aripiprazole, and seroquel are all approved for the treatment of bipolar disorder and may relieve symptoms of severe mania and psychosis (see www.nimh.nih.gov/publications/bipolar-disorder/complete-index.shtml). Electroconvulsive therapy (ECT) may also be used when medication and/or psychotherapy are not effective.

Patient and family education and support are essential, and the family must understand that the individual is not able to control mania and irritating behaviors because of a chemical imbalance in the brain. Treatment with medication and intensive psychotherapy, CBT interpersonal and rhythm therapy (improving relationships with others and managing regular daily routines), or family-focused therapy has been reported to be effective in decreasing relapses, preventing hospitalization, and improving adherence to treatment plans (National Institute of Mental Health [NIMH], 2009).

Depression

Depression is not a normal part of aging, and studies show that most older people are satisfied with their lives, despite physical problems. To understand depression, the nurse must understand the influence of late-life stressors and changes, culture, and the beliefs older people, society, and health professionals may have about depression and its treatment.

Prevalence and Consequences

Depression is the most common mental health problem of late life and among the most treatable, but it can be life-threatening if unrecognized and untreated. The prevalence of major depression in older adults (1% to 5%) is somewhat lower than that in the general population, but minor depression and depressive symptoms are experienced by a large number of older people (Evans, 2008). One in 10 older adults visiting a physician suffers from depression (see http://impact-uw.org/).

Estimates of prevalence vary widely depending on the qualitative variables being considered and the definition being used. The prevalence of major depression in home care recipients ranges from 12% to 26%, but depressive symptoms are present in as many as 57% of this population. Among homebound older adults, two thirds with clinically significant depression had not received treatment (Sirey et al., 2008). For older adults in nursing homes, the prevalence of depressive symptoms may be as high as 54%, and a recent study reported that 23% were not treated and only 2.5% received some form of behavioral therapy. Depression is a major reason why older people are admitted to nursing homes (Kurlowicz & Harvath, 2008a; Morley, 2010).

Depression and illness are likely to co-occur. Becoming sick doubles the probability of becoming depressed, and becoming depressed doubles the probability of becoming sick (Thielke et al., 2010). More than 15% of older adults with chronic physical conditions are depressed, and depression has been called "the unwanted cotraveler" accompanying many medical illnesses (Byrd, 2005, p. 132). Many medications that older people may take can also cause depression.

Depression is a major source of morbidity in older adults (Heller et al., 2010). Depression and depressive symptomatology are associated with negative consequences such as increased disability, delayed recovery from illness and surgery, excess use of health services, cognitive impairment, malnutrition, decreased quality of life, and increased suicide and non–suicide-related death (Evans, 2008; Kurlowicz & Harvath, 2008b). Depression remains underdiagnosed and undertreated, and major depressive disorder (MDD) is undiagnosed in approximately half of older persons with this disorder (Das et al., 2007).

The stigma associated with depression may be more prevalent in older people, and they may not acknowledge depressive symptoms or seek treatment. Many elders, particularly those who have survived the Great Depression, both world wars, the Holocaust, and other tragedies, may see depression as shameful, evidence of flawed character, self-centered, a spiritual weakness, and sin or retribution.

Health professionals often expect older people to be depressed and may not take appropriate action to assess for and treat depression. The differing presentation of depression in older people, as well as the increased prevalence of medical problems that may cause depressive symptoms, also contributes to inadequate recognition and treatment. Even if depression is identified, only about one half of Americans diagnosed with a major depression receive treatment for it, and even fewer, about one fifth, receive treatment consistent with current guidelines (Gonzalez et al., 2010).

Ethnic and Cultural Considerations

Depression diagnosis and treatment is an even greater concern for ethnically and culturally diverse elders. African Americans and African Caribbeans who experience a major depressive episode are more likely to be untreated, and they experience more disabling effects than non-Hispanic whites. Mexican-American and African-American individuals with depression have the lowest rates of depression care and treatment in accordance with accepted guidelines (Gonzalez et al., 2010). Nursing home patients who are female, black, or cognitively impaired are less likely to receive treatment for depression (Byrd, 2005; Kurlowicz & Harvath, 2008a).

Failure to treat depression increases morbidity and mortality. There is no evidence that current evidence-based treatments for geriatric depression, such as psychotherapy, psychosocial interventions, and medications, are any less effective as people age (Kurlowicz & Harvath, 2008a; Thielke et al., 2010). It is highly likely that nurses will encounter a large number of older people with depressive symptoms in all settings. Recognizing depression and enhancing access to appropriate mental health care are important nursing roles to improve outcomes for older people.

Etiology

The causes of depression in older adults are complex and must be examined in a biopsychosocial framework. Factors of health, gender, developmental needs, socioeconomics, environment, personality, losses, and functional decline are all significant to the development of depression in later life. Biologic causes, such as neurotransmitter imbalances or dysregulation of endocrine function, have also been proposed as factors influencing the development of depression in late life (Kurlowicz & Harvath, 2008a).

Some of the medical disorders that cause depression are cancers; cardiovascular disorders; endocrine disorders, such as thyroid problems and diabetes; neurological disorders, such as Alzheimer's disease, stroke, and Parkinson's disease; metabolic and nutritional disorders, such as vitamin B_{12} deficiency and malnutrition; viral infections, such as herpes zoster and hepatitis; and advanced macular degeneration. Among patients who have suffered a cerebral vascular accident, the incidence of major depressive disorder is approximately 25%, with rates being close to 40% in patients with Parkinson's disease (Das et al., 2007). Vascular depression is a term being used to describe a late-life depression associated with vascular changes in the brain and characterized by executive dysfunction (Thakur & Blazer, 2008).

Serious symptoms of depression occur in up to 50% of older adults with Alzheimer's disease and are associated with increased mortality, reduced quality of life, increase in caregiver burden and distress, and higher rates of institutionalization (Chang & Roberts, 2011; Gellis et al., 2009). Depression in individuals with Alzheimer's disease may be due to an awareness of progressive decline, but research suggests that there may be a biological connection between depression and Alzheimer's disease as well (Friedman et al., 2009; Kurlowicz & Harvath, 2008a; Morley, 2010).

Medications may also result in depressive symptoms including hypertensives, angiotensin-converting enzyme (ACE) inhibitors, methyldopa, reserpine, guanethidine, antidysrhythmics, anticholesteremics, antibiotics, analgesics, corticosteroids, digoxin, and L-dopa (Kurlowicz & Harvath, 2008b).

Other important factors influencing the development of depression are alcohol abuse, loss of a spouse or partner, loss of social supports, lower income level, caregiver stress (particularly caring for a person with dementia), and gender. Some psychological traits, such as neuroticism, pessimistic thinking, and being less open to new experiences, have been found to be associated with higher rates of depression and suicide (Das et al., 2007). Some common risk factors for depression are presented in Box 22-2.

Differing Presentation of Depression in Elders

The *DSM-IV* (American Psychiatric Association, 2000) provides criteria for the diagnosis of major depression, dysthymia, and minor (subsyndromal) depression. Depression can be considered a syndrome consisting of an array of affective, cognitive, and somatic or physiological symptoms. Depression may range in severity from mild symptoms to more severe forms, both of which can persist over long periods. Suicidal ideation and psychotic features (delusional thinking) accompany more severe depression (Kurlowicz & Harvath, 2008a).

Symptoms of depression are different in older people. Older people who are depressed report more somatic complaints, such as physical symptoms, insomnia, loss of appetite and weight loss, memory loss, or chronic pain. Somatic complaints may be even more prominent in individuals with limited education and no previous psychiatric history. The somatic complaints "are often difficult to distinguish from the physical symptoms associated with chronic physical

---

BOX 22-2 Risk Factors for Depression in Older Adults

- Chronic medical illnesses, disability, functional decline
- Alzheimer's disease and other dementias
- Bereavement
- Caregiving
- Female (2:1 risk)
- Lower SES
- Family history of depression
- Previous episode of depression

- Admission to long-term care or other change in environment
- Medications
- Alcohol or substance abuse
- Living alone
- Widowhood
- New stressful losses, including loss of autonomy; loss of privacy; loss of functional status; loss of independence; loss of body part; loss of family member, roommate, or pet

---

SES, Socioeconomic status.

illness" (Kurlowicz & Harvath, 2008a, p. 59). Hypochondriasis is also common, as are constant complaining and criticism, which may actually be expressions of depression.

Decreased energy and motivation, lack of ability to experience pleasure, hopelessness, increased dependency, poor grooming and difficulty completing activities of daily living (ADLs), withdrawal from people or activities enjoyed in the past, decreased sexual interest, and a preoccupation with death or "giving up" are also signs of depression in older people. Feelings of guilt and worthlessness, seen in younger depressed individuals, are less frequently seen in older people. Patients with late-life depression are also less likely to have a family history of depression than younger individuals (Das et al., 2007).

Individuals often present with complaints of memory problems, the "so-called pseudodementia (the dementia syndrome of depression) in which the patient has a memory loss and functional decline but of a generally more recent and abrupt onset than the more common progressive dementias. It is essential to differentiate between dementia and depression, and older people with memory impairment should be evaluated for depression. Symptoms such as agitated behavior and repetitive verbalizations in persons with dementia may be a symptom of depression (see Chapter 21). The Evidence-Based Practice box on page 344 presents evidence-based protocols for depression.

Implications for Gerontological Nursing and Healthy Aging

Assessment

Assessment involves a systematic and thorough evaluation using a depression screening instrument, interview, history and physical, functional assessment, cognitive assessment,

laboratory tests, medication review, determination of iatrogenic or medical causes, and family interview as indicated. Assessment for depressogenic medications and for related comorbid physical conditions that may contribute to or complicate treatment of depression must also be included.

Screening of all older adults for depression should be incorporated into routine health assessments across the continuum of care—in hospitals, primary care, long-term care, home care, and community-based settings (Kolanowski & Piven, 2006; Kurlowicz & Harvath, 2008a). The Geriatric Depression Scale (GDS) was developed specifically for screening older adults and has been tested extensively in a number of settings (Table 22-1).

The Center for Epidemiological Studies Depression Scale (CES-D) was developed for use in studies of depression with community samples and is frequently used in research. The Cornell Scale for Depression in Dementia (CSDD) was designed to identify major depressive disorders in persons who may have dementia. Since some persons with dementia can participate in the assessment, the person is first interviewed followed by an interview with an informant who knows the person's daily functioning. Interview results are corroborated by skilled observation. There are ample sources for this tool available on the Internet with a simple search for "Cornell Scale."

Interventions

If depression is diagnosed, treatment should begin as soon as possible, and appropriate follow-up should be provided. Depressed people are usually unable to follow through on their own, and without appropriate treatment and monitoring may be candidates for deeper depression or suicide. The most effective treatment is a combination of pharmacological therapy and psychotherapy or counseling. However,

TABLE 22-1	Geriatric Depression Scale (Short Form)		
Are you basically satisfied with your life?		Yes	No*
Have you dropped many of your activities and interests?		Yes*	No
Do you feel that your life is empty?		Yes*	No
Do you often get bored?		Yes*	No
Are you in good spirits most of the time?		Yes	No*
Are you afraid that something bad is going to happen to you?		Yes*	No
Do you feel happy most of the time?		Yes	No*
Do you often feel helpless?		Yes*	No
Do you prefer to stay at home, rather than going out and doing new things?		Yes*	No
Do you feel you have more problems with memory than most?		Yes*	No
Do you think it is wonderful to be alive?		Yes	No*
Do you feel pretty worthless the way you are now?		Yes*	No
Do you feel full of energy?		Yes	No*
Do you feel that your situation is hopeless?		Yes*	No
Do you think that most people are better off than you?		Yes*	No

*Each answer indicated by an asterisk counts as 1 point. Scores between 5 and 9 suggest depression; scores above 9 generally indicate depression.
From Yesavage J, Brink TL, Rose TL, et al: Development and validation of a Geriatric Depression Screening Scale: a preliminary report, *J Psychiatr Res* 17:37, 1982-1983.

as Morley (2010) noted, "behavioral interventions are at present underused and pharmaceutical approaches are overused" (p. 302). Interventions are individualized and are based on history, severity of symptoms, concomitant illnesses, and level of disability.

Generally, a stepped-care approach is recommended in which there are separate pathways for the management of mild to moderate and severe depression and the sequential application of different types of treatment, followed by monitoring progress and modifying treatment as indicated. Treatment for individuals with mild to moderate depression may involve self-help, counseling, and physical exercise. For those with severe depression, treatment would include antidepressants and psychotherapy (Seekles et al., 2009).

An interdisciplinary approach, collaborative models of care, clinic-based care, care management, and home-based depression care have all shown successful outcomes and lowered costs of care (USDHHS, 2012; Unützer et al., 2008). Many of these models involve nurses and services provided by psychiatric–mental health clinical nurse specialists in primary, home, and long-term care. Such models may be particularly effective in improving outcomes for depressed individuals and are well received by patients (Saur, et al., 2007; Morley, 2010).

Family and social support, education, grief management, exercise, humor, spirituality, CBT, brief psychodynamic therapy, interpersonal therapy, and problem-solving therapy have all been noted to be helpful in depression. Results of a recent study (Lavretsky et al., 2011) suggest that complementary use of a mind-body exercise, such as T'ai Chi Chih may provide additional improvements of clinical outcome in the pharmocological treatment of geriatric depression.

Reminiscence and Life Review

Reminiscence and life review therapy are other important therapeutic interventions that nurses can utilize in their work with older people who are depressed. Reminiscence can have many goals. It not only provides a pleasurable experience that improves quality of life, but also increases socialization and connectedness with others, provides cognitive stimulation, improves communication, and can significantly decrease depression scores (Haight & Burnside, 1993; Grabowski et al., 2010). The process of reminiscence can occur in individual conversations with older people, be structured as in a nursing history, or can occur in a group where each person shares his or her memories and listens to others sharing theirs. The nurse can learn much about a resident's history, communication style, relationships, coping mechanisms, strengths, fears, affect, and adaptive capacity by listening thoughtfully as the life story is constructed.

The work of several gerontological nursing leaders, including Irene Burnside, Priscilla Ebersole, and Barbara Haight, has contributed to the body of knowledge about reminiscence and its importance in nursing. The International Institute for Reminiscence and Life Review (University of Wisconsin, Superior, WI; www.reminiscenceandlifereview.org/), an interdisciplinary organization bringing together participants to study reminiscence and life review, is another valuable resource for nurses and members of other disciplines involved in research or practice. Box 22-3 provides some suggestions for encouraging reminiscence.

Life review was first noted and brought to public attention by Robert Butler (1963). Life review is a process that normally occurs in the older person as the realization of his or her approaching death creates a resurgence of unresolved conflicts. Life review occurs quite naturally for many persons during periods of crisis and transition. However, Butler (2002) noted that in old age, the process of putting one's life in order increases in intensity and emphasis. Life review occurs most frequently as an internal review of memories, an intensely private, soul-searching activity.

Life review is considered more of a formal therapy technique than reminiscence and takes a person through his or her life in a structured and chronological order. Life review therapy (Butler & Lewis, 1983), guided autobiography (Birren & Deutchman, 1991), and structured life review (Haight & Webster, 2002) are psychotherapeutic techniques based on the concept of life review.

BOX 22-3   Suggestions for Encouraging Reminiscence

- Listen without correction or criticism. Older adults are presenting their version of their reality; our version belongs to another generation.
- Encourage older adults to cover various ages and stages. Use questions such as "What was it like growing up on that farm?" "What did teenagers do for fun when you were young?" "What was WWII like for you?"
- Be patient with repetition. Sometimes people need to tell the same story often to come to terms with the experience, especially if it was meaningful to them. If they have a memory loss, it may be the only story they can remember, and it is important for them to be able to share it with others.
- Be attuned to signs of depression in conversation (dwelling on sad topics) or changes in physical status or behavior, and provide appropriate assessment and intervention.
- If a topic arises that the person does not want to discuss, change to another topic.
- If individuals are reluctant to share because they don't feel their life was interesting, reassure them that everyone's life is valuable and interesting and tell them how important their memories are to you and others.
- Keep in mind that reminiscing is not an orderly process. One memory triggers another in a way that may not seem related; it is not important to keep things in order or verify accuracy.
- Keep the conversation focused on the person reminiscing, but do not hesitate to share some of your own memories that relate to the situation being discussed. Participate as equals, and enjoy each other's contributions.

- Listen actively, maintain eye contact, and do not interrupt.
- Respond positively and give feedback by making caring, appropriate comments that encourage the person to continue.
- Use props and triggers such as photographs, memorabilia (e.g., a childhood toy or antique), short stories or poems about the past, and favorite foods.
- Use open-ended questions to encourage reminiscing. If working with a group, you can prepare questions ahead of time, or you can ask the group members to pick a topic that interests them. One question or topic may be enough for an entire group session.
- Consider using questions such as the following:
  How did your parents meet?
  What do you remember most about your mother? father? grandmother? grandfather?
  What are some of your favorite memories from childhood?
  What was the first house you remember?
  What were your favorite foods as a child?
  Did you have a pet as a child?
  Tell us about your first job?
  How did you celebrate birthdays or other holidays?
  If you were married, tell us about your wedding day.
  What was your greatest accomplishment or joy in your life?
  What advice did your parents give you? What advice did you give your children? What advice would you give to young people today?

Gerontological nurses participate with older adults in both reminiscence and life review, and it is important to acquire the skills to be effective in achieving the purposes of both. The most exciting aspect of working with older adults is being a part of the emergence of the life story: the shifting and blending patterns. When we are young, it is important for our emotional health and growth to look forward and plan for the future. As one ages, it becomes more important to look back, talk over experiences, review and make sense of it all, and end with a feeling of satisfaction with the life lived. This is important work and the major developmental task of older adulthood that Erik Erikson called *ego integrity versus despair* (see Chapter 6). Life review may be especially important for older people experiencing depressive symptoms and those facing death (Pot et al., 2010). The Hospice Foundation of America provides *A Guide for Recalling and Telling Your Life Story* (http://store. hospicefoundation.org/home.php?cat=5) that nurses and families may find helpful.

Life review should occur not only when we are old or facing death but also frequently throughout our lives. This process can assist us to examine where we are in life and change our course or set new goals. Butler (2002) commented that one might avoid the overwhelming feelings of despair that may surface when there is no time left to make changes if life review had been conducted throughout one's life. Box 22-4 presents additional suggestions for families and professionals caring for older adults with depression.

Medications

There are more than 20 antidepressants approved by the FDA for the treatment of depression in older adults. The most commonly prescribed are the SSRIs. These agents work selectively on neurotransmitters in the brain to alleviate depression. The SSRIs are generally well tolerated in older people. Common side effects include nausea, vomiting, dizziness, drowsiness, and hyponatremia. Choice of medication depends on comorbidities, drug side effects, and the type of effect desired. People with agitated depression and sleep disturbances may benefit from medications with a more sedating effect, whereas those who are not eating may do better taking medications that have an appetite-stimulating effect. If depression is immobilizing, psychostimulants may be used.

Medications must be closely monitored for side effects and therapeutic response. Side effects can be especially problematic for older people with comorbid conditions and complex drug regimens. It is important to carefully look for drug interactions and monitor for side effects when starting antidepressant medications. There are a wide range of antidepressant medications, and several may have to be evaluated. As with other medications for older people, doses should be lower at first and titrated as indicated while adequate treatment effect is ensured (Kurlowicz & Harvath, 2008b).

More severe depression complicated by psychosis or suicidal intent may necessitate lifelong medication therapy. Often, older people may be resistant to take medication for depression, and it is helpful to stress that while there may be

---

BOX 22-4   Interpersonal Support by Family and Professionals

- Provide relief from discomfort of physical illness.
- Enhance physical function (i.e., regular exercise and/or activity; physical, occupational, recreational therapies).
- Develop a daily activity schedule that includes pleasant activities.
- Increase opportunities for socialization and enhance social support.
- Provide opportunities for decision making and the exercise of control.
- Focus on spiritual renewal and rediscovery of meanings.
- Reactivate latent interests, or develop new ones.
- Validate depressed feelings as aiding recovery; do not try to bolster the person's mood or deny his or her despair.

- Help the person become aware of the presence of depression, the nature of the symptoms, and the time limitation of depression.
- Provide an accepting atmosphere and an empathic response.
- Share yourself.
- Demonstrate faith in the person's strengths.
- Praise any and all efforts at recovery, no matter how small.
- Assist in expressing and dealing with anger.
- Do not stifle the grief process; grief cannot be hurried.
- Create a hopeful environment in which self-esteem is fostered and life is meaningful.
- Assist in dealing with guilt, real or neurotic.
- Foster development of connections with others.

circumstances precipitating the depression, the final effect is a biochemical one that medications can correct (Ham et al., 2007).

ECT is considered an excellent, safe therapy for older people with depression that is resistant to other treatments and for patients at risk for serious harm because of psychotic depression, suicidal ideation, or severe malnutrition, with efficacy rates ranging from 60% to 80% (Morley, 2010; Unützer, 2007). ECT is much improved, but older people will need a careful explanation of the treatment since they may have many misconceptions.

Suicide

Elders compose only 13% of the U.S. population but account for 20% of the suicide deaths. The rate of suicide among older adults is higher than that for any other age group—and the suicide rate for persons 85 years of age and older is the highest of all—twice the overall national rate (Edelstein et al., 2009). Older non-Hispanic white men with mild depressive disorder are five times more likely to commit suicide than the general population (Das et al., 2007). Widowers are thought to be the most vulnerable because they often depended on their wives to maintain the comforts of home and the social network of family and friends. Despite these alarming statistics, there is little research on suicidal ideation and behavior among older adults. Suicide rates are increasing among middle-aged people and high rates of substance abuse and the onset of chronic illness are among the possible factors in this rising suicide rate (Phillips et al., 2010).

In most cases, depression and other mental health problems, including anxiety, contribute significantly to suicide risk. Eighty percent of suicides are related to depression (Das et al., 2007). Common precipitants of suicide include physical or mental illness, death of a spouse or partner, substance abuse, and pathological relationships. Suicide may have some familial tendencies, with estimates that a suicide of one parent in the family is associated with a six-fold increase of suicide in the children (Kennedy, 2008). One of the major differences in suicidal behavior in the old and the young is lethality of method. Eight out of 10 suicides for men older than 65 years of age were with firearms. Older people rarely threaten to commit suicide, they just do it.

Over 70 percent of older suicide victims visit their primary care physician within the month of their death (NIMH, 2009). Older people with suicidal ideation, or with other mental health concerns, often present with somatic complaints. The statistics suggest that opportunities

for assessment of suicidal risk are present, but the need for intervention is not seen as urgent or not even recognized. Consequently, it is very important for providers in all settings to inquire about recent life events, implement depression screening for all older people, evaluate for anxiety disorders, assess for suicidal thoughts and ideas based on depression assessment, and recognize warning signs and risk factors for suicide. Behavioral clues and risk and recovery factors are presented in Box 22-5.

Implications for Gerontological Nursing and Healthy Aging

Assessment

Older people with suicidal intent are encountered in many settings. It is our professional obligation to prevent, whenever possible, an impulsive destruction of life that may be a response to a crisis or a disintegrative reaction. The lethality potential of an elder must always be assessed when elements of depression, disease, and spousal loss are evident. Any direct, indirect, or enigmatic references to the ending of life must be taken seriously and discussed with the elder.

The most important consideration for the nurse is to establish a trusting and respectful relationship with the person. Since many older people have grown up in an era when suicide bore stigma and even criminal implications, they may not discuss their feelings in this area. The stigma related to mental illness also affects older people's willingness to share their feelings of sadness or anxiety. It is also important to remember that in older people, typical behavioral clues such as putting personal affairs in order, giving away possessions, and making wills and funeral plans are indications of maturity and good judgment in late life and cannot be construed as indicative of suicidal intent. Even statements such as "I won't be around long" or "I'm ready to die" may be only a realistic appraisal of the situation in old age.

If there is suspicion that the elder is suicidal, use direct and straightforward questions such as the following:

- Have you ever thought about killing yourself?
- How often have you had these thoughts?
- How would you kill yourself if you decided to do it?

Interventions

It is important to have a suicide protocol in place that clearly defines how the nurse will intervene if a positive response is obtained from any of the questions. The person

BOX 22-5   Suicide Risk and Recovery Factors

Risk Factors and Warning Signs

Male gender
Physical illness
Functional impairment
Depression
Alcohol and substance misuse and abuse
Major loss, such as the death of a spouse or partner
History of major losses
Recent suicide attempt
History of suicide attempts
Major crises or transitions, such as retirement or relocation
    to an assisted living or nursing facility
Major crises in the lives of family members
Social isolation
Preoccupation with death
Poorly controlled pain
Expression of the belief that one is in the way, a burden
Giving away favorite possessions, money

Recovery Factors

A capacity for the following:
    Understanding
    Relating
    Benefiting from experience
    Benefiting from knowledge
    Accepting help
    Being loving
    Expressing wisdom
    Displaying a sense of humor
    Having a social interest
    Accepting a caring and available family
    Accepting a caring and available social network
    Accepting a caring, available, and knowledgeable
        professional and health network

---

should never be left alone for any period of time until help arrives to assist and care for them. Patients at high risk should be hospitalized, especially if they have current psychological stressors and/or access to lethal means. Patients at moderate risk may be treated as outpatients provided they have adequate social support and no access to lethal means. Patients at low risk should have a full psychiatric evaluation and be followed up carefully (Das et al., 2007). The Evidence-Based Practice box on page 344 presents a protocol for suicide risk assessment. A toolkit for senior living communities for promotion of mental health and prevention of suicide is available at http://store.samhsa.gov/products/sma-4515.

Suicide is a taboo topic for most of us, and there is a lingering fear that the introduction of the topic will be suggestive to the patient and may incite suicidal action. Precisely the opposite is true. By introducing the topic, we demonstrate interest in the individual and open the door to honest human interaction and connection on the deep levels of psychological need. It is the nature of our concern and our ability to connect with the alienation and desperation of the individual that will make a difference. Working with isolated, depressed, and suicidal elders challenges the depths of nurses' ingenuity, patience, and self-knowledge.

Substance Misuse and Alcohol Use Disorders

Alcohol

Substance abuse often arises in old age as a coping mechanism to deal with loss, anxiety, depression, boredom, or pain associated with chronic illness. Misuse of alcohol and prescription medications appears to be a more common problem among older adults than abuse of illicit drugs. However, illicit drugs, such as cocaine and heroin, are becoming more prevalent with the aging of the baby boomer generation, who have a greater lifetime history of substance abuse (Evans, 2008).

Estimates are that the number of adults over age 50 with substance abuse problems will double by 2020. In 2020, approximately 50% of individuals 50 to 74 years of age will be in a high-risk group (use of alcohol and marijuana before 30 years of age) compared with less than 9% in 1999 (Wu & Blazer, 2011; Center for Behavioral Health Statistics and Quality, 2012). *Healthy People 2020* includes goals for reducing substance abuse that are directed more toward adolescents and do not specifically mention older adults. Objectives applicable to adults are presented in the Healthy People box.

HEALTHY PEOPLE 2020

Substance Abuse Objectives for Adults

- Increase the proportion of persons who need alcohol and/or illicit drug treatment and received specialty treatment for abuse or dependence in the past year
- Increase the proportion of persons who are referred for follow-up care for alcohol problems, drug problems after diagnosis, or treatment for one of these conditions in a hospital emergency department
- Increase the number of Level 1 and Level II trauma centers and primary care settings that implement evidence-based alcohol Screening and Brief Intervention (SBI)
- Reduce the proportion of adults who drank excessively in the previous 30 days
- Reduce average alcohol consumption
- Reduce the past-year nonmedical use of prescription drugs (pain relievers, tranquilizers, stimulants, sedatives, any psychotherapeutic drug)
- Decrease the number of deaths attributable to alcohol

From U.S. Department of Health and Human Services, Office of Disease Prevention and Health Promotion: *Healthy people 2020* (2012). Available at http://www.healthypeople.gov/2020.

The most common type of substance-use disorder is heavy drinking (Naegle, 2008). Alcohol-related problems in the elderly often go unrecognized, although the residual effects of alcohol abuse complicate the presentation and treatment of many chronic disorders of older people. Two thirds of elderly alcoholics are early-onset drinkers (alcohol use began at 30 or 40 years of age), and one third are late-onset drinkers (use began after 60 years of age). Late-onset drinking may be related to situational events such as illness, retirement, or death of a spouse and includes a higher number of women (Finfgeld-Connett, 2005).

Gender Issues
Although men (particularly older widowers) are four times more likely to abuse alcohol than women, prevalence in women may be underestimated. The number and impact of older female drinkers is expected to increase over the next 20 years as the disparity between men's and women's drinking decreases (Epstein et al., 2007). Women of all ages are significantly more vulnerable to the effects of alcohol misuse, including drug interactions, physical injury from alcohol-related falls and accidents, cognitive

impairment, and liver and heart disease. Older women are more susceptible to the effects of alcohol because they have less body water than men, less mean muscle mass, and lower levels of the enzyme that breaks down alcohol. Even low-risk drinking levels (no more than one standard drink/day) can be hazardous for older women (Epstein et al., 2007). Older women also experience unique barriers to detection of and treatment for alcohol problems. Health care providers often assume that older women do not drink problematically, so they do not screen for this. Often, alcohol abuse in women is undetected until the consequences are severe.

Drug Effects
Many drugs that elders use for chronic illnesses cause adverse effects when combined with alcohol. Alcohol interacts with at least 50% of prescription drugs (Naegle, 2008). Medications that interact with alcohol include analgesics, antibiotics, antidepressants, antipsychotics, benzodiazepines, histamine-2 (H_2) receptor antagonists, nonsteroidal antiinflammatory drugs (NSAIDs), and herbal medications (echinacea, valerian). Acetaminophen taken on a regular basis, when combined with alcohol, may lead to liver failure. Alcohol diminishes the effects of oral hypoglycemics, anticoagulants, and anticonvulsants. All older people should be given precise instructions regarding the interaction of alcohol with their medications.

Other effects of alcohol in older people include urinary incontinence, which results from rapid bladder filling and diminished neuromuscular control of the bladder; gait disturbances from alcohol-induced cerebellar degeneration and peripheral neuropathy; depression and suicide; sleep disturbances and insomnia; and dementia or delirium. Elders who drink to excess are susceptible to cognitive decline, physical decline, functional decline, and increased risk for injury.

Physiology
Older people develop higher blood alcohol levels because of age-related changes (increased body fat, decreased lean body mass and total body water content) that alter absorption and distribution of alcohol (Culberson, 2006a). Reduced liver and kidney function slow alcohol metabolism and elimination. A decrease in the gastric enzyme alcohol dehydrogenase results in slower metabolism of alcohol and higher blood levels for a longer time. Risks of gastrointestinal ulceration and bleeding may be higher in older people because of the decrease in gastric acidity that occurs in aging (Letizia & Reinboltz, 2005).

Implications for Gerontological Nursing and Healthy Aging

Assessment

Screening for alcohol and drug use (prescription or illicit) should be part of health visits for people over 60 years of age, but screening is not routinely conducted in primary, acute, or long-term care settings (Evans, 2008; Kolanowski & Piven, 2006). Reasons for the low rates of alcohol detection among older adults by health care professionals include poor symptom recognition, inadequate knowledge about screening instruments, lack of age-appropriate diagnostic criteria for abuse in older people, and ageism. Alcohol-related problems may be overlooked in older people because they do not disrupt their lives or are not clearly linked to physical disorders. Health care providers may also be pessimistic about the ability of older people to change long-standing problems (Naegle, 2008).

Alcoholism is a disease of denial and not easy to diagnose, particularly in older people with psychosocial and functional decline from other conditions that may mask decline caused by alcohol. Early signs such as weight loss, irritability, insomnia, and falls may not be recognized as indicators of possible alcohol problems and may be attributed to "just getting older." Box 22-6 presents signs and symptoms that may indicate the presence of alcohol problems in older adults.

The possible health benefits of alcohol in moderation have been reported in the literature (reduced risk of coronary artery disease, ischemic stroke, Alzheimer's disease, and vascular dementia). As a result, older people may not perceive alcohol use as potentially harmful, but clinically significant adverse effects can occur in some individuals consuming as little as two to three drinks per day over an extended period. Because of the increased risk of adverse effects from alcohol use, the National Institute on Alcohol Abuse and Alcoholism (NIAAA) has recommended that individuals over 65 years of age limit alcohol consumption to no more than one standard drink per day. Health professionals must share information with older people about safe drinking limits and the deleterious effects of alcohol intake.

Alcohol users often reject or deny the diagnosis, or they may take offense at the suggestion of it. Feelings of shame or disgrace may make elders reluctant to disclose a drinking problem. This may be especially true among ethnically or culturally diverse older women from a background in which alcohol use is highly discouraged (Finfgeld-Connett, 2004). Families of older people with substance abuse disorders,

---

BOX 22-6   Signs and Symptoms of Potential Alcohol Problems in Older Adults

Anxiety
Irritability (feeling worried or "crabby")
Blackouts
Dizziness
Indigestion
Heartburn
Sadness or depression
Chronic pain
Excessive mood swings
New problems making decisions
Lack of interest in usual activities
Falls
Bruises, burns, or other injuries
Family conflict, abuse
Headaches
Incontinence
Memory loss
Poor hygiene
Poor nutrition
Insomnia
Sleep apnea
Social isolation
Out of touch with family or friends
Unusual response to medications
Frequent physical complaints and physician visits
Financial problems

Adapted from National Institute on Alcohol Abuse and Alcoholism: *Older adults and alcohol problems: participant handout* (2005). Available at www.niaaa.nih.gov; Geriatric Mental Health Foundation: *Substance abuse and misuse among older adults: prevention, recognition, and help* (2006). Available at www.gmhfonline.org.

---

particularly their adult children, may be ashamed of the problem and choose not to address it. Health care providers may feel helpless over alcoholism or uncomfortable with direct questioning or may approach the person in a judgmental manner. Many of the traditional ways of dealing with alcoholism emphasize a confrontational or punitive approach that may have "little impact on a person who views him or herself at the final stage of life" (Naegle, 2008, p. 207). A caring and supportive approach that provides a safe and open atmosphere is the foundation for the therapeutic relationship. It is always important to search for the pain beneath the behavior.

Culberson (2006b) suggests that a simple question—"Have you had a drink containing alcohol within the past three months?"—be included in an assessment to identify clients in whom further screening is indicated. This may be followed by administration of a screening instrument such as the Michigan Alcoholism Screening Test—Geriatric Version (MAST-G) (see the Evidence-Based Practice box on p. 344) or the CAGE (Cut, Annoyed by others, feel Guilty, need Eye opener) Questionnaire (Evans, 2008; Naegle, 2008). Assessment of depression is also important. Alcohol and depression screenings should be offered routinely at health fairs and other sites where older people may seek health information and should be included as part of the annual assessment of all older adults. Screening should be done both before prescribing any new medications that may interact with alcohol and as needed after life-changing events (Epstein et al., 2007).

Interventions

Alcohol problems affect physical, mental, spiritual, and emotional health. Interventions must address quality of life in all of these spheres and be adapted to meet the unique needs of the older adult (Box 22-7). Abstinence from alcohol is seen as the desired goal, but a focus on education, alcohol reduction, and reducing harm is also appropriate. Increasing the awareness of older adults about the risks and benefits of alcohol consumption in the context of their own situation is an important goal (Merrick et al., 2008). Treatment and intervention strategies include cognitive-behavioral approaches, individual and group counseling, medical and psychiatric approaches, referral to Alcoholics Anonymous, family therapy, case management, community and home care services, and formalized substance abuse treatment. Treatment outcomes for older people have been shown to be equal to or better than those for younger people (Naegle, 2008).

Unless the person is in immediate danger, a stepped-care intervention approach beginning with brief interventions followed by more intensive therapies, if necessary, should be used. Brief interventions may range from one meeting to four or five short sessions. Brief intervention is a time-limited, patient-centered strategy focused on changing behavior and assessing patient readiness to change. Sessions can range from one meeting of 10 to 30 minutes to 4 or 5 short sessions. The goals of brief intervention are to (1) reduce or stop alcohol consumption, and (2) facilitate entry into formalized treatment if needed. Research results indicate that this type of intervention, with counseling by nurses in primary care settings, is effective for reducing alcohol consumption, and older people may be more likely to accept treatment given by their primary care provider (Culberson, 2006b; Jalbert et al., 2008).

Long-term self-help treatment programs for elders show high rates of success, especially when social outlets are emphasized and cohort supports are available. A significant concern is the lack of programs designed specifically for older people, particularly older women, whose concerns are very different from those of younger people who abuse drugs or alcohol. Health status, availability of transportation,

---

BOX 22-7   Adapting Alcohol Treatment Interventions for Older Adults

- Ensure treatment by staff experienced in working with older people.
- Accommodate for vision, hearing, and other functional impairments.
- Provide easy access and transportation if needed.
- Address issues older adults tend to face such as loss, grief, health problems.
- Including relevant topics to older adults such as worries about the future of independent living, grandparenting, retirement, fixed income.
- Consider using life review and reminiscence techniques.
- Use a respectful rather than confrontational approach.

- Slow the pace of treatment.
- Use case management and interdisciplinary approaches.
- Address spiritual needs.
- Tailor treatment to level of cognitive function.
- Provide opportunities for interesting activities and socialization opportunities that don't involve drinking.
- Focus on strengths and past coping skills used during hard times.
- Demonstrate faith in the person's ability to change, and avoid ageist attitudes.
- Consider groups designed for women only, since their needs are different.

Adapted from: Epstein E, Fischer-Elber K, Al-Otaiba Z: Women, aging, and alcohol use disorders, co-published simultaneously in *J Women Aging* 19 (1/2):31-48, 2007; Malatesta V, editor: *Mental health issues of older women: a comprehensive review for health care professionals*, Florence, KY, 2007, Routledge.

and mobility impairments may further limit access to treatment.

Epstein and colleagues (2007) suggest the development of treatment sites in senior centers, and assisted living facilities. Additional information on late-life addictions can be found in the Substance Abuse Among Older Adults Treatment Improvement Protocol (TIP), available at www.samhsa.gov. Videos about problem drinking in older adults are available at http://nihseniorhealth.gov/videolist.html.

Acute Alcohol Withdrawal

When there is significant physical dependence, withdrawal from alcohol can become a life-threatening emergency. Detoxification should be done in an inpatient setting because of the potential medical complications and because withdrawal symptoms in older adults can be prolonged. Older people who drink are at risk of experiencing acute alcohol withdrawal if admitted to the hospital for treatment of acute illnesses or emergencies. All patients admitted to acute care settings should be screened for alcohol use and assessed for signs and symptoms of alcohol-related problems. Older people with a long history of consuming excess alcohol, previous episodes of acute withdrawal, and/or a history of prior detoxification are at increased risk of acute alcohol withdrawal (Letizia & Reinboltz, 2005).

Symptoms of acute alcohol withdrawal vary but may be more severe and last longer in older people. Minor withdrawal (withdrawal tremulousness) begins 6 to 12 hours after a patient has consumed the last drink. Symptoms include tremor, anxiety, nausea, insomnia, tachycardia, and increased blood pressure and frequently may be mistaken for common problems in older adults. Major withdrawal is seen 10 to 72 hours after cessation of alcohol intake, and symptoms include vomiting, diaphoresis, hallucinations, tremors, and seizures (Letizia & Reinboltz, 2005).

Delirium tremens (DTs) is the term used to describe alcohol withdrawal delirium; it usually occurs 24 to 72 hours after the last drink but may occur up to 10 days later. DTs occur in 5% of patients with acute alcohol withdrawal and is considered a medical emergency, with a mortality rate from respiratory failure and cardiac arrhythmia as high as 15%. Other signs and symptoms include confusion, disorientation, hallucinations, hyperthermia, and hypertension. The Clinical Institute Withdrawal Assessment (CIWA) scale is recommended as a valid and reliable screening instrument (www.pubs.niaa.nih.gov) (Letizia & Reinboltz, 2005).

Recommended treatment is the use of short-acting benzodiazepines at one half to one third the normal dose around the clock or as needed during withdrawal. Disulfiram use in older adults to promote abstinence is not recommended because of the potential for serious cardiovascular complications. The use of oral or intravenous alcohol to prevent or treat withdrawal is not established.

The CIWA aids in medication adjustments. Other interventions include assessing mental status, monitoring vital signs, and maintaining fluid balance without overhydrating. Calm and quiet surroundings, no unnecessary stimuli, consistent caregivers, frequent reorientation, prevention of injury, and support and caring are additional suggested interventions. Nutritional assessment is indicated, as well as addition of a multivitamin containing folic acid, pyridoxine, niacin, vitamin A, and thiamine (Letizia & Reinboltz, 2005).

Other Substance Abuse Concerns

A more common concern seen among older people is the misuse of prescription and OTC medications. Drug misuse is defined as use of a drug for reasons other than those for which it was prescribed. Dependence on sedative, hypnotic, or anxiolytic drugs, often prescribed for anxiety or insomnia, and taken for many years with resulting dependence, is especially problematic for older women, who are more likely than men to receive prescriptions for these drugs (Epstein et al., 2007; Kolanowski & Piven, 2006). Benzodiazepines represent 17% to 23% of drugs prescribed to older adults (Morgan et al., 2005). Opiates are ranked second only to benzodiazepines among abused prescription drugs in the older adult population (Naegle, 2008). Increases in illness and mortality are associated with misusing prescription and nonprescription medications, although this is not considered a disorder by the *DSM-IV.*

Some of the reasons for the abuse of psychoactive prescription medications may be inappropriate prescribing and ineffective monitoring of response and follow-up. In many instances, older people are given prescriptions for benzodiazepines or sedatives because of complaints of insomnia (see Chapter 11) or nervousness, without adequate assessment for depression, anxiety, or other conditions that may be causing the symptoms. Older people may not be informed of the side effects of these medications, including interactions with alcohol, dependence, and withdrawal symptoms. More importantly, conditions such as anxiety and depression may not be recognized and treated appropriately.

Implications for Gerontological Nursing and Healthy Aging

Risk, prevention, assessment, and treatment of alcohol and substance abuse have not been sufficiently studied among older people. Diagnostic criteria to identify alcohol and prescription drug misuse among older adults, particularly older women and culturally and ethnically diverse elders, also need further investigation. Nurses in contact with older adults in all settings must be competent in assessment for mental health disorders as well as in screening, assessment, and counseling about the use of alcohol and prescribed, illicit, and OTC drug use. Providing education to older people and their families and referring to specialists and community resources are also important nursing roles and essential to best practices.

The development of holistic and humanistic models of care for elders experiencing mental health disturbances is critically important in gerontological nursing. Much of the distress associated with mental health disorders in late life can be relieved through competent, caring, and compassionate gerontological nursing care. Awareness of appropriate assessment and treatment of the distressing reactions that can occur in late life, as presented in this chapter, is a very important component of best practice care. However, knowing and appreciating each elder's uniqueness, his or her past and present experiences, and how they color the present may contribute far more to mental health and wellness than medications or therapy.

Believing in and supporting the strength and wisdom of older people restores self-confidence and feelings of worth, an important component of mental health and wellness. Appreciating the nature of loss and grief in old age means that gerontological nurses listen, *really listen,* and offer support to weather the storm. Our work must focus on the development of environments of care that enhance both physical and mental health and wellness, create conditions of hope, and support elders in the often difficult journey in late life.

Application of Maslow's Hierarchy

Using Maslow's Hierarchy of Needs model, satisfaction of basic needs is a significant component of mental health. Attention to basic needs of biological integrity, safety and security, belonging and attachment, self-esteem, and self-efficacy in the daily lives of elders is essential to mental health and wellness. The higher one rises in terms of needs met, the more likely one is to be mentally healthy.

KEY CONCEPTS

- Mental health in late life is difficult to determine because the accrual of life experiences makes for great variation. Mental health in late life must be determined by the gratification and satisfaction that individuals feel in their particular situations.

- Mental health is a fluctuating situation for most individuals, with peaks and valleys of happiness and pain.
- The prevalence of mental health disorders is expected to increase significantly with the aging of the baby boomers.
- Mental health disorders are underreported and underdiagnosed among older adults. Somatic complaints are often the presenting symptoms of mental health disorders, making diagnosis difficult.
- The incidence of psychotic disorders with late-life onset is low among older people, but psychotic manifestations can occur as secondary symptoms in a variety of disorders, the most common being Alzheimer's disease. Psychotic symptoms in Alzheimer's disease necessitate different assessment and treatment than do long-standing psychotic disorders.
- Anxiety disorders are common in late life and reestablishing feelings of adequacy and control is the heart of crisis resolution and stress management.
- PTSD is finally being recognized in older adults who have been subjected to extremely traumatic events.
- Depression is the most common emotional disorder of aging and likewise the most treatable. Unfortunately, it is often neglected or assumed to be a condition of aging that one must "learn to live with." An important nursing intervention is assessment of depression.
- Suicide is a significant problem among older men, particularly widowers. Many come to be seen by the health care professional with physical complaints shortly before they commit suicide and assessment of depression and suicidal intent is important.
- Substance abuse, particularly alcohol, and misuse of prescription drugs are often underrecognized and undertreated problems of older adults, particularly older women. Screening and appropriate assessment and intervention are important in all settings.
- Further research is needed to fully understand the cultural and ethnic differences in mental health concerns, as well as appropriate assessment and treatment in culturally and ethnically diverse older people.

ACTIVITIES AND DISCUSSION QUESTIONS

1. Discuss the three most common mental health disturbances that elders are likely to experience and describe appropriate assessment and treatment.
2. What is likely to be different in the appearance of depression in a person who is 70 years old compared to its appearance in a person who is 20 years old?

3. What behaviors are indicative of suicidal intent in an older adult? Discuss the methods of assessment and your reactions to these.

4. Discuss the various situations that may result in elder substance abuse and ways to effectively intervene.

5. What type of teaching would you provide to an older adult related to the use of alcohol and medications?

6. Formulate strategies that may be used to promote mental health and wellness in late life.

REFERENCES

American Psychiatric Association: *Diagnostic and statistical manual of mental disorders (DSM-IV),* ed 4, Washington, DC, 2000, The American Psychiatric Association.

American Psychological Association: *Growing mental and behavioral health concerns facing older Americans* (2012). Available at http://www.apa.org/about/gr/issues/aging/growing-concerns.aspx.

Ayers C, Loebach J, Wetherell E, et al: Treating late-life anxiety, *Psychiatr Times* 23:1–2, 2006.

Berry K, Barrowclough C: The needs of older adults with schizophrenia: implications for psychological interventions, *Clin Psychol Rev* 29:68, 2009.

Birren JE, Deutchman DE: *Guiding autobiography groups for older adults: exploring the fabric of life,* Baltimore, 1991, Johns Hopkins University Press.

Bludau J: Second institutionalization: impact of personal history on patients with dementia, *Caring for the Ages* 3(5):3–4, 2002.

Bormann J, Thorp S, Wetherell J, et al: A spirituality based group intervention for combat veterans with posttraumatic stress disorder: feasibility study, *J Holist Nurs* 26:109, 2008.

Bottche M, Kuwert P, Knaevelsrud C: Posttraumatic stress disorder in older adults: an overview of characteristics and treatment approaches, *Int J Geriatr Psychiatry* 27(3):230–239, 2012.

Burnside IM: Listen to the aged, *Am J Nurs* 75(10):1800–1803, 1975.

Butler R: The life review: an interpretation of reminiscence in the aged, *Psychiatry* 26:65, 1963.

Butler R: *Age, death and life review* (2002). Available at http://www.hospicefoundation.org/pages/page.asp?page_id=171322.

Butler R, Lewis M: *Aging and mental health: positive psychosocial approaches,* ed 3, St. Louis, 1983, Mosby.

Byers A, Yaffe K, Covinsky K, et al: High occurrence of mood and anxiety disorders among older adults, *Arch Gen Psychiatry* 67:489, 2010.

Byrd E: Nursing assessment and treatment of depressive disorders of late life. In Mellilo K, Houde S, editors: *Geropsychiatric and mental health nursing,* Sudbury, MA, 2005, Jones and Bartlett.

Center for Behavioral Health Statistics and Quality: *Data spotlight* (2012). Available at http://www.samhsa.gov/data/spotlight/WEB_SPOT_043/WEB_SPOT_043.pdf.

Chang CC, Roberts BL: Strategies for feeding patients with dementia, *Am J Nurs* 111(4):36–44, 2011.

Chaudhary M, Rabheru K: Paranoid symptoms among older adults, *Geriatr Aging* 11:143, 2008.

Culberson J: Alcohol use in the elderly: beyond the CAGE. Part 1 of 2: prevalence and patterns of problem drinking, *Geriatrics* 61(10):23–27, 2006a.

Culberson J: Alcohol use in the elderly: beyond the CAGE. Part 2 of 2: screening instruments and treatment strategies, *Geriatrics* 61(11):20–26, 2006b.

Das B, Greenspan M, Muralee S, et al: Late-life depression: a review, *Clin Geriatr* 15(10):35–44, 2007.

Edelstein B, Heisel M, McKee D, et al: Development and psychometric evaluation of the Reasons for Living—Older Adults Scale: A suicide risk assessment inventory, *Gerontologist* 49:736, 2009.

Epstein E, Fischer-Elber K, Al-Otaiba Z: Women, aging, and alcohol use disorders, *J Women Aging* 19(1–2):31–48, 2007.

Erikson EH, Erikson JM, Kivnick HQ: *Vital involvement in old age: the experience of old age in our time,* New York, 1986, WW Norton.

Evans L: *Mental health issues in aging* (2008). Available at http://hartfordign.org/uploads/File/gnec_state_of_science_papers/gnec_mental_health.pdf.

Finfgeld-Connett DL: Treatment of substance misuse in older women: using a brief intervention model, *J Gerontol Nurs* 30(8):31–37, 2004.

Finfgeld-Connett DL: Self-management of alcohol problems among older adults, *J Gerontol Nurs* 31(5):51–58, 2005.

Flood M, Buckwalter K: Recommendations for the mental health care of older adults: Part 1—an overview of depression and anxiety, *J Gerontol Nurs* 35:26, 2009.

Friedman M, Kennedy G, Williams K: Cognitive camouflage—how Alzheimer's can mask mental illness, *Aging Well* 2:16, 2009.

Gellis ZD, McClive-Reed KP, Brown E: Treatments for depression in older persons with dementia, *Ann Longterm Care,* 17(2):29–36, 2009.

Gonzalez H, Vega W, Williams D, et al: Depression care in the United States: too little too few, *Arch Gen Psychiatry* 67:37, 2010.

Gould R, Coulson M, Howard R: Efficacy of cognitive behavioral therapy for anxiety disorders in older people: a meta-analysis and meta-regression of randomized controlled trials, *J Am Geriatr Soc* 60(2):218–229, 2012.

Grabowski D, Aschbrenner K, Rome V, et al: Quality of mental health care for nursing home residents: a literature review, *Med Care Res Rev* 67(6):627–656, 2010.

Grossberg GT: Diagnosis and treatment of late-life psychosis in the elderly, *Long-Term Care Forum* 1(3):7, 2000.

Haight B, Burnside IM: Reminiscence and life review: explaining the differences, *Arch Psychiatr Nurs* 7:91, 1993.

Haight B, Webster J: *Critical advances in reminiscence work: from theory to application,* New York, 2002, Springer.

Ham R, Sloane P, Warshaw G, et al: *Primary care geriatrics: a case-based approach,* edition 5, St. Louis, 2007, Mosby.

Heller K, Viken R, Swindle R: Screening for depression in African American and Caucasian older women, *Aging Ment Health* 14:339, 2010.

Institute of Medicine [IOM]: *Retooling for an aging America: building the health care workforce,* Washington, DC, 2008, National Academies Press.

Jalbert J, Quilliam B, Lapane K: A profile of concurrent alcohol and alcohol-interactive prescription drug use in the US population, *J Gen Intern Med* 23:1318, 2008.

Kennedy GJ: Bipolar disorder in late life: depression, *Prim Psychiatry* 15(3):30–34, 2008.

Kolanowski A, Piven M: Geropsychiatric nursing: the state of the science, *J Am Psychiatr Nurs Assoc* 12:75, 2006.

Kurlowicz L, Harvath T: Depression. In Capezuti E, Swicker D, Mezey M, et al, editors: *Evidence-based geriatric nursing protocols for best practice*, ed 3, New York, 2008a, Springer.

Kurlowicz L, Harvath T: *Depression: nursing standard of practice protocol*, New York, 2008b, Hartford Institute for Geriatric Nursing. Available at www.consultgerirn.org.

Lavretsky H, Alstein LL, Olmstead RE, et al: Complementary use of tai chi chih augments escitalopram treatment of geriatric depression: a randomized controlled trial, *Am J Geriatr Psychiatry* 19(10):839–850, 2011.

Letizia M, Reinboltz M: Identifying and managing acute alcohol withdrawal in the elderly, *Geriatr Nurs* 26(3):176-183, 2005.

Leutwyler H, Wallhagen M: Understanding physical health of older adults with schizophrenia: building and eroding trust, *J Gerontol Nurs* 36:38, 2010.

Madhusoodanan S, Brenner R: Caring for the chronically mentally ill in nursing homes, *Ann Longterm Care* 15(9):29–32, 2007.

Mellilo K, Hoff L, Huff M: Geropsychiatric nursing as a subspecialty. In Mellilo K, Houde S, editors: *Geropsychiatric and mental health nursing*, Sudbury MA, 2005, Jones and Bartlett.

Mentes J, Bail J: Psychosis in older adults. In Mellilo K, Houde S, editors: *Geropsychiatric and mental health nursing,* Sudbury MA, 2005, Jones and Bartlett.

Merrick E, Hodgkins D, Garnick D, et al: Unhealthy drinking patterns in older adults: prevalence and associated characteristics, *J Am Geriatr Soc* 56(2):214–223, 2008.

Morgan B, White D, Wallace A: Substance abuse in older adults. In Mellilo K, Houde S, editors: *Geropsychiatric and mental health nursing,* Sudbury, MA, 2005, Jones and Bartlett.

Morley J: Depression in nursing home residents, *J Am Med Dir Assoc* 5:301, 2010.

Naegle M: Substance misuse and alcohol use disorders. In Capezuti E, Swicker D, Mezey M, et al, editors: *Evidence-based geriatric nursing protocols for best practice*, ed 3, New York, 2008, Springer.

National Institute of Mental Health [NIMH]: *Depression in elderly men* (2009). Available at http://www.nimh.nih.gov/health/publications/men-and-depression/depression-in-elderly-men.shtml.

Phillips J, Robin A, Nugent C, Idler E: Understanding recent changes in suicide rates among middle-aged: period or cohort effects, *Public Health Rep* 125(5):680–688, 2010.

Pietrzak R, Goldstein R, Southwick S, Grant B: Physical health conditions associated with posttraumatic stress disorder in U.S. older adults: results from wave 2 of the National Epidemiological Survey on Alcohol and Related Conditions, *J Am Geriatr Soc* 60(2):296-303, 2012.

Pot AM, Bohlmeijer ET, Onrust S, et al: The impact of life review on depression in older adults: a randomized controlled trial, *Int Psychogeriatr* 22(4):572–581, 2010.

Qualls S: Defining mental health in later life, *Generations* 26(7):9–13, 2002.

Qureshi S, Kimbrell T, Pyne J, et al: Greater prevalence and incidence of dementia in older veterans with posttraumatic stress disorder, *J Am Geriatr Soc* 58:1627, 2010.

Saur C, Steffens D, Harpole L, et al: Satisfaction and outcomes of depressed older adults with psychiatric clinical nurse specialists in primary care, *J Am Psychiatr Nurs Assoc* 13:62, 2007.

Schneider LS, Tariot P, Dagerman K, et al: Effectiveness of atypical antipsychotic drugs in patients with Alzheimer's disease, *N Engl J Med* 355(15):1525–1538, 2006.

Seekles W, van Straten A, Beekman A, et al: Stepped care for depression and anxiety: from primary care to specialized mental health care: a randomized controlled trial testing the effectiveness of a stepped care program among primary care patients with mood or anxiety disorders, *BMC Health Serv Res* 9:90, 2009.

Sherrod T, Quinlan-Colwell A, Lattimore T, et al: Older adults with bipolar disorder: guidelines for primary care providers, *J Gerontol Nurs* 36:20, 2010.

Sirey J, Bruce M, Carpenter M, et al: Depression symptoms and suicidal ideation among older adults receiving home delivering meals, *Int J Geriatr Psychiatry,* 23(12):1306–1311, 2008.

Smith M: Nursing assessment and treatment of anxiety in late life. In Mellilo K, Houde S, editors: *Geropsychiatric and mental health nursing,* Sudbury, MA, 2005, Jones and Bartlett.

Splete H: Mentally ill eclipse residents with dementia, *Caring for the Ages* 10(12):11, 2009.

Thakur M, Blazer D: Depression in long-term care, *J Am Med Dir Assoc* 9(2):82–87, 2008.

Thorp S, Ayers C, Nuevo R, et al: Meta-analysis comparing different behavioral treatments for late-life anxiety, *Am J Geriatr Psychiatry* 17:105, 2009.

Thielke S, Diehr P, Unützer J: Prevalence, incidence, and persistence of major depressive symptoms in the Cardiovascular Health Study, *Aging Ment Health* 14:168, 2010.

Unützer J: Clinical practice: late-life depression, *N Engl J Med* 357(22):2269–2276, 2007.

Unützer J, Katon W, Callahan C, et al: Long-term cost effects of collaborative care for late-life depression, *Am J Manag Care* 14(2):95–100, 2008.

U.S. Department of Health and Human Services [USDHHS], Office of Disease Prevention and Health Promotion: *Healthy people 2020* (2012). Available at http://www.healthypeople.gov/2020.

Wetherell J, Maser J, Balkom A: Anxiety disorders in the elderly: outdated beliefs and a research agenda, *Acta Psychiatr Scand* 111(6):401–402, 2005.

Wu L, Blazer D: Illicit and nonmedical drug use among older adults: a review, *J Aging Health* 23:481, 2011.

CHAPTER 23

Economic and Legal Issues

Kathleen F. Jett

evolve evolve.elsevier.com/Ebersole/gerontological

LEARNING OBJECTIVES

Upon completion of this chapter, the reader will be able to:
- Describe the major methods of financing health care for older adults.
- Compare the costs to the consumer between Medicare and Medicaid.
- Explain the fundamentals of Medicare, Medicaid, and TRICARE sufficiently to assist elders in accessing the services needed.
- Discuss the potential impact of health care financing in long-term and home health care.
- Describe the roles of the nurse as case and care managers.

GLOSSARY

CMS The Centers for Medicare and Medicaid Services, the federal agency under the U.S. Department of Health and Human Services responsible for the administration of Medicare and Medicaid.

Custodial care The provision of personal assistance related to a person's inability to perform the activities needed in daily living. This care may be provided informally by family and friends or formally by nursing assistants.

Prospective payment system (PPS) A system in which the payment of a health service is calculated in advance and based on a number of factors, including diagnosis and age of the patient rather than the actual costs and length of the care needed.

Skilled care The provision of a level of care that requires professional expertise and training, such as that provided by licensed nurses, physical therapists, or occupational therapists.

The Social Security Act The legislation passed in 1935 that provides regular income for older persons.

Title XVIII of the Social Security Act The federal legislation providing for Medicare for all eligible persons 65 years of age and over, the permanently disabled, and those with end-stage renal disease.

Title XIX of the Social Security Act The federal legislation providing for Medicaid to individuals at least 65 years of age and select others with very low incomes.

Title XVI of the Social Security Act The federal legislation that established Supplementary Security to elders with extremely low incomes and few assets.

THE LIVED EXPERIENCE

When I was growing up life was hard. We were so poor we couldn't do much but to hold on tight. When I was lucky I could get work plowing a field and make $1.00 an acre. You work hard, and you make do. There were not such things as going to a doctor or a hospital, you just did the best you could do and pray you don't get sick. Then when I turned 65 I got a little check from the government and a red, white, and blue insurance [Medicare] card. The check isn't much, only about $564 a month, but you know I just consider myself blessed and better off than ever before. And now I don't worry about my health, I will be taken care of.

Aida, age 74

People living in the United States represent all levels of education, experience, and income. However, all have in common the potential need for health care. It is rare to meet an older adult who does not have experience in some way with both the past and the present health care systems either in the United States or their country of origin. Today's system in the United States is in a state of flux and stress as we find a way to care for the ever increasing number of older adults in the face of skyrocketing costs and financial constraints. For gerontological nurses to provide the best care to older adults, it is helpful to have a basic understanding of the health care system and financing associated with the care they provide and a working knowledge of some of the legal issues older adults face.

This chapter will review the major mechanisms by which eligible elders in the United States receive a basic income and health insurance in place at the time of this writing. It will proceed to discuss common legal issues elders face that the nurse should know, and last offer a discussion of elder mistreatment.

It is recognized that the Affordable Care Act of the Obama administration has affected the health of older adults in at least two major ways already. The first is expanded access to preventive care (see Chapter 1) and the second is the tightening of the "donut hole" related to medication costs discussed later in this chapter. These may change in the near future or other aspects may evolve.

Social Security

The health care system of today and its financing began in 1935. There had been an exodus from the country and farms into the cities and the factories in the early 1900s, changing the social and financial basis of the family. In the country, an elder worked in some way until death, but this was not possible in cities given the exceedingly difficult work of the factories. For the first time people were retiring by reason of disability. The word *retiring*, which had meant "to withdraw from public" in the 1800s, now meant "no longer qualified," with dramatically different implications (Achenbaum, 1978).

The family, no longer able to provide all the care to their elders, looked to the federal government for help. In 1935 the Social Security Act was passed. The Social Security program, established at the time of the Great Depression, was considered by many to be one of the most successful federal programs. Its primary function was to provide monetary benefits to American citizens and legal residents at least 65 years of age to prevent their dependency on their families.

Social security (SS) was designed as a pay-as-you-go system. Payroll taxes collected from employees and employers are immediately distributed to beneficiaries (retirees, the disabled, or eligible spouses). In 2012 payroll taxes were collected on the first $110,100 of an individual's income. Social Security funds, although individually deposited by employers and employees, are not reserved for any one individual. No one has an account set aside in his or her name. All funds that are not immediately paid out to beneficiaries are "borrowed" by the federal government for regular operating expenses.

As long as the amount of contributions from the workers exceeds those paid to the beneficiaries, the program can continue as designed. At the time of its inception the system was constructed to transfer funds from those believed to be relatively well off (workers) to those believed to be relatively poor (retirees). Social security and a number of programs that followed were set up as "age-entitlement" programs. This meant that an individual could receive the benefits simply because of age and regardless of need. In other words, the monetary support is available to those persons at a certain age regardless of other sources of personal income or assets. They were and are, however, limited to United States citizens and legal residents older than a certain age who have previously earned the required amount of "credits" or married to someone who has. Earnings are translated into "credits," with one credit equivalent to $1130 in 2012. A minimum of 40 credits are required for all persons born in 1929 or later (U.S. Social Security Administration [SSA], 2012a).

At the same time, the amount of Social Security benefit is calculated in part on the person's average salary during 35 of his or her working years. If one did not work a total of 35 years, nonworking years count as zero in the calculation. This has been most beneficial to older white men, who are more likely to have worked the most consistently and at higher salaries than all other groups of workers. It has been most disadvantageous for persons of color and many women who took time off to care for a child or parent (Hooyman & Kiyak, 2008). The amount of benefit potentially increases each year on January 1 as a cost-of-living adjustment (COLA). In 2012 the COLA was 3.6% and the average SS retirement benefit was $1230 for the 39 million persons at least 65 years of age (SSA, 2012b). Twenty-two percent of all married elders and 43% of unmarried elders depend on Social Security for 90% of their income.

In an effort to save money the SS system has been increasing the age when one is eligible for full benefits. Those born in 1938 were eligible to begin receiving partial SS benefits at age 62; however, they had to wait until age 65 if they wanted to receive their full benefits. The age at which one becomes eligible is increasing slowly and will transition to at least 67 years of age for those born in 1960 or after (SSA, 1984).

Supplemental Security Income

Not all older persons living in the United States have Social Security benefits adequate to provide even the most basic necessities of life. This has been true especially for persons who have spent their lives employed in the agriculture industry or as domestic workers and were paid very low wages, often on a cash basis. Supplemental Security Income (SSI) was established in 1965 by Title XVI of the Social Security Act. SSI provides for a minimum level of economic support to older adults. Among the requirements is very low income. Income includes monetary gifts, food, and shelter provided by others. Federal SSI payments are calculated on total monthly income with potential supplementation to the maximum allowed by the state of residence. The Federal SSI benefit to about 2 million persons at least 65 years of age was $698 in 2012 (SSA, 2012c). If one's income or the contributions of others increases, the payment decreases accordingly.

Medicare and Medicaid

History

In 1934 President Franklin D. Roosevelt tried to create a plan to provide universal health insurance for the citizens in the United States. This was met with unbeatable opposition from groups such as the American Medical Association and, by poll, the majority of the American public (Cantril, 1951). Except for a few successful insurance plans for working people, health care was on a fee-for-service, out-of-pocket basis. This meant that each health care service could be purchased from one's own funds, or "pocket." When costs were reasonable, many older adults could continue to pay for their care. However, as people began to live longer with more health problems, and as technology advanced and costs rose, paying for the costs of health care out-of-pocket grew harder and even impossible for many older adults who were entirely dependent on the limited incomes of Social Security.

In 1965, through the efforts of President Lyndon B. Johnson, legislation (Title XVIII of the Social Security Act) was passed creating an insurance plan (Medicare A) covering the costs of hospitalization for all persons eligible for Social Security, SSI, or railroad retirement benefits. A

second subsidized insurance plan (Medicare B) could be purchased, to cover the costs of seeing health care providers and several other services. The costs of outpatient medications were not covered by Medicare until 2006, when Medicare D was created.

Medicare was meant to provide insurance coverage for medical care to the elderly and disabled regardless of their financial situation. Another amendment (Title XIX) to the Social Security Act created a second form of insurance for the elderly, the disabled, and children with low incomes, known as *Medicaid*. Medicaid was designed to help states defray expenses of the very poor; this included elders who did not qualify for or could not afford to purchase the supplemental health policy (Medicare B) or to pay the required copayments.

Medicare

Medicare is administered by the Centers for Medicare and Medicaid Services (CMS) (www.cms.gov) and is a part of the Department of Health and Human Services, a special Federal entity created to improve the administration of the programs. In 1966, just over 19 million people at least 62 years of age were enrolled in Medicare. In 2008 (latest data available) this number had increased to about 37.5 million over 62 and an additional 7.7 million younger, disabled persons (CMS, 2008).

To be eligible for Medicare today, one must be eligible for Social Security. Otherwise, coverage may be purchased. Medicare consists of four parts (Box 23-1). Medicare only covers select services and requires that these services be considered medically necessary. This means that the services are prescribed and are needed for the diagnosis or treatment of a medical condition, meet the standards of good medical practice, and are not performed for the convenience of the health care provider (CMS, 2011).

Medicare A

Unless previously disabled, a person first becomes eligible for Medicare A in the 6 months surrounding his or her 65th birthday (from 3 months before to 3 months after the birth month). If a person does not apply during that time, he or she has to wait for the next "open enrollment period" in the spring of each year with benefits beginning on July 1. Penalties may be charged (CMS, 2011). Medicare Part A is a hospital insurance plan covering acute care, acute and short-term rehabilitative care, and costs associated with hospice and home health care under certain circumstances.

In 2012 Part A is free to those who receive Social Security or can be purchased for a monthly fee of up to $440

BOX 23-1 **Medicare Basics**

Medicare A

A hospital insurance plan that is automatically provided for all persons who qualify, with no premium attached. Covers part of the costs of acute care, acute and short-term rehabilitative care, some costs associated with hospice care, and home health care under certain circumstances. There are copays and deductibles for most services.

Medicare B

A purchased insurance plan to cover some of the costs of services provided by physicians; nurse practitioners; outpatient services (e.g., lab work); qualified physical, speech, and occupational therapy; and skilled home and hospice care. It also covers a growing number of health screens with no or minimal copays. Annual prevention and health screening visits.* Persons can "opt out" of Medicare B and enroll in Medicare C.

Medicare C

Medicare C is also known as the Medicare Advantage Plan and includes covered services through either private PPO or MCPs, such as what are known as HMOs (e.g., United Health Care or Kaiser Permanente). The consumer "enrolls" to receive services from assigned specific locations and providers. In the MCP there are fewer out-of-pocket costs unless an individual decides to see a provider or seek a service without a referral or outside the system to which he or she has subscribed. While this has not always been the case, health services are expected to emphasize preventive health, comprehensive care, periodic physical examinations, and immunizations. In most geographic areas there are multiple plans from which one can select that will best meet their health and financial needs.

Medicare D

Medicare D is not one plan but is a designation for dozens of private medication payment plans that meet certain criteria and are approved by the Centers for Medicare and Medicaid Services. The premiums vary by company and reflect the range of medications covered. All Medicare D plans have an annual deductible and a certain amount of coverage until a cap occurs, with no coverage until the next cap and then significant coverage for the rest of the year. During the gap in coverage (called the "donut hole") prescriptions must be provided by pharmaceutical companies at reduced prices.* The deductibles and caps change every year.

HMO, Health maintenance organization; *MCP,* managed care plan; *PPO,* preferred provider organization.
See www.cms.gov for the latest information about covered services and associated costs. These are all subject to change.
* Part of the provisions of the Affordable Care Act, enacted but in debate at the time of this writing.

(CMS, 2011). The coverage and copayments under Medicare A vary by setting under the original fee-for-service plans. When acute care is needed, the patient responsibility can be quite high, including a deductible of $1156 (as of 2012) for days 1 to 60 and a copay of $289/day for days 61 to 90. Each beneficiary has a 60-day lifetime reserve at the copay cost of $578 per day; there is no coverage after 90 days. These copays are repeated every time the person is readmitted to an acute care facility with the exception of the lifetime reserve [2012 figures] (CMS, 2011).

Medicare A also pays 100% of the costs for the first 20 days in a skilled nursing facility if the purpose is for rehabilitation. There is a copay of $144.50 for days 21 to 100, and no coverage after that (CMS, 2011).

When the assistance needed is limited to personal care or medication supervision, it is not covered by Medicare at all. For home health care to be paid by Medicare, the care must be provided at the written direction of a physician. Ongoing supervision can be provided by either a physician or a nurse practitioner. It must be through a certified agency and for the purposes of active rehabilitation similar to that seen in the skilled nursing home setting. There are no copayments for home health care. Copays for hospice care are limited to 5% for inpatient short-term respite stays to provide temporary relief to the caregiver or for acute symptom management that cannot be handled at home (CMS, 2011).

Medicare B

A person who is eligible for Part A must apply for Part B through the local Social Security Administration office (www.socialsecurity.gov). At that time the person will be asked to choose either Medicare B or a Medicare C plan as an alternative plan that is available in the area. Medicare B covers the costs associated with the services provided by physicians; nurse practitioners; outpatient services (e.g., lab work); qualified physical, speech, and occupational therapy; and some home health care equiptment. Medicare C replaces Medicare B and is a managed care plan similar to what we know as a health maintenance organization (HMO).

Many older adults are being encouraged or directed to enroll in Medicare C plans rather than the Original Medicare.

The Original Medicare B Plan is based on a traditional fee-for-service arrangement; the patient receives services from a provider for a medical problem, a bill for the costs of the care is sent to Medicare (through a carrier) or to the patient, who can submit the claims, and the provider or the patient is reimbursed. In 2012, after a deductible of $140 a year, Medicare reimbursed physicians at a rate of 80% of what Medicare considers an "allowable charge" for necessary medical services (mental health is limited to 60%) (CMS, 2011). The patient is responsible for the remaining 20% (or 40%) of the charge. A provider who "accepts assignment" cannot charge a patient any more than the 20% of the "allowable charge." The number of physicians who accept assignment is decreasing rapidly.

A provider who does not accept assignment may charge the patient up to 15% above the allowable charge. With the Medicare B Plan, the patient is responsible for an annual deductible, copays, coinsurance charges, and a monthly premium based on income and marital status. The premium is usually deducted directly from the monthly Social Security check. In 2011 the average monthly premium for Original Medicare Part B was $115.40, with the premium increasing for those with adjusted gross incomes of greater than $214K for an individual or $428K for a couple (CMS, 2011).

The advantages of the Original Medicare Plan include choice and access. The person can seek the services of any provider of his or her choice, without a referral. Many people with the Original Plan purchase what are called Medigap policies to cover the deductibles and copays.

Medicare C

The type and availability of Medicare Advantage Plans (Medicare C) depends on location and may include a preferred provider organization (PPO) plan and/or any number of managed care plans (MCPs). Not all plans are offered at all locations. All provide extra benefits beyond those covered by the Original Medicare B; they may require only small copays but have special rules that must be followed, and they may charge extra premiums for the added services. Referrals for services are always required. Premiums vary by type.

The PPO plans work like the Original Medicare except that only specific providers can be used (those in the network) and the allowable charges are preset. Any additional services and fees or copays vary by plan. A patient may choose to be seen by a provider outside the PPO network for an additional charge.

In MCPs (also known as HMOs), the consumer "enrolls" to receive services from assigned specific locations and providers. There are fewer out-of-pocket costs unless an individual decides to see a provider or seek a service without a referral or outside the system to which he or she has subscribed. These are not usually covered at all. Medicare contracts with MCPs to provide comprehensive services, financed by Medicare premiums. The best of these are complete health care systems with highly trained physicians, nurse practitioners, and other health care professionals working out of single or regional completely equipped medical centers. Medical services are expected to emphasize preventive medicine, comprehensive care, periodic physical examinations, and immunizations.

Capitation is imposed on MCPs by Medicare; this means that the plan is paid a certain fixed amount each day for each enrollee regardless of the amount of care given, and with this amount all needed care must be provided. Although the intention of this design was to increase preventive care, in some cases, this has created abuses and horror stories in which elders were denied necessary treatments, presumably motivated by the plan's desire to lower its costs. Now patient protection laws allow consumers to lodge complaints and initiate legal action against the suspected abuse. The Center for Patient Advocacy supported a much needed bill that became law in October 1999, which allows appeals when an MCP denies care, guarantees access to specialists when needed, ensures that health-related decisions are made by health care providers rather than bureaucrats, and holds MCPs legally accountable for medical decisions that cause harm.

HMOs that have been granted Medicare capitation cannot refuse applicants based on preexisting health conditions. The supplemental services offered may save the participant a considerable amount in the costs of medications, assistive devices, and professional consultation charges. The negative aspects of HMOs and managed care are the access barriers to specialists and high-tech procedures and treatments. Some HMOs provide extensive health education services, support groups, and telephone support services to the homebound.

Medicare D

Medicare D was created as part of the Medicare Modernization Act of 2003 and is an optional prescription coverage plan. People must enroll within 6 months of initial Medicare eligibility. Otherwise they have to wait until the next open enrollment period, with a penalty based on the number of months they waited to enroll. Medicare D is not one plan but is a designation for dozens of private plans that meet certain criteria and are approved by the CMS.

The premiums vary by company, reflect the range of medications covered, and can be deducted from one's Social Security check. In 2012 the annual deductible was $320. For drug costs between $321 to $2930 there is approximately 75% coverage. Between $2930 and $4700 patients fall into what is referred to as the "donut hole" when there is no coverage. After $4700, coverage is at about 95%. While there is still no coverage in the donut hole, a provision of the Affordable Care Act is that pharmaceutical companies are required to provide a 50% discount for brand-name drugs and the person is responsible for 86% of costs of generic drugs during this period (CMS, 2011).

Medicaid

For elders with very low incomes (including all persons receiving SSI), Medicaid may be available to offset the high Medicare copays and deductibles, as well as to provide additional health benefits such as drug coverage.

In 2012 Medicaid provided health care insurance to 4.6 million persons at least 65 years of age or older at a cost of more than $15,869 per person. Nearly all of these persons were "dually eligible" or qualified for both Medicare and Medicaid. State Medicaid programs paid for 41% of all the nursing home and home health care in the United States in 2008. This included $47.7 billion ($29,533 per beneficiary) for 1.6 million of the people in nursing homes and $6.6 billion ($5789 per person) for 1.1 million at home (CMS, n.d.).

As of 2010 the minimum eligibility criteria for Medicaid for the elder living in the community was 133% of the Federal Poverty Level ($29,700 for a family of four). Other eligibility criteria include residency (usually five years in the U.S.) immigration status and documentation of citizenship (CMS, n.d.). Within the broad guidelines established by the federal government, each state establishes its own eligibility criteria, determines the types and extent of services to be covered, sets the payment rates to providers, and administers its own programs. States pay about 40% of the costs. This means that the Medicaid services available to the poorest of the elderly are dependent on the affluence and the policy of a given state. Alabama, with one of the highest percentages of poor residents, also has one of the lowest state incomes and therefore one of the lowest levels of Medicaid services. In most cases, Medicaid covers more services than Medicare, including custodial care in nursing homes.

More states are turning to Medicaid MCPs and HMOs and requiring persons who are dually eligible to enroll in these plans, in an attempt to control costs. Waiver programs, that is, alternative and sometime innovative models are used in some states to further control costs by helping keep Medicaid-eligible elders in their own homes and out of nursing homes with extra support. Medicaid does not help the near-poor, who cannot qualify for aid but cannot afford basic health care. In some states there have been "Medically Needy" and Medicare Saving Plans programs, with month-to-month Medicaid coverage the months the elders' medical expenses make them temporarily eligible for Medicaid. With the financial crisis that states have been experiencing, many of these programs have been abandoned and services under Medicaid have been reduced. The premise of Medicare and Medicaid managed care is that better outcomes will result from systems of care that integrate professionals in responsive teams, maximize the use of subacute care, and provide incentives to reduce the reliance on institutional acute care. Managed care systems are most effective for individuals enrolled over a long period who use ongoing primary care and preventive strategies to maintain health and avoid high-cost emergency services and intensive treatment.

Care For Veterans

The Veterans Health Administration (VA) system has long held a leadership role in gerontological research, medical care, and extended care. A great deal of the research that has guided gerontologists was generated through the VA system. In addition, the vast majority of geriatric fellowships have been provided through the Department of Veterans Affairs (VA) to physicians, nurse practitioners, and nurses. The VA system has been a model for continuity of care in the various care provider systems in place. Early on, this system provided VA-run nursing homes, home care and community-based primary care programs, respite care, blindness rehabilitation, mental health, and numerous other services in addition to acute medical-surgical provisions. As a result of a combination of budget cuts and growth of the covered population, services have become more restricted, but the needs of veterans, especially those who were active in a war zone, have remained a priority.

At one time, veterans' hospitals and services were available on an as-needed basis for anyone who had served at any time. It was not necessary for individuals to use their Medicare benefits. However, this system has undergone significant change. One of the first changes was restrictions placed on the use of veterans' hospitals and services. Instead of coverage for any health problems, priorities were set for those problems that were in some way deemed "service-connected"; in other words, the health care problem had to be linked to the time the person was on active duty. In addition, those with Medicare are expected to apply for and use that payment mechanism first before the

VA will cover the medical expenses, usually through TRICARE described later in this chapter.

For those veterans who served in a war zone and receive a military pension there is additional monetary support available to them if they need assistance with ADLs. The application process to the program called "Aid and Attendance Pension" is quite cumbersome but may be especially helpful for those who need custodial care at home or in an assisted living facility (see Chapter 3). The veteran may qualify (Box 23-2) for monetary help for their own care or that of a spouse, of up to $2022/month per couple depending on circumstances (2012 figures). Other benefits change from time to time, such as the recent availability of funds to reimburse a veteran for travel to and from a doctor's office. For those living in rural areas or dependent on companion transport services this can be quite helpful. The elder is encouraged to find out more about these and other programs on http://www.facebook.com/VANFSG#!/VeteransAffairs.

TRICARE for Life

TRICARE for Life (TFL) is the health care insurance program provided by the Department of Defense for active duty and retired military/uniformed service personnel and their dependents. This plan requires the person to enroll in both Medicare A and B and pay the premiums for Part B. As a Medigap policy, TFL covers those expenses not covered by Medicare, such as copays and prescription medicines. Dependent parents or parents-in-law may be eligible for pharmacy benefits if they turned 65 years of age on or after April 1, 2001 and are enrolled in Medicare B themselves. For more information, see www.tricare.osd.mil.

Long-Term Care Insurance

Some persons are electing to purchase additional insurance (long-term care insurance [LTCI]) for their potential long-term care needs. Ideally these policies cover both the expenses related to copays for nursing home and home care and for what is called custodial care, which is help with activities of daily living (ADLs). Traditionally these policies were limited to care in long-term care facilities, and provided a flat-rate reimbursement to residents for their costs. However, these policies are becoming more creative and innovative and may cover home care costs instead, or in addition, under some circumstances. Because they do not receive any governmental funding support, the premium costs can be prohibitive.

Many plans are being marketed at present, although many do not reach the ideal. The purchaser must be cautioned to read the policy carefully and understand all the details, limitations, and exclusions. There are particular concerns related to Alzheimer's disease because many policies exclude these individuals from home benefits and include very limited institutional benefits. The best LTCI packages have been negotiated by a large employer or state organization or association (see www.ANA.org). It is also advisable to check consumer reports of the particular insurance company and its claims paid history before purchasing a policy.

Implications for Gerontological Nursing and Healthy Aging

Nurses are increasingly at the frontlines of helping elders achieve the highest level of wellness possible. They also advocate for the best, most cost-effective care available.

Case and Care Management

Although the terms *case manager* and *care manager* have slightly different connotations, in real practice the roles are seldom that clear and there is much overlap. Both of these roles include that of advocate, broker, leader, manager, counselor, negotiator, administrator, and communicator. Ideally the care manager follows the person through the entire continuum of care. Care managers must be experts regarding community resources and understand how these can best be used to meet the person's needs. They are expected to make appropriate referrals within the person's expectations and abilities and to monitor the quality of any

---

BOX 23-2	Eligibility of VA Aid and Attendance Improved Pension

- War-time veteran with 90 days of active duty, at least 1 day beginning or ending during a period of war
- Eligible for, or receiving, a military pension
- Requires assistance with one or more activities of daily living due to physical or mental impairment or blindness
- Spouse of a war-time veteran in need of assistance
- May reside at home, in an assisted living facility, or in a nursing home
- Have on average less than $80,000 in assets, *excluding* home and vehicles

From Aid and Attendance Pension Eligibility. Available at http://www.veteranaid.org/eligibility.php.

arranged services. The care or case manager is a resource person whom the elder or caregiver can seek for advice and counsel and for brokering (negotiating, arranging) the flow of services. As a gatekeeper, the case or care manager controls the entrances and exits to services to make sure that the elder gets what is needed without wasting resources.

Care managers are usually paid privately. Those who cannot afford the out-of-pocket expenses of purchased case management services must rely on those available through Medicare-managed care plans or nonprofit community agencies, such as Catholic Senior Services, if available. Access to publicly funded programs varies by state and areas within the state and is dependent on state, county, and agency budgets and priorities. For further information see www.cmsa.org and www.rncasemanager.com.

Some frail and needy elders desire to remain in their homes even when few services and minimal assistance are available to them. This situation is often distressing to the nurse, but as competent adults, elders have a right to make their own life choices and may opt to stay home with less rather than going to a nursing home with more. However, nurses can continue to advocate for and support the elder in any way that is possible and acceptable to them.

Care that is well managed is believed to be a solution to both the spiraling cost and the fragmentation of care experienced by elders with multiple needs. The care manager works to optimize the resources and outcome for the client and the agency or community in which the person resides.

In response to the emergence of case management, the Case Management Society of America (CMSA), an international, nonprofit organization, was founded in 1990 (www.cmsa.org). The CMSA developed the Standards of Practice for Case Management and the Standards of Practice and Ethics Statement. Education, research, and networking to create professionalism and accountability are top priorities of the organization. These were last updated in 2010. The American Association of Managed Care Nurses (www.aamcn) provides significant opportunities for network and training for nurses in this practice.

Multidisciplinary Care Team Planning

The nurse also influences health outcomes and promotes healthy aging through participating in and leading multidisciplinary care team meetings. This can be part of his or her responsibility as the care or case manager, as a representative of an insurer, or as a health care provider (e.g., nurse in a nursing home). The basic case management team for the care of an individual and family involves a physician and/or nurse practitioner, licensed nurse, rehabilitation specialist, and social worker. It also may include

chaplains, dietitians, and certified nursing assistants. Patients and their significant others are also included.

As the health care system becomes more complex, the need for collaboration among these interested parties becomes more important. The special knowledge and skills of a dozen or more professionals may be required in working with a single elder and his or her family. A functioning multidisciplinary team will reduce care redundancy, fragmentation, and waste by making use of the resources available in a coordinated and cost-effective manner.

Ensuring Quality of Care

Nurses are also influential in and responsible for ensuring continuous quality improvement and quality management in all health care settings regardless of the financial arrangements. Funders, licensing agencies, accrediting bodies, and patients all depend on the nurse to make sure that the care provided is the care that is actually needed, and that the care is of high quality. Funding sources, especially the federal government through Medicare, have taken steps to ensure that their standards are met and that their monies are not wasted; this is accomplished through audits, the required documentation of care, and performance incentives.

Legal Issues in Gerontological Nursing

Basic knowledge of the most common legal issues that may arise when working with older adults is as important as the financial issues just discussed. Legal concerns are most often related to an individual's ability to make health care decisions and consent to treatment or research. While this section is not intended to provide legal advice or encourage nurses to do so; it is intended to provide background into common legal and protective issues the gerontological nurse will be exposed to in caring for older persons, especially those who are vulnerable.

Competence (Capacity)

Competence and *capacity* are interchangeable legal terms used to indicate the level of a person's ability to make decisions. This includes the ability to understand the consequences of one's actions and choices. This ability is presumed unless there is clear evidence indicating that the person cannot understand the information needed to make decisions.

Capacity is multifaceted. It includes the ability to handle finances and daily business, to take care of oneself, and, finally, to make medical and health-related decisions. Capacity includes the ability to agree to or to decline health care treatment and procedures. Giving consent to participate in research is more complex because it may or may not directly benefit the individual.

When the capacity of an individual to make informed decisions is believed to be impaired, only the courts can declare the person "incapacitated." He or she may be determined to have no or limited capacity in one area of his or her life but to have ability in another. For example, one may not be able to adequately take care of day-to-day personal business such as bill paying but may still be able to make personal health care decisions. For those who are unable to speak for themselves or not able to understand the consequences of their decisions for whatever reason, legal protection may be needed. However, every attempt should be made to match the level of protection to that which is needed. In other words, actions are taken that provide the needed protection at the lowest level of personal restriction.

Legal protection of the person with impaired capacity ranges from a general power of attorney, often limited to financial concerns, to guardianship, a mechanism in which the person becomes a "ward" under the complete protection of a guardian or conservator. Each is discussed in the following sections.

Power of Attorney

A *power of attorney* (POA) is a legal document in which one person designates another person (e.g., family member, friend) to act on his or her behalf. The two types are a general POA and a durable POA. The appointed person becomes known as the *attorney-in-fact*. The attorney-in-fact named in a general POA usually has the right to make financial decisions, pay bills, and so on, in defined circumstances but not necessarily to make decisions related to health care.

The attorney-in-fact appointed in a durable POA usually has additional rights and responsibilities to make health-related decisions for persons when they are unable to do so themselves. This person is known as the *health care surrogate or proxy*. A health care surrogate is expected to use "substituted judgment" in making decisions; that is, the decision is expected to be that which the person would have made for herself or himself if able to do so and not what the surrogate would make for herself or himself in the same situation. Therefore it is always advisable that the choice of the surrogate is someone who knows and is willing to uphold the wishes and preferences of the person. Whether the health care surrogate is allowed to make end-of-life decisions is determined by state statutes (see Chapter 25).

POAs are in effect only at the specific request of the elder or, in the case of the durable POA, in the event that he or she is unable to act on his or her own behalf. As soon as the person regains abilities, the POA is no longer in force unless the individual requests it to continue. The elder retains all of the rights and responsibilities afforded by usual law. This is the least restrictive form of protection and assistance, providing decision making for persons with impaired capacity. An important aspect of the POA is that persons who are given decision-making rights are those who have been chosen by the elder rather than by a court. This type of advance planning is generally recommended because it is the least restrictive and the most likely to ensure that the wishes of the person are followed.

Guardians and Conservators

Guardians and conservators are individuals, agencies, or corporations that have been appointed by the court to have care, custody, and control of a disabled person and manage his or her personal or financial affairs (or both) when the person has been found (adjudicated) to lack capacity.

Whereas a *conservator* is appointed specifically to control the finances of the ward, the person appointed to be responsible for the person is usually called the *guardian*, although these terms are sometimes used interchangeably. The conservator or guardian continues in that role until the court rescinds the order. The appointment is made at a court hearing in which someone demonstrates the incapacity of the elder. Often the elder is not present. The elder is declared *incapacitated* (formerly called *incompetent*). How this is handled differs by state. In many states the ward, as a person without any legal standing is called, is unable to petition the courts to have his or her rights restored.

In some states, limits are set according to the degree of protection needed. Total dependency means the person cannot meet basic needs for survival and is unable to manage the environment in any self-sustaining way. Some dependency means the person may be able to manage certain challenges of life; health or judgment may interfere with management of other needs. In the latter situation, a limited guardian may be appointed to protect the person in very specific ways. There are considerable pros and cons in the use of conservatorships and guardianships, including high risk for exploitation.

Implications for Gerontological Nursing and Healthy Aging

Although nursing has long recognized the need for gerontological specialization, the law and lawyers have only more recently done so. The National Elder Law Foundation (NELF) is one of the few specialty organizations that certify lawyers who have demonstrated knowledge pertinent to the legal needs of older adults (www.naela.org).

These categories of need relate to both legal and economic concerns of older adults and differ little from those with which nurses have been dealing for years as they care for their elderly clients. Gerontological nursing as a specialty has been evolving (see Chapter 2) and has become more important as the population of older adults has increased and their health care and other needs have been identified, been acknowledged, and become more complex. Nurses who are consulted by elders about legal issues should not attempt to provide legal advice, but instead should refer their clients to a NELF-certified attorney. The state or local bar association is a resource for nurses and for elders and their advocates.

Elder Mistreatment and Neglect

Unfortunately, a person in need of the assistance of others is at risk for harm and injury at the hands of a frustrated, angry, fraudulent, careless, or disturbed caregiver. Mistreatment of older frail and vulnerable adults is found in all socioeconomic, racial, and ethnic groups across the United States. Although cultural nuances exist in what is acceptable and what is not, mistreatment can be seen in any configuration of family and in every setting. Mistreatment includes several types of abuse and neglect. The most common types of abuse are physical, psychological, sexual, and financial (see Appendix 23-1 at the end of this chapter). Medical abuse is also seen, wherein the person is subjected to unwanted treatments or procedures, or medical neglect when desired treatment is withheld. Neglect implies that an identified caregiver has not met his or her obligation. Self-neglect is recognized when a person is not caring for herself or himself in the manner in which most peers would do so. In all cases the vulnerable person is harmed.

In recognition of the escalating problem of elder mistreatment across the globe, countries are busy defining the problem and establishing plans for prevention. Federal definitions of elder abuse, neglect, and exploitation appeared for the first time in the 1987 Amendments to the Older Americans Act. These definitions were provided in the law only as guidelines for identifying the problems and not for enforcement purposes. The specific definitions of elder abuse or mistreatment are now defined by state law and vary considerably from one jurisdiction to another. In 1992 the U.S. Congress passed the Family Violence Prevention and Services Act, mandating an analysis of the problem, and the Vulnerable Elder Rights Protection Act, which established the National Ombudsman Program (www.ltcombudsman.org). In December 2001, the first National Summit on Elder Abuse in the United States was held to identify future directions in the protection of abused elders. The National Center for Elder Abuse

(NCEA) provides detailed information on the state of elder abuse and related laws (www.elderabusecenter.org). In 2012 the Hartford Center for Geriatric Nursing at the University of Iowa published a compendium of evidence-based guidelines on the assessment of and intervention for elder abuse (Daly, 2011). And finally, on June 14, 2012, the White House held a first-ever Symposium on Elder Abuse. The extent of abuse is somewhat difficult to determine, however several studies have been done trying to estimate prevalence. In the most recent, 1 out of 10 respondents over 60 years of age reported being emotionally, physically, or sexually abused or potentially neglected in the past year (Daly, 2011). Most abuse occurs in the home setting, where the majority of caregiving occurs. Most abusers are spouses or adult children. The incidence of elder abuse is expected to increase with the increase in the numbers of persons in need of care, the increasingly conflicting demands on the caregivers' time, and the increased pressure to report suspicions of abuse (Gorbien & Eisenstein, 2005).

Elder abuse requires an abuser, an elder, and the context of caregiving and the expectation of trust (Lantz, 2006). The abuse tends to be episodic and recurrent rather than isolated. There are multiple risk factors for one to be or become an abuser or abused (Box 23-3). Persons who are abusing substances, have emotional or mental illnesses, or

BOX 23-3   Profiles of Abused and Abusers

Abused Elders
Married
Lower socioeducational level
Woman 80 years of age or older
Lives with abuser, but socially isolated
White
Has mental or physical disability
Is dependent on abuser
Reside in unsafe or inadequate housing

Abusers
Has mental health and substance abuse problems
Is stressed/frustrated with caregiving role
Is financially dependent on abused, has inadequate
    financial resources of their own
Has had or does have health problems
Has history of abuse and being abused

From Daly JM: Evidence-based guidelines: elder abuse prevention, *J Geriatr Nurs* 37(11):11-17, 2011.

have a history of abusing or being abused are more likely to be abusers, as are caregivers who are exhausted and frustrated. The abuser is usually the caregiver but may also be the care recipient. Caregivers, be they informal (e.g., spouses) or formal (e.g., nursing assistants), may be subjected to verbal and physical abuse by the person they are caring for. This may be a lifelong pattern that intensifies in the caregiving situation, or it may be the result of deepseated prejudices (Gorbien & Eisenstein, 2005).

Older women are at particular risk for mistreatment (Box 23-4). In a cross-sectional study of abuse among community-dwelling women older than 55 years of age, nearly half reported having experienced some type of abuse, and many of them reported repeated abuse (Fisher & Regan, 2006). This risk is intensified if they have been abused in the past or if their behavior is aggressive, combative, or provocative; that is, they are viewed as overly demanding or unappreciative (Gorbien & Eisenstein, 2005). The level of dependency is also a factor; the more dependent the elder, the more vulnerable he or she is to being abused. Men or women who had abused the caregiver earlier in life are at risk for retaliation.

Because both the majority of caregiving and the majority of abuse occur within the family, this is the context. Caregiver–care recipient relationships that were conflicted earlier in life will continue to be so. However, mistreatment and exploitation can also occur in any caregiving situation (Quinn & Zielke, 2005). When there are a number of providers, monitoring becomes especially difficult. Situations of potential formal caregiver abuse include those in which there is inadequate supervision of patient care, poor

coordination of services, inadequate staff training, theft and fraud, drug and alcohol abuse by staff, tardiness and absenteeism, unprofessional and criminal conduct, and inadequate record keeping. Exploitation includes what is referred to as "undue influence" when it is suspected that a caregiver, companion, or home care provider has influenced an impaired elder to transfer assets to them without consultation with those usually involved in care (Fitzwater & Puchta, 2010). These situations are being examined more carefully in the courts, and some states are activating legal protections against undue influence (Box 23-5). The nurse should pay particular attention to the caregiver, formal or informal, who is alone, with no support from others and no opportunities for respite.

Most often, older victims are unwilling or afraid to report the problem because of shame, embarrassment, intimidation, or fear of retaliation. The abuser may be the only caregiver available, and reporting or complaining could leave him or her without any care at all. The abuse may be part of a lifelong pattern in which the victim has always felt somewhat at fault and so he or she will remain in the situation.

Implications for Gerontological Nursing and Healthy Aging

Assessment

Nurses must be vigilant and sensitive to the potential for abuse, observing for signs and symptoms in all their interactions with vulnerable elders. In addition to the physical signs (see Appendix 23-1), the nurse looks for more subtle signals. Is there an unusual delay between the beginning of a health problem and when help is sought? Are appointments often missed without reasonable explanations? Are there inconsistencies between the history given by the elder and that by the caregiver?

There also may be behavioral indications suggestive of an abusive situation. Does the caregiver do all of the talking in a situation, even though the elder is capable? Does the caregiver appear angry, frustrated, or indifferent while the elder appears hesitant or frightened? Is the caregiver or the care recipient aggressive toward the other or the nurse?

If abuse is suspected, a full assessment should be done, including a determination of the safety of the victim and the desires of the victim if competent. Assessment of mistreatment involves several components. A detailed list of evidence-based assessment tools can be found in University of Iowa Hartford Center for Geriatric Nursing Excellence as well as the Hartford Geriatric Nursing Institute's websites (see the *Try This:* series and the Evolve website for this book).

BOX 23-4   Women and Abuse

A study conducted by Bonnie Fisher and Saundra Regan examined the types of abuse, repeated abuse, and the experiences of multiple abuse by women over 60 years of age. A telephone survey was responded to by 842 women living in the community. Almost half the women have experienced some type of abuse since the age of 55; many of these reported repeated abuse. The abused women were more likely than the nonabused women to complain of health problems, including bone and joint problems, digestive problems, depression or anxiety, chronic pain, high blood pressure, or heart problems.

Data from Fisher BS, Regan SL: The extent and frequency of abuse in the lives of older women and their relationship with health outcomes, *Gerontologist* 46(2):200-209, 2006.

BOX 23-5 Potential Indications of Undue Influence

- Elder takes actions inconsistent with his or her life history. Actions run counter to the person's previous long-time values and beliefs.
- Elder makes sudden changes with regard to financial management. Examples include cashing in insurance policies or changing titles on bank accounts or real property.
- Elder unexpectedly changes his or her will and previous disposition of assets.
- Elder is taken to practitioners different from those he or she has always trusted. Examples include bankers, stockbrokers, attorneys, physicians, and realtor.
- Elder is systematically isolated from or is continually monitored when with others who have been significant to him or her.
- Someone suddenly moves into the person's home, or the elder is moved into someone's home under the guise of providing better care.
- Someone attempts to get income checks directed differently from the usual arrangement.
- Documents are suddenly signed, frequently as the elder nears death.
- A history of mistrust exists in the elder's family, especially with financial affairs, and the elder places unusual trust in newfound acquaintances.

- Someone, especially previously uninvolved or unknown to others, promises to provide lifelong care in exchange for receipt of property on the elder's death.
- Statements of the elder and the alleged abuser vary concerning the elder's affairs or disposition of assets.
- A power imbalance exists between the parties in matters of finances or health.
- Someone shows unfairness to the weaker party in a transaction. The stronger person unduly benefits by the transaction.
- The elder is never left alone with anyone. No one is allowed to speak to the elder without the alleged abuser having a way of finding out about it.
- Unusual patterns arise in the elder's finances. For instance, numerous checks are written out to "cash," always in round numbers, and often in large amounts.
- The elder reports meeting a "wonderful new friend who makes me feel young again." The elder then becomes suspicious of family and begins to avoid family gatherings.
- The elder is pressed into a transaction without being given time to reflect or contact trusted advisors.

From Quinn M: Undue influence and elder abuse: recognition and intervention strategies, *Geriatr Nurs* 23(1):11-16, 2002.

Interventions

The goals of intervention are to stop mistreatment and neglect of elders, to protect the victim and society from inappropriate and illegal acts, to hold abusers accountable, to rehabilitate the offender, and to order restitution of property and payment for expenses incurred as a result of exploitation. However, most of these are beyond the nurse's usual scope of practice. The most important information for nurses to know is how to participate in the prevention and early recognition of potential abuse as well as the requirements for mandatory reporting in their states (Ziminski & Phillips, 2011).

Mandatory Reporting

In most states and U.S. jurisdictions, licensed nurses are required to report suspicions of abuse to the state, usually to a group called "adult protective services." Most often these reports are anonymous. Allegations of abuse should not be made on the basis of casual suspicion but on that of solid evidence. If the nurse believes the elder to be in immediate danger, the police must be notified and the person protected from harm. How the nurse accomplishes this varies with the work setting. In hospitals and nursing homes this is often first reported internally to the facility social worker or supervisor. In the home care setting, the report is made to the nursing supervisor. It would be very unusual for the nurse not to go through his or her employer. However, the nurse who is a neighbor, friend, or privately paid caregiver may be under obligation to make the report themselves. In the nursing home or licensed assisted living facility, the nurse has the additional resource of calling the state long-term care ombudsman for help. In each state, ombudsmen are either volunteers or paid state employees who are responsible for acting as advocates for vulnerable elders in institutions. All reports, either to the state ombudsman or to adult protective services, will be investigated. A unique aspect of elder abuse compared with child abuse is that the physically frail but mentally competent adult can refuse assessment and intervention and often does. Abused but competent elders cannot be removed from harmful situations without their permission, much to the frustration of the nurse and other health care providers. As discussed earlier, an older adult continues to have the right to make all personal decisions unless declared otherwise in a court of law.

Prevention of Mistreatment

In the ideal situation, gerontological nurses are alert to situations of risk for mistreatment of vulnerable elders and take steps to prevent the occurrence of abuse or neglect (see the Evidence-Based Practice box). In some situations the abuse may be preventable, and in others, it is not. If the abuse is the result of psychopathological conditions, especially if the situation is long-standing, the nurse is unlikely to be able to prevent the abuse. However, nurses can make sure that the potential victims know how to get help in an emergency and know what resources are available to them; nurses can provide support and encouragement that it is possible to leave the situation, if this is the case (Capezuti, 2011). Unfortunately there are very few shelters that will accept a frail older adult. The nurse can also work with the elder, the caregiver, and community supports to increase

EVIDENCE-BASED PRACTICE
Prevention of Elder Abuse and Mistreatment

- Learn how to assess for actual or potential abuse.
- Know your state statutes and regulations related to the nurse's role in elder abuse and reporting suspicions.
- Keep informed, attend related continuing education programs.
- Help caregivers find and obtain respite services for intermittent relief.
- Help caregivers and elders broaden their social support networks.
- Provide caregivers and elders with money management programs.
- Help families develop and nurture informal support systems.
- Link families with support groups.
- Teach families stress management techniques.
- Arrange comprehensive care resources.
- Provide counseling for troubled or high-risk families.

From Daly JM: Evidence-based guidelines: elder abuse prevention, *J Geriatr Nurs* 37(11):11-17, 2011.

the exposure of the elders to others. If the abusive behavior is learned or a response to stress, the situation may allow for change. Learned abuse, theoretically, can be unlearned and may respond to a close working relationship with a mentoring professional who can model positive problem solving and new ways of managing difficult situations including anger management.

If the abuse is based on the stress of caregiving, nurses can be very proactive and help all involved do things to lessen the stress. This may include finding respite services, changing the situation entirely (giving permission to the caregiver to give up the role), referring to support groups for ventilation of frustrations and peer support, teaching people how to use crisis hotlines, professional consultation, victim support groups, victim volunteer companions, and, above all, thoughtful and compassionate care for both.

It has become clear as we face the burgeoning population of very old survivors and the entry of the baby boomers into the ranks of older persons that many aspects of the health care system must be modified. Because nurses are pivotal players within the system and occupy diverse roles, there are abundant opportunities for professional growth and gratification in working with elders in our ever-shifting health care system. Nurses are case managers and primary care coordinators in the home. We expect that nurses will continue to occupy a pivotal role in home care as advocates and to carefully evaluate care plans, quality outcomes, and costs.

Application of Maslow's Hierarchy

At the most basic levels of Maslow's Hierarchy, nurses are expected to provide safety and security to the persons under their care to the extent possible regardless of the capacity of the person; this responsibility increases as the limitations of the elder increase. The nurse is often the one who provides much of the information that elders and their significant others need to make informed decisions. When doing so it is essential that this exchange is documented in the health care record (see Chapter 7). The nurse often deals with the difficult and problematic legal and ethical issues in the provision of culturally appropriate care. Providing culturally appropriate care within the context of a patient's changing cognitive capacity and judgment is at the core of many ethical and legal dilemmas in gerontological nursing.

KEY CONCEPTS

- Health care and its systems are undergoing profound changes, including the increase in the number of managed care organizations and changes in the roles of health care providers. All of these changes affect the care of the older adult.

- A combination of Social Security and Supplementary Security Income payments provides eligible persons with a regular income after the age of 65 or earlier if disabled. The total amount varies greatly and is dependent on qualified earned income during the working years.
- Medicare, Medicaid, and TRICARE are insurance plans for specific groups of people.
- Medicaid pays for a large portion of the cost associated with nursing home care.
- There may be substantial out-of-pocket costs associated with the receipt of health care today.
- In order for Medicare to pay for the expenses related to long-term care or home health care, strict criteria of medical necessity must be met.
- Good care management is that which considers cost, quality, and coordination of services.
- Nurses have key roles in the assurance of quality care to older adults.
- Protective measures are available for persons with limited or absent capacity through power-of-attorney, guardians, and conservators.
- The nurse has a responsibility to ensure the safety and security of those persons to whom care is provided. This responsibility does not change with the change in the persons' legal status or capacity.
- Elder abuse requires a situation of caregiving; however either the care recipient or the caregiver may be the perpetrator.
- In most jurisdictions the nurse is required to report suspicions of abuse of the elderly and any person who is vulnerable.

ACTIVITIES AND DISCUSSION QUESTIONS

1. Interview a nurse case manager, and ask about the components of the position that are gratifying and those that are the most difficult.
2. Discuss your thoughts about specific activities that are different for case managers and care managers.
3. Describe the role of the nurse-advocate in relation to health and consumer protections.
4. Explain the fundamentals of Medicare and Medicaid sufficiently to assist elders in obtaining more specific information.
5. Activity: Interview an elder in a rehabilitation center, adult day health or senior center and ask about his or her experience in the setting and across settings.
6. Activity: Identify a person at least 70 years of age who has Medicare. Interview them about how Medicare does or does not meet his or her needs. Write a brief summary, and present it to the class.

REFERENCES

Achenbaum WA: *Old age in a new land*, Baltimore, 1978, Johns Hopkins Press.

Cantril H: *Public opinion 1935–1946*, Princeton, NJ, 1951, Princeton University Press.

Capezuti E: Recognizing and referring suspected elder mistreatment, *Geriatr Nurs* 32(2), 209–211, 2011.

Center for Medicare and Medicaid Services [CMS]: *Medicare enrollment: national trends, 1966-2008* (2008). Available at http://www.cms.gov/Research-Statistics-Data-and-Systems/Statistics-Trends-and-Reports/MedicareEnrpts/downloads/HI08.pdf.

Center for Medicare and Medicaid Services [CMS]: *Medicare and you, 2012.* Baltimore, MD, 2011, CMS Product no. 10050-27.

Center for Medicare and Medicaid Services [CMS]: *Medicaid & CHIP program information: eligibility* (n.d.). Available at http://www.medicaid.gov/Medicaid-CHIP-Program-Information/By-Topics/Eligibility/Eligibility.html.

Daly JM: Evidence-Based guideline: Elder abuse prevention. *J Geriatr Nurs* 37(11):11–17, 2011.

Fisher BS, Regan SL: The extent and frequency of abuse in the lives of older women and their relationship with health outcomes, *Gerontologist* 46(2):200–209, 2006.

Fitzwater EL, Puchta C: Elder abuse and financial exploitation: Unlawful and just plain awful! *J Geriatr Nurs* 36(12): 3–5, 2010.

Gorbien MJ, Eisenstein AR: Elder abuse and neglect: an overview, *Clin Geriatr Med* 21(2):279–292, 2005.

Hooyman N, Kiyak H: *Social gerontology: a multidisciplinary approach*, New York, 2008, Pearson.

Lantz MS: Elder abuse and neglect: help starts with recognizing the problem, *Clin Geriatr* 14(9):10–13, 2006.

Quinn K, Zielke H: Elder abuse, neglect, and exploitation: policy issues, *Clin Geriatr Med* 21(2):440–457, 2005.

U.S. Social Security Administration [SSA]: *Summary of P.L. 98-21, (HR 1900)* (1984). Available at http://www.socialsecurity.gov/history/1983amend.html.

U.S. Social Security Administration [SSA]: *Earning Social Security credit* (2012a). Available at http://ssa-custhelp.ssa.gov/app/answers/detail/a_id/73/kw/credits.

U.S. Social Security Administration [SSA]: *Average monthly Social Security benefit for a retired worker* (2012b). Available at http://ssa.custhelp.ssa.gov/app/answers/detail/a_id/13/kw/retirement/session/L3RpbWUvMTMzNDcwMzkzOC9zaWQvYmt5aFVVVms%3D.

U.S. Social Security Administration [SSA]: *Understanding Supplementary Security Income (SSI) benefits* (2012c). Available at http://www.socialsecurity.gov/ssi/text-benefits-ussi.htm.

Ziminski CE, Phillips LR: The nursing role I reporting elder abuse: specific examples and interventions, *J Geriatr Nurs* 37(11), 19–23, 2011.

Definitions of Elder Abuse and Neglect

The following definitions of abuse, exploitation, and neglect pertain to elders. The perpetrator of this abuse may or may not be the caregiver of an elderly person or a member of the elderly person's family. Furthermore, some signs and symptoms are characteristic of several kinds of mistreatment and should be regarded as possible indicators. These are most important:

- An elder's frequent unexplained crying
- An elder's unexplained fear of or suspicion of a particular person(s)

Physical abuse is defined as the use of physical force that may result in bodily injury, physical pain, or impairment. Physical abuse may include but is not limited to such acts of violence as striking (with or without an object), hitting, beating, pushing, shoving, shaking, slapping, kicking, pinching, and burning. In addition, the inappropriate use of drugs and physical restraints, force-feeding, and physical punishment of any kind also are examples of physical abuse.

Signs and symptoms of physical abuse include but are not limited to the following:

- Bruises, black eyes, welts, lacerations, and rope marks
- Bone fractures, broken bones, and skull fractures
- Open wounds, cuts, punctures, untreated injuries, and injuries in various stages of healing
- Sprains, dislocations, and internal injuries or bleeding
- Broken eyeglasses or frames, physical signs of being subjected to punishment, and signs of being restrained
- Laboratory findings of medication overdose or under-utilization of prescribed drugs
- An elder's report of being hit, slapped, kicked, or mistreated
- An elder's sudden change in behavior
- The caregiver's refusal to allow visitors to see an elder alone

Sexual abuse is defined as nonconsensual sexual contact of any kind. Sexual contact with any person incapable of giving consent also is considered sexual abuse. It includes but is not limited to unwanted touching, all types of sexual assault or battery such as rape or sodomy, coerced nudity, and sexually explicit photographing.

Signs and symptoms of sexual abuse include but are not limited to the following:

- Bruises around the breasts or genital area
- Unexplained venereal disease or genital infections
- Unexplained vaginal or anal bleeding
- Torn, stained, or bloody underclothing
- An elder's report of being sexually assaulted or raped

Emotional or psychological abuse is defined as the infliction of anguish, pain, or distress through verbal or nonverbal acts. Emotional and/or psychological abuse includes but is not limited to verbal assaults, insults, threats, intimidation, humiliation, and harassment. In addition, treating an older person like an infant; isolating an elderly person from his or her family, friends, or regular activities; giving an older person a "silent treatment"; and enforced social isolation also are examples of emotional or psychological abuse.

Signs and symptoms of emotional and/or psychological abuse may manifest themselves in such behaviors of an elderly person as the following:

- Being emotionally upset or agitated
- Being extremely withdrawn and uncommunicative or unresponsive
- Unusual behavior usually attributed to dementia (e.g., sucking, biting, rocking)
- An elder's report of being verbally or emotionally mistreated

Neglect is defined as the refusal or failure to fulfill any part of a person's caregiving obligations or duties to an elder. Neglect may also pertain to a person who has fiduciary responsibilities to provide care for an elder (e.g., pay for necessary home care services), or to the failure on the part of an in-home service provider to provide necessary care. Neglect typically means the refusal or failure to provide an elderly person with such life necessities as food, water, clothing, shelter, personal hygiene, medicine, comfort, personal safety, and other essentials included in the responsibility or agreement to an elder.

Signs and symptoms of neglect include but are not limited to the following:

- Dehydration, malnutrition, untreated bedsores, and poor personal hygiene
- Unattended or untreated health problems
- Hazardous or unsafe living conditions or arrangements (e.g., improper wiring, no heat, or no running water)
- Unsanitary and unclean living conditions (e.g., dirt, fleas, lice on person, soiled bedding, fecal and/or urine smell, inadequate clothing)

Abandonment is defined as the desertion of an elderly person by an individual who has assumed responsibility for providing care for an elder, or by a person with physical custody of an elder.

Signs and symptoms of abandonment include but are not limited to the following:

- The desertion of an elder at a hospital, a nursing facility, or other similar institution
- The desertion of an elder at a shopping center or other public location
- An elder's own report of being abandoned

Self-neglect is characterized as the behaviors of the person that threaten his or her own health or safety. Self-neglect generally manifests itself in an older person's refusal or failure to provide himself or herself with adequate food, water, clothing, shelter, personal hygiene, medication (when indicated), and safety precautions. The definition of self-neglect excludes a situation in which a cognitively or mentally competent older person (who understands the consequences of his or her decisions) makes a conscious and voluntary decision to engage in acts that threaten his or her health or safety as a matter of personal preference.

Signs and symptoms of self-neglect include but are not limited to the following:

- Dehydration, malnutrition, untreated or improperly attended medical conditions, and poor personal hygiene
- Hazardous or unsafe living conditions or arrangements (e.g., improper wiring, no indoor plumbing, no heat or running water)
- Unsanitary or unclean living quarters (e.g., animal or insect infestation, no functioning toilet, fecal and/or urine smell)
- Inappropriate and/or inadequate clothing, lack of the necessary medical aids (e.g., eyeglasses, hearing aid, dentures)
- Grossly inadequate housing or homelessness

From National Center on Elder Abuse: *Major types of elder abuse,* 2007. Available at www.ncea.aoa.org/NCEAroot/main_site/FAQ/basics/Types_of_Abuse.aspx.

CHAPTER 24

Relationships, Roles, and Transitions

Theris A. Touhy

evolve evolve.elsevier.com/Ebersole/gerontological

LEARNING OBJECTIVES

Upon completion of this chapter, the reader will be able to:

- Identify the variations of relationships that people identify as constituting "family."
- Examine family relationships in later life.
- Describe the various roles of grandparents.
- Explain the issues involved in adapting to a major transition such as retirement or widowhood.
- Identify the range of caregiving situations and the potential challenges and opportunities of each.
- Discuss nursing responses with older adults and their families who are assuming caregiver roles or experiencing other transitions.
- Discuss intimacy and sexuality in late life and appropriate nursing responses.

GLOSSARY

Caregiving The act of providing assistance to those who are unable to care entirely for themselves. Caregivers may be *informal* (family, friends, and others who volunteer this service) or *formal* (those persons hired to provide the care).

Competent The status of being able to make some decisions independently. There is a wide range of levels of competence from minimal to complex.

Respite A relief in caregiving, providing benefit to both the caregiver and the care recipient.

THE LIVED EXPERIENCE

It is so irritating when Madge tries to help me do things. After all, I have lived 85 years and have done very well. I think she wants to put me away somewhere. I wish she would just leave me alone. I'm sure I could manage if she just wouldn't interfere.

John, the father

I just can't stand watching as my father becomes weaker and is unable to do the things he always did so naturally and well. Yesterday he got lost on his way to the market. He was always my guide and protector. I knew I could count on him no matter what. It makes me feel sort of alone in the world.

Madge, the daughter

Relationships, Roles, and Transitions

This chapter examines the various relationships, roles, and transitions that characteristically play a part in later life. Concepts of family structure and function, the transitions of retirement, widowhood, widowerhood, and caregiving, as well as intimacy and sexuality are examined. Nursing responses to support older adults in maintaining fulfilling roles and relationships and adapting to transitions are discussed.

Families

The idea of family evokes strong impressions of whatever an individual believes the typical family should be. Because everyone comes from a family, these impressions have powerful symbolic meanings. However, in today's world, the definition of family is in a state of flux. As recently as 100 years ago, the norm was the extended family made up of parents, their grown children, and the children's children, often living together and sharing resources, strengths, and challenges. As cities grew and adult children moved in pursuit of work, parents did not always come along, and the nuclear family evolved. The norm in the United States became two parents and their two children (nuclear family), or at least that was the norm in what has been considered mainstream America. This pattern was not as common among ethnically diverse families where the extended family is still the norm. However, families are changing and today, only about 23.5% of U.S. households are composed of nuclear families.

A decrease in fertility rates has reduced family size, and American families are smaller today than ever before (2.6 people in the nuclear family). A delay in the age of childbearing is more common, with the average age of first births now 25 years of age, and first births to women over 35 years of age increasing nearly eight times since 1970. The high divorce and remarriage rate results in households of blended families of children from previous marriages and the new marriage. Single-parent families, blended families, gay and lesbian families, childless families, and fewer families altogether are common.

Multigenerational families have grown by approximately 60% since 1990 (Hooyman & Kiyak, 2011). Growth of multigenerational households has accelerated during the economic downturn. Older people without families, either by choice or circumstance, have created their own "families" through communal living with siblings, friends, or others. Indeed, it is not unusual for childless persons residing in long-term care facilities to refer to the staff as their new "family."

Family members, however they are defined, form the nucleus of relationships for the majority of older adults and their support system if they become dependent. A long-standing myth in society is that families are alienated from their older family members and abandon their care to institutions. Nothing could be farther from the truth. Family relationships remain strong in old age, and most older people have frequent contact with their families. Most older adults possess a large intergenerational web of significant people, including sons, daughters, stepchildren, in-laws, nieces, nephews, grandchildren, and great-grandchildren, as well as partners and former partners of their offspring. Families provide the majority of care for older adults. Changes in family structure will have a significant impact on the availability of family members to provide care for older people in the future.

As families change, the roles of the members or expectations of one another may change as well. Grandparents may assume parental roles for their grandchildren if their children are unable to care for them; or grandparents and older aunts and uncles may assume temporary caregiving roles while the children, nieces, and nephews work. Adult children of any age may provide limited or extensive caregiving to their own parents or aging relatives who may become ill or impaired. A spouse, sibling, or grandchild may become a caregiver as well. This caregiving may be temporary or long term.

Close-knit families are more aware of the needs of their members and work to resolve problems and find ways to meet the needs of members, even if they are not always successful. Emotionally distant families are less available in times of need and have greater potential for conflict. If the family has never been close and supportive, it will not magically become so when members grow older. Resentments long buried may crop up and produce friction or psychological pain. Long-submerged conflicts and feelings may return if the needs of one family member exceed those of the others.

In coming to know the older adult, the gerontological nurse comes to know the family as well, learning of their special gifts and their life challenges. The nurse works with the elder within the unique culture of his or her family of origin, present family, and support networks, including friends.

Types of Families

Traditional Couples

The marital or partnered relationship in the United States is a critical source of support for older people, and nearly 55% of the population age 65 and older is married and lives with a spouse. Although this relationship is often the most binding if it extends into late life, the chance of a couple going through old age together is exceedingly slim. Women over 65 years of age are three times as likely as men of the same age to be widowed. Men who survive their spouse into old age ordinarily have multiple opportunities to remarry if they wish. Even among the oldest-old, the majority of men are married (Federal Interagency Forum on Aging, 2010). A woman is less likely to have an opportunity for remarriage in late life. Often, older couples live together but do not marry because of economic and inheritance reasons.

The needs, tasks, and expectations of couples in late life differ from those in earlier years. Some couples have been married more than 60 or 70 years. These years together may have been filled with love and companionship or abuse and resentment, or anything in between. However, in general, marital status (or the presence of a long-time partner) is positively related to health, life satisfaction, and well-being. For all couples, the normal physical and socio-logical circumstances in late life present challenges. Some of the issues that strain many of these relationships include (1) the deteriorating health of one or both partners, (2) limitations in income, (3) conflicts with children or other relatives, (4) incompatible sexual needs, and (5) mismatched needs for activity and socialization.

Divorce. In the past, divorce was considered a stigma-tizing event. Today, however, it is so common that a person is inclined to forget the ostracizing effects of divorce from 60 years ago. The divorce rate among people 50 years of age and older has doubled in the past 20 years. Older couples are becoming less likely to stay in an unsatisfactory mar-riage and with the aging of the baby boomers, divorce rates will continue to rise. Health care professionals must avoid making assumptions and be alert to the possibility of marital dissatisfaction in old age. Nurses should ask, "How would you describe your marriage?"

Long-term relationships are varied and complex, with many factors forming the glue that holds them together. Marital breakdown may be more devastating in old age because it is often unanticipated and may occur concur-rently with other significant losses. Health care workers must be concerned with supporting a client's decision to seek a divorce and with assisting him or her in seeking counseling in the transition. A nurse should alert the client that a divorce will bring on a grieving process similar to the death of a spouse and that a severe disruption in coping capacity may occur until the client adjusts to a new life. The grief may be more difficult to cope with because no socially sanctioned patterns have been established, as is the case with widowhood. In addition, tax and fiscal policies favor married couples, and many divorced elderly women are at a serious economic disadvantage in retirement.

Nontraditional Couples

As the variations in families grow, so do the types of coupled relationships. Among the types of couples we see today are lesbian, gay, bisexual, and transgender (LGBT) couples. Although the number of LGBT people of any age has remained elusive, an estimated 3 million Americans over 65 years of age are LGBT with projections that this figure is likely to double by 2030 (Gelo, 2008).

Many LGBT individuals are raising children, either alone or as part of a couple. Although these couples are less often seen in the aging population, they are still there but may not be obvious because of long-standing discrimina-tion and fear. It is important to recognize that there are considerable differences in the experiences of younger LGBT individuals when compared to those who are older. Older LGBT individuals did not have the benefit of antidiscrimination laws and support for same-sex partners. They were also more likely to keep their sexual orientation and relationships "hidden."

Many older LGBT individuals have been part of a live-in couple at some time during their life, but as they age, they are more likely to live alone. Some may have developed social networks of friends, members of their family of origin, and the larger community but many lack support. The continued legal and policy barriers faced by LGBT elders contribute to the challenges for those in domestic partnerships as they age. Organizations that serve LGBT elders in the community need to enhance outreach and support mechanisms to enable them to maintain independence and age safely and in good health. LGBT elders living in metropolitan areas may find organizations particularly designed for them, such as Senior Action in a Gay Environment (SAGE); New Leaf Outreach to Elders (formerly GLOE, San Francisco), and the Lesbian and Gay Aging Issues Network (LGAIN).

Increasing numbers of same-sex couples are choosing to have families, and this will call for greater understand-ing of these "new" types of families, young and old. The majority of research has involved gay and lesbian couples, and much less is known about bisexual and transgender relationships. Much more knowledge of cohort, cultural, and generational differences among age groups is needed to understand the dramatic changes in the lives of gay and lesbian individuals in family lifestyles. The National Resource Center on LGBT Aging is the country's first and only technical assistance resource center aimed at improv-ing the quality of services and supports offered to lesbian, gay, bisexual and transgender (LGBT) older adults (http://www.lgbtagingcenter.org/).

Elders and Their Adult Children

In adulthood, relationships between the generations become increasingly important for most people. Older parents enjoy being told about the various activities and successes of their offspring, and these adult children begin to see aspects of themselves that have developed from their parents. At times, the relationships may become strained because the younger adults are more concerned with their own spouses, partners, and children. The parents are no longer central to their lives, though offspring may be central to the lives of their parents. The most difficult situations occur when the elder parents are openly critical or judgmental about the lives of their offspring. In the best of situations, adult children shift to the role of friend, companion, and confidant to the elder, a concept known as filial maturity.

Most older people see their children on a regular basis, and even children who do not live close to their older parents maintain close connections, and *"intimacy at a distance"* can occur (Hooyman & Kiyak, 2011; Silverstein & Angelli, 1998). Approximately 50% of older people have daily contact with their adult children; nearly 80% see an adult child at least once a week; and more than 75% talk on the phone at least weekly with an adult child (Hooyman & Kiyak, 2011).

Never-Married Older Adults

Approximately 4% of older adults today have never married. Older people who have lived alone most of their lives often develop supportive networks with siblings, friends, and neighbors. Never-married older adults may demonstrate resilience to the challenges of aging as a result of their independence and may not feel lonely or isolated. Furthermore, they may have had longer lifetime employment and may enjoy greater financial security as they age. Single older adults will increase in the future because being single is increasingly more common in younger years (Hooyman & Kiyak, 2011).

Grandparents

The role of grandparenting, and increasingly great-grandparenthood, is experienced by most older adults. Eighty percent of those over 65 years of age, and 51% of those 50 to 64, have grandchildren. There are approximately 80 million grandparents in the United States today, spanning ages 30 to 110, with grandchildren that range from newborns to retirees. Fifty percent of grandparents are under 60 years of age, and some will experience grandparenthood for more than 40 years (Livingston & Parker, 2010; Legacy Project, n.d.). Sixty-eight percent of individuals born in 2000 will have four grandparents alive when they reach 18; and 76% will have at least one grandparent at 30 years of age (Hooyman & Kiyak, 2011). Great-grandparenthood will become more common in the future in light of projections of a healthier aging.

As the term implies, the "grands" are a step beyond parents in their concerns, exposure, and responsibility. The majority of grandparents derive great emotional satisfaction from their grandchildren. Historically, the emphasis has been on the progressive aging of the grandparent as it affects the relationship with the grandchild, but little has been said about the effects of the growth and maturation of the grandchild on the relationship. Many young adults who have had close contact with their grandparents report that this relationship was very meaningful in their lives. Growing numbers of adult grandchildren are assisting in caregiving for frail grandparents.

The age, vitality, and proximity of both grandchild and grandparent produce a kaleidoscope of possible activities and interactions as both progress through their aging processes. Approximately 80% of grandparents see a grandchild at least monthly, and nearly 50% do so weekly. Geographic distance does not significantly affect the quality of the relationship between grandparents and their grandchildren. The Internet is increasingly being used by distant grandparents as a way of staying involved in their grandchildren's lives and forging close bonds (Hooyman & Kiyak, 2011).

Younger grandparents typically live closer to their grandchildren and are more involved in child care and recreational activities (Box 24-1). Older grandparents with sufficient incomes may provide more financial assistance and other types of instrumental help. The need for support for adult children and grandchildren has the potential to increase during current economic conditions and may pose

---

BOX 24-1   A Grandmother as Seen by an 8-Year-Old Child

"A grandmother is a woman who has no children of her own. That is why she loves other people's children."

"Grandmothers have nothing to do. They are just there: when they take us for a walk they go slowly, like caterpillars along beautiful leaves. They never say, 'Come on, faster, hurry up!' "

"Everyone should try to have a grandmother, especially those who don't have a TV."

From *Ageing in Focus,* March 2006.

significant financial concerns for older people (American Association of Retired Persons, 2011). More than 60% of grandparents report taking care of their grandchildren on a regular basis, and 13% are primary caregivers. This phenomenon is discussed later in the chapter.

Siblings

Late-life sibling relationships are poorly understood and have been neglected by researchers. As individuals age, they often have more contact with siblings than they did in the years when family and work demands were more pressing. About 80% of older people have at least one sibling, and they are often strong sources of support in the lives of never-married older persons, widowed persons, and those without children. For many elders, these relationships become increasingly important because they have a long history of memories and are of the same generation and similar backgrounds. Sibling relationships become particularly important when they are part of the support system, especially among single or widowed elders living alone. The strongest of sibling bonds is thought to be the relationship between sisters. When blessed with survival, these relationships remain important into late old age. Service providers should inquire about sibling relationships of past and present significance.

The loss of siblings has a profound effect in terms of awareness of one's own mortality, particularly when those of the same gender die. When an elder reaches the age of the sibling who died, the reaction can be quite disruptive. Not only is grieving activated, but also rehearsal for one's own death may occur. In some cases in which an elder sibling survives younger ones, there may be not only a deep grief but also pangs of guilt: "Why them and not me?" (See Chapter 25.)

Other Kin

Interaction with collateral kin (i.e., cousins, aunts, uncles, nieces, nephews) generally depends on proximity, preference, and the general availability of primary kin. The quality of relationships varies but is still a potential source of joy, support, assistance, or conflict. Maternal kin (related through female bloodlines) may be emotionally closer than those in one's paternal line (Jett, 2002). These relatives may provide a reservoir of kin from which to find replacements for missing or lost intimate relationships for single or childless people as they grow older.

Fictive Kin

Fictive kin are nonblood kin who serve as "genuine fake families," as expressed by Virginia Satir. These non-relatives become surrogate family and take on some of the instrumental and affectional attributes of family. Fictive kin are important in the lives of many elders, especially those with no close or satisfying family relationships and those living alone or in institutions. Fictive kin includes both friends and, often, paid caregivers. Primary care providers, such as nursing assistants, nurses, or case managers, often become fictive kin. Professionals who work with older people need to recognize the instrumental and emotional support, as well as the mutually satisfying relationships, that occur between friends, neighbors, and other fictive kin who assist older adults who are dependent.

Later Life Transitions

Role transitions that occur in late life include retirement, grandparenthood, widowhood, and becoming a caregiver or recipient of care. These transitions may occur predictably or may be imposed by unanticipated events. Retirement is an example of a predictable event that can and should be planned long in advance, although for some, it can occur unexpectedly as a result of illness, disability, or being terminated from a job. To the degree that an event is perceived as expected and occurring at the right time, a role transition may be comfortable and even welcomed. Those persons who must retire "too early" or are widowed "too soon" will have more difficulty adapting than those who are at an age when these events are expected.

The speed and intensity of a major change may make the difference between a transitional crisis and a gradual and comfortable adaptation. Most difficult are the transitions that incorporate losses rather than gains in status, influence, and opportunity. The move from independence to dependence and becoming a care recipient is particularly difficult. Conditions that influence the outcome of transitions include personal meanings, expectations, level of knowledge, preplanning, and emotional and physical reserves. Cohort, cultural, and gender differences are inherent in all of life's major transitions. Those transitions that make use of past skills and adaptations may be less stressful. The ideal outcome is when gains in satisfaction and new roles offset losses.

Retirement

Retirement, as we formerly knew it, has changed. Retirement is no longer just a few years of rest from the rigors of work before death. It is a developmental stage that may occupy 30 or more years of one's life and involve many stages. The transitions are blurring, and the numerous patterns and styles of retiring have produced more varied experiences in retirement. With recent events that have seriously threatened pension security and portability, as well as a declining economy, more older people are remaining in the workforce. Forty-four percent of retirees work for pay at some point after retirement. Some do so because of economic need, whereas others have a desire to remain involved and productive. Obviously, health and financial status affect decisions and abilities to work or engage in new work opportunities. The baby boomers increasingly face the prospect of working longer, and 33% of this generation do not own assets and have little in savings or projected retirement income beyond Social Security. Eighty-three percent of baby boomers intend to keep working after retirement (Hooyman & Kiyak, 2011).

Retirement Planning

Current research suggests that retirement has positive effects on life satisfaction and health, although this may vary depending on the individual's circumstances. Predictors of retirement satisfaction are presented in Box 24-2. Decisions to retire are often based on financial resources, attitude toward work, family roles and responsibilities, the nature of the job, access to health insurance, chronological age, health, and self-perceptions of ability to adjust to retirement. Retirement planning is advisable during early adulthood and essential in middle age. However, people differ in their focus on the past, present, and future and their realistic ability to "put away something" for future needs.

Retirement preparation programs are usually aimed at employees with high levels of education and occupational

---

BOX 24-2 Predictors of Retirement Satisfaction

- Good health
- Functional abilities
- Adequate income
- Suitable living environment
- Strong social support system characterized by reciprocal relationships
- Decision to retire involved choice, autonomy, adequate preparation, higher-status job prior to retirement
- Retirement activities that offer an opportunity to feel useful, learn, grow, and enjoy oneself
- Positive outlook, sense of mastery, resilience, resourcefulness
- Good marital relationship if married
- Sharing similar interests to spouse/significant other

Data from Hooyman N, Kiyak H: *Social gerontology: a multidisciplinary perspective,* Boston, 2011, Allyn and Bacon.

---

status, those with private pension coverage, and government employees. Thus the people most in need of planning assistance may be those least likely to have any available, let alone the resources for an adequate retirement. Individuals who are retiring in poor health, culturally and racially diverse persons, and those in lower socioeconomic levels may experience greater concerns in retirement and may need specialized counseling. These groups are often neglected in retirement planning programs.

Working couples must plan together for retirement. Decisions will depend on their career goals, shared future interests, and the quality of their interpersonal relationship. The following are some questions one must weigh when deciding to retire or continue working:
- What do I want to do?
- Who needs me, and what are my best opportunities?
- What am I best able to do?
- What is the meaning of my life?
- What should my life accomplish or contribute?
- Am I financially secure for the rest of my life if I live 30 or more years?
- Can I afford to completely retire from paid work?

Retirement education plans are supplied through employers, group lectures, individual counseling, books, DVDs, and Internet resources. However, at this juncture and in light of the many hazards experienced by pre-retirees, planning is often insufficient. Many individuals have very high expectations for the final third of their lives. Although federal laws encourage increased participation in company-sponsored 401(k) plans, many of these plans are unreliable and rates of return have diminished considerably. The continued availability of Social Security is of great concern to current and future retirees (see Chapter 23).

The adequacy of retirement income depends not only on work history but also on marital history. The poverty rates of older women are excessively high. Couples who had previous marriages and divorces may have significantly lower economic resources available than those in first marriages. Child support, divorce settlements, and pension apportionment to ex-spouses may have diminished retirement income. This problem is an ever-increasing impediment to retirement because, among couples presently approaching retirement age, fewer than half are in a first marriage. Policies have been based on the traditional lifelong marriage, and this is no longer appropriate.

Special Considerations in Retirement

Retirement security depends on the "three-legged stool" of Social Security pensions, savings, and investments (Stanford & Usita, 2002). Older people with disabilities, those who have lacked access to education or held low-paying jobs with no benefits, and those not eligible for Social Security are at economic risk during retirement years. Culturally and racially diverse older persons, women—especially widows and those divorced or never married—immigrants, and gay and lesbian men and women often face greater challenges related to adequate income and benefits in retirement. Unmarried women, particularly African Americans, face the most negative prospects for retirement now and for at least the next 20 years (Hooyman & Kiyak, 2011).

Inadequate coverage for women in retirement is common because their work histories have been sporadic and diverse. Women are often called on to retire earlier than anticipated because of family needs. Whereas most men have always worked outside the home, it is only within the past 30 years that this has been the expectation of women. Therefore large cohort differences exist. Traditionally, the variability of women's work histories, interrupted careers, the residuals of sexist pension policies, Social Security inequities, and low-paying jobs created hazards for adequacy of income in retirement. The scene is gradually changing in many respects, but the gender bias remains.

Barriers to equal treatment for LGBT couples include job discrimination, unequal treatment under Social Security, pension plans, and 401(k) plans. LGBT couples are not eligible for Social Security survivor benefits, and unmarried partners cannot claim pension plan rights after the death of the pension plan participant. These policies definitely place LGBT elders at a disadvantage in retirement planning.

Implications for Gerontological Nursing and Healthy Aging

Successful retirement adjustment depends on socialization needs, energy levels, health, adequate income, variety of interests, amount of self-esteem derived from work, presence of intimate relationships, social support, and general adaptability. Nurses may have the opportunity to work with people in different phases of retirement or participate in retirement education and counseling programs (Box 24-3). Talking with clients older than age 50 about retirement plans, providing anticipatory guidance about the transition to retirement, identifying those who may be at risk for lowered income and health concerns, and referring to appropriate resources for retirement planning and support are important nursing interventions.

It is important to build on the strengths of the individuals' life experiences and coping skills and to provide appropriate counseling and support to assist older people to continue to grow and develop in meaningful ways during the transition from the work role. In ideal situations,

---

BOX 24-3   Phases of Retirement

Remote: Future anticipation with little real planning
Near: Preparation and fantasizing regarding retirement
Honeymoon: Euphoria and testing of the fantasies
Disenchantment: Letdown, boredom, sometimes depression
Reorientation: Developing a realistic and satisfactory lifestyle
Stability: Personal investment in meaningful activities
Termination: Loss of role resulting from illness or return to work

---

retirement offers the opportunity to pursue interests that may have been neglected while fulfilling other obligations. However, for too many older people, retirement presents challenges that affect both health and well-being, and nurses must be advocates for policies and conditions that allow all older people to maintain quality of life in retirement.

Death of a Spouse

Losing a partner after a long, close, and satisfying relationship is the most difficult adjustment one can face, aside from the loss of a child. The loss of a spouse is a stage in the life course that can be anticipated but seldom is. Seventy-six percent of women over 85 years of age are widowed compared with 38% of men (Federal Interagency Forum on Aging, 2010). The death of a life partner is essentially a loss of self. The mourning is as much for oneself as for the individual who has died. A core part of oneself has died with the partner, and even with satisfactory grief resolution, that aspect of self will never return. Even those widows and widowers who reorganize their lives and invest in family, friends, and activities often find that many years later they still miss their "other half" profoundly.

With the loss of the intimate partner, several changes occur simultaneously that involve social status, economics, and self-image. Individuals who have been self-confident and resilient seem to fare best. The transitional phase of grief, if handled appropriately, leads to the confirmation of a new identity, the end of one stage of life and the beginning of another. Seldom in life is there such an abrupt and distinct breach that creates intense pain but offers the opportunity for the emergence of a new identity.

Gender differences are found in the literature on widowhood. Bereaved husbands may be more socially and emotionally vulnerable (see Chapter 22). Suicide risk is highest among men over 80 years of age who have experienced the death of a spouse. Widowers adapt more slowly than widows to the loss of a spouse and often remarry quickly. Loneliness and the need to be cared for is a factor influencing widowers to seek out new partners. Association with family and friends, being members of a church community, and continuing to work or engage in activities can all be helpful in the adjustment period following the death of a wife.

Implications for Gerontological Nursing and Healthy Aging

Assessment

Feelings of the bereaved one are not orderly or progressive; they are conflicted, ambivalent, suicidal, full of rage, and often suspicious. Widows and widowers may exhibit personality disorganization that would be considered mentally aberrant or frankly psychotic under other circumstances. Some people handle grief with less apparent decompensation. Grief reactions must be accepted as personally valid and useful evidences of healing. DeVries (2001) discusses the signs of ongoing bonds and connections with the deceased (e.g., dreaming of the deceased, ongoing daily communication, "checking in") that persist long after death and counsels professionals to reexamine the idea that there is a timetable for "resolution" of grief. There are several tools that can be used to assess aspects of the bereavement process including coping, grief symptomatology, personal growth, continuing bonds, and health risk assessment (Minton & Barron, 2008).

Interventions

Nurses will interact with bereaved older people in many settings. Knowing the stages of transition to a new role as a widow or widower will be useful in determining interventions, although each individual is unique in this respect. Individuals respond to losses in ways that reflect the nature and meaning of the relationships as well as the unique characteristics of the bereaved. Patterns of adjustment are presented in Box 24-4. With adequate support, reintegration can be expected in 2 to 4 years. People with few familial or social supports may need professional help

---

BOX 24-4   Patterns of Adjustment to Widowhood

Stage One: Reactionary
(First Few Weeks)
Early responses of disbelief, anger, indecision, detachment, and inability to communicate in a logical, sustained manner are common. Searching for the mate, visions, hallucinations, and depersonalization may be experienced.
Intervention: Support, validate, be available, listen to talk about mate, reduce expectations.

Stage Two: Withdrawal
(First Few Months)
Depression, apathy, physiological vulnerability occur; movement and cognition are slowed; insomnia, unpredictable waves of grief, sighing, and anorexia occur.
Intervention: Protect against suicide, and involve in support groups.

Stage Three: Recuperation
(Second 6 Months)
Periods of depression are interspersed with characteristic capability. Feelings of personal control begin to return.

Intervention: Support accustomed lifestyle patterns that sustain and assist person to explore new possibilities.

Stage Four: Exploration
(Second Year)
Individual begins new ventures, testing suitability of new roles; anniversaries or holidays, birthdays, and date of death may be especially difficult.
Intervention: Prepare individual for unexpected reactions during anniversaries. Encourage and support new trial roles.

Stage Five: Integration
(Fifth Year)
Individual will feel fully integrated into new and satisfying roles if grief has been resolved in a healthy manner.
Intervention: Assist individual to recognize and share own pattern of growth through the trauma of loss.

to get through the early months of grief in a way that will facilitate recovery. To support the grieving person, it is necessary to extend one's own self to reconnect the severed person with a world of warmth and caring. No one nurse or family member can accomplish this task alone. Hundreds of small, caring gestures build strength and confidence in the grieving person's ability and willingness to survive. Additional information about dying, death, and grief can be found in Chapter 25.

Caregiving

Rosalyn Carter said: *"There are four kinds of people in the world: those who have been caregivers, those who are currently caregivers, those who will be caregivers, and those who will need caregivers"* (National Family Caregivers Association [NFCA], 2012).

Family caregiving has become a normative experience (similar to marriage, working, or retirement) for many of America's families and cuts across racial, ethnic, and social class distinctions. Gerontological nurses are most likely to encounter elders with their family and friends in situations relating to caregiving of some kind. Family members and other unpaid caregivers provide 80% of care for older adults in the United States. More than 65 million people, nearly 29% of the U.S. population, provide care for a chronically ill, disabled, or older family member or friend during any given year. Caregivers are present in one of every five households, and seven out of ten caregivers are caring for loved ones over 50 years of age. Informal caregivers may also include friends, paid and unpaid workers, or volunteers in the home, but current trends suggest that the use of paid, formal care by older persons with disabilities in the community has been decreasing, while their sole reliance on family caregivers has been increasing (NFCA, 2012).

Approximately 66% of family caregivers are women, and the typical family caregiver is a 49-year-old woman caring for a widowed mother who does not live with her. Middle-aged caregivers, *"the sandwich generation,"* often struggle to balance the demands of work and parenting with caregiving for an older relative. Caregiving can also present financial burdens, and women who are family caregivers are 2.5 times more likely than non-caregivers to live in poverty. Even though generally considered a women's issue, in more and more cases, male caregivers, including those other than spouses (e.g., brothers, nephews, sons), are assuming a full range of caregiving roles. Thirty-nine percent of caregivers are men, and this area needs further research to uncover their special needs and challenges.

Additionally, 1.4 million children 8 to 18 years of age provide care for an adult relative, and 73% are caring for a parent or grandparent. This is another area that requires more investigation (NFCA, 2012).

Caregivers spend an average of 20 hours per week providing care for their loved ones, and the value of these services is estimated to be $375 billion annually—more than twice as much as is spent on home care and nursing home care combined, and exceeding Medicaid long-term care spending in all states. Without family caregivers, the present level of long-term care could not be sustained. Supporting family caregivers and their ability to provide care at home or in the community is crucial to our long-term care system.

Caregiving is considered a major public health issue, and attention to the physical and mental health of caregivers is receiving increased attention. The aging of the population, medical advances, shorter hospital stays, limited discharge planning by hospitals, and expansion of home care technology will increase the demand for family caregivers in the future. It is estimated that the number of family caregivers will increase by 85% from 2000 to 2050. However, the number of family members who are available to provide care will decrease substantially in that same time period (Centers for Disease Control and Prevention [CDC] and the Kimberly-Clark Corporation, 2008). Recruitment and retention of all levels of health care workers for long-term care services is also a significant problem. The Institute of Medicine report (2008) states that "unless action is taken immediately, the health care workforce will lack the capacity (in both size and ability) to meet the needs of older patients in the future" (p. 23).

Impact of Caregiving

Although caregiving is a means to "give back" to a loved one and can be a source of joy in the giving, it is also stressful. Caregivers are considered to be *"the hidden patient"* (Schulz & Beach, 1999, p. 2216). Family caregiving has been associated with increased levels of depression and anxiety, poorer self-reported physical health, compromised immune function, and increased mortality (CDC and the Kimberly-Clark Corporation, 2008). "Caregiving is a very complex issue, and assuming a caregiving role is "a time of transition that requires a restructuring of one's goals, behaviors, and responsibilities. It requires taking on something new but it is also about loss—of what was and what could have been" (Lund, 2005, p. 152).

Whereas not all caregivers experience consequential stress, the circumstances that are more likely to cause problems with caregiving include competing role responsibilities (e.g., work, home), advanced age of the caregiver,

---

BOX 24-5   Suggestions to Reduce Caregiver Stress

To reduce caregiver stress, nurses are advised to use all means and resources at their disposal to do the following:

Restore a sense of control and effectiveness in the situation.

Reinforce any social supports that are available to the caregiver.

Find opportunities for group participation with other caregivers.

Advise routine times of respite, and assist caregiver in finding respite sources.

Tailor programs and services to the unique situation of caregiver and care recipient.

Urge the caregiver to take care of self.

Encourage caregiver to maintain activities important to his or her well-being.

Allow the caregiver to express negative and angry feelings they may have about the care recipient and the caregiving experience.

Encourage the caregiver's efforts to use all available resources and assistance.

Include all directly involved parties in decisions about care.

Praise whatever is being done well, and encourage letting go of things that have not gone well.

From Schmall VL, Stiehl R: *Coping with caregiving: How to manage stress when caring for older relatives*, Corvallis, Ore, 2003, Pacific Northwest Extension. Available at http://extension.oregonstate.edu/catalog/PDF/PNW/PNW315.pdf.

---

high-intensity caregiving needs, insufficient resources, poor self-reported health, living in the same household with the care recipient, dementia of the care recipient, and prior relational conflicts between the caregiver and care recipient. Suggestions to reduce caregiver stress are presented in Box 24-5. Lack of adequate long-term care services and financial difficulty have been reported to be the most consistent predictors of health and psychosocial outcomes (Robison et al., 2009). Caregivers of persons with dementia may experience even greater emotional and physical stress than other caregivers (see Chapter 21).

Cultural differences have been reported in caregiving burden and stress, and further research is needed in light of the increasing numbers of racially and culturally diverse elders and their unique needs. Some studies suggest that perceived caregiver stress and burden may be less in African-American caregivers as a result of the use of more cognitive and emotion-focused coping strategies and reliance on faith and spirituality. However, the effect of caregiving on physical health in this population is often overlooked and may be significant. Culturally diverse caregivers are also reported to rely less on formal support and have more available informal support networks to assist in caregiving. Some of these findings may be attributed to inadequate outreach to these populations as a result of our belief that "they take care of their own," as well as a lack of culturally competent formal services (Pinquart & Sorensen, 2005; Skarupski et al., 2009; Siefert et al., 2008).

The positive benefits of caregiving have been given more attention in recent years, but further research is needed to help understand what factors influence how caregivers perceive the experience. Positive benefits of caregiving may include enhanced self-esteem and well-being, personal growth and satisfaction, and finding or making meaning through caregiving. Most attention in caregiving research has been given to the caregiver and less to the care recipient or to the relationship between the caregiver and care recipient.

Patricia Archbold and colleagues studied caregiving as a role and examined how the relationships between the caregiver and care recipient (mutuality) and the preparation of the caregiver (preparedness) influence reactions to caregiving (Archbold et al., 1990). Caregivers who have a positive relationship with the care recipient experience less stress and find caregiving more meaningful. Nursing interventions to assist in preparing the caregiver for the caregiving role, particularly at the time of discharge from the hospital, also seem to prevent or reduce role strain. Further research is needed to understand the complexities of the caregiving and care receiving role and provide a theory base for nursing interventions. Boxes 24-6 and 24-7 present caregiver needs and suggestions for caregivers.

Spousal Caregiving

Of family caregivers over 60 years of age, spouses provide the most care, and 80% of persons who live with spouses with disabilities provide care for them. Many may have significant health problems that are neglected in deference to the greater needs of the incapacitated partner. The disabled spouse may need physical care that

BOX 24-6   Caregiver Needs

- Finding time for myself
- Keeping the person I care for safe
- Balancing work and family responsibilities
- Managing emotional and physical stress
- Finding easy and satisfying activities to do with the care recipient
- Learning how to talk to physicians
- Making end-of-life decisions
- Moving or lifting the care recipient; bathing and dressing
- Managing the challenging behaviors of the care recipient
- Negotiating health care and home and community-based services
- Managing complex medication schedules or high-tech medical equipment
- Choosing a home health agency, assisted living or skilled nursing facility
- Managing incontinence or toileting problems
- Finding non-English educational material

From Curry L, et al: Educational needs of employed family caregivers of older adults: evaluation of a workplace project, *Geriatr Nurs* 27(3): 166-173, 2006; Family Caregiver Alliance: *Caregiver assessment: principles, guidelines and strategies for change. Report from a National Consensus Development Conference* (vol 1), San Francisco, 2006, The Alliance.

BOX 24-7   Suggestions for Caregivers

- Educate yourself about the disease or medical condition.
- Find a health care professional who understands the disease.
- Consult with other experts to help plan for the future (legal, financial).
- Tap your social resources for assistance.
- Find a confidante.
- Take time for relaxation and exercise.
- Use community resources.
- Maintain your sense of humor.
- Explore religious beliefs and spiritual values.
- Set realistic goals.

From U.S. Department of Health and Human Services, Administration on Aging, National Family Caregiver Support Program Resources: *Taking care of yourself,* Available at www.aoa.gov.

is beyond the capabilities of the spousal caregiver. Spousal caregivers provide more intensive, time-consuming care than other family caregivers, as much as 56 hours of care per week on average. They also are less likely to receive assistance from other family members. Older spouses are at greater risk for negative consequences and often take on greater burdens than they can reasonably handle and wait longer for outside help, using formal services as a last resort. Spousal caregivers are more prone to loneliness, depression, increased risk of stroke (particularly among African-American male caregivers), and have a 63% greater chance of dying than people of the same age who are not caring for spouses (Ostwald, 2009). More wives than husbands provide care, but this is expected to change as life expectancy for men increases.

Older spouses caring for disabled partners also face many role changes. Older women may need to learn to drive, manage money, or make decisions by themselves. Male caregivers may need to learn how to cook, shop, do laundry, and provide personal care to their wives. Spousal caregivers also deal with the added responsibilities of caregiving while at the same time dealing with the anticipated loss of their spouse. Nurses should be alert to situations in which health care personnel may be able to provide supports and resources that make it possible for an individual to assume new responsibilities without being totally overwhelmed. Adult day programs, respite care services, or periodic assistance from a home health aide or homemaker may make it possible for the couple to continue to live together. It is important to pay attention to the physical and mental health needs of the caregiver as well as the care recipient.

Aging Parents Caring for Developmentally Disabled Children

Although we tend to think of caregivers as middle-aged adults caring for elders, an unknown number of elders are caring for their middle-aged children who are physically and mentally disabled. In the past century, developmentally disabled children usually died before reaching adulthood; now, with improved care, they are surviving. For the first time in history, individuals with developmental disabilities are outliving their parents.

With increased survival, these adults with developmental disabilities are also at risk for developing chronic illness and will need more care and services. For example, individuals with Down's syndrome are more likely to develop dementia. Often, the burden of caring for a developmentally disabled child has been carried by parents for their entire adult life and will end only with the death of the parent or the adult child. Parental caregivers who are aging face changes in their financial resources and health that affects their continued caregiving ability.

A major worry is how their child will be cared for if they develop a debilitating illness or when they die. The phenomenon of an aging parent caring for an aging child is beginning to receive attention by both organizations for aging and organizations for developmentally disabled individuals. The Planned Lifetime Assistance Network (PLAN), available in some states through the National Alliance for the Mentally Ill, provides lifetime assistance to individuals with disabilities whose parents or other family members are deceased or can no longer provide for their care (www.nami.org). The Alzheimer's Association and other aging organizations offer education and support programs for both parents and their developmentally disabled adult children in some communities. There is a continued need for more community-based care and housing for developmentally disabled adults who are aging (Hooyman & Kiyak, 2011).

Grandparents Raising Grandchildren

In recent years, more grandparents have become, by default, the primary caregivers of grandchildren because the parents are unable to provide the care needed as a result of child abuse, teen pregnancy, imprisonment, joblessness, military deployment, drug and alcohol addictions, illness, death, and other social problems. Over 2 million grandparents are providing primary care (custodial grandparents) for grandchildren in the United States. In the United States, 1 out of every 10 children lives with a grandparent, and 41% of those children are being raised primarily by that grandparent. More than two thirds of grandparent primary caregivers are younger than 60 years of age, and 62% are female. Nearly one in five are living below the poverty line (Livingston & Parker, 2010; Smith et al., 2008). The phenomenon of grandparents serving as primary caregivers is more common among African Americans and Hispanics than whites, but the increase in grandparent primary caregiving across the last decade has been much more pronounced among whites (a 19% increase) (Livingston & Parker, 2010).

Research is lacking related to the effect of grandparent caregiving on health status (Smith et al., 2008). For many, it is a life-changing decision to dedicate one's life to raising a child at a time in life when one may be looking forward to more leisure and less responsibility. Often, crisis situations precipitate the decision, and time for preparation is not available. In many cases, grandparents assume care so

that their grandchildren's care is not taken over by the public care system (delBene, 2010). The unexpected career of caregiving for grandchildren and the "off timing" of this family role transition contributes to the challenges faced (Musil et al., 2011). As with other types of caregiving, there are both blessings and burdens. The experience of children who have been raised by a grandparent also needs to be investigated.

For many grandparents, however, economic, health, and social challenges associated with caregiving may include limited income and financial support through the welfare system, lack of informal support systems, loss of leisure and social activities in retirement, and shame or guilt related to their children's inability to parent. Too often, both the children and their grandparents are in need of help. Approximately twice as many children cared for by a custodial grandparent have emotional or behavioral problems compared to those in two-parent families. Physical and mental stressors are also greater when grandparents are raising a chronically ill or special-needs child (delBene, 2010; Hooyman & Kiyak, 2011).

Routine screening and monitoring of the psychological distress of primary care grandparents and offering support, advice, and referral to reduce stressors is important (Smith et al., 2009). Education and training programs and support groups are valuable resources that should be available in communities. Nurses can be instrumental in developing and conducting these types of interventions. Suggestions for nursing interventions with older adults providing primary care to their grandchildren are presented in Box 24-8.

BOX 24-8 **Suggested Nursing Interventions with Grandparent Caregivers**

- Early identification of at-risk grandparents
- Comprehensive assessment of physical, psychosocial, and environmental factors affecting those in the caregiving role for grandchildren
- Anticipatory guidance and counseling about child growth and development and other child-raising issues
- Referral to resources for support, counseling, and financial assistance
- Advocacy for policies supportive of grandparents who have assumed a caregiving role

The U.S. government has recognized that increasing numbers of older adults are raising grandchildren, great-grandchildren, and other younger relatives. The Temporary Assistance for Needy Families Program (TANF) provides assistance but is limited to benefits for the child only. No funds are provided for financial support of the grandparent or for child care. Legal options for primary care grandparents include guardianship, custody, adoption, and informal and formal foster parenthood (Hooyman & Kiyak, 2011). However, there is a continued need to develop services that support grandparents as sole caregivers and that attend to the physical and mental health of primary care (custodial) grandparents. The National Family Caregiver Support Program (NFCSP), under the Older Americans Act program, provides support services, education and training, counseling, and respite care. Nurses can refer the grandparents to their local area agency on aging to inquire about available resources.

Long-Distance Caregiving

Because of the increasing mobility of today's society, more children move away from home for education or employment and do not return home. When the parent needs help, it must be provided "long distance." This is perhaps one of the most difficult situations, and it presents unique challenges. Issues that need to be considered include identifying a local person who will be available quickly in emergency situations; identifying reliable individuals or services that will provide daily monitoring if necessary; identifying acceptable facilities for assisted living if that becomes necessary; determining which family member is most likely to be free to travel to the elder if needed; and being sure that legalities regarding advance directives, a will, and power of attorney (for health care and financial) have been established.

A profession and industry have emerged to assist the geographically distant family member to ensure that an older relative will receive care. This profession is made up of geriatric care managers, some of whom are nurses or social workers. A care manager can be hired to do everything a family member would do if able, from being available in an emergency, to helping with estate planning, to making arrangements for a move to a nursing home. Often care managers know of resources that can assist the elder to remain independent and yet assure the family that safety and other needs are being met. These services are available primarily to those who are able to pay for them because they are not covered by private insurance, Medicare, or any public agencies. Although these services are expensive, they are far less expensive than alternative living arrangements or institutional placement.

Similar services may be available for persons with very low incomes by asking the local area agency on aging about local "Community Care for the Elderly" programs. Some states also have nursing home diversion projects to provide home support to those who would otherwise qualify for Medicaid coverage for nursing home care. When incomes are too high to qualify for Medicaid and too low to pay for private care managers, the persons and their families must do the best they can. Long-distance care then depends on the goodness of neighbors, local friends, and apartment managers and frequent trips by the long-distance caregiver to the elder.

Implications for Gerontological Nursing and Healthy Aging

Nurses are often the primary care providers and care managers for elders and their families both in the home and in the institutional setting. The nurse monitors progress and manages chronic disorders of the elder within the context of the family.

Assessment

Family Assessment

A comprehensive assessment of the elder includes assessment of the family: Who are the members? What is the family history? What are their usual roles and their strengths, contributions, and deterrents to the function of the family unit? Assessing the family's needs and strengths, as well as its sources of stress, particular methods of coping, meaning of caregiving, cultural values, support system, and family dynamics, will help the nurse know the family and design responses that may strengthen the family unit.

Often, nurses see families in times of crisis when an older family member needs care. It is important to encourage the expression of feelings from all involved family members, as well as the older person, and maintain a nonjudgmental attitude. It is important for the nurse to be aware of his or her vision of what a "family" should be and what a "family" should do. Our values should not enter into assessment and intervention with clients. Meiner (2011, p. 113) reminds us that we should not "label families as 'dysfunctional.' It is necessary to identify the strengths within each family and to build on those strengths while recognizing the family's limitations in providing support and caregiving." Thus, the nurse's role is to teach, monitor, and strengthen the family system so as to maintain health and wellness of the entire family structure.

Caregiver Assessment

Family members who assume the caregiving role experience both stressors and benefits. The stresses, expectations of future needs and problems, and the positive aspects of the caregiving situation should be explored. Caregiver assessment includes how the family member can help the care recipient and how the health care team can help the person providing care. In light of the physical and emotional stressors often associated with the caregiving role, nurses need to monitor the physical and emotional health of both the caregiver and the care recipient and provide support as necessary. A partnership model, combining the "nurse's professional expertise with the caregiver's knowledge of the family member, is recommended" (Schumacher et al., 2006, p. 47). A Nursing Standard of Practice Protocol: Family Caregiving (Messecar, 2012) is available at http://consultgerirn.org/topics/family_caregiving/want_to_know_more. Box 24-9 presents a research-based model to guide nursing interventions with caregivers.

Principles to guide caregiver assessment include the following: (1) caregiver assessment should include the needs and preferences of both the care recipient and the family caregiver; (2) caregiver assessment should reflect culturally competent practice; (3) caregiver assessment should be multidimensional and conducted with an interprofessional approach; and (4) caregiver assessment should

result in a plan of care developed collaboratively with the caregiver that specifies the provision of services and intended measurable outcomes (Family Caregiver Alliance, 2006). Several validated caregiver assessment instruments are available, including the Preparedness for Caregiving Scale and the Mutuality Scale (Archbold et al., 1990), the Caregiver Strain Index developed by Robinson (1983), and the Modified Caregiver Strain Index (http://consultgerirn.org/topics/family_caregiving/want_to_know_more).

Interventions

Research over the past several decades has provided a wealth of information on interventions to support caregivers and improve their health and well-being. The Centers for Disease Control and Prevention (CDC) provide extensive information about putting evidence-based programs into practice (http://www.cdc.gov/Features/Caregiving/). As part of the Affordable Health Care Act, $68 million in grants are to be awarded to states, territories, tribal, and community-based organizations to help older people and their caregivers better understand and navigate their health and long-term care options.

Intervention programs should include risk assessment, education about caregiving and stress, caregiver health and home safety, support groups, linkages to ongoing telephone or e-mail support, counseling, resource identification, and stress management. Linking caregivers to community resources, such as respite care, adult day programs, and financial support resources, is important. Respite care allows the caregiver to take a break from caregiving for various periods of time. Respite care may be provided in institutions, in the home, or in other community settings. Nurses should be aware of respite care resources in their communities and the local Area Agency on Aging can provide information on respite care and other caregiver services. These interventions, when available, can alleviate much of the stress of caregiving.

Interventions with caregivers must always consider the great variability in family structures, resources, traditions, and history. The range of adaptations is enormous, and the goal is always to restore the balance of the system to the greatest extent possible and support caregivers in their caring. The family can be visualized as a mobile with many parts, and when one part is touched, each part shifts to regain the balance. The intrusion of professionals in a family system will temporarily unbalance the system and may provide an opportunity to restore the balance in a healthier manner, sometimes by adding an element or increasing the weight of one or decreasing the weight of another. Further research is needed to provide the foundation for nursing interventions

---

| BOX 24-9 | **Nursing Actions to Create and Sustain a Partnership with Caregivers** |

- Surveillance and ongoing monitoring
- Coaching: helping caregivers apply knowledge and develop skills
- Teaching: providing information and instruction
- Fostering partnerships: fostering communication and collaboration between the caregiver and the care recipient and between them and the nurse
- Providing psychosocial support: attending to psychosocial well-being
- Rescuing: providing a safety net by stepping in to provide direct care and making clinical decisions
- Coordinating: orchestrating the work of other health care team members and the activities of the caregiver

Data from Eilers J, Heermann J, Wilson M, et al: Independent nursing actions in cooperative care, *Oncol Nurs Forum* 32(4):849-855, 2005; Schumacher K, Beck C, Marren J: Family caregivers: caring for older adults working with their families, *Am J Nurs* 106(8):40-49, 2006.

with family caregivers, particularly among racially and ethnically diverse families and nontraditional families.

Intimacy and Sexuality

Intimacy

Although intimacy is often thought of in the context of sexual performance, it encompasses more than sexuality and includes five major relational components: commitment, affective intimacy, cognitive intimacy, physical intimacy, and interdependence (Youngkin, 2004). "Intimacy is from a Greek word meaning 'closest to; inner lining of blood vessels'" (Steinke, 2005, p. 40). It is a warm, meaningful feeling of joy. Intimacy includes the need for close friendships; relationships with family, friends, and formal caregivers; spiritual connections; knowing that one matters in someone else's life; and the ability to form satisfying social relationships with others (Steinke, 2005).

Youngkin (2004) points out that older people may be concerned about changes in sexual intimacy but "social relationships with people important in their lives, the ability to interact intellectually with people who share similar interests, the supportive love that grows between human beings (whether romantic or platonic), and physical non-sexual intimacy are equally—and in many instances more—important than the physical intimacy of direct sexual relations. All of these facets of intimate life are integrally woven into the fabric of aging, along with other influences that can make life rewarding" (p. 46). Intimacy needs change over time, but the need for intimacy and satisfying social relationships remains an important component of healthy aging.

Sexuality

Sexuality is defined as a central aspect of being human and encompasses sex, gender identities and roles, sexual orientation, eroticism, pleasure, intimacy, and reproduction (World Health Organization [WHO], 2004). As a major aspect of intimacy, sexuality includes the physical act of intercourse, as well as many other types of intimate activity. Sexuality provides the opportunity to express passion, affection, admiration, and loyalty. It can also enhance personal growth and communication. Sexuality also allows a general affirmation of life (especially joy) and a continuing opportunity to search for new growth and experience.

Sexuality, similar to food and water, is a basic human need, yet it goes beyond the biological realm to include psychological, social, and moral dimensions (Waite et al., 2009) (Figure 24-1). The constant interaction among these

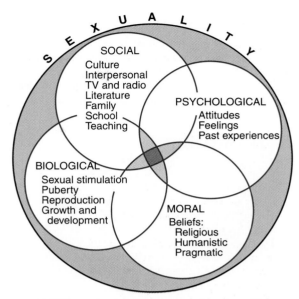

FIGURE 24-1 Interrelationship of dimensions of sexuality.

spheres of sexuality work to produce harmony. The linkage of the four dimensions composes the holistic quality of an individual's sexuality.

The *social* sphere of sexuality is the sum of cultural factors that influence the individual's thoughts and actions related to interpersonal relationships, as well as sexuality related to ideas and learned behavior. Television, radio, literature, and the more traditional sources of family, school, and religious teachings combine to influence social sexuality. The belief of that which constitutes masculine and feminine is deeply rooted in the individual's exposure to cultural factors.

The *psychological* domain of sexuality reflects a person's attitudes, feelings toward self and others, and learning from experiences. Beginning with birth, the individual is bombarded with cues and signals of how a person should act and think about the use of "dirty words" or body parts. Conversation is self-censored in the presence of or in discussion with certain people. The *moral* aspect of sexuality, the "I should" or "I shouldn't," makes a difference that is based in religious beliefs or in a pragmatic or humanistic outlook.

The final dimension, *biological* sexuality, is reflected in physiological responses to sexual stimulation, reproduction, puberty, and growth and development. Because of the interrelatedness, these dimensions affect each other directly or indirectly whenever an aspect of sexuality is out of harmony.

Sexuality is a vital aspect to consider in the care of the older person regardless of the setting. Sexuality exists throughout life in one form or another in everyone. All older people have a need to express sexual feelings, whether the individuals are healthy and active or frail. Sexuality is linked with the person's personality and identity and has a significant role in promoting better life adaptation.

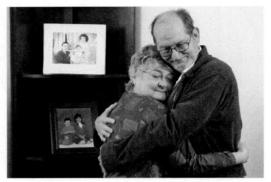

Love and affection are important to older persons. (From Sorrentino SA, Gorek B: *Mosby's textbook for long-term care assistants,* ed 5, St. Louis, 2007, Mosby.)

Sexual Health

The World Health Organization defines sexual health as a state of physical, emotional, mental, and social well-being related to sexuality (WHO, 2004). "Sexual health, as with physical health, is not simply the absence of sexual dysfunction or disease, but, rather a state of sexual well-being that includes a positive approach to a sexual relationship and anticipation of a pleasurable experience without fear, shame, or coercion" (Rheaume & Mitty, 2008, p. 342).

These interpretations speak of the multifaceted nature of the biological, psychosocial, cultural, and spiritual components of sexuality and imply that sexual behavior is the capacity to enhance self and others. Sexual health is individually defined and wholesome if it leads to intimacy (not necessarily coitus) and enriches the involved parties.

Factors Influencing Sexual Health

Expectations. A large number of cultural, biological, psychosocial, and environmental factors influence the sexual behavior of older adults. The older person may be confronted with barriers to the expression of his or her sexuality by reflected attitudes, health, culture, economics, opportunity, and historic trends. Factors affecting a person's attitudes on intimacy and sexuality include family dynamics and upbringing and cultural and religious beliefs.

Older people often internalize the broad cultural proscriptions of sexual behavior in late life that hinder the continuance of sexual expression. Much sexual behavior stems from incorporating other people's reactions. Older people do not feel old until they are faced with the fact that others around them consider them old. Similarly, older adults do not feel asexual until they are continually treated as such.

American society continues to struggle with open acceptance of sexual expression for the young but continues to remain hostile to the attempts of older people to do the same. Sexual interest and activity in older adults are sometimes regarded as deviant behavior and described in such terms as "dirty old man," "lecher," and "old biddy." The same activity attempted by a younger person would be viewed as appropriate. An often quoted statement by Alex Comfort (1974) sums it up nicely: "In our experiences, old folks stop having sex for the same reasons they stop riding a bicycle—general infirmity, thinking it looks ridiculous, no bicycle." Box 24-10 presents some of the myths about sexuality in older women that may be held by older people themselves and by society in general.

Activity Levels. For both heterosexual and homosexual individuals, research supports that liberal and positive attitudes toward sexuality, greater sexual knowledge, satisfaction with a long-term relationship or a current intimate relationship, good social networks, psychological well-being, and a sense of self-worth are associated with greater sexual interest, activity, and satisfaction. Both early studies of sexual behavior in older adults, and more recent ones, indicate that

---

BOX 24-10 Sexuality and Aging Women: Common Myths

- Masturbation is an immature activity of youngsters and adolescents, not older women.
- Sexual prowess and desire wane during the climacteric, and menopause is the death of a woman's sexuality.
- Hysterectomy creates a physical disability that results in the inability to function sexually.
- Sex has no role in the lives of older adults, except as perversion or remembrance of times past.
- Sexual expression in old age is taboo.
- Older people are too old and frail to engage in sex.
- The young are considered lusty and virile; older adults are considered lecherous.
- Sex is unimportant or over.
- Older women do not wish to discuss their sexuality with professionals.

men and women remain sexually active and find their sexual lives satisfying. Determinants of sexual activity and functioning include the interaction of each partner's sexual capacity, motivation, conduct, and attitudes, as well as the quality of the dyadic relationship (Waite et al., 2009). Patterns of sexual activity in earlier years are the major predictor of sexual activity in later life, and individuals with higher levels of sexual activity in middle age show less decline with advanced age (Kennedy et al., 2010).

The National Social Life, Health, and Aging Project (NSHAP) is a national probability survey of 3005 men and women between 57 and 85 years of age that is focused on intimate social relationships, including marriage, social ties, and sexuality. The central hypothesis of the study is that individuals with high-quality intimate social and sexual relationships will age better in terms of health and well-being than those with poor-quality relationships or those who lack social relationships (Lindau et al., 2007; Lindau & Gavrilova, 2010; Suzman, 2009). Findings from this survey revealed that about three quarters of individuals 57 to 85 years of age are married or living with a partner and three quarters of those are sexually active. The prevalence of sexual activity declined with age: 73% of people between 57 and 64 years of age reported being sexually active; 53% of those between 65 and 74; and 26% of those between 75 and 85.

Sexual activity was closely tied to overall health, and people whose health was rated as excellent or very good were nearly twice as likely to be sexually active as those who rated their health as poorer. The most common reason for sexual inactivity among those with a partner was the male partner's health. Men are more sexually active than women, most likely because women live longer and may not have a partner. Women, especially those not in a relationship, were more likely than men to report lack of interest in sex (Lindau et al., 2007; Lindau & Gavrilova, 2010).

Cohort and Cultural Influences. The era in which a person was born influences attitudes about sexuality. Women in their 80s today may have been strongly influenced by the prudish, Victorian atmosphere of their youth and may have experienced difficult marital adjustments and serious sexual problems early in their marriages. Sexuality was not openly expressed or discussed, and this was a time when "pleasurable sex was for men only; women engaged in sexual activity to satisfy their husbands and to make babies" (Rheaume & Mitty, 2008, p. 344). These kinds of experiences shape beliefs and knowledge about sexual expression as well as comfort with sexuality, particularly for older women. It is important to come to know and understand the older person within his or her social and

cultural background and not make judgments based on one's own belief system.

The next generation of older people ("baby boomers") has experienced other influences, including more liberal attitudes toward sexuality, the women's movement, a higher number of divorced adults, the human immunodeficiency virus (HIV) epidemic, and increased numbers of gay and lesbian couples, that will affect their views and attitudes as they age. The baby boomers and beyond, as they find themselves experiencing sexuality beyond the age they had assigned to their elders, may alter current perceptions.

Most of what is known about sexuality in aging has been gained through research with well-educated, healthy, white older adults. Further research is needed among culturally, socially, and ethnically diverse older people; those with chronic illness; and gay, lesbian, and bisexual older people.

Biological Changes with Age. Acknowledgement and understanding of the age changes that influence sexual physiology, anatomy, and the stages of sexual response may partially explain alteration in sexual behavior to accommodate these changes and facilitate continued pleasurable sex. Characteristic physiological changes during the sexual response cycle do occur with aging, but these vary from individual to individual depending on general health factors. The changes occur abruptly in women starting with menopause but more gradually in men, a phenomenon called *andropause* (Kennedy et al., 2010). The "use it or lose it" phenomenon also applies here: the more sexually active the person is, the fewer changes he or she is likely to experience in the pattern of sexual response. Changes in the appearance of the body (wrinkles, sagging skin) may also affect the older person's security about his or her sexual attractiveness (Arena & Wallace, 2008). Table 24-1 summarizes physical changes in the sexual response cycle.

Older people who do not understand the physical changes that affect sexual activity become concerned that their sex life is approaching its natural conclusion with the onset of menopause or, for men, when they discover a change in the firmness of their erection or the decreased need for ejaculation with each orgasm or when the refractory period is extended between episodes of intercourse. A major nursing role is to provide information about these changes, as well as appropriate assessment and counseling within the context of the individual's needs.

Sexual Dysfunction

Sexual dysfunction is defined as impairment in normal sexual functioning and can have many causes, both physical and psychological. Sexual disorders in older people have not been well studied, but generally, the following

TABLE 24-1	Physical Changes in Sexual Response in Old Age
Female	**Male**

Female	Male
Excitation Phase	
Diminished or delayed lubrication (1-3 min may be required for adequate amounts to appear)	Less intense and slower erection (but can be maintained longer without ejaculation)
Diminished flattening and separation of labia majora	Increased difficulty regaining an erection if lost
Disappearance of elevation of labia majora	Less vasocongestion of scrotal sac
Decreased vasocongestion of labia minora	Less pronounced elevation and congestion of testicles
Decreased elastic expansion of vagina (depth and breadth)	
Breasts not as engorged	
Sex flush absent	
Plateau Phase	
Slower and less prominent uterine elevation or tenting	Decreased muscle tension
Nipple erection and sexual flush less often	No color change at coronal edge of penis
Decreased capacity for vasocongestion	Slower penile erection pattern
Decreased areolar engorgement	Delayed or diminished erectal and testicular elevation
Labial color change less evident	
Less intense swelling or orgasmic platform	
Less sexual flush	
Decreased secretions of Bartholin glands	
Orgasmic Phase	
Fewer number and less intense orgasmic contractions	Decreased or absent secretory activity (lubrication) by Cowper gland before ejaculation
Rectal sphincter contraction with severe tension only	Fewer penile contractions
	Fewer rectal sphincter contractions
	Decreased force of ejaculation (approximately 50%) with decreased amount of semen (if ejaculation is long, seepage of semen occurs)
Resolution Phase	
Observably slower loss of nipple erection	Vasocongestion of nipples and scrotum slowly subsides
Vasocongestion of clitoris and orgasmic platform	Very rapid loss of erection and descent of testicles shortly after ejaculation
	Refractory time extended (time required before another erection ranges from several to 24 hours, occasionally longer)

four categories are described: hypoactive sexual desire disorder; sexual arousal disorder; orgasmic disorder; and sexual pain disorders (Arena & Wallace, 2008).

Male Dysfunction. Erectile dysfunction (ED) is the most prevalent sexual problem in men. In the NSHAP study, ED was reported by 31% of men 57 to 65 years of age and by about 44% of those over 65 years of age (Waite et al., 2009). ED is defined as the inability to achieve and sustain an erection sufficient for satisfactory sexual intercourse in at least 50% or more attempts. When discussing ED with older men, it is important to provide education about normal age-related changes as well. Older men

require more physical penile stimulation and a longer time to achieve erection, and the duration of orgasm may be shorter and less intense (Rheaume & Mitty, 2008).

An erection is governed by the interaction among the hormonal, vascular, and nervous systems. A problem in any of these systems can cause ED. Of course, multiple causes exist for this problem in older men. Nearly one third of ED is a complication of diabetes. Alcoholism, medications, depression, and prostate cancer and treatment are also causes of ED in older men. The new nerve-sparing microsurgical techniques used for prostatectomies often spare erectile function. Testosterone levels have little to do with ED but can have a major effect on libido (sexual desire).

The use of phosphodiesterase type 5 (PDE-5) inhibitors such as sildenafil (Viagra), vardenafil (Levitra), and tadalafil (Cialis) has revolutionized treatment for ED regardless of cause. Some have commented that this can be called "the Viagratization of the older population." Contraindications to the use of these medications include nitrate therapy, heart failure with low blood pressure, certain antihypertensive regimens, and other medications and cardiovascular conditions. If a man with ED responds poorly to PDE-5 inhibitors, it may be important to measure serum testosterone levels. If decreased, testosterone replacement may be indicated in addition to medication (Janeway & Baum, 2012).

Before the availability of these medications, intracavernosal injections with the drugs papaverine and phentolamine, vasoactive agents that reduce resistance of arteriolar and cavernosal smooth muscle tissue of the penis, were used. Penile implants of the semirigid, adjustable-malleable, or hinged and inflatable types are available when impotence does not respond to other treatments or is irreversible. The hinged and inflatable types, which are inserted in the testicular area, are the most popular. Another alternative is the vacuum pump device, which works by creating a vacuum that draws blood into the penis, causing an erection. Vacuum pumps are available in manual and battery-operated versions and may be covered by Medicare if deemed medically necessary (Rheaume & Mitty, 2008).

Female Dysfunction. Female dysfunction is considered "persistent impediment to a person's normal pattern of sexual interest, response, or both" (Kaiser, 2000, p. 1174). Female sexual function can be influenced by factors such as culture, ethnicity, emotional state, age, and previous sexual experiences, as well as age-related changes in sexual response. For heterosexual women, frequency of intercourse depends more on the age, health, and sexual function of the partner or the availability of a partner rather than on their own sexual capacity.

Postmenopausal changes in the urinary or genital tract as a result of lower estrogen levels can make sexual activity less pleasurable (Rheaume & Mitty, 2008). Dyspareunia, resulting from vaginal dryness and thinning of the vaginal tissue, occurs in one third of women older than age 65. In many instances, using water-soluble lubricants such as K-Y, Astroglide, Slip, and HR lubricating jelly during foreplay or intercourse can resolve the difficulty. Topical low-dose estrogen creams, rings, or pills that are introduced into the vagina may also help to plump tissues and restore lubrication, with less absorption than oral hormones (Kennedy et al., 2010; Rheaume & Mitty, 2008).

Women can experience arousal disorders resulting from drugs such as anticholinergics, antidepressants, and chemotherapeutic agents and from lack of lubrication from radiation, surgery, and stress. Orgasmic disorders also may result from drugs used to treat depression. Unlike ED, studies of vascular insufficiency are less clear in women with sexual dysfunction. Prolapse of the uterus, rectoceles, and cystoceles can be surgically repaired to facilitate continued sexual activity. Pelvic organ prolapse has a prevalence rate of 41% among women with an intact uterus (Janeway et al., 2012). Urinary incontinence (UI) is another condition that may affect sexual activity for both men and women. Appropriate assessment and treatment are important because many causes of UI are treatable (see Chapter 10).

Alternative Sexual Lifestyles: Lesbian, Gay, Bixexual, and Transgender

Older LGBT individuals are as diverse as the remainder of the heterosexual elder population. Many age successfully, are healthy, and are active with satisfied lives. Some are coupled, have children, and are open about their sexual orientation, and some are not. Some of these individuals have only recently "come out"; others have been "out" most of their lives; and some find themselves isolated in the larger society. Older gay and lesbian individuals are more likely to have kept their relationships hidden than those who grew up in the modern-day gay liberation movement. Transgender and bisexual individuals are less likely to "be out" (American Society on Aging and MetLife, 2010).

LGBT older adults are much less likely than their heterosexual peers to access needed health and social services or identify themselves as gay or lesbian to health care providers (Services and Advocacy for Gay, Lesbian, Bisexual, and Transgender Elders [SAGE] and Movement Advancement Project [MAP], 2010). Health care providers may assume that their LGBT patients are heterosexual and neglect to obtain a sexual history, discuss sexuality, or be aware of their particular medical needs. *Healthy People 2020* includes a new section on LGBT health and efforts to improve health and address health disparities (U.S. Department of Health and Human Services [USDHHS], 2012).

Providers receive little education and training in the needs of this population and may lack sensitivity when caring for older LGBT individuals (Gelo, 2008). Sensitivity is of utmost importance when attempting to obtain a health history. Using open-ended questions such as "Who is most important to you?" or "Do you have a significant other?" is much better than asking "Are you married?" This form of the question allows the nurse to look beyond the rigid category of family.

Euphemisms are frequently used for a life partner (e.g., roommate, close friend). Asking individuals if they consider themselves as primarily heterosexual, homosexual, or bisexual is also better. This question conveys recognition of sexual variety. An older lesbian woman in a health care situation may refer to herself indirectly by saying "people like us." Nurses need to become more aware of these nuances and try to understand the fear of discovery that is apparent in the older gay man and lesbian woman. These elders are of a generation in which they were, and may still be, closeted because of the homophobic experiences they had throughout their younger years.

Better support and care services for LGBT individuals by care providers should include working through homophobic attitudes and discomfort discussing sexuality, learning about special issues facing older gay men and lesbians, and becoming aware of the gay and lesbian resources in the community. Facilities or agencies already in the community need to be assessed from the perspective of the client, patient, or resident who may be gay, lesbian, bisexual, or transgender. Ninety-six percent of America's social service and caregiving agencies for older adults offer no services specifically designed for LGBT older adults, and 46% of them indicated that LGBT older people would be unwelcome at senior centers if their sexual orientation were known (Gelo, 2008). Medicare recently finalized new rules to require equal visitation rights for all hospital patients, including a visitor who is a same-sex domestic partner. Programs to increase awareness of the needs of LGBT elders and reduce discrimination are necessary especially in light of the anticipated increase in older LGBT individuals.

Intimacy and Chronic Illness

Chronic illnesses and their related treatments may bring many challenges to intimacy and sexual activity. Some research has been done on the effects of myocardial infarction on sexual function; less information is available for patients with heart failure, implantable cardioverter-defibrillators (ICDs), hypertension, arthritis, chronic pain, or chronic obstructive pulmonary disease (COPD) (Steinke, 2005).

Often, patients and their partners are given little or no information about the effect of illnesses on sexual activity or strategies to continue sexual activity within functional limitations. Timing of intercourse (mornings or when energy level is highest), oral or anal sex, masturbation, appropriate pain relief, and different sexual positions are all strategies that may assist in continued sexual activity. If pain due to arthritis is a concern, taking pain medications or a warm bath prior to lovemaking may be helpful. Alternate sexual positions such as side-by-side, back-to-belly (spoon), or the cross-wise sex position with one partner supine and the other on his or her side, require less flexion of hip and knee, and these positions may reduce the pressure of body weight associated with the missionary position (Kennedy et al., 2010). Table 24-2 presents other suggestions for individuals with chronic illness.

Intimacy and Sexuality in Long-Term Care Facilities

Research is needed on sexuality in residential care facilities and nursing homes, but surveys suggest that a significant

TABLE 24-2	Chronic Illness and Sexual Function: Effects and Interventions	
Condition	**Effects/Problems**	**Interventions**
Arthritis	Pain, fatigue, limited motion Steroid therapy may decrease sexual interest or desire	Advise patient to perform sexual activity at time of day when less fatigued and most relaxed Suggest use of analgesics and other pain-relief methods before sexual activity Encourage use of relaxation techniques before sexual activity such as a warm bath or shower, application of hot packs to affected joints Advise patient to maintain optimum health through a balance of good nutrition, proper rest, and activity Suggest that he or she experiment with different positions, use pillows for comfort and support Recommend use of a vibrator if massage ability is limited Suggest use of water-soluble jelly for vaginal lubrication

TABLE 24-2	**Chronic Illness and Sexual Function: Effects and Interventions—cont'd**	
Condition	**Effects/Problems**	**Interventions**
Cardiovascular disease	Most men have no change in physical effects on sexual function; one fourth may not return to pre–heart attack function; one fourth may not resume sexual activity Women do not experience sexual dysfunction after heart attack Fear of another heart attack or death during sex Shortness of breath	Encourage counseling on realistic restrictions that may be necessary Instruct patient and spouse on alternative positions to avoid strain Suggest that patient avoid large meals several hours before sex Advise patient to relax; plan medications for effectiveness during sex
Cerebrovascular accident (stroke)	Depression May or may not have sexual activity changes Often erectile disorders occur; decrease in frequency of intercourse and sexual relations Change in role and function of partners Decreased physical endurance, fatigue Mobility and sensory deficits Perceptual and visual deficits Communication deficit Cognitive and behavioral deficits Fear of relapse or sudden death	Encourage counseling Instruct patient to use alternative positions Suggest use of a vibrator if massage ability is limited Suggest use of pillows for positioning and support Suggest use of water-soluble jelly for lubrication Instruct patient to use alternative forms of sexual expression
Chronic obstructive pulmonary disease (COPD)	No direct impairment of sexual activity although affected by coughing, exertional dyspnea, positions, and activity intolerance Medications may lead to erectile difficulties	Encourage patient to plan sexual activity when energy is highest Instruct patient to use alternative positions Advise patient to plan sexual activity at time medications are most effective Suggest use of oxygen before, during, or after sex, depending on when it provides the most benefit
Diabetes	Sexual desire and interest unaffected Neuropathy and/or vascular damage may interfere with erectile ability. About 50% to 75% of men have erectile disorders; a small portion have retrograde ejaculation Some men regain function if diagnosis of diabetes is well accepted, if diabetes is well controlled, or both Women have less sexual desire and vaginal lubrication Decrease in orgasms/absence of orgasm can occur; less frequent sexual activity; local genital infections	Recommend possible candidates for penile prosthesis Instruct patient to use alternative forms of sexual expression Recommend immediate treatment of genital infections
Cancers Breast	No direct physical effect. There is a strong psychological effect: loss of sexual desire, body image change, depression, reaction of partner	Encourage individual or group counseling
Most other cancers	Men and women may lose sexual desire temporarily Men may have erectile dysfunction; dry ejaculation; retrograde ejaculation Women may have vaginal dryness, dyspareunia Both men and women may experience anxiety, depression, pain, nausea from chemotherapy, radiation, pelvic surgery, hormone therapy, nerve damage from pelvic surgery	

number of older people living in these settings might choose to be sexually active if they had privacy and a sexual partner (Messinger-Rapport et al., 2003). Intimacy and sexuality among residents includes the opportunity to have not only coitus but also other forms of intimate expressions, such as hugging, kissing, hand holding, and masturbation. Wallace (2003) commented that the sexual needs of older adults in long-term care facilities should be addressed with the same priority as nutrition, hydration, and other well-accepted needs. The institutionalized older person has the same rights as noninstitutionalized elders to engage in or refrain from sexual activity.

Nursing homes are required by federal regulation to allow married spouses to share a room if they desire, but no other requirements related to sexual activity in nursing homes exist. However, what about unmarried individuals in intimate relationships or gay and lesbian partners? In research with older gay and lesbian individuals and their families, participants reported being terrified of going into care facilities and having to hide their relationships or lose their partners and friends (Brotman et al., 2003). One lesbian couple, who had been living together for several decades, was separated by health care professionals and family members who were not aware of the nature of their partnership. Another partner in a lesbian relationship changed her last name to her partner's so that they would be taken for sisters and put in the same room.

Privacy is a major issue in nursing homes that can prevent fulfillment of intimacy and sexual needs. Suggestions for providing privacy and an atmosphere accepting of sexual activity include the availability of a private room, not interrupting when doors are closed and sexual activity is taking place, allowing residents to have sexually explicit materials in their rooms, and providing adaptive equipment, such as siderails or trapezes and double beds. In one facility where the author worked, the staff would assist one of the female residents to be freshly showered, perfumed, and in a lovely nightgown when she and her partner wanted to have sexual relations.

Attitudes about intimacy and sexuality among long-term care staff and, often, family members may reflect general societal attitudes that older people do not have sexual needs or that sexual activity is inappropriate. Families may have difficulty understanding that their older relative may want to have a new relationship. Caregivers often view residents' sexual acts as problems rather than as expressions of the need for love and intimacy. Reactions may include disapproval, discomfort, and embarrassment, and caregivers may explicitly or implicitly discourage or deny intimacy needs.

Staff, family, and resident education programs to promote awareness, provide education on sexuality and intimacy in later life, involve residents in discussions of sexuality, and discuss interventions to respond to residents' needs are important in long-term care settings. Staff education should include the opportunity to discuss personal feelings about sexuality, changes associated with aging, the impact of diseases and medications on sexual function, as well as role playing and skill training in sexual assessment and intervention.

Intimacy, Sexuality, and Dementia

Intimacy and sexuality remain important in the lives of persons with dementia and their partners throughout the illness. Intimacy and sexuality may "serve as a nonverbal form of communication and intimacy when other cognitive skills and functions have declined" (Agronin, 2004, p. 13). As dementia progresses, particularly in persons living in long-term care facilities, intimacy and sexuality issues may present challenges, especially regarding the impaired person's ability to consent to sexual activity, and require accurate assessment and documentation.

Determination of a cognitively impaired person's ability to consent to participation in a sexual activity involves concepts of voluntary participation, mental competence, and an understanding of the risks and benefits. It is important for the person to understand the potential physical risks but also the "psychological risks including risk of loss through transfer, death, or discharge of his or her partner" (Messinger-Rapport et al., 2003, p. 52).

The Hebrew Home for the Aged in Riverdale, New York, initiated model sexual policies in 1995 that have been used to develop a guide for long-term care facilities for intimacy, sexuality, and sexual behavior for older people with dementia. These guidelines can be found at www.fhs.mcmaster.ca/mcah/cgec/toolkit.pdf.

Inappropriate sexual behavior (exposing oneself, masturbating in public, or making inappropriate sexual advances or sexual comments) may also occur in long-term care settings. These behaviors are most distressing to staff and to other residents. Rheaume and Mitty (2008) suggest an interdisciplinary sexual assessment to determine the underlying need that the person is expressing and how it might be addressed is important. These kinds of behaviors may be triggered by unmet intimacy needs or may be symptoms of an underlying physical problem, such as a urinary tract or vaginal infection.

Encouraging family and friends to touch, hug, kiss, and hold hands when visiting may help to meet touch and intimacy needs and decrease inappropriate sexual behavior. Also, allowing the person to stroke a pet or hold a stuffed animal may be helpful. Aggressive or violent behavior may require limit setting, working with the resident and family, providing for sexual expression in a nonharmful manner, and pharmacological treatment if indicated (Messinger-Rapport et al., 2003). Staff will need opportunities for discussion and assistance with interventions.

HIV/AIDS and Older Adults

About 15% of new HIV infections occur in individuals aged 50 years or older, and 31% of those living with HIV are in this age group. By 2015, half of all Americans with HIV will be 50 years of age or older. Between 2003 and 2007, the annual estimated number of individuals age 50 and older living with acquired immunodeficiency syndrome (AIDS) increased more than 60% (Population Reference Bureau, 2009). The racial/ethnic disparities in HIV/AIDS among older people parallel trends among all age groups. Rates of HIV/AIDS among older African Americans are 12 times higher than for Caucasian older people, and the rates for Hispanic older adults are 5 times as high as those of Caucasian older adults (Emlet et al., 2009). Men who have sex with men continue to have the highest rates of both incidence and prevalence of HIV (Fredriksen-Goldsen & Emlet, n.d.).

Women older than 60 years of age make up one of the fastest-growing risk groups, and the rise in cases in women of color over 50 has been especially steep. Most got the virus from sex with infected partners (National Institute on Aging [NIA], 2009). In the last decade, AIDS cases in women over 50 years of age are reported to have tripled, while heterosexual transmission rates in this age group may have increased as much as 106% (HIV Wisdom for Older Women, 2010).

The incidence of HIV in older people is rising faster among the older population than it is in those 24 years of age and younger. Incidence is expected to continue to increase as more individuals become infected later in life, and those who were infected in early adulthood live longer as a result of advances in disease treatment. The compromised immune system of an older individual makes him or her even more susceptible to HIV or AIDS than a younger person.

AIDS in older adults has been called the "Great Imitator" because many of the symptoms such as fatigue, weakness, weight loss, and anorexia are common to other disease conditions and may be attributed to normal aging. Older adults with HIV may also be at more risk for cognitive decline and may be misdiagnosed with Alzheimer's disease (AD) instead of AIDS. In addition, the idea that elders are not sexually active limits physicians' and other care providers' objectivity to recognize HIV/AIDS as a possible diagnosis.

Older adults who are sexually active are at risk for HIV/AIDS and other sexually transmitted diseases. People older than 50 years of age are about one sixth as likely to use condoms during sex. Older women who are sexually active are at

high risk for HIV/AIDS (and other sexually transmitted infections) from an infected partner, resulting, in part, from normal age changes of the vaginal tissue—a thinner, drier, friable vaginal lining that makes viral entry more efficient.

Lack of awareness about HIV in older people often results in late diagnosis and treatment. Older people may have the virus for years before being tested. By the time of diagnosis, the virus may be in the late stages (NIA, 2009). Older adults are also at higher risk of HIV-medication toxicity (Vance et al., 2009). Mortality rates are higher for older adults with HIV, and survival time after diagnosis is shorter (Population Reference Bureau, 2009).

In general, elders lack adequate knowledge about HIV/AIDS and believe that it "just does not happen in my generation." This view places elders at high risk for HIV and AIDS. Further, older people may have limited access to HIV tests and age-appropriate information. Only 16% of older adults over 65 years of age have been tested for HIV, compared to 40% of those 50 to 64, 61% of those 30 to 49, and 54% of people 18 to 29 (University of Connecticut Health Center, 2010). Older adults, especially older women, have also not been included in research and drug trials on HIV/AIDS.

In 2010, Medicare began covering HIV screening for beneficiaries who are at increased risk or who request it. The CDC has also revised HIV-screening recommendations to include provisions for testing adults 65 years of age and older. In addition to screening for HIV, assessment and screening for other sexually transmitted diseases (STDs) (gonorrhea, chlamydia, syphilis, trichomonas, human papillomavirus [HPV]) should also be a part of primary care for sexually active elders. Medicare is considering providing coverage for STD screenings as well as related behavioral counseling for older adults.

Healthy People 2020 (USDHHS, 2012) includes STDs as a topic area with the goal of promoting healthy sexual behaviors, strengthening community capacity, and increasing access to quality services to prevent STDs and their complications. While the objectives are aimed more toward younger people, cases of STDs are increasing significantly among older adults.

Educational materials and programs tailored for older adults need to be developed that include information about HIV/AIDS and how it is transmitted, the need to use condoms for protection when engaging in sexual activity, symptoms of which to be aware, and the treatments that are available. Jane Fowler, director of the National HIV Wisdom for Older Women (WOW) program, suggests that HIV/AIDS educational campaigns and programs are not targeted to older individuals and asks, "How often does a wrinkled face appear on a prevention poster?" (HIV Wisdom for Older Women, 2010). Only 15 out of 50 states have HIV publications for older adults. Easily accessible educational materials for older adults are available at http://aoa.gov/AoARoot/AoA_Programs/HPW/HIV_AIDS/toolkit.aspx and http://www.healthinaging.org/files/documents/tipsheets/safe_sex_for_seniors.pdf.

Physicians, nurse practitioners, and other health professionals need to increase their knowledge of HIV in older adults and become comfortable taking a complete sexual history and talking about sex with older adults. In addition, the myth that elders do not engage in sexual activity must be put to rest.

Implications for Gerontological Nursing and Healthy Aging

Nurses have multiple roles in the area of sexuality and older people. The nurse is a facilitator of a milieu that is conducive to the older person asking questions and expressing his or her sexuality. The nurse has the responsibility to help maintain the sexuality of older people by offering opportunity for discussion. Some older people remain or want to remain sexually active, whereas others do not see this as an important part of their life. Nurses should open the door to discussions of sexual concerns in a nonjudgmental manner, helping those who want to continue to be sexually active, and making it clear that stopping sex is an acceptable option for others (Lindau et al., 2007). The nurse should be an educator and provide information and guidance to older people who need it.

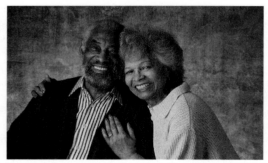

Sexuality is an important need in late life; it affects pleasure, adaptation, and a general feeling of well-being. (Copyright © Getty Images.)

Assessment

To assist and support older people in their sexual needs, nurses should be aware of their own feelings about sexuality and their attitudes toward intimacy and sexuality in older people (single, married, and LGBT). Only after confronting one's own attitudes, values, and beliefs can the nurse provide support without being judgmental. Rarely are sexual histories elicited from the older adult. Physical examinations often do not include the reproductive system unless it is directly involved in the present illness. However, when questions about sexual issues are asked or when the older adult is examined, the nurse needs to be particularly cognizant of the era and culture in which the individual has lived to understand the factors affecting conduct.

Older persons should be asked about their sexual satisfaction, because they may not mention it voluntarily. Anticipation of problems in older individuals' sexual experiences can ward off anxiety, misconceptions, and an arbitrary cessation of sexual pleasure. Validation of the normalcy of sexual activity or a discussion of the physiological changes that occur either with age or illness is important.

Because of professionals' discomfort discussing sexuality or lack of knowledge about sexuality in older people, medications are often prescribed to both older men and women without attention to the sexual side effects. If medications that affect sexual function are necessary, adjustment of doses, use of alternative agents, and prescription of antidotes to reverse the sexual side effects are important. For a complete listing of medications that can affect sexual functioning and suggestions for management, see http://www.netdoctor.co.uk/menshealth/feature/medicinessex.htm. Counseling may also be needed for the older person to adapt to natural physiological changes, illness, and image-altering surgical procedures. The nurse may also be a consultant and counselor to others who give care to older people.

The PLISSIT model (Annon, 1976) is a helpful guide for discussion of sexuality (Box 24-11). A Nursing Standard of Practice Protocol: Sexuality in Older Adults (Kazer, 2012) is available at http://consultgerirn.org/uploads/File/trythis/try_this_10.pdf. The CDC provides a guide

---

BOX 24-11   PLISSIT Model

P   **P**ermission from the client to initiate sexual discussion
LI Providing the **L**imited **I**nformation needed to function sexually
SS Giving **S**pecific **S**uggestions for the individual to proceed with sexual relations
IT Providing **I**ntensive **T**herapy surrounding the issues of sexuality for the clients (may mean referral to specialist)

From Annon J: The PLISSIT model: a proposed conceptual theme for behavioral treatment of sexual problems, *J Sex Educ Ther* 2(2):1-15, 1976; Wallace M: Best practices in nursing care to older adults: sexuality, *Dermatol Nurs* 15(6):570-571, 2003; Youngkin E: The myths and truths of mature intimacy: mature guidance for nurse practitioners, *Adv Nurse Pract* 12(9):45-48, 2004.

for taking a sexual history (http://www.cdc.gov/std/see/HealthCareProviders/SexualHistory.pdf).

Youngkin (2004) provides suggestions for use of the PLISSIT model with older people:

- **Permission:** Obtain permission from the client to initiate sexual discussion. Allow the person to discuss concerns related to sexual issues, and gather information about what might have changed in the person's life to affect sexual needs and response. Questions such as the following can be used: "What concerns or questions do you have about fulfilling your sexual needs?" or "In this era of HIV and other sexually transmitted infections, I ask all my patients about sexual practices and concerns. Are there any questions I can answer for you?"
- **Limited Information:** Provide the limited information to function sexually (Wallace, 2003). Offer teaching about the normal age-associated changes that affect sexual performance or how illness may affect sexuality. Encourage the person to learn more about the concern from books and other sources.
- **Specific Suggestions:** Offer suggestions for dealing with problems such as lubricants for atrophic vaginitis; use of condoms to prevent sexually transmitted infections; proper use of ED medications; how to communicate sexual and other needs; ways to increase comfort with coitus or ways to be intimate without coital relations.
- **Intensive Therapy:** Refer as appropriate for complex problems that require specialist intervention.

Interventions

Interventions will vary depending on the needs identified from the assessment data. Following a comprehensive assessment, interventions may center on the following categories: (1) education regarding age-associated change in sexual function; (2) compensating for age-associated changes; (3) effective management of acute and chronic illness affecting sexual function; (4) removal of barriers associated with fulfilling sexual needs; and (5) special interventions to promote sexual health in cognitively impaired older adults (Arena & Wallace, 2008). Education about prevention of HIV and STDs is also important in sexually active older adults.

KEY CONCEPTS

- Ability to successfully negotiate transitions and develop new and gratifying roles depends on personal and environmental supports, timing, clarity of expectations, personality, and degree of change required.
- Elders and their family members carry a long history. Current family dynamics must be understood within the context of family history.

- Loss of a spouse is the role change that has the greatest potential for life disruption, and nursing support can make a positive difference in the transition.
- Grandparenting is a significant role among elders. In an increasing number of families, grandparents are increasingly assuming primary caregiving roles with grandchildren.
- Caregiving activities are one of the most major social issues of our time as well as a significant public health problem. Most spouses will spend some time caring for one another, and most adult children will spend some time caring for older parents.
- Sexuality is love, sharing, trust, and warmth, as well as physical acts. Sexuality provides an individual with self-identity and affirmation of life.
- Sexuality continues in late life, though adaptations are needed for the age-related changes and the effects of chronic illness.
- Further research is needed to promote knowledge and understanding of the sexual health of older adults with alternative lifestyles, such as gay men, lesbians, and bisexual and transgender individuals.
- AIDS awareness and the practice of safe sex among older adults is still lacking. Older adults and health professionals may not consider older adults at risk for AIDS or STDs even though the incidence of these diseases in the older population is rapidly increasing.
- The major roles of the nurse in older adult sexuality in the community or long-term care setting are education and counseling about sexual function; adaptations for age-related changes and chronic conditions; prevention of HIV/AIDS and STDs in sexually active older adults; and the maintenance of sexuality for the older adult who desires this.

ACTIVITIES AND DISCUSSION QUESTIONS

1. Discuss your position in the family and how that has affected your relationship with siblings and parents.
2. What do you suppose your role will be when your parent or parents need help?
3. Write a brief essay discussing the ways in which your grandparents have affected your life.
4. What would you find most difficult in regard to assisting your older parent?
5. With a classmate, role play how you would conduct a review of systems in the area of sexual health with an older adult. What would be the most important factors to consider when providing education about sexuality and sexual health?
6. What resources are available for older LGBT individuals in your community?

REFERENCES

Agronin M: Sexuality and aging: an introduction, *CNS Long-Term Care* Summer:12–13, 2004.

American Association of Retired Persons, Public Policy Institute: *Fact sheet: multigenerational householders are increasing.* Fact sheet 221 (2011).

American Society on Aging and MetLife: Still out, still aging (2010). Available at http://www.metlife.com/assets/cao/mmi/publications/studies/2010/mmi-still-out-still-aging.pdf.

Annon J: The PLISSIT model: a proposed conceptual scheme for behavioral treatment of sexual problems, *J Sex Educ Ther* 2(2):1–15, 1976.

Archbold PG, Stewart BJ, Greenlick MR, et al: Mutuality and preparedness as predictors of caregiver role strain, *Res Nurs Health* 13(6):375–384, 1990.

Arena J, Wallace M: Issues regarding sexuality. In Capezuti E, Swicker D, Mezey M, et al, editors: *Evidence-based geriatric nursing protocols for best practice,* New York, 2008, Springer.

Brotman S, Ryan B, Cormier R: The health and social service needs of gay and lesbian elders and their families in Canada, *Gerontologist* 43(2):172–202, 2003.

Centers for Disease Control and Prevention [CDC] and the Kimberly-Clark Corporation: *Assuring healthy caregivers, a public health approach to translating research into practice: the RE-AIM framework* (2008). Available at www.cdc.gov/aging/caregiving/assuring.htm.

Comfort A: Sexuality in old age, *J Am Geriatr Soc* 22(10):440–442, 1974.

delBene S: African American grandmothers raising grandchildren: a phenomenological perspective of marginalized women, *J Gerontol Nurs* 36:32, 2010.

DeVries B: Grief: intimacy's reflection, *Generations* 25(2):75-79, 2001.

Emlet C, Gerkin A, Orel N: The graying of HIV/AIDS: Preparedness and needs of the aging network in a changing epidemic, *J Gerontol Soc Work* 52:803, 2009.

Family Caregiver Alliance: Caregiver assessment: principles, guidelines and strategies for change. Report from a National Consensus Development Conference (Vol 1), San Francisco: The Alliance, 2006.

Federal Interagency Forum on Aging: *Older Americans 2010: key indicators of well-being.* Federal Interagency Forum on Aging-Related Statistics, Washington, DC, 2010, U.S. Government Printing Office. Available at http://www.agingstats.gov/agingstatsdotnet/Main_Site/Data/2010_Documents/Docs/OA_2010.pdf.

Fredriksen-Goldsen K, Emlet C: *Research note: health disparities among LGBT older adults living with HIV* (n.d.). Available at http://www.asaging.org/blog/research-note-health-disparities-among-lgbt-older-adults-living-hiv.

Gelo F: Invisible individuals—LGBT elders, *Aging Well* 1:36, 2008.

HIV Wisdom for Older Women: Things you should know about HIV and older women (2010). Available at http://www.hivwisdom.org/facts.html.

Hooyman N, Kiyak H: *Social gerontology: a multidisciplinary perspective,* ed 9, Boston, 2011, Allyn & Bacon.

Institute of Medicine: *Retooling for an aging America: building the healthcare workforce* (2008). Available at http://www.iom.edu/Reports/2008/Retooling-for-an-Aging-America-Building-the-Health-Care-Workforce.aspx.

Janeway M, Baum N: Sexual dysfunction in older men, *Clin Geriatr* 20(10):14–19, 2012.

Janeway M, Baum N, Smith R: Sexual dysfunction in older women, *Clin Geriatr* 20(11):16–20, 2012.

Jett KF: Making the connection: seeking and receiving help by elderly African Americans, *J Qual Health Res* 12(3):373–387, 2002.

Kaiser F: Sexual function and the older woman, *Clin Geriatr Med* 19(3):463–472, 2000.

Kazer M: Issues regarding sexuality. In Boltz M, Capezuti E, Fulmer T, Zwicker D, editors: *Evidence-based geriatric nursing protocols for best practice,* New York, Springer, 2012.

Kennedy G, Martinez M, Garo N: Sex and mental health in old age, *Prim Psychiatry* 17:21, 2010.

Legacy Project: *Fast facts on grandparenting and intergenerational mentoring* (n.d.). Available at www.legacyproject.org/specialreports/fastfacts.html.

Lindau S, Gavrilova N: Sex, health, and years of sexually active life gained due to good health: evidence from two US population based cross sectional surveys of ageing, *BMJ* 340, 2010.

Lindau ST, Schumm LP, Laumann EO, et al: A study of sexuality and health among older adults in the United States, *N Engl J Med* 357(8):762–744, 2007.

Livingston G, Parker K: Since the start of the great recession, more children raised by grandparents (2010). Available at http://pewresearch.org/pubs/1724/sharp-increase-children-with-grandparents-caregivers.

Lund M: Caregiver, take care, *Geriatr Nurs* 26(3):152–153, 2005.

Meiner S: *Gerontological nursing,* ed 4, St. Louis, 2011, Mosby.

Messecar D: Family caregiving. In Boltz M, Capezuti E, Fulmer T, Zwicker D, editors: *Evidence-based geriatric nursing protocols for best practice,* New York, 2012, Springer.

Messinger-Rapport B, Sandhu SK, Hujer ME: Sex and sexuality: is it over after 60? *Clin Geriatr* 11(10):45–53, 2003.

Minton M, Barron C: Spousal bereavement assessment: a review of bereavement-specific measures, *J Gerontol Nurs* 34:34, 2008.

Musil CM, Gordon NL, Warner CB, et al: Grandmothers and caregiving to grandchildren: continuity, change, and outcomes over 24 months, *Gerontologist* 51(1):86–100, 2011.

National Family Caregivers Association [NFCA]: *Who are America's family caregivers?* (2012). Available at www.nfcacares.org/who_are_family caregivers/care_giving_statistics.htm.

National Institute on Aging: HIV, AIDS, and older people (2009). Available at http://www.nia.nih.gov/health/publication/hiv-aids-and-older-people.

Ostwald S: Who is caring for the caregiver? Promoting spousal caregiver's health, *Fam Community Health* 32:S5, 2009.

Pinquart M, Sorensen S: Ethnic differences in stressors, resources, and psychological outcomes of family caregiving: a meta-analysis, *Gerontologist* 45(1):90–106, 2005.

Population Reference Bureau: HIV/AIDS and older adults in the United States, *Today's Research on Aging* 18:1–7, 2009. Available at http://www.prb.org/pdf09/TodaysResearchAging18.pdf.

Rheaume C, Mitty E: Sexuality and intimacy in older adults, *Geriatr Nurs* 29:342, 2008.

Robinson B: Validation of a caregiver strain index, *J Gerontol* 38(3):344, 1983.

Robison J, Fortinsky R, Kleppinger A, et al: A broader view of family caregiving: effects of caregiving and caregiver conditions on depressive symptoms, health, work, and social isolation, *J Gerontol B Psychol Sci Soc Sci* 64(6):788–798, 2009.

Services and Advocacy for Gay, Lesbian, Bisexual, and Transgender Elders [SAGE] and Movement Advancement Project [MAP]: *Improving the lives of LGBT older adults* (2012). Available at https:sageusa.org/resources/resource_view.cfm?resource=183.

Schulz R, Beach SR: Caregiving as a risk factor for mortality: the Caregiver Health Effects Study, *JAMA* 282(23):2215–2219, 1999.

Schumacher K, Beck C, Marren J, et al: Family caregivers: caring for older adults, working with their families, *Am J Nurs* 106(8):40–49, 2006.

Siefert ML, Williams AL, Dowd MF, et al: The caregiving experience in a racially diverse sample of cancer family caregivers, *Cancer Nurs* 31(5):399–407, 2008.

Silverstein M, Angelli J: Older parents' expectations of moving closer to their children, *J Gerontol B Psychol Sci Soc Sci* 53B:S153, 1998.

Skarupski K, McCann J, Bienias J, et al: Race differences in emotional adaptation of family caregivers, *Aging Ment Health* 13:715, 2009.

Smith G, Palmieri P, Hancock G, et al: Custodial grandmothers' psychological distress, dysfunctional parenting, and grandchildren's adjustment, *Int J Aging Hum Dev* 67:327, 2008.

Stanford P, Usita P: Retirement: who is at risk? *Generations* 26(11):45–48, 2002.

Steinke E: Intimacy needs and chronic illness, *J Gerontol Nurs* 31(5):40–50, 2005.

Suzman R: The National Social Life, Health, and Aging Project: an introduction, *J Gerontol B Psychol Sci Soc Sci* 64B:i5, 2009.

University of Connecticut Health Center: *Medicare to help with screening for HIV in older Americans* (2010). Available at http://today.uchc.edu/headlines/2010/jan10/hiv.html.

U.S. Department of Health and Human Services [USDHHS], Office of Disease Prevention and Health Promotion: *Healthy people 2020* (2012). Available at http://www.healthypeople.gov/2020.

Vance D, Childs G, Moneyham L, et al: Successful aging with HIV, *J Gerontol Nurs* 35:19, 2009.

Waite L, Laumann E, Das A, et al: Sexuality: measures of partnerships, practices, attitudes, and problems in the National Social Life, Health and Aging Study, *J Gerontol B Psychol Sci Soc Sci* 64B(suppl 1):156–166, 2009.

Wallace M: Best practices in nursing care to older adults: sexuality, *Dermatol Nurs* 15(6):570–571, 2003.

World Health Organization [WHO]: Sexual health: a new focus for WHO, progress in reproductive health research (2004). Available at www.who.int/en/.

Youngkin E: The myths and truths of mature intimacy, *Adv Nurse Pract* 12(9):45–48, 2004.

CHAPTER 25

Loss, Death, and Palliative Care

Kathleen F. Jett

evolve evolve.elsevier.com/Ebersole/gerontological

LEARNING OBJECTIVES

Upon completion of this chapter, the reader will be able to:

- Differentiate between loss and grief.
- Explain the different types of grief and the dynamics of the grieving process.
- Explain the characteristics required of the nurse to be able to effectively care for those who are grieving.
- Propose palliative measures when comfort is the goal of care.
- Explain the role and responsibility of the nurse in advance directives.
- Explain the difference between passive and active euthanasia.

GLOSSARY

Bereavement overload A number of grief situations in a short period of time.

Euthanasia Death that is unrelated to the natural life processes or random accident.

Grief An emotional response to loss.

Mourning The process by which grief is expressed.

Palliative care Care which is directed toward maximizing comfort rather than achieving a cure.

THE LIVED EXPERIENCE

When we were in our sixties my friends and I met over cards, went on trips, and experienced all the joys of retirement. We didn't have much time to worry about aches and pains. In our seventies we had less time to play because we were busy visiting one another in the hospital or nursing home. In our eighties we met frequently again, but it was usually at our friends' funerals, leaving little time for cards or travel. Now that I am in my nineties hardly any of my friends are still alive; you know it gets kind of lonely, so you just have to make new younger friends!

Theresa, age 93

Life is like a pinwheel, a thing of beauty and change. Loss, like the wind, sets it in motion, beginning the life-changing process of grieving. Throughout one's life the winds of loss will gently stir recurrent episodes of grief through sights, sounds, smells, anniversary dates, and other triggers. The arms of the pinwheel suggest movement by the bereaved, reaching out of the experience of grief by surrendering through resting, or lowering one's defenses toward life and being open to reality, or the acceptance of the life event and reaching out to others and rejoining life through change. Each gust of wind may generate a resurgence of grief, but the pinwheel will never lose its beauty.

Loss, dying, and death are universal, incontestable events of the human experience. Some loss is associated with the normal changes with aging, such as the loss of flexibility in the joints (see Chapter 5). Some is related to the normal changes in everyday life and life transitions, such as moving and retirement. Other losses are those of loved ones through death. Some deaths are considered normative and expected, such as older parents and friends. Other deaths are considered non-normative and unexpected, such as the death of adult children or grandchildren.

Regardless of the type of loss, each one has the potential to trigger grief and a process we call bereavement or mourning. Grieving and mourning are usually used synonymously. However, grieving is an individual's response to a loss and mourning is an active and evolving process that includes those behaviors used to incorporate the loss experience into one's life after the loss. Mourning behaviors are strongly influenced by social and cultural norms that prescribe the appropriate ways of both reacting to the loss and coping with it (Chow et al., 2007; Gerdner et al., 2007). For example, in much of the world, widows are expected to wear black after the death of their husbands, but in India the traditional dress is a white sari for the remainder of the time the woman remains a widow. There is no single way to grieve or respond to loss; each person grieves in his or her own way.

Although there are cultural expectations related to grief behaviors for loss through death, there are no guidelines for behavior when the loss is of another type. For example, an individual who moves to a nursing home (loses one's home), or who retires (willingly or unwillingly) may be very sad, irritable, and forgetful. The person may be suspected of developing dementia when he or she is actually grieving. When the losses accumulate in quick succession, a state of bereavement overload may result. The griever may become incapacitated and require careful and skilled support and guidance.

Gerontological nurses need to have basic knowledge of the grieving process and how to comfort and care for grievers, including one another. Additional knowledge and skills are related to care of the dying person and his or her survivors including those needed to provide quality care. And finally nurses caring for the dying must be comfortable with their own mortality. In this chapter we hope to provide the basic information necessary to promote effective grieving, peaceful dying, and good and appropriate deaths.

The Grieving Process

Researchers have tried for years to understand the grieving process. Their efforts have resulted in a number of models proposed to explain and predict the experience. The majority of the models developed between the early 1970s and early 1980s influence what caregivers and society in general have been taught about grief. Although intended to describe death-related grief, these same models can be applied to any of the losses in the lives of older adults that are significant or meaningful to that person.

All models recognize similar physical and psychological manifestations of acute grief (when it is first felt), a middle period in which the manifestations of grief (e.g., despair, depression) affect the person's day-to-day functioning, and an ending phase where the person learns to adjust to life in a new way without that which has been lost or in anticipation of their pending deaths. At the same time it is also recognized that the grieving process is not rigidly structured and that a predictable pattern of responses does not always occur.

A Loss Response Model

Jett's Loss Response Model is a modification of that proposed by Barbara Giacquinta for families facing cancer (Giacquinta, 1977). It incorporates Betty Newman's System Model (Parker & Smith, 2010) that leads to a framework for the design of nursing interventions.

When loss occurs within a system, such as a family, the impact is experienced as acute grief. The system's equilibrium is in chaos and is seen as a *functional disruption*; that is, the system cannot perform its usual activities. Either the person or the members are in a state of disequilibrium. The loss seems unreal. The grieving family searches for meaning: why did this happen? How will they survive the loss? If an elder is reacting to the loss of a child or a grandchild, thoughts of "why wasn't it me?" are common. If it is the loss of one's health or a move out of one's home, the question "how could this happen to me?" could arise. The family or elder then may become active in *informing others*. Each time the story is repeated, the loss becomes more real and the system moves toward a new steady state. The story may be different each time it is told, as it is told from a new perspective. Informing others involves *engaging emotions* that may have been previously withheld or subdued because of the shock of the impact. The expression of emotions can be quite powerful: anger, frustration or even relief. They can release energy that can be used to *reorganize the family structure*. As roles change, adaptation and accommodation are necessary. Someone else steps in to perform the roles of the person who is now absent or to complete the tasks no longer possible in the presence of the loss. For example, when the elder patriarch dies, the eldest son may step up and assume some of his father's roles and responsibilities. Finally, if the system is to survive, it will need to redefine itself. One of the ways that it does this is by *reframing its memories;* that is, families accept that portraits and reunions are still possible, just different than they were before the loss; or they accept that a person can still be vital, active, and

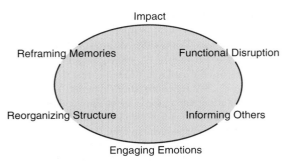

FIGURE 25-1 The Loss Response Model. (From Jett KF: The loss response model, unpublished manuscript, 2004. Adapted from Giacquinta B: Helping families face the crisis of cancer, *Am J Nurs* 77(10):1585-1588, 1977.)

important even after the loss of the ability to drive a car, to walk unassisted, or to live alone (Figure 25-1).

Types of Grief

Grieving takes enormous amounts of physical and emotional energy. It is the hardest thing anyone can do and may be especially hard for older adults who must simultaneously face other challenges discussed throughout this book. Emotions can be intense, and this intensity may manifest as confusion, depression, or preoccupation with thoughts of the deceased or the loss. This reaction may be mistaken for other conditions, such as dementia, when it probably is a type of delirium, a temporary change in mental status, something that requires careful assessment and care (see Chapter 21). The gerontological nurse is most likely to work with elders who are experiencing anticipatory grief, acute grief, or chronic grief. A fourth type, disenfranchised grief, may be hidden, but when it occurs it is nonetheless significant.

Anticipatory Grief

Anticipatory grief is the response to a real or perceived loss before it actually occurs, a dress rehearsal, so to speak. One observes this grief in preparation for potential loss, such as loss of belongings (e.g., selling of a home), moving (e.g., into a nursing home), or knowing that a body part or function is going to change (e.g., a mastectomy), or in anticipation of the loss of a spouse or oneself either through dementia or through death. Behaviors that may signal anticipatory grief include preoccupation with the loss, unusually detailed planning, or a sudden change in attitude toward the thing or person to be lost (Lewis & McBride, 2004). End-of-life communication has been found to be associated with anticipatory grief and improved bereavement-related outcomes (Metzger & Gray, 2008).

The grieving process described by the models may occur in the context of anticipatory grief with one significant difference: the loss has not yet occurred. If the loss is certain but no one can say when it will occur, or if it does not occur when or as expected, those awaiting the actual loss or death may become irritable, hostile, or impatient, not because they want the loss to occur but in response to the emotional ups and downs of the waiting. Researchers Glaser and Strauss (1968) described what they call an interruption in the sentimental order of a nursing unit when this occurs—no one quite knows how to behave. Professionals who are grieving, such as nurses, as well as family and friends, usually deal much more easily with anticipated losses when they occur at an expected time or in a set manner.

Anticipatory grief can result in the phenomenon of premature detachment from an individual who is dying or detachment of the dying person from the environment. Pattison (1977) called the premature withdrawal of others sociological death, and the premature withdrawal of the person, psychological death. In either case, the person who is dying is no longer involved in day-to-day activities of living and essentially suffers a premature death.

Acute Grief

Acute grief is a crisis. It has a definitive syndrome of somatic and psychological symptoms of distress that occur in waves lasting varying periods of time. These symptoms may occur every time the loss is acknowledged, others are informed, or even when another person offers condolences. Preoccupation with the loss is a phenomenon similar to daydreaming and is accompanied by a sense of unreality. Depending on the situation, feelings of self-blame or guilt may be present and manifest themselves as hostility or anger toward friends, depression, or withdrawal. A formerly bad relationship may be idealized and confusing to others.

It is often difficult for persons who are acutely grieving to accomplish their usual activities of daily living or meet other responsibilities (functional disruption). Even if the tasks are accomplished, the person may complain of feeling distracted, restless, and "at loose ends." Common, simple activities such as deciding what to wear may seem too complex a task. Fortunately the signs and symptoms of acute grief do not last forever, or else none of us could survive. Acute grief is most intense in the months immediately following the loss, especially the first 3 months, with the intensity of feelings lessening over time (Taylor et al., 2008). A griever may cry in the first months any time that which is lost is mentioned. Later, the person will still be grieving, but the tears are replaced with a surging sense of loss and sadness, and still later by more fleeting reactions.

Chronic and Complicated Grief

Grief may temporarily inhibit some activity but is considered a normal response. The intermittent pain of grief is often exacerbated on anniversary dates (birthdays, holidays, and wedding anniversaries). For the survivors of tragedies, such as war, the Oklahoma City bombing, the 9/11 or some other terrorist attack, the grief may never completely go away. In some cases this takes the form of post-traumatic stress disorder (PTSD) and for others there is a lingering grief described as "shadow grief," or that which resurfaces from time to time in the form of a fleeting grief response, usually triggered by a sight, smell, or sound (Coryell, 2007) (Box 25-1).

Some chronic grief is more than that of shadow grief and crosses the boundary to what we call impaired, pathological, abnormal, dysfunctional, or maladaptive grief. It has been thought that pathological chronic grief begins with normal grief responses, whose normal evolution toward adjustment, toward the reestablishment of equilibrium, is blocked by some obstacle. The memories resist being reframed. Reactions are exaggerated, and memories are experienced as recurrent acute grief—over and over again, months and years later. Signs of possible pathological grief include excessive and irrational anger, outbursts in social settings, and insomnia that lingers for an extended time or surfaces months or years later, or a grief episode that triggers a major depressive episode. The families who have had a loved one who has committed suicide have been found to be among those who have a greater risk for complicated, chronic grief (Sveen & Walby, 2008). This type of grief necessitates the professional intervention of a grief counselor, a psychiatric nurse practitioner, or a psychologist who has skills at helping grieving elders and their loved ones.

BOX 25-1   The Carved Birds

One day as I was browsing at an art show, I came across a booth of carved birds, a favorite design of my beloved mother. I turned to remark to her. Except she was not there: she had died 15 years earlier in my home. Sadness passed over me like a cloud, and I wished she were there—I would buy her one as a special gift. Instead, I turned to my husband and shared reminiscences as I had done before, and he listened patiently. As the wind blows, so did the cloud pass, and I moved on, enjoying the day.

Kathleen Jett at 40

Disenfranchised Grief

Disenfranchised grief is experienced by persons whose loss cannot be openly acknowledged or publicly mourned. The grief is socially disallowed or unsupported (Doka, 2002). The person does not have a socially recognized right to be perceived or function as a bereaved person. In other words, a relationship is not recognized; the loss is not sanctioned, or the griever is not recognized or cannot be made public. Disenfranchised grief has frequently been associated with domestic partnerships in which the family of the deceased does not acknowledge the partner or in secret relationships in which the involved party cannot tell others of the meaning or depth of the attachment. Disenfranchised grief can also occur in situations of family discord in which a member of the family is considered the "black sheep." It has also been recognized in combat veterans who must integrate their own roles in killing in a war zone (Aloi, 2011). Older adults can experience this disenfranchisement when persons close to them do not understand the full meaning of the loss such as retirement or the death of a pet. Families coping with a member who has Alzheimer's disease may also experience disenfranchised or chronic grief, particularly when others perceive the death of the elder as a blessing and fail to support the griever or caregiver who has struggled for years with anticipatory grief and now must cope with the acute grief of the actual death (Doka, 2002; Paun & Farran, 2011).

Factors Affecting Coping with Loss

Coping as it relates to loss and grief is the ability of the individual or family to find ways to deal with the stress. In the language of the Loss Response Model, it is the ability to move from a state of chaos and disequilibrium to one of renewed order, equilibrium, and peace. Many factors affect the ability to cope with loss and grief (Box 25-2).

Those at special risk for significantly adverse effects of grief are older spouses and life partners of any kind. Intense grief may cause a temporary decrease in cognitive function that can be misinterpreted as dementia, isolating the griever (Ward et al., 2007).

A classic authority on death and dying was psychiatrist Avery Weisman (1979). He described those who are more likely to effectively deal with loss as "good copers" (p. 42). These are individuals or families who have experience with the successful management of crisis; they are resourceful and are able to draw on coping strategies that have worked in the past. Weisman (1979, pp. 42-43) found persons who cope effectively with cancer do the following:

- Avoid avoidance
- Confront realities, and take appropriate action
- Focus on solutions

BOX 25-2   Factors Influencing the Grieving Process

- If the illness causes a number of losses
- If each loss can be identified
- How important the loss is to the person
- If psychotropic drugs are used appropriately
- Level of health and fitness before the loss (e.g., nutritional status, sleep, and exercise)
- Coping skills and types of coping responses available to the person
- Past experience with loss or death
- Immediate circumstances surrounding loss
- Timing of the loss
- Number, type, and quality of secondary losses occurring at the same time

Additional Factors Specific to Dying and Death

- Role that deceased occupied in family or social system
- Amount of unfinished business
- Perception of deceased's fulfillment in life
- Immediate circumstances surrounding death
- Length of illness before death
- Anticipatory grief and involvement with dying patient

Modified from Hess PA: Loss, grief, and dying. In Beare PG, Myers JL, editors: *Principles and practice of adult health nursing*, ed 2, St. Louis, 1994, Mosby.

- Redefine problems
- Consider alternatives
- Have good communication
- Seek and use constructive help
- Accept support when offered
- Can keep up their morale

In other words, the effective copers are those who can acknowledge the loss and try to make sense of it. They are able to generally use good judgment, and are able to remain optimistic without denying the loss. These good copers seek guidance when they need it.

In contrast, those who cope less effectively have few if any of these abilities. They tend to be more rigid and pessimistic, are demanding, and are given to emotional extremes. They may be dogmatic and expect perfection from themselves and others. Ineffective copers are also more likely to be individuals who live alone, socialize little, and have few close friends or an ineffective support

network. They may have a history of mental illness, or they may have guilt, anger, and ambivalence toward the individual who has died or that which has been lost. Those at risk for pathological grief will more likely have unresolved past conflicts or be facing the loss and other, secondary stressors simultaneously. They will have fewer opportunities as a result of the loss. They are the elders who are most in need of the expert interventions of grief counselors and skilled psychiatric gerontological nurse practitioners (Weisman, 1979).

Implications for Gerontological Nursing and Healthy Aging

The goal of the nurse is not to prevent grief but to support those who are grieving. Although the loss will never change, the potential long-term detrimental effects can be lessened. Working with grieving elders is part of the normal workday of gerontological nurses, who are professional grievers in our own way. It is one of the few areas in nursing where small actions can make a large difference in the quality of life for the person to whom we provide care and with whom we work.

Assessment

The goal of the grief assessment is to differentiate those who are likely to cope effectively from those who are at risk for ineffective coping, so that appropriate interventions can be planned. A grief assessment is based on knowledge of the grieving process and the subsequent mourning. Data are obtained through observation of behavior of the individual and are assessed within the context of the person's culture (National Cancer Institute [NCI], 2006).

A thorough grief assessment includes questions about recent significant life events, life or religious values, and relationship to that which has been lost. How many other stressful or demanding events or circumstances are going on in the griever's life? This information will help determine who is at most risk for impaired grieving. The more concurrent stressors in the person's life, the more he or she will need the nurse or other grief specialists. The nurse determines what stress management techniques have been used in the past, and whether they were helpful (e.g., talking) or potentially harmful (e.g., substance use or abuse). Was the griever's identity closely tied to that which is lost, such as a lifelong athlete who is faced with never walking again? If the loss is of a partner, how was the relationship? The loss of an abusive or controlling partner may liberate the survivor, who may feel guilty for not feeling the amount of grief that is expected. For many older women who have been dependent financially on their spouses, death may leave them impoverished, significantly complicating their grief. Knowing more about the loss and the effect of the loss on the elder's life will enable the nurse to construct and implement appropriate and caring responses.

Interventions

One goal of intervention is to assist the individual (or family) in attaining a healthy adjustment to the loss experience and reestablishing equilibrium. Memories are *reframed* so that they can account for the loss without diminishing the value of that which has been lost thus minimizing the risk for complicated grief (Maccallum & Bryant, 2011). Actions that can meet these goals are basic and simple; however, the emotional overlay makes the simple difficult. For the new nurse who is confronted with a person's grief for the first time, there may be discomfort, fear, and insecurity. The tendency is to be sympathetic rather than empathetic. Questions arise in one's mind: What do I say? Should I be cheerful or serious? Should I talk about or even mention the dead person's name?

Nursing interventions, especially when elders are in crisis, begin with the gentle establishment of rapport. Nurses introduce themselves, explain the nature of their roles (e.g., charge nurse, staff nurse, medication nurse) and the time available. If it is the time of *impact* (e.g., just after a new serious diagnosis, at the death of a family member, or upon becoming a new but resistant resident of a long-term care facility), the most we can do is to provide support and a safe environment and ensure that basic needs, such as meals, are met. The nurse can soften the despair by fostering reasonable hope, such as, "You will make it through this time, one moment at a time, and I will be here to help."

Nurses observe for *functional disruption* and offer support and direction. They may have to help the family figure out what has to be done immediately and find ways to do it—either the nurse offers to complete the task or finds a friend or family member who can step in so the disruption does not have any deleterious effects.

As grievers *search for meaning,* they may need help finding what they are looking for if this is possible. Sometimes it is information about a disease, a situation, or a person. Sometimes it is a spiritual search and help in finding a source of comfort such as a priest, rabbi, or medicine person or a place of peace, such as the chapel or mosque. Often what is needed most is someone to listen to the "whys" and "hows"—questions that cannot be answered.

Sometimes nurses offer to contact others for those who are grieving, thinking that this is something that will help.

However, it is far more therapeutic for grievers to be the ones who *inform others* because it helps the reality of the loss become real. The nurse can offer to find a phone number or hold the griever's hand during the conversation or just "be there" when the news is being shared. In this way the nurse can be available to provide support when the griever's *emotions engage* and move toward wellness and equilibrium.

As the elder moves forward in adjusting to the loss, such as a move from home to a nursing home, the nurse can help the person *reorganize the structure* of life. The nurse talks with the elder about what was most valued about living at home and what habits were comforting, and finds ways to incorporate these in a new way into the new environment. If the elder does not have access to a kitchen and always had a cup of tea before bed, this can become part of the individualized plan of care.

According to the Loss Response Model, *memories are reframed* in order for the cycle of grieving to be completed. The grandmother who had always hosted her eldest daughter's birthday party can still do that even if she is now a resident in a long-term care facility. When the nurse has the information about this important ritual, she or he can help the person reserve a private space, send out invitations, and have the birthday party as always, just reframed in that it is catered by the facility in the elder's new "home."

Countercoping

Avery Weisman (1979) described the work of health care professionals related to grief as "countercoping." Although he was speaking of working with people with cancer, it is equally applicable to working with people who are grieving for any loss and for families coping with the pending or past loss. "Countercoping is like counterpoint in music, which blends melodies together into a basic harmony. The patient copes; the therapist [nurse] countercopes; together they work out a better fit" (Weisman, 1979, p. 109). Weisman suggests four very specific types of interventions or countercoping strategies: (1) clarification and control, (2) collaboration, (3) directed relief, and (4) cooling off.

Clarification and Control. The nurse helps griever(s) cope with loss by helping them confront it by getting or receiving information, considering alternatives, and finding a way to make the grief manageable. The nurse helps persons resume control by encouraging them to avoid acting on impulse. It may be necessary to say, "No, this is probably not a good time to make any major decisions."

Collaboration. The nurse collaborates by encouraging grievers to share stories with others and repeat the stories as often as is necessary as they "talk it out." The nurse as a collaborator is more directive than usual; it may be acceptable to say, "Yes—this is a good time to talk."

Directed Relief. Some temporary directed relief may be necessary, especially during acute grief. Catharsis may be helpful. In many instances it is the nurse who encourages the griever to cry or otherwise express feelings such as hurt or anger which is culturally acceptable to them. The nurse may have to say something like, "Expressing your feelings might help." Activity may also be recommended as a natural extension of feelings. Intense physical activity gives one emotional relief. In some cultures, people may tear their clothes or cut their hair. Today, there are numerous ways of acting out feelings—from throwing things, to taking a walk, to busying oneself with tasks, to expressing feelings through creative works.

Cooling Off. From time to time grievers might need to be encouraged to temporarily avoid active mourning through diversions that worked in the past during times of stress, especially when things have to be done or decisions have to be made. The nurse may need to suggest new tactics that may prove helpful. Although there is considerable cultural variation, cooling off also means encouraging the person to modulate emotional extremes at times and to think about ways to make sense of the loss, to build a new sense of self-esteem after the loss, and help reestablish life patterns.

In all interventions related to grief, the nurse must have skills in therapeutic communication. Active listening is greatly preferable to giving advice. When listening, the nurse soon discovers that it is often not the actual loss that is of utmost concern, but rather the fear associated with the loss. If the nurse listens carefully to both the stated and the implied, what will be heard may be expressions such as the following: "How will I go on?" "What will I do now?" "What will become of me?" "What will happen to my loved ones, pets, etc.?" "I don't know what to do." "How could he (she) do this to me?" Because the nurse knows there will be resolution of some kind, such comments may seem exaggerated or melodramatic, but to the one who is acutely grieving there seems to be no resolution. The person cannot yet look ahead and know that the despair and other feelings will lessen. Like good copers, good gerontological nurses must be flexible, practical, resourceful, and abundantly optimistic.

Dying, Death, and Palliative Care

Many people have said that death is not the problem, it is the dying that takes the work. This is true for all involved: the person who is dying, the loved ones, and the professional caregivers, such as nurses and, in long-term care facilities, nursing assistants (Anderson & Gaugler, 2006-2007).

Dying is both a challenging life experience and a private one. How one deals with dying is a reflection of one's culture and the way the person has handled earlier losses and stressors. Most people probably do die as they have lived. Although not all older adults have had fulfilling lives or have a sense of completion, transcendence, or self-actualization, their deaths at the age or after that of their parents are considered normative. If the dying process is particularly long or the death occurs after a painful illness, we may rationalize it or view it as a relief, at least in part. Death at a younger age or as the result of trauma or catastrophe is viewed as tragic and sometimes incomprehensible. After the Indonesian tsunami or the blowing up of the World Trade Centers in New York City on 9/11 no one rationalized the deaths of the older victims as a relief; all deaths were considered an unacceptable loss of human potential.

Conceptual Models

As models have been proposed to explain the grieving process, so have they been proposed for the process of dying. One of the most well known has been that of Dr. Elizabeth Kübler-Ross. In her book *On Death and Dying* (1969) she reported on her observations of inpatients on the psychiatric ward where she did her psychiatry residency. She proposed the stages of dying as denial, anger, bargaining, depression, and acceptance. Nurses and many others have tried to help the dying work through denial to achieve acceptance before their deaths. However, we have come to realize that the "stages" are actually types of emotional reactions to dying that people experience rather than a stepwise progression. An alternative model that has been very useful to nursing practice is presented next.

The Living-Dying Interval

As proposed by the theories of aging (Chapter 5) we begin dying early at the time of birth; yet in realistic terms dying begins at a moment called the "crisis knowledge of death" (Pattison, 1977, p. 44) and ends at the moment of physiological death. Pattison (1977) calls the time between these two points the living-dying interval, made up of the acute, chronic, and terminal phases (Figure 25-2). The chronological time of the living-dying interval is accordion-like because of remissions and exacerbations in the terminal diagnosis; it may last days, weeks, months, or years. The manner in which one faces dying is an expression of personality, circumstances, illness, and culture.

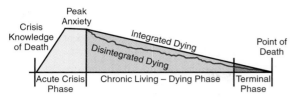

FIGURE 25-2 The living-dying interval. (From Pattison EM: *The experience of dying,* Englewood Cliffs, NJ, 1977, Prentice-Hall.)

The "crisis knowledge of death" occurs when someone receives the information that he or she will not live as long as previously anticipated. Certainly it would appear that the greater the discrepancy between the previously assumed length of life and the newly projected length of life, the greater the difficulties in adjustment and perhaps the intensity of the grief experienced. The point of crisis is a moment in time that is followed by an acute phase. It is a peak time of stress and anxiety since the life and future of the individual and the family is thrown into disequilibrium. Crisis intervention is most effective here because the individual, the family, and the caregivers are struggling to come to terms with the knowledge. A significant amount of anticipatory grieving may be observed.

Because no one can withstand a crisis indefinitely, most of the dying time is spent in the chronic phase when functional disruption must be compensated for. During this time the dying and those about them are forced to resume some sense of normalcy. Bills still need to be paid, dishes still need to be done, and life can still be lived (Box 25-3). The challenge for persons with terminal diagnoses and their families is to work toward living while dying and not

---

BOX 25-3   Functional Disruption: The Dirty Dishes

During a visit to the home of a woman who was in the last months of her life, I noticed that there was a stack of dirty dishes in the sink. She had gotten progressively weaker to the point she was no longer able to stand except briefly. Her husband sat watching TV. Using the best therapeutic conversation I learned in nursing school I asked about the dishes. They both started crying. He said he did not know how to load the dishwasher – she had always done it and she didn't know how to tell him they needed to be done. My "nursing intervention" that day was a lesson on loading a dishwasher.

---

dying while still living. Entertainment, work, and relationships can be maintained as normally as the individual's condition permits. Life goes on despite the anticipation of its end.

The terminal phase is reached when the speed of the physical dying is accelerated and the person no longer has the energy to maintain the activities of everyday life. The person may withdraw or turn away from the outside world; or the person may engage in coded communication, such as giving away cherished possessions as gifts, or urgently contacting friends and relatives with whom he or she has not communicated for a long time or saying "good-bye" instead of the usual "good night." The focus then turns to preserving energy and completing life's journey. In some cultures this period of time is called the "death watch" and is associated with prescribed rituals.

The living-dying interval can reflect an integrated or disintegrated trajectory (Pattison, 1977). The interval is integrated when as each new crisis occurs, it is dealt with effectively, and the quality of life while dying is preserved. The interval is described as disintegrated when one crisis tumbles on to the next one without any effective resolution and the quality of life while dying is compromised.

Implications for Gerontological Nursing

The needs of the dying are like threads in a piece of cloth. Each thread is individual but necessary to the integrity and completeness of the fabric. If one thread is pulled, it affects the other threads, and the material's appearance, the thread placement, and the stability of the cloth. When one need is unmet it will affect all others because they are interdependent and interwoven.

A good and appropriate death is one that a person would choose if choosing were possible. A good and appropriate death is one in which one's needs are met to the extent possible. The responsibility of the nurse is to provide safe conduct as the dying and their families navigate through unknown waters to a good and appropriate death. There are several ways the nurse can intervene to promote healthy aging along the living dying interval; one of these is to apply Weisman's six *C*'s approach (1984).

The Six *C*'s Approach

Weisman (1984) identified six needs of the dying: care, control, composure, communication, continuity, and closure. While they are most applicable to those of northern European descent, when combined with the work of Pattison (1977), they can provide a place to begin to think about caring for persons from all cultures.

Care

Persons who are dying should have the best care possible; this includes expert management of symptoms and support at all times. Care includes the adequate treatment of pain (see Chapter 15). Care also goes beyond the physical to psychological pain, induced by depression, anxiety, fear, and unresolved emotional concerns that are just as strong and just as real. When emotional needs are not met, the total pain experience is intensified. Medication alone cannot relieve pain. Instead, empathic listening and allowing the person to verbalize his or her thoughts is an important intervention. If tears and sadness are present, gentleness of touch, closeness, and sitting near the person may be helpful, when culturally appropriate. As an advocate, the gerontological nurse makes sure that the medical care that is needed is received.

Other common symptoms requiring management are breathlessness and fatigue. These are often interrelated. Caring for the dying means helping the person conserve energy; fatigue is an almost universal problem (Glare et al., 2011). Dying calls for great amounts of energy to cope with the emotional and physical assault of illness on the body. How much can the individual do without becoming physically and emotionally taxed? Is there something in particular that causes more or less shortness of breath? Would having oxygen available provide comfort? What activities of daily living are most important for the person to do independently? How much energy is needed for the patient to be able to talk with visitors or staff without becoming exhausted? Only the person can answer these questions and the nurse can advocate for the person to be given the opportunity to do so; and in doing so, the patient is able to remain in better control and maintain composure.

A detailed discussion of common symptoms addressed in palliative care can be found at http://consultgerirn.org, a service of the Hartford Institute for Geriatric Nursing.

Control

As persons proceed along the living-dying interval they are in the process of losing everything they have every known or will ever know. The potential loss of identity, independence, and control over body functions can lead to a sense of having lost control and self-esteem. The person may begin to feel ashamed, humiliated, and like a "burden." Control is the need to remain in a collaborative role relating to one's own living and dying and as active a participant in one's care to the extent desired. Once nurses know what the elder's preferences are, they can help the person meet these needs by taking every opportunity to return this level of control and in doing so bolster the person's self-esteem. Whenever possible the nurse can have the person decide when to groom, eat, wake, sleep, and so forth. The nurse never has the right to determine the activities of the individual, especially in relation to visitors and how time is spent (Box 25-4).

Composure

The need for composure is that which enables the person to modulate emotional extremes, the degree to which is appropriate within cultural norms. In some cultures it is a time of great emotional expression, in others a time of stoicism. The goal of composure is not to avoid the sadness but to have moments of relief. The nurse may use many of the countercoping techniques discussed earlier to help persons meet this need.

Communication

The need for communication is broad, from the need for information to make decisions to the need to share information. Although the type and content of communication that is acceptable to the person varies by culture, the nurse has a responsibility to make sure that the dying person has an opportunity for the communication he or she desires.

In a study of communication among the patient, family, and hospital staff about terminal illness, Glaser and Strauss (1963) identified four types: *closed awareness, suspected awareness, mutual pretense,* and *open awareness.* Each of these influences the work on the nursing home or hospital unit and the care of the patient.

- *Closed awareness* is described as "keeping the secret." Hospital staff and the family and friends know that the patient is dying, but the patient does not know it or knows and keeps the secret as well. Generally, caregivers invent a fictitious future for the patient to believe in, in hopes that it will boost the patient's morale. Although this happens less today because of legislation related to patients' rights, it still occurs. In some cultures, such as in many Latino families, it is expected.

- In *suspected awareness,* the person suspects he or she is dying, but since it is not discussed it cannot be confirmed. Inquiries on the part of the person are indirect or avoided by others. Hints are bandied back and forth, and a contest ensues for control of the information.

BOX 25-4   Having Some Control

I asked, "Is there anything else I can do for you?"—to which she replied, "Can you help me tell my husband that I do not want his sister to visit? I have never liked her and I have so little time left."

- *Mutual pretense* is a situation of "let's pretend." Everyone knows the patient has a terminal illness, but no one talks about it—real feelings are kept hidden.
- *Open awareness* occurs when the patient, family, friends, nurses, and physicians openly acknowledge the eventual death of the patient. The patient may ask, "Will I die?" and "How and when will I die?" The patient becomes resigned to dying, and the family grieves with the patient rather than for the patient. The nurse can encourage open awareness whenever possible while at the same time respecting the patient's culture. In some cultures, talking about an anticipated death is deemed helpful. In others, one can be aware of the dying but talking about it openly may be taboo, such as in the Haitian culture.

Continuity

The need for continuity equates to preserving as normal a life as possible while dying and transcending the present by leaving a legacy for the future. Too often a dying patient can feel shut off from the rest of the world at a time when he or she is still capable of being involved and active in some way. Loneliness is the result of a loss of continuity with one's life. The nurse may ask about the person's life and those things most valued, and work with the family and the patient or resident on a plan to remain engaged in as many of the activities and past roles as possible. A father who watches a certain ballgame with his son every Sunday can continue to do this regardless of the need to be in a hospital, a nursing home, or an inpatient hospice unit. If the person is at home and is bedridden, it may make more sense to have the bed in a central area rather than in a distant room. Treating the person who is dying as an intelligent adult, holding a hand, or putting an arm around a shoulder if culturally acceptable says, "I care" and "You're not alone" and "You are important."

One approach people have taken to obtain continuity of their lives after death is in the establishment of legacies. Legacies can take many different forms and may range from memories that will live on in the minds of others to bequeathed fortunes. A grandmother who is likely to die before a favorite grandchild's wedding can create a legacy when she participates with planning, regardless of the age of the grandchild if this is important to her, thereby leaving an enduring and special legacy.

Closure

The need for closure corresponds to an opportunity for reconciliation and transcendence, the highest of Maslow's Hierarchy. Reminiscence is one way of putting one's life in order, to evaluate the pluses and minuses of a life lived. It is a means of resolving conflicts, giving up possessions, and making final good-byes. Learning to say "good-bye" today leaves open the possibility of many more "hellos." Pain and other symptoms that are not well controlled may interfere with this reconciliation, making appropriate interventions by the nurse especially important.

For some, closure means coming to terms with their spiritual selves, with Jesus, God, Allah, or Buddha. If the expressions of the patient have spiritual overtones, arranging for pastoral care may be offered but should never be done without the person's permission. The nurse can foster transcendence by providing patients with the time and privacy for self-reflection as well as an opportunity to talk about whatever they need to talk about, especially about the meanings of their lives and the meanings of their deaths.

Care, control, composure, communication, continuity, and closure create the borders necessary to complete the fabric of needs of the dying. Their influence is omnipresent in the other needs. Without them, the cloth can fray, and attempts to meet the needs will be limited.

The Family

The nurse is often present and supporting the family at the time of death and in the moments preceding it. Regardless of the age of the surviving family members, as spouse, partner, children, or friends, they too have needs, and nurses have a responsibility to care for them. In a now classic study, newly bereaved persons were asked what they had found most helpful (Richter, 1987). They most appreciated nurses who did the following:

- Kept me informed
- Asked how I was doing and offered support
- Put an arm around me when I cried
- Brought me food
- Knew my name
- Cried with me
- Brought a bed and encouraged me to stay in the room with my dying husband
- Told me to hold my husband's hand while he was dying
- Held my hand
- Got the chaplain for me
- Let me take care of my husband
- Stayed with me after their shift was over

Similar findings have been found more recently (Lee et al., 2012). Although these will not provide comfort to all, nor are all these behaviors always possible, they can be used as starting points.

Dying and the Nurse

Nurses are professional grievers. We invest time and caring, and if working with older adults, especially those who are frail and in acute and long-term care settings, we experience the death of patients and residents over and over again. Some consider the death of a patient as a failure, that they have "lost" the person they cared for; yet, when they are good deaths, they can be viewed as professional successes each time we share the special and very personal experience of providing safe conduct for elders while dying and gentle caring for their survivors. We can use the reminders of our own mortality as motivation to live the best we can with what we have. Nurses can seek support and give it to one another. As grievers, we too may need to tell the story of the dying, or the person, to those professionals around us, either in formal or informal support groups; and we must listen to those stories of our colleagues over and over again until they become part of the fabric of our colleagues' lives as well.

Caring for older adults requires knowledge of the grieving and dying processes as well as skills in providing relief of symptoms or palliative care. However, it is also acknowledged that working with the grieving or dying day in and day out is an art. The development of the art calls for inner strength and coping skills. The most important coping skills for nurses may be meaning-making and the ability to disengage (Desbiens & Fillion, 2007). The effective gerontological nurse has developed a personal philosophy of life and of death. Although this can and does change over time, it will help when times are difficult. Emotional maturity allows the nurse to deal with disappointment and postponement of immediate wants or desires. Maturity means that the nurse can reach out for help when needed. Finally, in order to provide comfort to grieving persons, nurses must be comfortable with their own lives or at least be able to set aside their own sadness and grief while working with the sadness and grief of others.

Palliative Care

Nurses routinely care for elders who have irreversible and progressive conditions, such as Alzheimer's disease and Parkinson's disease. Other elders have exhausted all treatment options for conditions such as cancer or end-stage heart or renal disease. A nursing home resident may elect to remain at the facility rather than return (ever) to a hospital, even if faced with an acute event, such as a myocardial infarction (MI) or stroke. They are receiving a type of care called *palliative care*, or that which focuses on comfort rather than cure, on the treatment of symptoms rather than disease, on quality of life left rather than quantity of life lived. Palliative care comprises much of what is done in gerontological nursing and may indeed be the heart of caring. Some type of palliative care can be provided anywhere by anyone sharing these goals and skills. It can even be provided at the same time a person is receiving curative care for something else, such as receiving treatment for a bladder infection while terminally ill with heart disease (Batchelor, 2010).

The scope and specialty of palliative care has grown considerably over the years; research has been conducted, professional organizations have been formed, and standardized curricula have been developed. With the support of the American Association of Colleges of Nursing and City of Hope Medical Center a broad initiative was initiated in 1999 to train nurses through the End of Life Nursing Consortium (ANA-ELNEC) (www.aacn.nche.edu/ELNEC). It is hoped that by training nurses and faculty, nursing as a profession can provide the highest level of palliative care.

Whereas initially palliative care was the specialty of community-based organizations referred to as hospices, specialized units and staff are now seen in long-term care and acute care facilities across the United States. Palliative care was originally not well reimbursed, but since a hospice benefit was added to Medicare in the 1980s, some level of skilled palliative care is usually a covered service under most insurance plans (see Chapter 23).

Hospice

The term *hospice* refers to a formalized structure from which a significant amount of the palliative care in the United States is delivered. It gets its meaning from the medieval concept of hospitality in which a community assisted a traveler at dangerous points along his or her journey. Hospice has been a vehicle to help return nursing to its roots—as humane compassionate care, an ideal that has been the basis of nursing for centuries. The dying are indeed travelers—travelers along the continuum of life—and the community consists of friends; family; and specially prepared people to care, the hospice team.

The concept of the contemporary hospice was made famous by Dr. Cicely Saunders, founder of Saint Christopher's Hospice in London more than 30 years ago. Both for-profit and not-for-profit hospice organizations are now all over the United States and provide comprehensive and interdisciplinary care to persons assessed to be in the last 6 months of life. Under Medicare, a hospice organization must provide medical, nursing, nursing assistant, chaplain, social work, and volunteer support 24 hours per day. Additional services may include massage, music, art, and pet therapy and others. Hospices provide care not only to the dying but also to their families and friends through support before and after the death of loved ones.

The majority of hospice care is provided at home. The home becomes the primary center of care, provided by family members or friends, who are taught basic nursing care and how to administer the medication needed to provide comfort for their loved one who is dying. A growing number of inpatient hospice facilities exist as well. These are often free-standing, small inpatient facilities for those with symptoms that could not be managed at home, those without caregivers, or to provide short periods of rest from caring (respite) for the caregivers. Hospice nurses and others may also see patients who are residents in long-term care facilities and work with the staff to supplement care and provide expertise in symptom management. Special units in acute care hospitals and some long-term care facilities may also provide palliative care services guided by traditional hospice principles. Pain control and the opportunity to die at home are the key ideas and activities that people associate with hospice services. In actuality, hospice represents much more. It supports and guides the family in patient care and ensures that the patient will not die alone and that the family will not be abandoned. Bereavement services for the family extend for a period of time on an emergency and regular basis after the death of the patient. In contrast to palliative care, hospice services are limited to the time when one's life expectancy is anticipated to be 6 months or less.

The Nurse's Role in Palliative Care

The nurse provides much of the direct palliative care including that which is provided by hospice programs. Nurses function in a variety of roles: as staff nurse giving direct care, as coordinator implementing the plan of the interdisciplinary team or as executive officer responsible for clinical care, and as an advocate for humane care for persons who are dying and their families.

The American Nurses Association's *Standards and Scope of Hospice and Palliative Nursing Practice* (2002) enumerates the special skills, knowledge, and abilities needed by a nurse who provides end-of-life care:

1. Thorough knowledge of anatomy and physiology and considerable familiarity with pathophysiological causes of numerous diseases
2. Well-grounded skill in physical assessment and in various nursing procedures, such as catheterization and colostomy and traction care

3. Above-average knowledge of pharmacology, especially of analgesics, narcotics, antiemetics, tranquilizers, antibiotics, hormone therapy, steroids, cardiotonic agents, and cancer chemotherapy
4. Skill in using psychological principles in individual and group situations
5. Great sensitivity in human relationships
6. Personal characteristics such as stamina, emotional stability, flexibility, cooperativeness, and a life philosophy or faith
7. Knowledge of measures to comfort the dying in the last hours

The National Hospice Organization and the Hospice and Palliative Care Nurses Association also provide guidance in end-of-life care. These guidelines bring gerontological theory, nursing concepts, and knowledge of medical management of acute and chronic conditions of elders together to provide the most sensitive and comprehensive care possible (www.hpna.org).

Decision Making at the End of Life

Decision making at the end of life has become a legal, ethical, medical, and personal concern. The lines between living and dying are blurred as a direct result of technological advances. This results in ambivalence concerning whether death is to be delayed, fought, or accepted.

The issue of who has the authority to make end-of-life decisions and for whom, has been the subject of research, debate, and federal legislation. An adult who has not been adjudicated to lack capacity (see Chapter 23) is recognized as the decision maker; however, this assumption is based on a very Euro-American or Western perspective. Persons who are from non-Western traditions place less emphasis on the individual and more on the needs of the family or community (Mazanec & Tyler, 2003). Nurses have an obligation to know the legal requirements in their jurisdictions and then work with the elder and the family to determine how these will fit with their cultural patterns and needs as they relate to end-of-life decisions.

Advance Directives

Whereas people have always had opinions about their wishes, their right to refuse medical treatment was legislated in the United States by the Patient Self-Determination Act (PSDA) in 1990 and implemented in all states in 1991. Under the PSDA, the adult was recognized as the ultimate authority to accept or reject medical care, including the decision to forego life-sustaining treatment. Through the legislation related to the PSDA, adults were granted the legal authority to complete what are known as advance health care directives (AHCD)—or statements about their wishes, or directions to others—before the need for a decision arises. These directives may be as vague as "no treatment if I am terminally ill" to as detailed with a breakdown of decisions about dialysis, antibiotics, tube feedings, cardiopulmonary resuscitation (CPR), and so on. The AHCD provides a mechanism for an adult to appoint another adult of his or her choosing to make decisions if he or she is unable to do so (see Chapter 23).

The common forms of advance directives are known as living wills, durable powers of attorney for health care (DPAHC), and medical powers of attorney (Gittler, 2011). In each of these the persons creating it (called a principle) appoints an agent or proxy or surrogate to act on their behalf should a time come when they are unable to do so themselves. A living will is usually restricted to represent a person's wishes specific to the condition of a terminal illness. In contrast, a person appointed in a DPAHC can speak for the other in most or all matters of health care. In many states, advance directives are legally binding documents that nurses, physicians, and health care institutions are required to respect. Both the proxy and the health care surrogate are expected to use what is known as *substituted judgment.* Substituted judgment means that the decision made on behalf of the other is believed to be the decision that the principle would make if he or she were able to do so (Box 25-5)

All agencies in the United States that receive Medicare and Medicaid funds are required to disseminate PSDA information to their clients and inquire as to the existence of advance directives. Hospitals and long-term care facilities are responsible for providing written information at the time of admission about the individual's rights under law to both refuse medical and surgical care and to provide this decision in writing and in advance. Health maintenance organizations (HMOs) are required to do the same at the time of member enrollment, as are home health agencies before the patient comes under the care of the agency. Hospices are obliged to inform patients of their self-determination rights on the initial visit. Providers (physicians and nurse practitioners) are encouraged but are not under obligation to provide this same information to their patients.

Although the exact format and signature (e.g., notarization) requirements vary from state to state, the PSDA is a federal mandate and applies to persons in all jurisdictions. There are several clearinghouses of related information, including www.fivewishes.com which has a downloadable document acceptable in most states. For information about advanced directive information by state see www.noah-health.org/en/rights/endoflife/adforms.html.

Although the nurse cannot provide legal information, she or he does serve as a resource person ready to answer many of the questions people have about end-of-life decision making. The nurse may be called not only to inquire about the presence of an existing advance directive, but also to ensure that the directive still reflects the person's wishes and advocate for the wishes to be followed. The nurse also has the responsibility to make sure that existing or newly created advance directives are available in the appropriate locations in the medical record.

Euthanasia

The recognition of a patient's right to refuse life-sustaining medical measures renewed age-old questions over the patient's right to make decisions about the continuation of natural life. Some people, especially those who are suffering unremitting pain from a terminal illness, have ended their lives. Others have asked for assistance in accomplishing this in the most painless way possible (Box 25-6).

BOX 25-5 **Characteristics of an Appropriate and Helpful Health Care Surrogate**

- Willing and able to discuss this sensitive and difficult subject with the principle
- Agrees to act on behalf of the principle when needed
- Agrees to uphold the wishes of the principle
- Able to handle conflicts between family members and health care personnel if needed

Adapted from Gittler J: Advance care planning and surrogate health care decision making for older adults, *J Gerontol Nurs* 37(5):15-19, 2011.

BOX 25-6 **Can I Help You?**

As a nurse practitioner, I visited a nursing home resident. One day when checking on a woman with end-stage pulmonary disease, I asked, "Is there anything I can do for you at this time?" She responded quickly asking if I knew how she could reach Dr. Kevorkian, a physician known for assisted suicide. I knew that I had to be much more proactive in finding ways to make her more comfortable while she waited for death.

Kathleen Jett at 40

As early as May 1992 the *Journal of the American Medical Association* reported that 73% of the general public in a large sample approved of some form of euthanasia. *Physician-assisted death, physician-assisted suicide, physician aid in dying,* and *passive* and *active euthanasia* are all terms that are heard. An example of physician-assisted suicide or death or physician aid in dying might be the physician providing the patient with sleeping pills. If instructions about a lethal dose are provided but not administered it is considered passive euthanasia. If the dose is administered by the physician, even at the request of the patient this would be considered active euthanasia.

As of 2012 there were three states in which physician-assisted suicide in the form of passive euthanasia is legal. In 1994 and again in 1997, voters in the state of Oregon passed the Death with Dignity Law, and Oregon became the first state to legalize a form of passive euthanasia (see the Legislative report found at www.leg.state.vt.us/reports/05Death/Death_With_Dignity_Report.htm#Section1). In March 2009 the Death with Dignity Law was finalized in Washington State. In both Oregon and Washington adults who are residents of the states with life expectancies of 6 months or less may obtain a lethal dose of a medication (usually secobarbital or phenobarbital) to self-administer after considerable other requirements have been met (Box 25-7). The person then decides if and when the dose is taken. In the State of Oregon it cannot be taken in the presence of the prescribing physician (State of Oregon, 2011). In December 2009 the Montana Supreme Court ruled that physicians in the state could legally prescribe medications for terminally patients

to use to end their lives (Byock, 2010). Physician-assisted suicide is permitted in the Netherlands, Belgium, and Switzerland as well (Steinbrook, 2008).

After a slow but steady increase to the year 2002, the number of persons who took lethal doses of medications has remained relatively steady in Oregon with a total of 308 men and 288 women since 1997 and 71 all together in 2011. They are most often over 60 years of age, have cancer, are married, enrolled in hospice programs, and are college educated. They are almost exclusively white (Oregon Health Authority, 2011). The statistics are almost identical in Washington. In 2010, 87 persons were provided with prescriptions, and 72 died; however, only 51 of the deaths were known to be after ingestion of the medications (Washington State Department of Health, 2010). The laws have not been shown to significantly increase the number of deaths, and they have resulted in the establishment of programs such as the POLST (Physician Orders for Life-Sustaining Treatment) program. Originating in Oregon in the 1990s, the POLST program supports effective communication of patient desires and respect for these wishes in end-of-life care (http://www.ohsu.edu/polst).

Nurses have had strong opinions both for and against euthanasia. The American Nurses Association leaders as well as those from the End-of-Life Care Center at Johns Hopkins continue to examine this evolving issue. The nurse is involved in many end-of-life care situations because she or he is the primary care provider who implements the decisions of others around end-of-life care. However, such advice should not mean patients who want to end their lives should be abandoned.

BOX 25-7   Select Requirements for Those Requesting Physician-Assisted Suicide in Oregon or Washington

- Documented resident of the state.
- At least 18 years of age.
- An attending physician and one other consulting physician must certify the diagnosis, the prognosis (less than 6 months), the person's competency, and the voluntary nature of the request.
- Two oral requests for assistance, 15 days apart.
- A written request, witnessed by two persons, one of whom is not a relative or person who can benefit in any way from the death.

- At least 48 hours between the written request and receipt of prescription.
- The prescribing physician may request but not require that the person notify next-of-kin of the decision.
- The individual must be counseled on alternatives and receive counseling from a pharmacist.
- All persons must be fully informed of the alternatives and encouraged to notify their next-of-kin of their decision.

From Oregon State Statute 127.800 s.1.01. Available at http://public.health.oregon.gov/ProviderPartnerResources/EvaluationResearch/DeathwithDignityAct/Pages/ors.aspx; Washington State Statute RCW 70.245. Available at http://www.doh.wa.gov/dwda/.

Considerable confusion exists regarding terminology and interpretation of what effects the nurse's role may have. Many nurses believe that turning off the ventilator, turning off tube feedings, stopping intravenous fluids, or giving as much pain medication as is needed, if a potential side effect is death, constitutes assisted suicide. Another perspective is that providing the level of comfort necessary or the withdrawal of such devices is allowing natural death to occur, which is very different from actively doing something to cause death. Nurses individually and collectively must consider the implication of this for themselves and our profession.

KEY CONCEPTS

- Grief is an emotional and behavioral response to loss. Grief responses are individual; what is appropriate for a person from one ethnic group may be considered inappropriate by another.
- One never completely resolves grief. Instead, the individual incorporates the loss as a part of his or her life through mourning.
- Dying is a multifaceted, active process. It affects all involved: the one who is dying, the family, and the professional caregivers.
- The "stages" or "phases of dying" and the type of coping are not obligatory and do not prescribe the way one should die. Such expectations place an added burden on the one who is dying.
- The dying older adult is a living person with all the same needs for good and natural relationships with people as others.
- Hospice is both a concept and a health care program that focuses on care rather than cure and on the provision of comfort for the person who is dying and for significant others.
- Advance directives allow an individual control over life and death decisions by written communication and the appointment of a person (a proxy) to be the individual's advocate when he or she is not able to personally communicate his or her desires.

ACTIVITIES AND DISCUSSION QUESTIONS

1. Explore your response to being given a terminal diagnosis. What coping mechanisms work for you? With which awareness approach would you be comfortable?
2. Describe how you would deal with a dying person and his or her family when they are especially protective of one another.
3. Describe and strategize how you would bring up the topic of advance directives.
4. What advance directive is legally recognized in your state?
5. Describe how you would introduce the topic of dying with a patient who is critically ill and not expected to live.

REFERENCES

Aloi JA: A theoretical study of the hidden wounds of war: disenfranchised grief and the impact on nursing practice, *ISRN Nurs*: 954081, Apr 2011. [Epub.]

American Nurses Association: *Standards and scope of hospice and palliative nursing practice*, Kansas City, MO, 2002, American Nurses Association. Available at www.ana.org.

Anderson KA, Gaugler JE: The grief experiences of certified nursing assistants: personal growth and complicated grief. *Omega (Westport)* 54(4):301–318, 2006–2007.

Batchelor NH: Palliative or hospice care? understanding the similarities and differences, *Rehabil Nurs* 35(2):60–64, 2010.

Byock I: Dying with dignity, *Hastings Ctr Rpt* 40(2): inside back cover.

Chow A, Chan C, Ho S: Social sharing of bereavement experience by Chinese bereaved persons in Hong Kong, *Death Stud* 31(7):601–618, 2007.

Coryell D: *Good grief: healing through the shadow of grief,* Rochester, VT, 2007, Healing Arts Press.

Desbiens J, Fillion L: Coping strategies, emotional outcomes and spiritual quality of life in palliative care nurses, *Int J Palliat Nurs* 13(6):291–300, 2007.

Doka KJ: *Disenfranchised grief: new direction, challenges, and strategies for practice,* Champaign, IL, 2002, Research Press.

Gerdner LA, Yang D, Cha D, et al: The circle of life, *J Gerontol Nurs* 33(5):20–31, 2007.

Giacquinta B: Helping families face the crisis of cancer, *Am J Nurs* 77(10):1585–1588, 1977.

Gittler J: Advance care planning and surrogate health care decision making for older adults, *J Geriatr Nurs* 37(5):15–19, 2011.

Glare P, Miller J, Nikolova T, et al: Treating nausea and vomiting in palliative care: a review, *Clin Interv Aging* 6:243–259, 2011.

Glaser BG, Strauss AL: *Awareness of dying*, Chicago, 1963, Aldine.

Glaser BG, Strauss AL: *Time for dying*, Chicago, 1968, Aldine.

Kübler-Ross E: *On death and dying*, New York, 1969, Macmillan.

Lee GL, Woo IM, Goh C: Understanding the concept of a "good death" among bereaved family caregivers of cancer patients in Singapore, *Palliat Support Care* Mar 1:1–10, 2012.

Lewis ID, McBride M: Anticipatory grief and chronicity: elders and families in racial/ethnic minority groups, *Geriatr Nurs* 25(1):44–47, 2004.

Maccallum F, Bryant RA: Imagining the future in complicated grief, *Depress Anxiety* 28(8):658–665, 2011.

Mazanec P, Tyler MK: Cultural considerations in end-of-life care: how ethnicity, age and spirituality affect decisions when death is imminent, *Am J Nurs* 103(3):50–59, 2003.

Metzger PL, Gray MJ: End-of-life communication and adjustment: pre-loss communication as a predictor of bereavement-related outcomes, *Death Stud* 32(4):301–325, 2008.

National Cancer Institute [NCI]: *Culture and response to grief and mourning* (2006). Available at www.cancer.gov/cancertopics/pdq/supportivecare/bereavement/Patient/page10.

Oregon Health Authority: *Oregon's Death with Dignity Act—2011* (2011). Available at http://public.health.oregon.gov/ProviderPartnerResources/EvaluationResearch/DeathwithDignityAct/Pages/index.aspx.

Parker ME, Smith MC: *Nursing theories and nursing practice*, Philadelphia, 2010, F.A. Davis.

Pattison EM: The experience of dying. In Pattison EM, editor: *The experience of dying*, Englewood Cliffs, NJ, 1977, Prentice-Hall.

Paun O, Farran CJ: Chronic grief management for dementia caregivers in transition. *JGN* 37(12): 28–35.

Richter JM: Support: a resource during crisis of mate loss, *J Gerontol Nurs* 13(11):18–22, 1987.

Steinbrook R: Physician assisted suicide: From Oregon to Washington State, *NEJM* 359:2513-15, 2008.

Sveen CA, Walby FA: Suicide survivors' mental health and grief reactions: a systematic review of controlled studies, *Suicide Life Threat Behav* 38(1):13–29. 2008.

Taylor DH Jr, Kuchibhatla M, Ostbye T, et al: The effect of spousal caregiving and bereavement on depressive symptoms, *Aging Ment Health* 12(1):100–107, 2008.

Ward L, Mathias JL, Hitchings SE: Relationships between bereavement and cognitive functioning in older adults, Gerontology 53(6):362–372, 2007.

Washington State Department of Health: *2010 Death with Dignity Act report* (2010). Available at http://www.doh.wa.gov/portals/1/Documents/5300/DWDA2010.pdf.

Weisman A: *Coping with cancer*, New York, 1979, McGraw-Hill.

Weisman A: *The coping capacity: on the nature of being mortal*, New York, 1984, Human Sciences Press.

Index